ANNUAL PROGRESS IN CHILD PSYCHIATRY AND CHILD DEVELOPMENT 1992

Edited by

MARGARET E. HERTZIG, M.D.

Associate Professor of Psychiatry
Cornell University Medical College

and

ELLEN A. FARBER, PH.D.

Assistant Professor of Psychology in Psychiatry
Cornell University Medical College

BRUNNER/MAZEL, *Publishers* ● New York

Library of Congress Card No. 68-23452
ISBN 0-87630-692-X
ISSN 0066-4030

Published by
BRUNNER/MAZEL, Inc.
19 Union Square
New York, New York 10003

Manufactured in the United States of America
10 9 8 7 6 5 4 3 2 1

CONTENTS

iii

PREFACE

The first volume of the *Annual Progress in Child Psychiatry and Child Development* was published in 1968 under the editorship of Drs. Stella Chess and Alexander Thomas. For the next 20 years, these two distinguished investigators and clinicians admirably fulfilled their original purpose in compiling a yearly collection of outstanding contributions to the literature of value to workers in the field, both for immediate information and for long-term reference. In 1987, I was privileged to be invited by Drs. Chess and Thomas to assist in the preparation of the 20th anniversary volume. My initiation into the task of surveying a rapidly growing body of literature was an exciting learning experience as I sought to emulate Drs. Chess and Thomas' skill in identifying what contributions were at the cutting edge of advances in our field.

Although Dr. Thomas officially retired from the editorial board in 1989, his wisdom continued to inform the selection process on an informal basis over the next three years. With this, the 1992 volume, Dr. Chess also has retired, and joining me in its preparation is Dr. Ellen A. Farber. Dr. Farber, currently Assistant Professor of Psychology in Psychiatry at Cornell University Medical College, is an investigator and clinician with interests in the areas of developmental psychopathology, attachment, parent–child interaction, high-risk families, child abuse, social competence, primary prevention, and social policy. She brings to the position of editor highly developed critical skills and investigative competence in areas that have long been prominently featured in the *Annual Progress*.

Together, Dr. Farber and I have followed the guidelines established by Drs. Chess and Thomas. Over 100 journals published in the English language during 1991 have been surveyed. Selections fall into two major categories: (1) original work that holds promise of making a contribution to progress, and (2) review articles, which although not reporting new work, present a clear, thoughtful, and systematic picture of the present state of knowledge in an important area. Articles were chosen for their intrinsic merit rather than to fill a quota of predetermined topics. A broad range of studies is included, but the selection by no means represents all of the major subdivisions of child psychiatry and child development. Dr. Farber and I have searched the literature extensively and have sought to apply our selection criteria as objectively as possible. We recognize that we have missed some valuable publications, and that our personal interests and experience also have, to some degree, influenced our judgments. To insure that the price of *Annual Progress* remains within the reach of our readership we have had to limit the length of the volume.

In particular, we would like to direct the attention of our readers to three meritorious papers that we were unable to include. In the second part of a two-part article, Bregman (Bregman, J.D. Current developments in the understanding of mental retardation Part II: Psychopathology. *Journal of the American Academy of Child and Adolescent Psychiatry,* 1991, Vol. 30, No. 6, 861–872) considers the problems of psychiatric illness among the retarded. Increasingly, standardized assessment procedures and diagnostic criteria are being used in defining the clinical characteristics of this group of patients. As associations between distinct genetic syndromes and specific patterns of psychopathology are identified, generic treatments are giving way to multidisciplinary approaches, including environmental change, behavioral strategies, psychotherapy, and family interventions, as well as pharmacotherapy, with the aim of ameliorating specific psychiatric symptoms and/or disorders.

Fletcher and co-workers (Fletcher, J.M., Francis, D.J., Penuegnat, W., Raudenbush, S.W., Bornstein, M.H., Schmitt, F., Brouwers, P., and Stover, E. Neurobehavioral outcomes in diseases of children. *American Psychologist,* 1991, Vol. 46, No. 122, 1267–1277) describe a methodologic approach for studying the effects of HIV and AIDS on development. The paper details the individual growth approach as a viable option for studying neurobehavioral outcomes in children, particularly as they relate to disease progression, recovery, and treatment—which can be applied to studies of other chronic diseases as well.

Amato and Keith (Amato, P.R. and Keith, B. Parental divorce and the well-being of children: A meta-analysis. *Psychological Bulletin,* 1991, Vol. 110, No., 1, 26–26) examine research on the impact of divorce on chidren through the use of meta-analysis. The results of studies of children living in single-parent and two-parent intact families are compared. The evidence suggests that effects are more the result of family conflict than of parental absence and economic disadvantage, although all three are relevant factors. Moreover, the effects of divorce may be more significant for the life choices of adolescents and adults than for younger children. Meta-analytic techniques are being applied with increasing frequency to a wide range of issues of clinical interest, and this clear and thorough description provides a sound introduction to the procedures involved.

Drs. Chess and Thomas have set a high editorial standard for the *Annual Progress.* I look forward to many years of fruitful collaboration with Dr. Farber in continuing to bring papers that document advances in the fields of child psychiatry and child development to our readership on a yearly basis.

MARGARET E. HERTZIG, M.D.

Part I
DEVELOPMENTAL STUDIES

The articles in this section span a range of developmental topics, including the development of emotions, socioemotional relationships, cognition, and visual preferences.

The first paper presented examines social-cognitive development within the mother–child–sibling family unit. During the preschool years, there is a marked change in childern's ability to understand "other's minds" and to understand that people's actions are based on their own belief systems. Dunn, Brown, Slomkowski, Tesla, and Youngblade attempt to tie individual differences in children's social-cognitive abilities to family discourse about feeling states, sibling interaction, and parent–child behavior. Using a short-term longitudinal design, they observed parent–child–sibling interaction and discourse in the home. Seven months later, they administered affective perspective-taking and false-belief tasks to the preschoolers. The content of family conversations proved to be more important than overall quantity of verbal exchange. Families in which discourse about causality and feelings was observed were more likely to have children who could explain feelings and actions of characters. Cooperative interactions with older siblings were also predictive of social cognition. Not surprising, but rarely studied, is the finding that children learn not only from actions directed toward themselves, but from observing parent–sibling exchanges.

This study is interesting in that it raises many questions for further investigation into the nature of individual differences in social-cognitive development and social skills. The direction of causality needs to be examined. Do children with greater skills of understanding others cooperate more with siblings and peers or does such cooperation lead to enhanced understanding?

The next paper, by Langlois and her colleagues, adds to her already significant body of work on attractiveness and infant visual preferences. A series of three studies revealed that 6-month-old infants can discriminate attractive from unattractive faces and that they visually prefer attractive ones. Attractiveness ratings were made by adults and the diverse stimuli included white male and female, black female, and infant faces. The authors suggest that attractiveness preferences are not learned through lengthy cultural exposure, but rather may be innate or acquired with only minimal experience with faces.

The third paper deals with continuity and lawful discontinuity in development. The focus is on infant temperament in the first year of life. Belsky, Fish, and Isabella examine the dimensions of positive and negative emotionality. Using a

longitudinal design, they examined the influence of distal factors (prenatal parental personality, marital quality, and newborn behavior) and proximal factors
(parent–child interaction at 3 months) on changes in emotionality from 3 to 9
months and the association of changes in emotionality with attachment security.
Results indicate that limited stability found on temperament measures reflects lawful discontinuity. Changes to lower levels of negative emotionality and higher
levels of positive emotionality were associated with psychologically healthier parents, more positive marriages, and more complementary mother–infant interaction patterns. It was harder to predict changes in positive than in negative
emotionality. Changes in infant emotionality were predictive of attachment security. Of note in this study was the inclusion of fathers, a group often unavailable
to researchers. Consistent with other studies, mothers and fathers were found to
have differential impacts on child behavior.

In recent years, the notion of internal working models has been used to extend
attachment research from a focus on early childhood to adult models of relationships, marital relationships, and adolescent personality. This has led to increased
interest by clinicians and researchers in attachment theory. The next paper elaborates on the measurement of adult attachment and the concept of measuring
"state of mind" with respect to relationships. Bowlby proposed that working
models of one's self and of one's parents developed in childhood play a major part
in the intergenerational transmission of relationship patterns and subsequently in
the "inheritance" of mental health and mental illness. Evidence of
intergenerational continuity in attachment relationships has thus far relied on concurrent or retrospective research designs; that is, the mother's attachment model
was assessed at the same time as or several years subsequent to the assessment
of the child in the Strange Situation. In the first published prospective study,
Fonagy, Steele, and Steele examine the prediction of quality of the infant–mother
attachment relationship based on the mother's "state of mind" during pregnancy
as documented by the adult attachment interview (AAI). They administered the
AAI to 100 middle-class primiparous women during the last trimester of pregnancy. When the infants were 12 to 13 months, Strange Situation assessments
were conducted. The concordance for mothers' AAI classifications and infants'
security of attachment to the mother was significantly higher than one would
expect by chance alone. Of critical importance in this type of predictive study is
understanding the misses or intergenerational discontinuities. The authors examine
these from both directions—infants who look better and those who look worse
than one would expect based on their mothers' internal models.

In the next paper, Dr. Goldberg presents a concise review of the concepts
underlying attachment theory and a brief history of attachment research. She summarizes the antecedents and sequelae of infant-parent attachment relationships, as
well as the extension of attachment measurement and research throughout the life

span. The possibilities and limitations of incorporating attachment measures into clinical practice are described.The current measures all require extensive training for coding, and it is unlikely that they will be used by clinicians. One methodological issue omitted from this article is the use of the attachment Q-sort for infants and preschoolers. This ultimately may prove an easier, although not simple, measure for assessing quality of attachment.

The Hoffman paper focuses on siblings. In a thoughtful review, she considers the evidence from both behavioral genetics and developmental psychology to examine sibling similarity and dissimilarity. She proposes that the notion that siblings are not very similar may reflect limitations in methodology and in the range of outcome variables. For example, on one hand, values and interests are often ignored in favor of personality traits. On the other hand, from developmental psychology the transactional model would predict that each child brings a unique contribution and creates his or her own environment.

The final paper in this section deals with the topic of children's understanding of death. Much of the literature on death deals with the bereavement process. Lazar and Torney-Purta investigated children's understanding of four subconcepts of death: irreversibility, cessation, causality, and inevitability. This study demonstrated one of the difficulties in examining children's understanding of death; only 30% of the parents gave permission for their children to be interviewed. Nonetheless, using a short-term longitudinal design, they assessed 99 first and second graders in the fall and then again in the spring. Using a standard questionnaire, they found significant changes in children's understanding of the four subconcepts during the seven-month interval. Many of the children had mastered the subconcepts of death by the second interview despite the fact that parents generally reported not discussing death with their children. Examining the developmental hierarchy of the subconcepts revealed that the understanding of cessation and causality were not dependent on each other, but were dependent on the understanding of irreversibility and inevitability.

There are important clinical implications for understanding children's notions of death from a developmental perspective. Suicide may occur when a child does not understand the irreversibility of death. Cognitive developmental state will also affect adjustment to death of a parent or relative. Finally, at a time when many young children are shooting other children, the understanding of children's concepts of death and violence, guns, and retribution seems a fruitful area for further investigation. Helping children to understand the consequences (e.g., irreversibility) of aggressive actions might be incorporated into community and school-based prevention programs.

1

Young Children's Understanding of Other People's Feelings and Beliefs: Individual Differences and Their Antecedents

Judy Dunn, Jane Brown, Cheryl Slomkowski,
Caroline Tesla, and Lise Youngblade
Pennsylvania State University, University Park

Individual differences in young children's understanding of other's feelings and in their ability to explain human action in terms of beliefs, and the earlier correlates of these differences, were studied with 50 children observed at home with mother and sibling at 33 months, then tested at 40 months on affective-labeling, perspective-taking, and false-belief tasks. Individual differences in social understanding were marked; a third of the children offered explanations of actions in terms of false belief, though few predicted actions on the basis of beliefs. These differences were associated with participation in family discourse about feelings and causality 7 months earlier, verbal fluency of mother and child, and cooperative interaction with the sibling. Differences in understanding feelings were also associated with the discourse measures, the quality of mother-sibling interaction, SES, and gender, with girls more successful than boys. The results support the view that discourse about the social world may in part mediate the key conceptual advances reflected in the social cognition tasks; interaction between child and sibling and the relationships between other family members are also implicated in the growth of social understanding.

The very early stages of children's understanding of other minds and others' feel-

Reprinted with permission from *Child Development*, 1991, Vol 62, 1352–1366. Copyright 1991 by the Society for Research in Child Development, Inc.

This study was supported by an NIH grant (HD 23158-02); we are very grateful to the families who participated in the study, and to Susan Evans, Stephanie McGhee, and Clare Stocker for their contributions to the project.

ings have in the last few years received rapidly growing attention (Astington, Harris, & Olson, 1988; Frye & Moore, 1990; Whiten, 1990); particular interest has been shown in the question of when young children are aware of mental states and of the psychological causes of behavior (Miller & Aloise, 1989). Research strategies have included the documentation of the recognition and differentiation of emotions by infants (Harris, 1989); the development of children's use of, first, feeling state terms and, later, mental terms (Bretherton, McNew, & Beeghly-Smith, 1981; Ridgeway, Waters, & Kuczaj, 1985; Shatz, Wellman, & Silber, 1983); the distinctions very young children make between the mental and physical worlds involving knowledge states (Wellman, 1985); and their ability to reason about and explain human action in terms of beliefs and desires. A focus of special interest has been the development of children's ability to predict and explain actions that are premised on mistaken or false beliefs, in terms of what another person thinks or believes (Olson, Astington, & Harris, 1988). As Bartsch and Wellman (1989) put it, "Understanding actions in terms of beliefs and desires is fundamental to understanding people and to social action. A central question for developmental research, therefore, concerns when we are able to participate in this system of reasoning." The issue of interest here is not so much children's understanding of false belief per se—their grasp of the idea that people can believe something that is not true—but rather their growing understanding of how belief or desire influences behavior.

In this burst of productive research on children's "theories of mind," the focus has been on describing with cross-sectional studies the ages at which particular abilities are manifest and on delineating the nature of the limitations and problems children have in conceiving of others' mental states and in understanding false beliefs as a basis for action. Although there is considerable disagreement about the earliest stages of this understanding, it is generally agreed that between 3 and 5 years children's ability to reflect on other minds and their understanding of the psychological bases of human action change markedly in nature.

Within this research on children's understanding of "other minds" there has been no consideration, as yet, of individual differences in the abilities of children to conceive of mental states or in their grasp of the basis of people's actions in terms of beliefs. Yet if the growth of this ability is such a central aspect of human development, the question of what influences differences in its developmental course is surely important, as is the matter of the prognostic significance of individual differences in the timing of its early appearance. To date, we have no information on either issue. We do not know whether differences are related primarily to individual differences in, for example, children's verbal intelligence, or children's experience of participation in discussions of *why* people behave as they do, or the quality of their family relationships more broadly considered.

In contrast, studies of the recognition and understanding of emotions in preschool children have included a number of investigations of individual differences, such as studies of individual differences in response to distress (Cummings, Hollenbeck, Ianotti, Radke-Yarrow, & Zahn-Waxler, 1986; Denham & Couchoud, 1990; Main & George, 1985), in talk about emotions (Dunn, Bretherton, & Munn, 1987), in comforting (Murphy, 1937) and hurting (Dunn & Kendrick, 1982), and in understanding the situational causes of another's emotion (Denham, 1986). Among the variables thought to influence these individual differences, the following have been cited: parental socialization techniques (Denham & Couchoud, 1990), parental verbal explanation, discourse about emotions and moral messages (Dunn et al., 1987; Zahn-Waxler, Radke-Yarrow, & King, 1979), children's perspective-taking ability (Stewart & Marvin, 1984), and individual differences in children's sociability or assertiveness (Murphy, 1937). With children of 5 and above, individual differences in emotional understanding have been linked to their sociometric status and social competence with peers (Cassidy & Parke, 1990; Gnepp, 1989; Rothenberg, 1970), to the emotional expressiveness of their parents (Cassidy & Parke, 1990), to parent-child discourse about feeling states (Dunn, Brown, & Beardsall, 1991), and to cognitive ability (Rothenberg, 1970).

The relative importance of these various potential influences on the development of children's emotional understanding remains to be established with young children. One study reports, for instance, associations between frequency of family discourse about feeling states in the preschool period and children's ability in middle childhood to make judgments about emotions in an affective perspective-taking task (Dunn et al., 1991). However, it remains possible that differences between families in such discourse are correlated with other differences in family interaction, and no inferences about the unique contribution of discourse in the development of understanding are possible until both discourse *and* family interaction variables are considered together. The possible role of such variables in contributing to individual differences in children's understanding of mental states has not yet been examined. It is not known whether such differences are attributable to differences in cognitive or verbal ability, or whether interactional experiences within the family also play a role in their development. The issue of how far language experiences are related to the conceptual development reflected in children's growing understanding of "other minds" remains to be explored. It is a reasonable hypothesis that family conversations about why people behave the way they do may foster the development of children's understanding of the connection between others' thoughts and beliefs and their behavior. It is also compatible with Wellman's (1988) proposal that 3-year-olds' understanding of human action is based on an everyday folk psychology in which actions are explained in terms of the wishes, hopes, beliefs, and intentions of the actor. However, such a possibility has not yet been tested.

In this article, such an examination is carried out, with data from a longitudinal study in which children were first observed within their families at 33 months, and then tested at 40 months on their understanding of others, with two types of assessment. An assessment of their understanding of how another person's beliefs will affect his or her behavior, developed by Bartsch and Wellman (1989), was conducted. In this series of tasks the focus is specifically on the children's ability to explain the actions taken by another when those actions are the consequence of a belief the child knows to be incorrect, and their ability to predict the behavior of another who is in possession of a belief that the child knows to be false. An assessment of affective perspective-taking developed by Denham (1986) was also employed: this involves a series of scenarios enacted with puppets in which the children's understanding of the situational determinants of another's feelings is assessed.

The first goal of the article is to describe individual differences in children's understanding of feelings and of how people's actions are premised on their beliefs at a stage when, according to current work on children's theory of mind, some but not all children are able to reflect on mental states and to explain behavior in terms of beliefs.

The second goal is to examine associations between such individual differences in understanding others and a number of variables from children's family experiences 7 months earlier. First, we were interested in the possibility that differences in children's experiences of family discourse about feeling states, and about the causes of behavior and events, might be linked to later individual differences in understanding others' feelings and in comprehending the connections between beliefs and behavior. As already noted, family conversations about feelings have been found to relate to later affective perspective-taking assessments (Dunn et al., 1991). The potential significance of family discourse about causality lies in the opportunity that such discourse provides for children to enquire, argue, and reflect about why people behave the way that they do. Children's participation in conversation about cause is focused especially on psychological causality (Hood & Bloom, 1979); the hypothesis is examined here that differences in such participation in causal talk and feeling state talk are associated with later differences in understanding of belief as the basis for action.

Second, we considered the possibility that differences in the quality of relationships between different family members may be implicated in the development of differences in social understanding. Here, we wished to examine not only the quality of relations between mother and child, widely considered to be important in the development of social understanding, but also the possibility that the relations between other family members (mother to sibling, sibling to mother) may also be implicated in the development of social understanding. Children are sensitive observers of the emotional exchanges between others (Cummings, Zahn-Waxler, & Radke-Yarrow, 1981; Dunn & Munn, 1985); they may well, as family members, learn from observing the interactions between others. The relations between child and sibling were also included as a focus of interest: work on older children indicates that differences in emotional understanding are related to children's experiences with peers (e.g., Cassidy & Parke, 1990). Third, we examined the possibility that differences in children's social understanding, as reflected in assessments that depend on verbal answers, are primarily related to differences in verbal ability, the educational and social background of the family, or the child's gender.

The third goal of the paper is to examine how much of the variance in these aspects of children's social understanding could be explained by combinations of these family and background variables, and what independent contribution to the variance was made by the discourse, relationship, and background variables, respectively.

METHOD

Subjects

The subjects were 50 second-born children, participating with their older siblings and their mothers in a longitudinal study in central Pennsylvania. There were 23 boys (13 with older brothers, 10 with older sisters) and 27 girls (10 with older sisters and 17 with older brothers). The mean age gap between the siblings was 43 months (range 16–73). The families, recruited from sequential birth announcements in the local newspaper, included a wide range of backgrounds; the occupational status of the fathers was assessed with the National Opinion Research Corporation prestige ratings based on the 1970 census (Hauser & Featherman, 1977): the mean paternal prestige rating was 51.5 (SD = 16.3), the range from 15 to 88. For the U.S. white labor force, the mean NORC rating is 41.7 (SD = 13.9); thus although the Pennsylvania sample has a higher occupational prestige rating than the working U.S. population, the variance is similar. Mean values for parental education were 14.7 (SD = 2.4) years and 15.4 (SD = 2.9) years for mothers and fathers, respectively.

Procedures

The families were visited at home, at two time points: when the children were 33 months old (time 1), and 40 months old (time 2).
Time 1 Observations At time 1, two observations, each of 1 hour 15 min, were carried out 1 week apart. The observations were unstructured and carried out by a single observer. To reduce the intrusive effect of the observer's presence, the same observer visited the family on each occasion, and did not begin recording until at least 15 min after her arrival. We emphasized to the mothers that we wished to study "normal" interaction between the siblings and to disrupt family patterns of interaction as little as possible. The mothers continued to carry out their usual

domestic routine while we were present. Family conversation during the observation was recorded on a portable audiotape recorder, and paper-and-pencil recording methods were used (see Dunn & Munn, 1987, for similar methods). The observer targeted her observations on the second-born child and noted in a lined notebook who was present with the child, recording the time that different family members entered or left the room in which the target child was; a narrative record was kept in which details of the context and affect of family members were noted. Context details included, for example, the actions that led to a dispute, the details of pretend or cooperative play, and nonverbal behavior such as provocative physical teasing. Shortly after the observation the observer prepared a detailed transcript of the observation, including all family talk and the nonverbal record. Following the observation, the observer rated each family member's behavior toward each other family member in a series of rating scales, focusing on the mother's responsiveness, attention, control, and affection to the child and to the sibling, and on the child's and the sibling's conflict, cooperation, control, competition, and attention toward each other (see Stocker, Dunn, & Plomin, 1989). The data from the observations reported here concern children's conversations with their mothers and siblings (specifically, their conversations concerning feeling states and concerning causality) and the ratings of family members' interaction. Details of the discourse measures used, and these rating scales, are given below.

Time 2 Social Cognition Tasks At time 2, two visits were made in which the sociocognitive assessments considered in this article, the false belief tasks (Bartsch & Wellman, 1989), and the affective perspective-taking tasks (Denham, 1986), were conducted. On the first visit, the false belief tasks were carried out with the children. A questionnaire was also administered to mothers to decide on appropriate content for the affective perspective-taking task for each child (see below). On the second visit, the affective perspective-taking task was carried out; information on the parents' occupations and education was obtained from an interview with the mother. Six observers were involved in the data collection.

Measures

Conversational Measures The transcripts provided a data base of on average 316 child speaker turns, 356 turns of mother and sibling to the child (Table 1). A speaker turn was defined as all of one speaker's utterances bounded by the utterances of another speaker. The correlations between the measures on the first and second visits at time 1 gave an estimate of test-retest reliability for the different speaker turns; these were as follows: child to mother $r(50) = .69$, mother to child $r(50) = .74$, child to sibling $r(50) = .68$, sibling to child $r(50) = .68$, all significant at $p < .05$.

Mean Length of Utterance The mean length and the upperbound mean length of each child's utterances were coded following standard procedures (Shatz & Gelman, 1973) from the 100 consecutive child utterances that followed the child's first 10 conversational turns. The number of words in the 10 longest of these utterances was used to determine the upperbound MLU. The mothers' MLU and upperbound MLU were similarly calculated. The MLU and upperbound MLU were positively correlated for both mothers and children, $r(50) = .86$ and $.85$, for mothers and for children, respectively, both $p < .001$, and the pattern of correlations with these measures and the other time 1 measures to be reported was very similar. In the analyses that follow we therefore report just the results for the upperbound MLU.

Feeling State Talk A coding system was designed for the analysis of conversations in which family members referred to feeling states (see Dunn et al., 1991). References included conversational turns in which the speaker used a feeling state term (e.g., "sad" or "happy"), those in which the speaker used a phrase that connoted a feeling state (e.g., "made a fuss"), and those in which an expletive was used that connoted a particular feeling state (e.g., "Yuck!" [disgust]). Nonspecific expletives (e.g., "Aha!"), crying, or laughter were not included in this coding scheme. Statements of a moral or evaluative nature were included only if their content specifically denoted or connoted a feeling state on the part of the speaker or person referred to (e.g., "That's disgusting!"). The term "like" was included only when it referred to a state of enjoyment or dislike, not when it indicated desire or volition, as in the example "Would you like to have this toy?" Terms that projected feeling states as attributes onto the persons or objects that elicited them (e.g., "scary" or "poor") were included.

A conversational turn referring to feeling states was defined as all of one speaker's utterances bounded by the utterances of another speaker in which an explicit reference to a feeling state was made. If an individual's utterances within one conversational turn referred to more than one emotional theme, or to more than one individual's feelings, each reference was coded separately. Each conversational turn that referred to a feeling state was coded in terms of a number of variables (speaker, addressee, theme, dispute, causal reference, pragmatic context). In the present article, we consider the categories of speaker and addressee, and employ measures of total feeling state turns. In our initial examination of the data we employed three measures: *total child feeling state turns* (i.e., child to mother + child to sibling feeling state turns) as an index of the child's participation in family talk about feelings; *total feeling state turns to child* (i.e., mother to child + sibling to child feeling state turns) as an index of the talk directly addressed to the target child concerning feelings; *mother-child total feeling state turns* (i.e., mother to child + child to mother feeling state turns) as an index of the conversations between mother and child about feelings; this was included because the previous study had found mother-child conversational turns about feeling states to be the most powerful predictor

TABLE 1
Means and Standard Deviation of Discourse Measures

SPEAKERS	TOTAL TURNS		FEELING STATE TURNS (%)		CAUSAL TURNS (%)	
	Mean	SD	Mean	SD	Mean	SD
Child to mother and sib	316.4	162.5	4.1	2.7	2.7	2.3
Mother and sib to child	355.9	166.4	7.8	3.3	7.4	3.1
Mother and child conversation	441.5	286.3	6.4	3.0	5.9	3.1

	MLU		UPPERBOUND MLU	
	Mean	SD	Mean	SD
Child	3.67	.82	7.17	1.53
Mother to child	5.38	.78	11.93	2.20

of later affective perspective taking. Frequencies of these measures, and of the total turns in the observations, are shown in Table 1.

Talk about Causality A second coding system was designed for the analysis of conversations about causality, in which speaker turns wherein a causal relationship was discussed were included. It should be noted that in those analyses in which both feeling state talk and causal talk turns were entered, those speaker turns that included both causal and feeling state references were entered only once. The turn could be related to the causal component of the conversation as either the antecedent or consequent of the causal reference ("You broke my glass [antecedent] and that makes me sad" [consequent]). The criteria used to determine whether a causal inference was made were based on those developed by Hood and Bloom (1979). Causal statements by young children and indeed also adults do not invariably contain causal connectives (see Hood & Bloom, 1979); thus turns coded as causal included, in addition to those in which an explicit causal term was used (e.g., "why" or "because"), turns in which a reference was made to two events or states that had a conditional relationship (e.g., "Don't jump, you'll break that!"). Measures of causal talk paralleled those of the feeling state talk, and included *total child causal turns* (i.e., child causal turns to mother + child causal turns to sibling, expressed as percentage of total child turns to mother and sibling); *total causal turns to child* (i.e., mother causal turns to child + sibling causal turns to child, as percentage of total mother and sibling turns to child); *total mother and child causal turns* (i.e., mother to child and child to mother causal turns). As with the feeling state coding, if more

TABLE 2
Means, Standard Deviations, Inter-rater Agreement,
and Test-Retest Correlations of Rating Scales

Rating Scales	Mean	SD	Interrater Agreement	Test-Retest Correlation
Mother to child:				
Responsiveness	3.87	.88	.82*	.74*
Attention	3.28	.92	.80*	.73*
Control	3.13	.77	.80*	.19
Affection	3.57	1.02	.83*	.80*
Mother to sibling:				
Responsiveness	3.48	.89	.82*	.76*
Attention	2.86	.80	.80*	.58*
Control	2.32	.87	.80*	.42*
Affection	3.03	.94	.83*	.59*
Child to sibling:				
Conflict	2.52	.77	.84*	.34*
Cooperation	2.81	.86	.79*	.58*
Control	2.11	.90	.76*	.52*
Competition	1.98	.82	.95*	.58*
Affection	2.86	1.11	.85*	.66*
Sibling to child:				
Conflict	2.73	.83	.84*	.39*
Cooperation	2.88	.94	.79*	.55*
Control	3.22	1.02	.76*	.60*
Competition	2.41	.99	.95*	.57*
Affection	2.89	1.15	.85*	.63*

* $p < .05$.

than one causal reference occurred within a speaker turn it was coded separately. All discussions of cause were coded; it should be noted, however, that as with other studies of causal conversations with children of this age period (e.g., Hood & Bloom, 1979), discussion of psychological/behavioral causality predominated.

Intercoder agreement on the discourse coding was assessed by coders coding the same 20 transcripts. Intraclass correlation for the coders' categorization of the total number of feeling state turns was .97, of the total number of causal turns was .86, both significant at $p < .05$.

Rating Scales The rating scales employed were developed in a previous study of mothers and siblings (Stocker et al., 1989). Means and standard deviation of scores are shown in Table 2.

Mother's interaction with child and with sibling. Four 5-point scales were used: *responsiveness, attention, control/intrusiveness,* and *affection.* Taking affection as an example, the scale ranged from (1) many negative remarks, no physical affection, more negative than positive remarks, negative tone of voice even if content is neutral, through (3) some praise and positive comments, some smiles and laughter with child, some comments made with warm tone of voice, to (5) many positive comments, many smiles, affectionate physical contact, tone of voice very warm and friendly, praise, and positive evaluation.

Child's interaction with sibling, and sibling with child. Five 5-point scales were used: *cooperation, control/dominance, competition,* and *affection.* Taking cooperation as an example, the scale ranged from (1) no attempts to cooperate, no innovatory suggestions for joint activity, refusal to cooperate with other's suggestions, ignores other's conversational attempts, through (3) follows suggestions, occasional tentative attempts at cooperation, shares and helps if requested, responds to questions and comments on most occasions but may fail to reply on occasion, brief sustained conversations, to (5) frequent attempts to cooperate, responds promptly to suggestions or questions, frequent sustained conversation, makes innovatory suggestions for cooperative play, friendly imitation, may praise sib, let sib win in games, spontaneously helps or shares. (Details of all scales are available from authors.)

Interobserver agreement among the six individuals who conducted the observations was assessed from videotapes of 10 families using Finn's *r* (shown in Table 2). This is an appropriate index of reliability when there is reduced variance in ratings (Finn, 1970, 1972; see also Tinsley & Weiss, 1975), which takes account of chance agreement and gives similar results to the intraclass correlation (Finn, 1970, 1972). The videotaped families were not part of the main study but were from similar backgrounds. Test-retest reliabilities of these scales were assessed by comparing the ratings given on visits 1 and 2 and are shown in Table 2.

Affective Labeling The two procedures reported in Denham (1986) were followed. First, children examined four faces made of felt on which the expressions of happy, sad, angry, and afraid were drawn. They were then asked to identify these expressions, first expressively with a verbal label, and then receptively, by pointing to the appropriate face when the experimenter asked, "Which is the happy/sad/angry/afraid face?" They received 2 points for correct expressive, 2 points for correct receptive, and 1 point for expressively or receptively identifying positive/negative dimensions (e.g., "He feels bad" rather than "He feels angry/sad/afraid" would be given a 1-point score [total correct = 16]).

Affective Perspective-Taking The puppets enacted 16 vignettes centered on emotion-inducing situations such as making an unexpected visit to the zoo, a new bicycle, having a frightening dream, seeing a parent off on a trip, being punched by a sibling, and being threatened with punishment for a naughty act. Each vignette was accompanied by vocal and visual affective cues emitted by the puppet/observer. In eight of these vignettes the puppet felt the way most people would feel (e.g., fear during a nightmare; see Borke, 1971); in eight the puppet felt the opposite of what the mothers had reported in the questionnaire administered at the previous visit that their child would probably feel. This questionnaire focused on situations in which children's emotional reactions differ, such as arrival at preschool, meeting a big though friendly dog, or seeing a parent off on a trip. In the second portion of the puppet tasks, the puppet in these same situations expressed an emotion that was different from that which the child (according to her mother's report) herself expressed in that situation; thus, the task was designed to require inference about the puppet who was expressing an emotion different from the emotion typical for the child in that situation, but also within the realm of the child's everyday experience. For example, mothers indicated whether their child would be happy or sad to come to day-care and whether they would be happy about or fearful of big dogs, and the puppet then enacted the emotion that the child would *not* express in that situation. After each of the vignettes, the children were asked "How does the puppet feel?" and encouraged to fix the relevant face on the puppet. Scoring proceeded as in the affective labeling task. A total score for the 16 vignettes was created (total correct = 32). As Denham (1986) found, scores on the labeling and perspective-taking tasks were correlated, $r(50)$ = .69, $p < .05$. They showed very similar patterns of correlations with the other time 1 measures, and an affective aggregate score was therefore created by combining the scores of the two sets of tasks (total score = 48). Cronbach's alpha for the affective aggregate was .91.

False Belief Tasks The children's understanding of false belief was tested in a series of tasks that required them to predict how a puppet would behave given a false belief, and also to give an explanation of a puppet's behavior given a false belief (Bartsch & Wellman, 1989). The procedures described by Bartsch and Wellman (1989) were followed. For each task, the child was shown two small closed boxes, one marked with a familiar and obvious picture (e.g., a Band-Aid box), and the other a plain unmarked box of the same size and color. At the beginning of the session, the experimenter told the child, "Pick the box that you think has Band-Aids in it." The child picked one of the boxes (almost always the marked container) and was told to look inside it. The marked container was empty. The child was then told to look inside the other (plain) box, which was full of Band-Aids. The purpose of this part of the task was to demonstrate that the marked box was empty and the unmarked box was full. Both boxes were then closed.

The child was then introduced to a series of hand puppets and given both prediction and explanation tasks. In the prediction task, the child was told, for example, "Look, here's Pam. Pam has a cut, see? And she wants a Band-Aid. Where do you think she'll look for Band-Aids?" The child's response, either pointing or verbally indicating one of the two boxes, was recorded. Then the puppet was made to start to look in the predicted location, and the observer asked, "Will she/he find [Band-Aids]?" In the explanation tasks, the child was introduced to the puppet and watched as the puppet started to look in the marked, but empty, container. Then the observer asked the child to explain the puppet's action. For example, "Look, here's Bill. Bill has a cut, see? And he wants a Band-Aid." (Bill approaches the Band-Aid box and starts to open it, without revealing its contents.) "Why do you think he's looking in there?" If the child failed to respond or mentioned only something other than the puppet's beliefs, the observer prompted with: "What does Bill think?" If a false belief was mentioned, the child was asked, "Are the Band-Aids there really?" to be certain that the child had not forgotten the actual contents of the container.

Four types of marked containers were used: a Band-Aid box, a crayon box, a Play-Doh box, and a raisin box. Each unmarked box was of the same dimensions as its paired marked box, but of a solid color. The different pairs of containers were used to sample a variety of situations and to keep children from becoming bored. Each pair was introduced immediately prior to the scenario in which it was used. Three of the four types of containers were used to present each child with the nine total tasks. The remaining type of container was used for a filler task, designed to prevent children from thinking simply that all of these boxes were deceptive (the marked box actually contained the item).

Children were given a total of four prediction and five explanation tasks. The presentation of tasks was counterbalanced: Prediction and explanation questions were presented in an alternating format for each child, and half the children received a prediction task first, while the other half received an explanation task first. The presentation of stimuli was also counterbalanced.

Scoring. On each of the four prediction tasks, children's responses were scored as being either correct (predicting that the puppet would search in the marked but empty box) or incorrect (predicting that the puppet would search in the unmarked but full box). The child received one credit for each correct prediction in the four stories; total possible correct predictions was four. To allow for chance correct replies, a child needed three or more correct predictions to "succeed"; two or less correct predictions were coded as "failed."

On the five explanation tasks, correct answers were explanations that attributed a false belief to the character, as in Bartsch and Wellman (1989). For example, after seeing the puppet start to look in the empty Band-Aid box, each child was asked, "Why do you think he's looking there?" One child answered, "Because he thinks there's Band-Aids in it," pointing to the Band-Aid box. Another child responded to this question with "Don't know." In this case the observer asked, "What does he think?" and the child replied, "That there's Band-Aids in there." In conjunction with the invariably correct responses to the control question ("Are there really?"), both of these answers, unprompted and prompted, were coded as false belief attributions. Children giving one or more explanations of the puppet's action in terms of the puppet's false belief, prompted or unprompted, were coded as *offering explanations* in terms of false belief; that is, the variable offering explanations was dichotomized 0 = no explanation, 1 = one or more explanations.

RESULTS

The results of the analyses are presented in three sections. First, the individual differences in performance on the false belief and affective perspective-taking tasks are reported and the relation between children's scores on these measures presented. Second, correlations between these time 2 measures and the measures from time 1 (discourse measures, SES, ratings of family interaction) are examined. Third, the variance in the social cognition measures at time 2 that was explained jointly by the time 1 variables and the individual contribution of the various time 1 measures is examined with multiple regression analyses.

Time 2: Affective Aggregate There was a wide range of individual differences in the children's performance on the Denham tasks. For the affective aggregate, scores ranged from 9 to 47; the mean was 32.2 (SD 10.4).

False Belief Tasks There were marked individual differences in the children's success on the various sections of the false belief tasks. First, it should be noted that only seven children succeeded on the prediction tasks. Fourteen children offered at least one explanation in terms of false belief. Given the small number of children who predicted actions in terms of false belief (a finding in agreement with those of Bartsch & Wellman, 1989), in the analyses that follow we omit the prediction measure; the explanation measure is retained in view of the theoretical interest in children's explanations in false belief tasks.

The relations between scores on the affective understanding tasks and on the false belief tasks were next examined. Correlation between the affective aggregate and the false belief measure did not reach significance at the $p < .05$ level, $r(50) = .25$.

Correlations Between Scores on Time 2 Social Cognitive Tasks and Measures from Time 1

Correlations were next conducted between the two social cognition measures from time 2 and (*a*) total number of talk turns per hour of observation and the measures of feeling state talk and causal talk during the time 1 observations; (*b*) mother's education, father's occupation, gender of the child, and the upperbound MLU of child and mother; and (*c*) the rating scales of family members' interaction with each other.

There was no significant relation between total talk and the two social cognition measures. Table 3 shows the correlations for the discourse measures, the MLU measures, gender, the education and SES measures, and the significant correlations with the rating scales. For the affective aggregate score, significant correlations were found with the child's talk about feelings and about causality in the observations 7 months earlier, and with mother-child conversations about feelings and the total talk to the child about feelings. The score was also related to the children's

TABLE 3
Correlations Between Time 1 Measures and Time 2 Social
Understanding Measures

	Affective Aggregate	False Belief Explanations
Feeling state talk:		
Child total	.45*	.31*
Total to child	.29*	.14
Mother-child	.36*	.28*
Causal talk:		
Child total	.42*	.19
Total to child	.06	.22
Mother-child	.20	.42*
Child upperbound MLU	.51*	.20
Mother upperbound MLU	.35*	.33*
Mother education	.26	.14
Father occupational prestige	.45*	.24
Gender (girls = 1; boys = 2).	−.36*	−.18
Rating scales:[a]		
Mother to sibling:		
Responsiveness	.31*	.09
Attention	.28*	−.06
Control	.26	.34*
Affection	.25	.08
Child to sibling:		
Conflict	−.15	−.16
Cooperation	.51*	.38*
Control	.04	−.10
Competition	.06	.04
Affection	.33*	.18
Sibling to child:		
Conflict	−.06	−.04
Cooperation	.27*	.15
Control	.26	.15
Competition	−.03	−.03
Affection	.35*	.20

[a] Note that correlations for rating scales of mother to child are not included in the table; all were nonsignificant.
* $p < .05$.

and mothers' upperbound MLU and the SES level, as reflected in the fathers' occupational prestige scores, and to gender. Girls scores higher on the affective understanding measure.

Offering explanations in the false belief tasks was related to the child's talk about feeling states and to mother-child conversations about feeling states and about causality at the earlier time point. Mothers' upperbound MLU was correlated with explanations in the false belief tasks, but the SES, mothers' education, child MLU, and gender associations did not reach significance.

The relations between the social cognition scores and the rating scales of family members' interaction were examined next.

Mother-to-Child Ratings The four maternal rating scales (responsiveness, attention, control/intrusiveness, affection) were each correlated with the two social cognition measures from time 2. Of the eight correlations, none was significant.

Mother-to-Sibling Ratings Three of the eight correlations between mother-to-sibling rating scales and the social cognition measures were significant at $p < .05$ (see Table 3). The attention and responsiveness that the mothers showed toward the sibling was correlated with the children's affective aggregate score at the later time point, and the mothers' control/intrusiveness toward the sibling was related to the children offering explanations in the false belief tasks.

Child-to-Sibling Ratings Three of the 10 correlations between the five child-to-sibling scales and the two social cognition measures were significant (see Table 3): The social cognition measures were related to the cooperation shown toward the sibling 7 months earlier, and affection to the sibling was also related to the affective tasks.

Sibling-to-Child Ratings Of the 10 correlations between the five scales and the two social cognition scores, two were significant; sibling affection and cooperation were related to the child's later score on the affective aggregate measure.

Multivariate Analyses of the Correlates of the Social Cognition Measures

The analyses conducted so far indicate that discourse about feelings and about causality, SES, and parental education, ratings of mothers' behavior to the sibling, and ratings of child-sibling interaction are each related to some of the individual differences in the outcome measures of social cognition. However, the interpretation of these univariate associations is complicated by the relations between the variables from time 1. For instance, it cannot be assumed that the discourse measures were related to outcome independently of SES or parental education. In the third set of analyses, we examine (*a*) the variance in each of the social cognition measures that could be explained jointly by these different sets of variables and (*b*) the unique variance in each outcome measure accounted for by each set of predictors.

Affective Aggregate Given the relatively small sample size, we limited the variables to be entered to four sets. On the basis of the preceding correlational analyses, the variables selected to enter in the multiple regression for this variable were the rating of child-to-sibling cooperation, father's occupational prestige, the upperbound MLU of child and mother entered as one step, and the discourse variables child talk about causality and child talk about feelings (minus those turns in which cause was discussed) entered as one step. Table 4 shows that together these variables accounted for 56% of the variance in the affective aggregate measure. By next conducting separate hierarchical multiple regression analyses systematically excluding each of the four sets of variables in turn, the unique variance contributed by each variable was determined. Table 4 shows that for the affective aggregate variable, the discourse variables independently contributed 10% of the variance, the child-sibling cooperation rating 7%, the SES variable a further 4%, and the child and mother upperbound MLU 5%

On the issue of gender, as noted earlier, boys and girls differed on average on the affective aggregate measure. However, we are concerned here with the question of whether these associations between the predictors and affective understanding interact with gender. That is, does discourse about feelings and causality, for instance, relate to affective understanding differently for boys and girls? With a sample of 50, power to detect such gender interactions is very limited. However, in order to explore the possibility of gender interactions, we conducted the multiple regressions separately for boys and girls. None of the differences between the standardized beta weights for boys and girls approached significance.

Explanation in the False Belief Task On the basis of the previous correlational analyses, the variables selected for the multiple regressions for the measure of *explanation* in the false belief tasks were as follows: the child-sibling cooperation rating, the mother-child causal and child feeling state talk, the mother's upperbound MLU, and the mother-sibling control rating. Table 4 shows that together these variables accounted for 39% of the variance in the explanation measure. The ratings of child-sibling cooperation and of the mother's controlling/intrusive behavior with the sibling independently contributed 11% and 7% to the prediction of this measure, and the discourse variables 4% independent of the shared variance.

DISCUSSION

At 40 months, the children in this study differed widely in their understanding of the situational determinants of others' feelings, and while some were able to explain actions in terms of false beliefs, the majority were not. While any direct comparison of performance on the explanation and prediction tasks would be inappropriate—with one a forced-choice and the other an open-ended task—it is worth noting that twice as many children provided explanations linking action to beliefs as those who made predictions successfully in the forced-choice tasks. We take these results to support the argument of Bartsch and Wellman (1989) that some children of this age can understand belief constructs and can engage in belief-desire reasoning, even though they fail traditional forced-choice false belief prediction tasks that present a conflict between what would satisfy the actor's desire and what she believes (see, however, Moses & Flavell, 1990, for an interpretation of children's explanations that differ in some respects). In this conflict, it appears that 3-year-olds weigh the satisfaction of desire over belief; they seem unlikely to suppose that some-

TABLE 4

Variance in Social Understanding Measures Explained by Discourse Measures, Ratings of Interaction, SES, Upperbound MLU

Social Understanding Measure	R^2	F	df	Discourse Measures	Change in R^2	Ratings	Change in R^2	SES	Change in R^2	Upperbound MLU	Change in R^2
Affective aggregate	.56*	10.99	5.44	Child feeling state[a] + child causal	.10*	Child cooperate with sib	.07*	Father prestige	.04+	Child and mother	.05+
False belief task: explanations	.39*	7.08	4.45	Mother-child causal + child feeling state[a]	.04+	Child cooperate with sib Mother control sib	.11* .07*			Mother	.01

[a] Child feeling state talk minus causal turns.
+ $p < .10$.
* $p < .05$.

one will act in a way that will not satisfy their desires. Moreover, in everyday conversation it is likely that children are witnesses to, or participants in, conversations in which explanations for behavior in terms of belief are given more often than predictions about how belief will influence action. For example, during the observations mothers frequently attempted to sort out disagreements between siblings by explaining how the other child's (often mistaken) beliefs governed his or her actions: "He thought you had finished yours"; "She didn't know I had promised it to you"; "He thought it was his turn."

The exploration of the earlier correlates of these abilities showed that children who grew up in families in which they engaged in conversations about feelings and about causality were better able 7 months later to explain the feelings and actions of the puppet characters in the task situations. While the large number of correlations conducted suggests caution about generalizing from these data, the results do indicate the usefulness of studying not only global aspects of family relationships but also the content of family conversations. Each of these aspects of family interaction raises its own set of issues about the development of individual differences. First, it is possible that in the pattern of findings for family discourse and affective perspective taking we may be picking up a pattern of continuity, in *child differences*, rather than evidence for an association between parental or sibling talk and later child outcome. Second, the continuity between the discourse measures and the abilities assessed 7 months later was not explained by the children's verbal fluency, nor by the amount of talk in the family. We should, of course, be very cautious about suggesting causal links from these correlational data; the results, however, do support the view that the conceptual development reflected in the abilities revealed in the affective perspective-taking and false belief tasks may have been encouraged through the conversations in which the children participated—that is, that language specific in content may have in part mediated the conceptual development. It is of course equally possible that children's participation in conversations about causality and feelings and their later performance on sociocognitive tasks both reflect some common underlying ability rather than any direct causal link. Third, a larger number of correlations were found for talk about feelings than talk about causality. This may reflect the fact that the causal talk category was not limited to behavioral or psychological causality but included a broad range of causal discussion.

The results from the analysis of the ratings of family interaction raise four further issues. First, associations were found between the children's cooperation with their siblings and their later performance on the social cognition tasks. Again, it would be inappropriate to draw conclusions about directional cause-effect links. It could be that through cooperation and play with the sibling children gain insights into the thoughts, actions, and feelings of the other child—who is of course closer in interests and feelings to the child than a parent would be. Such a view is compatible with the arguments for the significance of peer interaction in sociocognitive development (Hartup, 1983). However, it is also possible that with greater skills of understanding others, children are able to cooperate and play more effectively; here the pattern of results would be seen as reflecting a continuity in differences between children. Such an argument would be supported by the evidence for a positive relation between emotional understanding and children's relationships with peers (Cassidy & Parke, 1990; Denham, McKinley, Couchoud, & Holt, 1990; Rothenberg, 1970). In common sense terms, it seems likely that both processes may operate. Second, the lack of association between ratings of mother-child interaction and the social cognition tasks should be noted. Connections might well have been expected here, especially in light of the associations between mother-child discourse and the outcome measures. This failure to demonstrate connections could reflect insensitivity of the ratings of maternal behavior (though the findings on mother-to-sibling ratings decrease the plausibility of this interpretation). It could also be—as we have noted—that it is child differences, rather than differences in maternal behavior, that are key to the connection between the discourse and social cognition measures, at least within the range of differences within this sample.

The third point concerns the question of why there should be a clearer pattern of association between the family measures and the children's affective perspective-taking measure than the false belief measure. It could be that this is primarily a statistical matter, which reflects differences in the distribution of scores in the two outcome measures—with a greater range of individual variation in the affective perspective-taking measure. Such a difference reflects in part the different developmental course of the growth of these two aspects of social understanding: Understanding of emotions appears earlier in childhood than the ability to understand other minds and to relate actions to beliefs. However, an intriguing issue for future investigation is the question of whether these two domains of social understanding are in fact influenced to differing degrees by the features of family relationships and discourse that were considered here. Is emotional understanding influenced to a greater extent by patterns of family interaction than the development of the ability to grasp the links between thoughts, beliefs, and action? The relation between these two aspects of social understanding deserves further study.

The final point raised by the analysis of the ratings concern the links found between mother-sibling interaction and the children's social cognitive sophistication. Children who grew up in families in which their mothers engaged in relatively frequent controlling behavior with the older sibling were more likely to be able to give explanations in the false belief task; they also tended to be better at affective labeling and perspective taking if their mothers had been highly responsive and affectionate with the sibling than children whose mothers and siblings were not involved in this way. These results alert us to the importance of recognizing that children grow up as *family members*, and that the salient influences on children's development include more than the behavior or language directed directly to them. Children are extremely interested in what happens between their siblings and their parents, monitoring closely both the language (Dunn & Shatz, 1989) and the emotions expressed (Dunn & Kendrick, 1982; Dunn & Munn, 1985). It is of course highly adaptive for children who are born into a social group—the family—to attend to and begin to make sense of the interaction between those other family members early in their own development. The findings of the present study remind us that the appropriate framework in which we should study developmental influences is that of the family, rather than solely that of a parent-child dyad. Promising next steps in the investigation of individual differences in understanding others will be to examine in more detail the nature of interaction between siblings implicated, to clarify which particular aspects of discourse about others are most important, to pursue the issue of gender differences in early understanding of other people, and to conduct longitudinal studies to explore the prognostic significance of these early differences in understanding other minds.

REFERENCES

Astington, J. W., Harris, P. L., & Olson, D. R. (1988). *Developing theories of mind.* Cambridge: Cambridge University Press.

Bartsch, K., & Wellman, H. (1989). Young children's attribution of action to beliefs and desires. *Child Development, 60,* 946–964.

Borke, H. (1971). Interpersonal perception of young children: Egocentrism or empathy? *Developmental Psychology, 60,* 263–269.

Bretherton, I., McNew, S., & Beeghly-Smith, M. (1981). Early person knowledge as expressed in gestural and verbal communication: When do infants acquire a "theory of mind"? In M. E. Lamb & L. R. Sherrod (Eds.), *Infant social cognition* (pp. 333–373). Hillsdale, NJ: Erlbaum.

Cassidy, J., & Parke, R. (1990). *Family-peer connections: The roles of parental emotional expressiveness and children's understanding of emotions.* Manuscript submitted for publication.

Cummings, E. M., Hollenbeck, B., Ianotti, R., Radke-Yarrow, M., & Zahn-Waxler, C. (1986). Early organization of altruism and aggression: Developmental patterns and individual differences. In C. Zahn-Waxler, E. M. Cummings, & R. Ianotti (Eds.), *Altruism and aggression* (pp. 165–188). Cambridge: Cambridge University Press.

Cummings, E. M., Zahn-Waxler, C., & Radke-Yarrow, M. (1981). Young children's responses to expressions of anger and affection by others in the family. *Child Development, 52,* 1274–1282.

Denham, S. A. (1986). Social cognition, prosocial behavior, and emotion in preschoolers: Contextual validation. *Child Development, 57,* 194–201.

Denham, S. A., & Couchoud, E. A. (1990). *Knowledge about emotions: Relations with socialization and social behavior.* Manuscript submitted for publication.

Denham, S. A., McKinley, M., Couchoud, E. A., & Holt, R. (1990). Emotional and behavioral predictors of preschool peer ratings. *Child Development, 61*, 1145–1152.

Dunn, J., Bretherton, I., & Munn, P. (1987). Conversations about feeling states between mothers and their young children. *Developmental Psychology, 23*, 791–798.

Dunn, J., Brown, J., & Beardsall, L. (1991). Family talk about emotions, and children's later understanding of others' emotions. *Developmental Psychology, 27*, 448–455.

Dunn, J., & Kendrick, C. (1982). *Siblings: Love, envy and understanding.* Cambridge, MA: Harvard University Press.

Dunn, J., & Munn, P. (1985). Becoming a family member: Family conflict and the development of social understanding in the second year. *Child Development, 56*, 764–774.

Dunn, J., & Munn, P. (1987). The development of justification in disputes. *Developmental Psychology, 23*, 791–798.

Dunn, J., & Shatz, M. (1989). Becoming a conversationalist despite (or because of) having a sibling. *Child Development, 60*, 399–410.

Finn, R. H. (1970). A note on estimating the reliability of categorical data. *Educational and Psychological Measurement, 30*, 71–76.

Finn, R. H. (1972). Effects of some variations in rating scale characteristics on the means and reliabilities of ratings. *Educational and Psychological Measurement, 35*, 255–265.

Frye, D., & Moore, C. (Eds.). (1990). *Children's theories of mind.* Hillsdale, NJ: Erlbaum.

Gnepp, J. (1989). Personalized inferences of emotions and appraisals: Component processes and correlates. *Developmental Psychology, 25*, 277–288.

Harris, P. L. (1989). *Children and emotion.* Oxford: Basil Blackwell.

Hartup, W. W. (1983). Peer relations. In E. M. Hetherington (Ed.), P. H. Mussen (Series Ed.), *Handbook of child psychology: Vol. 4. Socialization, personality, and social development* (pp. 103–196). New York: Wiley.

Hauser, R. M., & Featherman, D. L. (1977). *The process of stratification: Trends and analysis.* New York: Academic Press.

Hood, L., & Bloom, L. (1979). What, when, and how about why: A longitudinal study of early expressions of causality. *Monographs of the Society for Research in Child Development, 44*(6, Serial No. 181).

Main, M., & George, S. (1985). Responses of abused and disadvantaged toddlers to distress in agemates: A study in the daycare setting. *Developmental Psychology, 21*, 407–412.

Miller, P. H., & Aloise, P. A. (1989). Young children's understanding of the psychological causes of behavior: A review. *Child Development, 60*, 257–285.

Moses, L. J., & Flavell, J. H. (1990). Inferring false beliefs from actions and reactions. *Child Development, 61*, 929–945.

Murphy, L. B. (1937). *Social behavior and child personality.* New York: Columbia University Press.

Olson, D. R., Astington, J. R., & Harris, P. L. (1988). Introduction. In J. W. Astington, P. L. Harris, & D. R. Olson (Eds.), *Developing theories of mind* (pp. 1–15). Cambridge: Cambridge University Press.

Ridgeway, D., Waters, E., & Kuczaj, S. A. (1985). The acquisition of emotion descriptive language: Receptive and productive vocabulary norms for ages 18 months to 6 years. *Developmental Psychology, 21*, 901–908.

Rothenberg, B. (1970). Children's social sensitivity and the relationship to interpersonal competence, intrapersonal comfort and intellectual level. *Developmental Psychology, 2*, 335–350.

Shatz, M., & Gelman, R. (1973). The development of communication skills: Modification in the speech of young children as a function of listener. *Monographs of the Society for Research in Child Development, 38*(5, Serial No. 152).

Shatz, M., Wellman, H. M., & Silber, S. (1983). The acquisition of mental verbs: A systematic investigation of the first reference to mental state. *Cognition, 14*, 301–321.

Stewart, R. B., & Marvin, R. S. (1984). Sibling relations: The role of conceptual perspective-taking in the ontogeny of sibling caregiving. *Child Development, 55*, 1322–1332.

Stocker, C., Dunn, J., & Plomin, R. (1989). Sibling relationships: Links with child temperament, maternal behavior, and family structure. *Child Development, 60*, 715–727.

Tinsley, H. E. A., & Weiss, D. J. (1975). Inter-rater reliability and agreement of subjective judgments. *Journal of Counselling Psychology, 22*, 358–376.

Wellman, H. M. (1985). The origins of metacognition. In D. Forrest-Pressley, C. McKinnon, & T. Waller (Eds.), *Metacognition, cognition and human performance.* New York: Academic Press.

Wellman, H. M. (1988). First steps in the child's theorizing about the mind. In J. W. Astington, P. L. Harris, & D. R. Olson (Eds.), *Developing theories of mind* (pp. 64–92). Cambridge: Cambridge University Press.

Whiten, A. (Ed.). (1990). *Natural theories of mind.* Oxford: Basil Blackwell.

Zahn-Waxler, C., Radke-Yarrow, M., & King, R. A. (1979). Child rearing and children's prosocial initiations towards victims of distress. *Child Development, 48*, 319–330.

2

Facial Diversity and Infant Preferences for Attractive Faces

Judith H. Langlois

University of Texas at Austin

Jean M. Ritter

California State University at Fresno

Lori A. Roggman

Utah State University, Logan

Lesley S. Vaughn

Three studies examined infant preferences for attractive faces in four types of faces: White adult male and female faces, Black adult female faces, and infant faces. Infants viewed pairs of faces, previously rated for attractiveness by adults, in a visual preference paradigm. Significant preferences were found for attractive faces across all facial types. The results confirm earlier reports of this phenomenon and extend those results by showing that infant preferences for attractive faces generalize across faces differing in race, gender, and age. Two potential explanations for these observed infant preferences are discussed.

We recently reported several studies showing that young infants visually discriminate among adult female faces based on the adult-judged attractiveness of the faces and that infants exhibit both visual and behavioral preferences for attractive compared with unattractive female faces (Langlois et al., 1987; Langlois, Roggman, & Rieser-Danner, 1990). These results were surprising to many people because infants were not expected to be able to make such subtle discriminations. In addition, most researchers interested in the effects of physical attractiveness have assumed that preferences for attractiveness are only gradually learned through a

Reprinted with permission from *Developmental Psychology*, 1991, Vol. 27, No. 1, 79–84. Copyright 1991 by the American Psychological Association, Inc. This research was supported by Grant HD 21332 from the National Institute of Child Health and Human Development to Judith H. Langlois.

lengthy period of cultural transmission and through exposure to the standards of attractiveness extant in the contemporary media and society. However, these behaviors of young infants suggested that preferences for attractiveness in faces are present much earlier than has been assumed.

Other researchers have also found that infants look longer at and seem to prefer attractive compared with unattractive female faces. Samuels and Ewy (1985) and Shapiro, Hazan, and Haith (1984) showed both adult male and adult female faces that were rated as high or low in attractiveness by adult judges to infants ranging from 3 to 6 months of age. The infants in these studies looked significantly longer at both the male and the female attractive faces compared with unattractive faces. Although some methodological limitations of these two studies prevent a clear-cut interpretation of their results, they at least suggest that infants can discriminate attractiveness in two different types of faces, male and female.

Given the challenge that these findings from infants pose to the widely accepted assumptions about the origins of preferences for attractiveness (Langlois et al., 1987), it is important to investigate the generality of these preferences across different types of faces. Demonstrating infant preferences for attractive faces across different types of faces would extend the phenomenon to the class of faces in general and would serve as an important replication of the work with female faces.

The purpose of the present studies was therefore to replicate our previous results with adult female faces and to determine if infant preferences for attractive faces extend beyond adult female faces to other types of faces. Specifically, we used a visual preference paradigm to investigate infant preferences for attractiveness in male and female adult White faces, in Black adult female faces, and in the faces of other young infants.

STUDY 1

Our purposes in conducting this study were, first, to replicate our previous results with adult female facial stimuli (Langlois et al., 1987), second, to extend the results to male facial stimuli, and, third, to investigate whether the manner in which male and female faces are presented influences infant preferences. Shapiro et al. (1984), for example, noted that infant interest in male faces was significantly reduced when these faces were presented separately compared with when they were alternated with female faces. Because Samuels and Ewy (1985) also presented male faces alternating with female faces, it is not clear whether infants preferred attractive male faces themselves or whether the female faces somehow "primed" the preferences of the infants in these two studies. Therefore, in addition to presenting both male and female faces, we included two methods of presentation. In one condition, infants viewed separate sets of attractive and unattractive male and female faces; in the other condition, infants viewed alternating pairs of attractive and unattractive male and female faces, similar to the procedures of Samuels and Ewy (1985) and of Shapiro et al. (1984).

Method

Subjects. One hundred ten 6-month-old infants were recruited from the subject pool at the Children's Research Lab at the University of Texas at Austin. Fifty infants were eliminated from the final sample for the following reasons: 41 for fussing,[1] 3 for computer or equipment failure, 3 for experimenter error, 2 because the mother looked at the slides, and 1 because the infant was 1 month premature. The 60 remaining infants (35 boys and 25 girls) were healthy, full-term infants from middle-class families, with an average age of 6 months, 6 days. Fifty-three infants were White, 5 were Hispanic, 1 was Black, and 1 was Asian. All of the infants were tested within 3 weeks of their 6-month birthday.

Stimuli. Each infant saw color slides of 16 adult women and 16 adult men; half of the slides of each sex depicted attractive faces, the other half unattractive faces. The slides of the women's faces had been used in a previous study of infant preferences for attractive faces (Langlois et al., 1987). The slides were selected from a pool of 275 women's and 165 men's faces that were rated for attractiveness by at least 40 undergraduate men and women using a 5-point Likert-type scale (range of mean attractiveness for women = 1.05 to 4.02, M = 2.26, SD = 0.68; range for men = 1.11 to 4.06, M = 2.42, SD = 0.56). The reliabilities of these ratings were .97 for the women's faces and .95 for the men's faces, as assessed by coefficient alphas.

Slides with high and low attractiveness ratings from the pools of male and female faces were identified as potential stimuli. The final stimuli were selected so that facial expression, hair length, and hair color were equally distributed across attractiveness conditions within sex of slides. All of the male faces were clean-shaven. Clothing cues were masked and all of the faces were posed with neutral expressions. The mean attractiveness ratings for the stimulus faces were 3.46 for the attractive women, 3.35 for the attractive men, 1.44 for the unattractive women, and 1.40 for the unattractive men. Both the attractive female and the attractive male stimuli were significantly more attractive than the mean of the larger pool of photographs for each group, $t(274) = 4.99, p < .001$, for the women and $t(164) = 4.70, p < .001$, for the men. Likewise, the unattractive women and men were significantly less attractive than the mean group, $t(274) = -3.41, p < .001$, for the women and $t(164) = -4.34, p < .001$, for the men. There were no significant differences

---

[1]The very large number of trials in this procedure ($N = 32$) relative to the typical infant visual preference study contributed to the high rate of fussing and, thus, attrition. In addition, a relatively strict criterion of fussing was required: Infants who fussed on any trial during the procedure were not included in the data analysis because fussing interfered with their looking behavior.

between the attractive male and the attractive female faces or between the unattractive male and the unattractive female faces.

Procedure. A standard visual preference technique was used in which two faces, one attractive and one unattractive, were simultaneously rear-projected onto a screen. The infant was seated on the parent's lap approximately 35 cm from the screen. The parent wore occluded glasses to prevent him or her from viewing the faces so that parental preferences could not be communicated to the infant. A light and a buzzing noise were used to capture the infant's attention at the center of the screen before the beginning of each trial. When the infant looked at the center of the screen, the next pair of slides was displayed. A trial began when the infant first looked at one of the slides; each trial lasted for 10 s. During intertrial intervals, filtered light was displayed to keep the level of brightness on the screen consistent throughout the procedure.

The stimuli were presented in two sets of 16 slides. Each set was divided into eight trial blocks of two slides each. To control for infant side biases, each trial block consisted of two consecutive 10-s trials in which a slide pair was presented in a right-left position for the first trial and the reversed left-right position for the second trial. Slides were always paired within sex so that infants viewed only pairs of women or pairs of men. In one condition of presentation (alternating), the infants observed alternating pairs of males and females. In the other condition (grouped), infants saw all the women's slides together and all the men's slides together. The infants were given a 5-10-min break after eight trial blocks to alleviate fatigue. Order of set presentation, order of slide-pair presentation within sets (within the constraints of the set), and order of slide pairing were randomized across subjects so that a particular slide of an attractive face could be paired with any slide of an unattractive face of the same sex for any given subject. Trial length, slide advance, and recording of the data were controlled by a laboratory computer.

The experimenter observed the infants' visual fixations on a video monitor connected to a video camera mounted just under the projection screen. Direction and duration of looks were recorded on the keyboard of a laboratory computer that functioned as an event recorder. Using the televised image of the infant to observe visual fixation ensured that the experimenter could not see the displayed slides and was therefore blind to the attractiveness level of the slides the infant was observing. Reliability of the visual-fixation scoring was obtained by having each experimenter score randomly selected videotaped sessions periodically throughout data collection. An intraclass correlation, which allows generalization to other populations of experimenters and infants, was used to assess reliability. The resulting intraclass correlations for the average of the reliabilities of the individual experimenters ranged from .97 to .99.

Because some infants were excluded from the analysis for fussing, it was impor-

TABLE 1
Mean Fixation Times for High- and Low-Attractiveness Slides

Type of face	High attractiveness		Low attractiveness	
	M	SD	M	SD
Male and female faces (Study 1)	7.82	1.35	7.57	1.27
Black female faces (Study 2)	7.05	1.83	6.52	1.92
Baby faces (Study 3)	7.16	1.97	6.62	1.83

tant to establish agreement among experimenters on infant fussing. Using video-taped sessions, the agreement among experimenters' judgments of fussing on each trial in a session was evaluated using coefficient kappa, a conservative estimate of agreement that takes the probability of chance into account. The kappas for fussing ranged from .60 to 1.0, with a mean kappa of .82.

To determine whether the infants' preferences for faces might be influenced by the attractiveness of the mothers, photographs were taken of the mothers.[2] These photographs were rated for attractiveness by 72 undergraduates (29 men, 43 women), who judged attractiveness using a 5-point Likert-type scale. The reliability of these ratings was .98 as assessed by coefficient alpha.

Results

Looking time. Each infant's total looking time at each stimulus slide was obtained by summing looking time at the right- and the left-side presentations of the slides. Looking time was then subjected to a four-way repeated-measures multivariate analysis of variance (MANOVA), using the regression approach to control for the unequal numbers of male and female infants (Langlois et al., 1987; McCall & Appelbaum, 1973). Infant sex was the between-subjects factor; condition of presentation (slides of the same sex grouped together or alternating with the other sex), sex of face, attractiveness level (attractive or unattractive), and trial were within-subjects factors.

The results indicated that infants looked longer at the attractive faces than the unattractive faces, $F(1,58) = 4.73, p = .03$ (see Table 1). This main effect for attractiveness did not interact with sex of face, indicating that infant preferences for attractive faces were evident for both adult male and adult female faces.

[2]Eleven mothers were not photographed because of equipment failure or experimenter error.

TABLE 2
Mean Fixation Times for Sex of Infant × Sex of Face Interaction

	Male face		Female face	
Sex of infant	M	SD	M	SD
Male	7.95	1.45	7.36	1.31
Female	7.69	1.35	7.81	1.33

Condition of presentation was not significant and did not interact with any other factors.

A Sex of Infant × Sex of Stimulus Face interaction was also obtained, $F(1,58)$ = 4.34, p = .04. Univariate analyses indicated that boys looked at male faces longer than at female faces, $F(1,34)$ = 7.66, $p < .01$ (Table 2). The girls also looked longer at same-sex faces, although the difference was not significant. Finally, a main effect for trial was found, $F(3,56)$ = 24.46, $p < .001$. The univariate analyses of this trial effect revealed that infant looking time decreased over the session.

Maternal attractiveness. The relationship between maternal attractiveness and infant preferences for faces based on attractiveness and sex was also examined. A median split was performed on maternal attractiveness, and infants were divided into two groups depending on whether their mothers were in the upper or lower half of the range of maternal attractiveness (Langlois et al., 1987). A MANOVA was performed on infant looking time, with mother attractiveness and sex of infant as between-subjects factors and sex of stimulus face and attractiveness of stimulus face as within-subject factors. No significant relationships were found between mother attractiveness and infant sex, sex of stimulus face, or attractiveness of stimulus face.

STUDY 2

To extend the findings to non-White faces, a second study was conducted, in which infants were shown faces of Black adult women. The faces were rated for attractiveness by both Black and Caucasian adult judges.

Method

Subjects. Forty-three 6-month-old infants selected from the Children's Research Lab subject pool were tested. Two infants were excluded from the analysis because of fussing, and 1 was excluded because of equipment failure. The remaining 40 infants (15 boys and 25 girls) were healthy, full-term infants with an average age of 6 months, 5 days. Thirty-six babies were White, 2 were Black, and 2 were Hispanic.

Stimuli. The infants were shown color slides of the faces of 16 adult Black women selected from a pool of 127 photographs that had been rated for attractiveness by 98 White and 41 Black undergraduate men and women using a 5-point Likert-type scale. The reliability of the ratings of this pool was .99 for the White raters and .97 for the Black raters as assessed by coefficient alpha. The correlation between the mean ratings from the White judges and those from the Black judges for each photo was quite substantial, $r(127) = .93, p < .001$. The mean attractiveness ratings for the pool of faces ranged from 1.16 to 3.92 for the White raters ($M = 2.15$, $SD = 0.61$) and from 1.29 to 3.83 for the Black raters ($M = 2.18, SD = 0.62$). Eight of the slides that had been rated as attractive and eight rated as unattractive were selected as stimuli. Clothing cues were masked and all of the faces had neutral expressions. Amount of hair and skin color were equally distributed across attractiveness conditions. The mean attractiveness rating for the attractive women was 3.41 as assessed by the White raters and 3.42 as assessed by the Black raters. For both White and Black raters, these attractiveness ratings were significantly above the mean for the pool, $t(126) = 5.84, p < .001$, for White raters and $t(126) = 5.66, p < .001$ for Black raters. The mean attractiveness rating for the unattractive women was 1.44 as assessed by the White raters and 1.54 as assessed by the Black raters. Both White and Black raters evaluated these stimuli as significantly less attractive than the mean of the larger pool, $t(126) = -3.29, p < .01$, for White raters and $t(126) = -2.92, p < .01$, for Black raters.

Procedure. A visual preference technique similar to the one described in Study 1 was used to assess infants' preferences. However, we did not include a condition of presentation factor (grouped vs. alternating), and we reduced the number of trials required for each infant in order to lessen fatigue and attrition. Each infant saw four of the eight attractive slides paired with four of the eight unattractive slides presented in four trial blocks. As in Study 1, each slide pair was presented twice; the second presentation was in the reversed right-left position from the first presentation. The pairing of slides varied randomly, the only restriction being that slides had to be paired with slides of the other level of attractiveness. Across infants, all eight attractive and all eight unattractive faces were presented. The intraclass correlation calculated to assess reliability for looking time ranged from .95 to .97. Kappas assessing the agreement of fussing judgments ranged from .89 to 1.0, with a mean kappa of .93.

To determine whether the infants' preferences were influenced by the attractiveness of the mother, photographs were taken of the mothers. These photographs were rated for attractiveness by 49 undergraduates (27 men, 22 women), who judged attractiveness using a 5-point Likert-type scale. The reliability of these ratings was .97 as assessed by coefficient alpha.

Results

Looking time. Each infant's total looking time at each slide was obtained by summing the right- and the left-side presentations of that slide. Looking time was then subjected to a two-way repeated-measures MANOVA using the regression approach, with infant sex as a between-subjects factor. The within-subjects factors were attractiveness of stimulus face (attractive or unattractive) and trial.

The analyses indicated that 6-month-old infants looked longer at the attractive Black women's faces than at the unattractive faces, $F(1.38) = 4.34$, $p < .05$ (see Table 1). In addition, a main effect for trial was found, $F(3,36) = 15.81$, $p < .001$. The univariate analyses revealed that infants looked longer in the first two trials than in subsequent trials. There was no interaction between stimulus attractiveness and trial, and sex of infant was not significant and did not interact with any of the within-subjects factors.

Maternal attractiveness. The relationship between maternal attractiveness and infant preferences for faces was examined using the same procedures as in Study 1. Like Study 1, no significant relationships were found between maternal attractiveness and either infant sex or attractiveness of stimulus face.

STUDY 3

To extend the results obtained when infants look at adult faces, we conducted a third study using stimulus faces of babies varying in attractiveness.

Method

Subjects. Fifty-two 6-month-old infants selected from the same subject pool as in Studies 1 and 2 were tested. Eleven infants were excluded from the analysis because of fussing, and 2 infants were excluded because they were not tested within 3 weeks of their 6-month birthday. The 39 remaining infants (19 boys and 20 girls) were healthy, full-term infants from middle-class families, with an average age of 6 months, 15 days. Thirty-seven of the infants were Caucasian; 2 were Hispanic.

Stimuli. The infants were shown color slides of the faces of sixteen 3-month-old male and female infants selected from a pool of photographs of 60 boys and 62 girls that had been rated for attractiveness by at least 40 undergraduate men and women using a 5-point Likert-type scale. The reliability of the ratings of these larger pools was .97 for the male infants' faces and .96 for the female infants' faces as assessed by coefficient alpha. Attractiveness ratings, averaged across raters, ranged from 1.22 to 4.21 for the male infants and 1.37 to 3.98 for the female infants. Four male and 4 female slides that had been rated as attractive and 4 male and 4 female slides rated as unattractive were selected as stimuli. Clothing cues were masked and all faces had neutral expressions. Amount of hair was equally distributed across attractiveness conditions. The mean attractiveness ratings were 3.02 for the attractive babies and 1.69 for the unattractive babies. When compared with the mean rating (2.44) of the larger pool from which they came, the attractive set was significantly more attractive, $t(121) = 2.56, p < .05$, and the unattractive set was significantly less attractive, $t(121) = -3.31, p < .01$.

Procedure. A visual preference technique identical to the one used in Study 2 was used. The intraclass correlation calculated to assess reliability for looking time ranged from .95 to .97. Kappas assessing reliability for fussing ranged from .85 to 1.00, with a mean kappa of .92. Because we did not find any significant effects of the attractiveness of the mother on infant preferences in Studies 1 and 2 and because it seemed unlikely that the attractiveness of the mother would influence preferences for baby faces, maternal attractiveness was not evaluated in this study.

Results

As in the previous two studies, each infant's total looking time was obtained by summing the right- and the left-side presentations of the slides. Looking time was then subjected to a two-way repeated-measures MANOVA, with infant sex as a between-subjects factor. The within-subjects factors were attractiveness of stimulus face and trial.

The analyses indicated that 6-month-old infants looked longer at the attractive babies' faces than at the unattractive faces, $F(1.37) = 4.85, p = .034$. In addition, a main effect for trial was found, $F(3,35) = 7.53, p < .001$. The univariate analyses revealed that infants looked longer in the first two trials than in subsequent trials. There was no interaction between stimulus attractiveness and trial, and sex of infant was not significant and did not interact with any of the within-subjects factors.[3]

GENERAL DISCUSSION

The results of these three studies unambiguously show that 6-month-old infants can discriminate attractive from unattractive faces and that they visually prefer attractive faces of diverse types. These results represent more than just replications of previous findings of infant preferences for the faces of attractive women. Rather,

---

[3]Although same-sex preferences were obtained in Study 1 with adult faces, we considered it unlikely that such preferences would be observed with the faces of 3-month-old infants as stimuli. Indeed, when asked to guess the sex of the stimulus infants, 10 adults performed at chance levels. The results of an analysis that included sex of stimulus infant as a factor confirmed our suspicion: Neither sex of stimulus nor the Sex of Stimulus Infant × Sex of Subject interaction were significant. $Fs(1,37) = 1.66$ and 0.17, respectively, both *ns*.

these results are important because they show that infants treat attractive faces as distinctive regardless of the sex, age, and race of the stimulus faces, even though most of the infants had little experience with some of the types of faces they viewed (e.g., the faces of Black women and of 3-month-old infants) and even though the infants had little experience with cultural transmission of standards of beauty. The ability of young infants to discriminate attractiveness in such diverse faces is all the more remarkable given the rather substantial differences in the structure of male and female, Black and White, and adult and infant faces (e.g., Farkas, 1981). Thus, the facial cues that yield judgments of attractiveness seem to be invariant across different types of faces, and even young infants seem to be able to perceive them. Other research has shown that there are important behavioral concomitants of these laboratory-derived visual preferences, at least in slightly older infants: twelve-month-olds interact differently with attractive and unattractive faces and show more positive affect, less withdrawal, and more play involvement with an attractive compared with an unattractive unfamiliar adult (Langlois et al., 1990).

Why are attractive faces special to infants and why do infants prefer them to less attractive faces? And why is it that, contrary to common assumption, recent cross-cultural investigations have demonstrated surprisingly high (e.g., .66-.93) interrater reliabilities in judgments of attractiveness (Bernstein, Lin, & McClellan, 1982; Cunningham, 1986; Johnson, Dannenbring, Anderson, & Villa, 1983; Maret, 1983; Maret & Harling, 1985; McArthur & Berry, 1987; Richardson, Goodman, Hastorf, & Dornbusch, 1961; Thakerar & Iwawaki, 1979; Weisfeld, Weisfeld, & Callaghan, 1984)? For example, Cunningham (1986) assembled an international sample of photographs of female faces, had the faces rated for attractiveness, and measured various features of the faces. As in other cross-cultural studies, and like our own samples of Black and White judges, raters agreed about the attractiveness of this international sample of faces. Furthermore, the facial measurements showed that although Black, White, and Oriental faces possessed ethnically distinct features, there was considerable similarity in facial features associated with attractiveness across racial groups. Thus, ethnically diverse faces possess both distinct and similar, perhaps even universal, structural features. These features seem to be perceived as attractive regardless of the age and the racial and cultural background of the perceiver.

Perhaps, then, attractive faces are preferred by infants and adults from different cultures because they are more prototypic of the category of faces. One definition of a prototype includes exemplars of a category that represent the averaged members of the class of objects comprising the category (e.g., Reed, 1972; Rosch, 1978; Strauss, 1979). We recently reported data showing that prototypical, or "average," faces, created by digitizing and then mathematically averaging a series of individual faces, were rated as highly attractive (Langlois & Roggman, 1990). The averaged faces were not at all average in facial attractiveness, but, in fact, were rated as significantly more attractive than digitized images of the individual faces that were averaged together. Furthermore, averaged faces became even more attractive as more faces were added. This phenomenon held true for several samples of both male and female faces and for several samples of raters.

Given that "averageness" seems to be an important ingredient of facial attractiveness, two explanations seem viable for our findings showing that even young infants prefer attractive faces. Evidence already exists demonstrating that the average value of the members of a class of objects can be prototypical, that infants are capable of forming prototypes by averaging features, and that infants assign prototypes special status even when they have not seen them before (e.g., Bomba & Siqueland, 1983; Cohen & Younger, 1983; Posner & Keele, 1968; Strauss, 1979). Strauss (1979), for example, showed schematic faces to infants and demonstrated that young infants recognized facial prototypes made from the averaged values of previously viewed facial features and that they responded to these prototypical or averaged schematics as distinctive, even though they had never seen them before. In contrast, infants did not treat schematics made from the most frequently seen features as special. Although our data did not demonstrate that attractive faces are perceived as prototypes by infants, they did show that infants have remarkable capabilities to respond differentially to attractive versus unattractive faces with greater visual attention. The perception by adults of prototypes or averaged faces as attractive supports an interpretation of infant preferences for attractive faces as part of a categorical social response to prototypic members of the category of faces.

Another explanation for the preferences of infants for attractive faces, although also resting on the notion that an attractive face is an averaged member of the category of faces, depends on a very different literature and theoretical rationale than that of cognitive abstraction of facial stimuli. Evolutionary biologists would account for infant preferences for attractive faces as an innate tendency to prefer average values of the population of faces. In normalizing or stabilizing selection, evolutionary pressures operate in favor of the average of the population and against the extremes of the population (e.g., Bumpas, 1899; Dobzhansky, 1970; Schmalhausen, 1949; Symons, 1979). Thus, the average values of many anatomical features should be preferred in the population because individuals close to the mean for the population are less likely to carry harmful genetic mutations. Symons (1979) specifically proposed an innate mechanism of perception that detects the population mean of anatomical features by averaging observed faces. Because of stabilizing selection pressures, these "average" faces are preferred by the species over faces more distant from the mean, according to Symons.

Although the date currently available do not allow us to choose between the cognitive and the evolutionary explanations, both perspectives bring coherence and reason to data showing preferences for attractive faces during infancy, long before any significant cultural input is possible, and to the cross-cultural data showing more similarities than differences in cross-cultural preferences for attractive faces. Although studies demonstrating an innate preference for attractive faces would be difficult to conduct because of the limitations of the visual system of the newborn (e.g., Banks & Salapatek, 1983), studies showing that infants perceive attractive faces as prototypical are, in principle, possible and are now called for to further explicate infants' preferences for attractive faces.

As we have noted in other reports, the preferences of the infants who participated in these three studies, although quite reliable and consistent across studies, were not strong. Infants do not refuse to look at unattractive faces in exclusive preference to attractive faces. Furthermore, differences in looking time toward attractive and unattractive faces may be obtained only for unfamiliar faces; it seems unlikely that attractiveness would influence infant behavior toward familiar caregivers given the importance of the attachment system to the survival of the infant. At the same time, however, differential responsiveness toward unfamiliar attractive and unattractive faces would perhaps be even greater than that obtained here if faces more extreme in appearance were used as stimuli. We also note that the faces viewed by the infants in these three studies were always presented in contrasting pairs. Thus, we cannot assume from these data that infants prefer attractive faces in the absence of a contrasting face, although 6-month-old infants in our earlier study (Langlois et al., 1987) did exhibit preferences for attractive faces both when the attractive faces were presented with contrasting unattractive faces and when they were not.

Several factors that may have limited or moderated in some way the preferences of the infants were examined. However, these variables did not interact with or influence infants' preferences for attractiveness. The attractiveness of the mother was not related, in either Study 1 or Study 2, to the infants' preferences for attractive male or female, Black or White faces. Nor was maternal attractiveness related to infant preferences for attractive faces in our earlier study (Langlois et al., 1987). The method of presenting faces to infants, either in groups or alternating male and female faces, did not interact with or influence infants' preferences for attractive male or female faces. Thus, infant preferences for attractive faces seem robust and are not merely a function of the appearance of the infant's own mother or of the method used to present the faces in a visual preference paradigm.

An interesting serendipitous finding obtained from Study 1 concerns the Sex of Infant × Sex of Face interaction. Both male and female infants preferred to look at same-sex adult faces (although the pattern for girls was not statistically significant) compared with faces of the other sex. Although previous work has suggested that young infants are capable of discriminating gender in faces (Fagan & Singer, 1979; Kagan & Lewis, 1965; Leinbach & Fagot, 1986), no work of which we are aware has examined infants as young as these for their visual preferences of the faces of one gender over the other. Other work has shown, however, that older infants (12 to 18 months old) display similar same-sex preferences when presented with photographs of male and female same-age infants (Lewis & Brooks-Gunn, 1979). The fact that our 6-month-old infants did not display same-sex preferences toward photographs of male and female 3-month-olds is not surprising given that even adults could not discriminate the sex of these very young infants (see footnote 3). Perhaps same-sex preferences would be observed in 6-month-olds if they were allowed to view photographs of older infants. It is intriguing to speculate that the preferences of young infants for same-sex adult faces may be the rudiments of the strong and possibly even universal same-sex preferences found in older children (Edwards & Whiting, 1988; Maccoby, 1988). Research specifically designed to systematically investigate the gender preferences of young infants merits attention in the future.

The results of these three studies and those of other studies with infants (Langlois et al., 1987, 1990; Samuels & Ewy, 1985; Shapiro et al., 1984) are convincing in demonstrating that preferences for attractiveness appear very early in life, are consistent across various types of faces, and generalize beyond visual behaviors to social and play behaviors. Exposure to cultural media does not seem to account for these preferences; rather, preferences for attractiveness are either innate or acquired with only minimal experience with faces in the environment. The basis for preferences for attractive faces may be that attractive faces are prototypical of the category of faces. Contrary to the common proverb that "beauty is merely in the eye of the beholder," it may well be that the majority of perceivers at any age and from any culture can detect and prefer a particular type of face (e.g., one that is "average" for that population) as attractive.

REFERENCES

Banks, M. S., & Salapatek, P. (1983). Infant visual perception. In P. H. Mussen, M. M. Haith, & J. J. Campos (Eds.), *Infancy and developmental psychobiology* (pp. 435–571). New York: Wiley.

Bernstein, I. H., Lin, T., & McClellan, P. (1982). Cross- vs. within-racial judgments of attractiveness. *Perception & Psychophysics, 32*, 495–503.

Bomba, P. C., & Siqueland, E. R. (1983). The nature and structure of infant form categories. *Journal of Experimental Child Psychology, 35*, 294–328.

Bumpas, H. C. (1899). The elimination of the unfit as illustrated by the introduced sparrow. *Biology Lectures in Marine Biology at Woods Hole, Massachusetts, 11*, 109–226.

Cohen, L. B., & Younger, B. A. (1983). Perceptual categorization in the infant. In E. K. Scholnik (Ed.), *New trends in conceptual representation: Challenges to Piaget's theory?* (pp. 197–220). Hillsdale, NJ: Erlbaum.

Cunningham, M. R. (1986). Measuring the physical in physical attractiveness: Quasi-experiments on the sociobiology of female facial beauty. *Journal of Personality and Social Psychology, 50*, 925–935.

Dobzhansky, T. (1970). *Genetics of the evolutionary process.* New York: Columbia University Press.

Edwards, C. P., & Whiting, B. B. (1988). *Children of different worlds.* Cambridge: Harvard University Press.

Fagan, J. F., & Singer, L. T. (1979). The role of single feature differences in infant recognition of faces. *Infant Behavior and Development, 2,* 39–45.

Farkas, L. G. (1981). *Anthropometry of the head and face in medicine.* New York: Elsevier North-Holland.

Johnson, R. W., Dannenbring, G. L., Anderson, N. R., & Villa, R. E. (1983). How different cultural and geographic groups perceive the attractiveness of active and inactive feminists. *The Journal of Social Psychology, 119,* 111–117.

Kagan, J., & Lewis, M. (1965). Studies of attention in the human infant. *Merrill-Palmer Quarterly, 11,* 95–127.

Langlois, J. H., & Roggman, L. A. (1990). Attractive faces are only average. *Psychological Science, 1,* 115–121.

Langlois, J. H., Roggman, L. A., Casey, R. J., Ritter, J. M., Rieser-Danner, L. A., & Jenkins, V. Y. (1987). Infant preferences for attractive faces: Rudiments of a stereotype? *Developmental Psychology, 23,* 363–369.

Langlois, J. H., Roggman, L. A., & Rieser-Danner, L. A. (1990). Infants' differential social responses to attractive and unattractive faces. *Developmental Psychology, 26,* 153–159.

Leinbach, M. D., & Fagot, B. I. (1986, April). *Gender-schematic processing by one-year-olds: Categorical habituation to male and female faces.* Paper presented at the International Conference on Infant Studies, Los Angeles.

Lewis, M., & Brooks-Gunn, J. (1979). *Social cognition and the acquisition of self.* New York: Plenum Press.

Maccoby, E. E. (1988). Gender as a social category. *Developmental Psychology, 24,* 755–765.

Maret, S. M. (1983). Attractiveness ratings of photographs of Blacks by Cruzans and Americans. *Journal of Psychology, 115,* 113–116.

Maret, S. M., & Harling, G. A. (1985). Cross-cultural perceptions of physical attractiveness: Ratings of photos of whites by Cruzans and Americans. *Perceptual Motor Skills, 60,* 163–166.

McArthur, L. Z., & Berry, D. S. (1987). Cross-cultural agreement in perceptions of babyfaced adults. *Journal of Cross-Cultural Psychology, 18,* 165–192.

McCall, R. B., & Appelbaum, M. I. (1973). Bias in the analysis of repeated-measures designs: Some alternative approaches. *Child Development, 44,* 401–415.

Posner, M. I., & Keele, S. W. (1968). On the genesis of abstract ideas. *Journal of Experimental Psychology, 77,* 353–363.

Reed, S. K. (1972). Pattern recognition and categorization. *Cognitive Psychology, 3,* 382–407.

Richardson, S. A., Goodman, N., Hastorf, A. H., & Dornbusch, S. M. (1961). Cultural uniformity in reaction to physical disabilities. *American Sociological Review, 26,* 241–247.

Rosch, E. (1978). Principles of categorization. In E. Rosch & B. B. Lloyd (Eds.), *Cognition and categorization* (pp. 27–47). Hillsdale, NJ: Erlbaum.

Samuels, C. A., & Ewy, R. (1985). Aesthetic perception of faces during infancy. *British Journal of Developmental Psychology, 3*, 221–228.

Schmalhausen, I. I. (1949). *Factors of evolution: The theory of stabilizing selection.* Philadelphia: Blakiston.

Shapiro, B. A., Hazan, C., & Haith, M. (1984, March). *Do infants differentiate attractiveness and expressiveness in faces?* Paper presented at the meeting of the Southwestern Society for Research in Human Development, Denver, CO.

Strauss, M. S. (1979). Abstraction of prototypical information by adults and 10-month-old infants. *Journal of Experimental Psychology: Human Learning and Memory, 5*, 618–632.

Symons, D. (1979). *The evolution of human sexuality.* New York: Oxford University Press.

Thakerar, J. N., & Iwawaki, S. (1979). Cross-cultural comparisons in interpersonal attraction of females toward males. *Journal of Social Psychology, 108*, 121–122.

Weisfeld, G. E., Weisfeld, C. C., & Callaghan, J. W. (1984). Peer and self perceptions in Hopi and Afro-American third- and sixth-graders. *Ethos, 12*, 64–83.

3

Continuity and Discontinuity in Infant Negative and Positive Emotionality: Family Antecedents and Attachment Consequences

Jay Belsky and Margaret Fish

Pennsylvania State University, University Park

Russell Isabella

University of Utah, Salt Lake City

This study was based on the premise that much of the instability evident in research on infant emotionality/temperament is a function not so much of measurement error (as typically presumed) but of lawful discontinuity. Infants who changed from high to low and from low to high levels of negative or positive emotionality between 3 and 9 months of age were compared with infants who remained stable during the period on distal measures of the family environment (prenatally and neonatally measured) and proximal measures of parent-infant interaction (3 months) thought to account for stability and change in infant emotionality and on 1-year infant-mother attachment security. Results revealed more success in forecasting stability and change in negative emotionality than positive emotionality; maternal personality and marital factors and mother-infant interaction accounted for why infants highly negative at 3 months changed, and comparable father factors and processes accounted for why infants initially low in negativity changed. Attachment-related analyses revealed change in positive emotionality to be more related to 1-year security than change in negative emotionality, but it was also the case

Reprinted with permission from *Developmental Psychology*, 1991, Vol. 27, No. 3, 421–431. Copyright ©1991 by the American Psychological Association, Inc.

Work on this article was supported by National Institute of Child Health and Human Development Grant RO1HD15496 and National Institute of Mental Health Research Scientist Development Award K02MH00486 to Jay Belsky.

> *that continuity and discontinuity in both positivity and negativity*
> *interacted to forecast attachment security.*

Individual differences in temperament, that is, variation in behavioral style thought to influence children's interactions with their environments, has been a fertile area of investigation for more than three decades (Campos, Barrett, Lamb, Goldsmith, & Stenberg, 1983). Despite a continued lack of consensus on defining dimensions of individuality (Bates, 1987; Goldsmith & Campos, 1986), the expression of emotionality plays a prominent role in all current conceptualizations of temperament. Meta-analysis of parent-report measures (Goldsmith & Rieser-Danner, 1986) suggests that the two temperamental dimensions that most often show stability are activity level and some manifestation of negative affect (i.e., either irritability/difficulty or fear/withdrawal). Of these two dimensions, negative emotionality has been the focus of more study; attention to difficult temperament and its possible links to subsequent problematic behavior and parent-child relationships have dominated research in infant temperament since the original publications of Thomas, Chess, and Birch (1968).

Like the other dimensions of temperament (Bates, 1987), difficultness has been defined in various ways by investigators. Thomas et al. (1968) originally characterized as difficult those children who withdraw from new experiences, adapt slowly, have irregular biological functions and intense emotional reactions, and are negative in mood. Buss and Plomin (1975, 1984) defined their emotionality dimension in terms of strong arousal and negative affect, whereas Bates (1987) specified crying and social demandingness as the defining features of difficult temperament. Researchers who tried to measure temperament by means of naturalistic observations tended to focus on irritability (i.e., fuss/cry behavior; Belsky, Rovine, & Taylor, 1984; Crockenberg & Smith, 1982). The common element in these approaches, whether focused on difficulty, emotionality, or irritability, is that they share a concern for the expression of negative emotion.

A major empirical issue in research on infant temperament concerns the stability of individual differences (Bates, 1987). Not surprisingly, the degree of continuity that characterizes temperament during infancy appears to vary according to the dimension examined and the measurement approach used. Greater stability has been found for aggregated scores, particularly those reflecting difficultness (Belsky, Rovine, & Fish, 1989; Lee & Bates, 1985) or emotionality (Matheny, Riese, & Wilson, 1985; Riese, 1987), and for parent-report questionnaires (as opposed to behavioral observations; Belsky et al., 1989; Isabella, Ward, & Belsky, 1985; Pettit & Bates, 1984).

In considering the stability of individual differences in temperament, it must be acknowledged that even when stability coefficients achieve conventional levels of significance, there remains noteworthy instability of individual rankings. Lee and

Bates (1985) observed, for example, that the continuity of classification of a child in their sample as temperamentally difficult, although significant, was only about 50% from 6 to 24 months, and other researchers reported similar findings (McNeil & Persson-Blennow, 1982). Consider in this regard the .37 ($p<.05$) stability coefficient that Matheny, Wilson, and Nuss (1984) generated when composite measures of tractability at 12 and 18 months were correlated in one of the best efforts to date to create a multimeasure index of temperament based on infant behavior observed in the laboratory under controlled conditions. It is findings such as these, which are quite representative of those reported in the literature, that lead us to take issue with Campos, Campos, and Barrett's (1989, p. 400) recent statement that "the conclusion is *clear* that irritability and negative emotionality show *impressive* continuity throughout infancy and early childhood" (emphasis added).

Several explanations have been advanced to account for what can best be described as modest stability of individual differences in infant negative emotionality, particularly in the first year of life. These include problems in conceptualizing and measuring infant temperament (Hubert, Wachs, Peters-Martin, & Gandour, 1982) and stage-determined changes in the expression of temperament (Riese, 1987). Another possibility is that negative emotionality may simply be unstable. Indeed modest stability coefficients may reflect the fact that while some children remain high or low over time on a particular dimension of temperament, others change on that same dimension. To the extent that the nature of the care that the child experiences in the family accounts for such variability, as Crockenberg (1986) suggested, it seems appropriate to speak in terms of lawful discontinuity rather than to presume that instability is exclusively a function of measurement error (Belsky & Pensky, 1988).

The identification of family conditions associated with continuity and discontinuity poses an important challenge for developmental theory and research. As Thomas (1984) noted some time ago, "rather than the simple question of whether temperament is or is not consistent over time, the more significant issue would appear to be the identification of the factors which may influence continuity or discontinuity" (p. 105). This point was reiterated recently by Coll and her colleagues (1989), who, on finding modest stability between 3 and 7 months in infant negative and positive emotionality, highlighted "the need to investigate . . . the determinants of change in temperamental characteristics over time" (p. 6). Despite the theoretical and practical importance of understanding why sameness characterizes the emotional proclivities of some infants, whereas change characteristics that of others, it is surprising how little research on this topic has been performed, particularly in view of the extensive work focused on stability. As Clarke-Stewart (1988) recently noted, "for most contemporary researchers who have studied temperament . . . this [stability] is all that matters" (p. 48).

Particularly interesting, therefore, are the rather consistent findings that emerge from the few investigations that have sought to illuminate the conditions of continuity and discontinuity in infant negative emotionality. The most systematic and extensive research is that of Matheny (1986), which indicates that even though temperament was significantly stable from 12 to 24 months, infants who became less negative, more attentive, and more socially oriented (i.e., more tractable) had mothers who were more expressive and involved with them and came from families that were more emotionally cohesive. Similarly, Washington, Minde, and Goldberg (1986) found that preterm babies who became less difficult over time had mothers who were more sensitive to their needs than were mothers whose premature infants became more difficult. Finally, Engfer (1986) reported that German mothers who perceived their infants as becoming more difficult between 4 and 18 months experienced more marital problems and were judged less sensitive in their mothering, whereas mothers who described their infants as becoming less difficult were more relaxed and optimistic and less irritable. Of course, the infant's capacity to regulate his or her negative emotionality—with or without parental and family support—will also influence parental and family functioning. Thus, even though these studies highlight the role of parent factors and family processes in affecting infant emotionality, we should not lose sight of the effect of the changing infant on the family.

Nevertheless, it is noteworthy that findings from all these studies suggest that, under conditions of general family stress, the quality of maternal care deteriorates (Belsky, 1984) and, as a result, so does the infant's capacity to regulate his or her negative emotionality. Conversely, when marital and general family processes promote maternal sensitivity, this serves to facilitate the self-regulatory capacity of the infant and leads to positive change in negative emotionality. This conclusion, like the findings on which it is based, is consistent with the view of Ainsworth and other attachment researchers that quality of maternal care influences infant crying (Ainsworth, Blehar, Waters, & Wall, 1978).

Although not extensive, the evidence reviewed clearly implicates parental personality and marital quality as distal conditions and parent-infant interactions as more proximal conditions of continuity and discontinuity in infant negative emotionality. A primary purpose of the current investigation is to extend work in this area by examining not only such distal and proximal conditions that seem to play a role in accounting for why some infants evince high or low negativity over time whereas others change, but also to examine father factors as well as mother factors. The general hypothesis guiding this inquiry is that negative emotionality will decrease over time when parents are psychologically healthy, are involved in satisfying marriages, and interact with their infants in a sensitive, supportive manner, whereas negative emotionality will increase over time when the opposite conditions exist.

This report also seeks to extend research by considering the conditions of continuity and discontinuity in positive emotionality/social responsiveness as well as the more extensively investigated negative emotionality. The importance of focusing on positive affect and social orientation as a separate and distinct dimension of individuality is suggested by a growing body of evidence that indicates, at least in the case of adults, that this dimension of affective functioning is independent of negative emotionality at both the state (Eysenck & Eysenck, 1969; McCrae & Costa, 1984) and trait (Watson & Clark, 1984; Watson, Clark, & Tellegan, 1988; Watson & Tellegan, 1985) levels, and that, in the case of infants, different hemispheres of the brain are responsible for processing positive and negative affective experience (Fox & Davidson, 1988). A further impetus for studying positive emotionality derives from recent research indicating that low sociability and decline in the expression of positive affect over the first year are associated with increased risk of insecure infant-mother attachment (Bates, Maslin, & Frankel, 1985; Malatesta, Culver, Tesman, & Shepard, 1989; Wille, 1989). It is just such evidence that leads us to examine relations between infant-mother attachment security and continuity and discontinuity in infant positive emotionality and negative emotionality. A general hypothesis guiding our inquiry is that risk of insecure attachment will increase when infants remain high in negative emotionality or change from low to high or remain low in positive emotionality or change from high to low. In other words, insecure attachment to mother is expected to be associated with stable high or increasing levels of negativity over time or with stable low or decreasing levels of positivity.

To address the issues raised, we relied on data collected during the course of a multicohort longitudinal study of infant and family development. Observational and parent-report indexes of positive and negative emotionality were used to create composite measures of these constructs when infants are 3 and 9 months of age, so that four groups of infants were constituted with respect to each dimension of emotionality: subjects who scored high or low at both times of measurement (high-high, low-low) and those that changed (high-low, low-high). Working with such groups, we specifically sought to determine why infants who look similar in terms of their expressed emotionality early in the first year look decidedly different 6 months later. Thus, we compared infants who, at 3 and 9 months, scored high on the dimension of emotionality in question (negativity, positivity) with infants who changed from high to low across the 6-month period (HH vs. HL) and infants who remained low over time with those who changed from low to high (LL vs. LH). The first set of comparisons to be made involved distal factors measured prenatally (parent personality, marital quality) and neonatally (newborn behavior, gender), whereas the second set focused on proximal processes of mother-infant and father-infant interaction measured during the course of dyadic (mother-infant) and triadic (mother-father-infant) home observations when infants were 3 months of age and thus before any change in measured positive and negative emotionality. It should be noted that analyses of data collected at 3 months is dictated principally by the design of our longitudinal study rather than by any presumption that this is a point of particular plasticity in emotionality. As a final set of analyses, groups that changed or stayed the same with respect to positive and negative emotionality are compared in terms of attachment security. In this way, we sought to illuminate both the family antecedents and attachment consequences of continuity and discontinuity in infant negative and positive emotionality.

METHOD

Subjects

The subjects of this investigation were 148 firstborn infants (88 boys and 60 girls) and their parents participating in the second and third cohorts of the Pennsylvania Infant and Family Development Project (Belsky, Gilstrap, & Rovine, 1984; Belsky et al., 1989). Parents-to-be were recruited to participate in this longitudinal study during the last trimester of pregnancy, and families were studied intensively through the infant's first year of life. All parents were White, predominantly of middle- and working-class socioeconomic status. At time of enrollment, average family income was $24,500 (range = $13,000-$80,000) and couples had been married an average of 3.8 years (range = <1-13). The mean ages of husbands and wives, respectively, were 28.7 years (range = 18-41 years) and 26.8 years (range = 18-35 years); and the two spouses averaged 16.3 (range = 10-22 years) and 15.1 years (range = 12-21 years) of education, respectively.

Design and Procedures

As part of the Infant and Family Development Project's longitudinal study of marriage, parenting, and infant development, data were gathered at several points in time, beginning in the last trimester of pregnancy and continuing through the child's first birthday (Belsky, Gilstrap, et al., 1984; Belsky et al, 1989). This report uses data collected at several points in time. Information on so-called distal conditions of continuity and discontinuity in infant emotionality, including data on parent personality and marital quality, was obtained during the last trimester of pregnancy and during the first 10 days of the infant's life (Brazelton Behavioral Assessments). Information on proximal conditions of continuity and discontinuity, namely that pertaining to actual experiences that infants had with their parents, was obtained during two separate, 1-hr, naturalistic home observations of mother-infant and mother-father-infant interactions performed when infants were 3 months of age. Information on the consequences of continuity and discontinuity in emotionality, specifically security of infant-mother attachment, was obtained during strange-situation assessments when infants were 12 months of age. Finally, home observational data and maternal report data obtained when infants were 3 months and 9 months of age were used to define high and low negative- and positive-emotionality groups at each time of measurement.

Measuring Continuity and Discontinuity in Emotionality

High and low negative- and positive-emotionality groups of infants at 3 months and 9 months of age were identified by rescaling and aggregating three different sources of information relevant to negative and to positive emotionality at each time of measurement. For purposes of assessing negative emotionality, we relied on (a) scores of the number of 15-s intervals that infants cried during the 1-hr observation of the mother-infant dyad (Belsky, Taylor, & Rovine, 1984; Isabella, Belsky, & von Eye, 1989), (b) scores of the number of 15-s intervals that infants cried during the 1-hour observation of the mother-father-infant triad (Belsky, Gilstrap, et al., 1984; Belsky et al., 1989), and (c) the fussy/difficult subscale from the Infant Characteristics Questionnaire (Bates, Freeland, & Lounsbury, 1979), which mothers completed when infants were 3 months and 9 months of age. These independent indicators were, as expected, only moderately positively correlated (mean $r = .28$).

For purposes of assessing positive emotionality/social responsiveness, we relied on observational scores reflecting (a) the number of 15-s intervals in which infants vocalized during the mother-infant dyadic observation, (b) the number of intervals infants smiled, laughed, or evinced excitement in some other way during the mother-father-infant triadic observation, and (c) a summary of four items taken from the Infant Characteristics Questionnaire that explicitly tapped positive emotionality/social responsiveness ("How much does your baby smile and make happy sounds?"; "How much does your baby enjoy playing little games with you?"; "How excited does your baby become when people play with or talk to him?"; and "What kind of mood is your baby generally in?"). These three component indicators were also only modestly positively correlated with one another (mean $r = .24$). They were composited to create an aggregate index of positive emotionality/social responsiveness in light research on both infants (Bates et al., 1985) and adults (McCrae & Costa, 1984), indicating that positive emotionality and social responsiveness are positively correlated. As anticipated, the negative and positive aggregated scores were independent of each other at both 3 months ($r = .10$, ns) and 9 months ($r = -.09, ns$). The negative-affect composite demonstrated only modest stability across this 6-month period ($r = .21, p < .01$), whereas the positive-affect composite was not stable from 3 to 9 months ($r = .09$, ns).[1]

As a second step toward creating high and low negative- and positive-

---

[1]The limited stability of positive emotionality did not derive from including emotion and social responsivity components in the composite.

emotionality subgroups at 3 months and 9 months, each of the three negative- and three positive-emotionality component scores was divided in thirds and rescored 0, 1, and 2 to reflect low, medium, and high levels, respectively, of the emotionality dimension in question. The three negative-emotionality items and the three positive-emotionality items were then separately summed to create composite negative- and positive-emotionality scores, each of which could range from 0 to 6 at each time of measurement. This was done for two reasons: (a) to ensure that the two observational and single maternal-report components that made up each aggregate measure contributed equally to the final aggregate score, and (b) to facilitate categorization of infants into high- and low-emotionality subgroups. It is noteworthy that rescaling had little effect on the stability of negative emotionality ($r = .19$, $p< .05$) but increased to a significant degree the stability of positive emotionality ($r = .26, p<. 001$). Even with rescaling, the positive- and negative-emotionality composites remained unrelated at 3 months ($r =-.13$) and 9 months ($r = .16$).

Infants whose rescaled composite scores at 3 months or 9 months fell into the 0 to 2 range were classified as low on the dimension of emotionality in question, whereas those whose scores fell in the 4 to 6 range were classified as high on that dimension. All subjects who received intermediate composite scores of 3 at either 3 months or 9 months were excluded from analysis (36% negative emotionality, 36% positive emotionality). This was done for two reasons: (a) to decrease the likelihood that a child who was low or high in the emotionality dimension would be erroneously subgrouped because she or he fell at or near the midpoint of the distribution, and (b) to amplify what were expected to be weak or modest effects.

Once infants were classified at each time of measurement, the 3-month and 9-month classifications on a particular dimension of emotionality were cross-classified to identify stable high (HH) and stable low (LL) groups and groups that changed from high to low (HL) and from low to high (LH). In the case of negative emotionality, this procedure resulted in 33 HH subjects, 26 LL subjects, 19 HL subjects, and 16 LH subjects. The number of positive-emotionality subjects were 29, 29, 19, and 19, respectively.

Measuring Family Antecedents of Continuity and Discontinuity

Two types of measurements were conceptualized as potential family antecedents of continuity and discontinuity for purposes of this investigation. Distal factors were indexes of parental personality and marital quality obtained before the infant's birth as well as infant gender and assessments of neonatal functioning. Proximal processes were measures of mother-infant and father-infant interaction obtained during the 3-month home observations of the mother-infant dyad and the mother-father-infant triad.

Distal factors. As part of a lengthy questionnaire completed by each parent in the last trimester of pregnancy, assessments of personality and marital quality were obtained. Specifically, each parent completed the Interpersonal Affect Scale (assessing orientation toward the feelings of others), the Self-Esteem scale from the Jackson (1976) Personality Inventory, and the Ego Strength scale (assessing emotional maturity and flexibility) from the Cattell 16PF (Cattell, Eber, & Tatsuoka, 1970). These scales were selected for inclusion in the longitudinal study because of their presumed relevance to relationship functioning and their documented reliability and validity. As a result of scoring conventions, low scores reflect psychologically healthier functioning.

On the basis of prior factor analyses (Isabella & Belsky, 1985), four subscales derived from Braiker and Kelley's (1979) questionnaire assessing intimate relations were composited to create measures of positive (love and maintenance) and negative (conflict and ambivalence) marital activities and sentiments. Past analyses of these measures reveal them to be internally consistent, sensitive to stability and change in marital quality across the transition to parenthood (Belsky et al., 1989), and related to infant-mother attachment security (Belsky et al., 1989; Isabella & Belsky, 1985) and parent and child behavior when children are 3 years of age (Belsky, Youngblade, Rovine, & Volling, in press)[2]

Within the first 10 days of the infant's birth, each child was assessed by a trained examiner on the Brazelton (1973) Neonatal Behavioral Assessment Scale (NBAS). Items were composited according to conventions proposed by Jacobson, Fein, Jacobson, and Schwartz (1984) to create measures of orientation, autonomic stability, range of state, regulation of state, and motor maturity (for details, see Belsky & Rovine, 1987). To reduce the number of variables subject to analysis, these measures were composited to create a total score reflecting the behavioral integrity of the organism.[3]

---

[2]In view of the fact that the same mothers/wives who completed the infant temperament report at 3 months and 9 months, which contributed to the creation of positive- and negative-emotionality scores, also completed personality and marital scales, which will be used to distinguish emotionality groups, it was necessary to determine whether these two sets of maternal reports were related. To the extent that they were, then any capacity of the wife personality and marriage scales to distinguish the emotionality groups might simply be a function of the fact that the same individual contributed to the measurement of independent and dependent variables in a particular analysis. This turned out not to be a concern, because the maternal report scores of infant fussy/difficult and social responsiveness at both 3 months and 4 months were unrelated to the three personality and two marital measures obtained prenatally (mean $r3$ = .04; range = −.07–.16).

[3]Following the scoring conventions of Jacobson et al. (1984), high scores on the orientation, autonomic-stability, regulation-of-state, and motor-maturity dimensions indicate more optimal newborn functioning, whereas a high score on range of state reflects high irritability, arousal, and state lability. Therefore, to create a composite score indicating well-functioning neonatal behavior, the first four dimensions were added and the range-of-state score subtracted from the sum. Once analyses reported in this article were completed, the newborn composite was decomposed to determine whether results would be different using individual component scores. In no case did individual dimension scores prove to discriminate between groups that changed and that remained the same in negative or positive emotionality.

Proximal Processes

The two 1-hr home observations conducted at 3 months provided several indexes of parent-infant interaction used in this study. Measures obtained from the dyadic and triadic observations were totally different because these two home observations used entirely different behavior-recording systems. In particular, the triadic system was far more molar and less microanalytic because it was designed to capture interaction in three separate dyads—mother-infant, father-infant, and husband-wife (Belsky, Gilstrap, & Rovine, 1984)—rather than in a single one (i.e., mother-infant).

With respect to the measurement of mother-infant interaction in the dyadic observations, we relied on a procedure outlined in detail by Isabella et al. (1989) and derived from theory and research highlighting the role of sensitive, harmonious, and appropriately responsive interactions in promoting attachment security (e.g., Ainsworth et al., 1978; Belsky, Rovine, & Taylor, 1984; Smith & Pedersen, 1988). Mother and infant behaviors recorded as present (vs. absent) within continuous 15-s sampling intervals were recoded such that every 15-s episode within the 1-hr observation was represented by a cross-classification of 11 infant behaviors (vertical axis) and 12 maternal behaviors (horizontal axis) in a contingency table. Thereafter, each co-occurrence within a 15-s sampling period was judged a priori as reflecting either sensitive/complimentary, insensitive/poorly coordinated, or neutral (i.e., neither sensitive nor insensitive) exchanges.

In general, the 31 co-occurrences characterized as sensitive/complimentary were those in which the behavior displayed by both members of the dyad reflected an obvious exchange of behaviors (e.g., mother stimulate-baby response/explore) or the behavior of at least one member of the dyad was judged as being appropriately responsive to the behavior of the other (e.g., infant fuss/cry-mother soothe). The 31 co-occurrences characterized as insensitive-poorly coordinated were those in which one member of the dyad engaged in behavior that either was not responded to by the other (e.g., infant fuss/cry-mother attend to the infant) or was enjoined by behavior of the other member so that the combination of behaviors was not considered representative of a mutual and reciprocal exchange (e.g., infant fuss/cry-mother stimulate). (Note that of the 70 co-occurrences not accounted for by this delineation, 21 were classified as neutral [e.g., infant explorer-mother leisure]; the remaining 49, by definition, could not occur [e.g., infant sleep-mother responsively vocalize; infant explore-mother soothe].) The a priori judgments guiding this characterization of interaction were theoretically based, and the utility of this scoring system in distinguishing the interactional histories of secure and insecure dyads has been demonstrated (Isabella, et al., 1989) and replicated (Isabella & Belsky, 1990): Dyads subsequently classified as securely attached in the strange situation are disproportionately likely to experience harmonious, complimentary, and appro-

priately responsive exchanges, whereas those classified as insecure are disproportionately likely to experience unresponsive and poorly coordinated interactions.

In addition to the measurements derived from the observations of the mother-
infant dyad, summary mother-infant and father-infant engagement scores obtained
during the observations of the mother-father-infant triad also were used in this study.
At the end of each 15-s sampling period during these observations, mother-infant
and father-infant interactions were rated on a 4-point scale (0 = no interaction;
3 = intense, reciprocal exchange; for further details, see Belsky, Gilstrap, & Rovine,
1984). Ratings per sampling period were summed to create total engagement scores.
Previous publications reveal that these ratings were made reliably; and that they
are sensitive to differences in maternal and paternal involvement and to changes
in infant development (Belsky, Gilstrap, & Rovine, 1984; Belsky et al., 1989)[4]

Consequences of Continuity/Discontinuity in Emotionality

Assessments of security of infant-mother attachment obtained when infants were
1 year of age were available as part of the longitudinal study. The standard strange
situation (Ainsworth & Wittig, 1969) was used, and well-trained, reliable coders
classified attachment relationships as secure or insecure using standard scoring conventions (for additional details, see Belsky & Rovine, 1987).

RESULTS

The first set of analyses examines the family antecedents of continuity and discontinuity in negative emotionality with regard to both distal factors and proximal
processes. The second set of analyses addresses the same issue with respect to positive emotionality. Because the principal focus of this inquiry was to determine
why infants who looked similar in their expressed emotionality (positive or negative) at 3 months looked different at 9 months, comparisons were made (a) between
groups that started high and remained high (HH) or changed to low (HL), and (b)
between groups that started low and remained low (LL) or changed to high (LH).
The third and final set of analyses examines the relation between attachment security and continuity and discontinuity in negative and positive emotionality.

---

[4]Because these proximal indexes of parent-infant interaction and the measures of crying and social
responsiveness (which contributed to the negativity and positivity composites) derived form the same
sets of observations, it was necessary to determine whether these two sets of measures were related.
To the extent that they were, it would confound any possible interpretation that proximal interactional
processes between parents and infants at 3 months contributed to stability and change in infant emotionality from 3 months to 9 months. As it turned out, this did not prove to be an empirical concern,
because neither of the engagement scores from the triadic observations or the harmony-complementarity
scores from the dyadic observation at 3 months were significantly related to the observational indexes
of crying and social responsiveness, which contributed to the negative and positive emotionality scores,
respectively.

Family Antecedents of Continuity/Discontinuity in Negative Emotionality

To examine the family antecedents of continuity and discontinuity in negative emotionality, we proceeded in three steps with respect to both the HH versus HL and LL versus LH comparisons. First, a discriminant function analysis was conducted to determine how well the multivariate set of distal factors (personality, marriage, and infant gender, but not NBAS scores because of missing data on 41 subjects) collectively distinguished groups.[5] If groups that were compared could be reliably discriminated at the multivariate level, we proceed in Step 2 of the analysis to conduct univariate *t* tests comparing groups on all of the distal factors (including NBAS scores). Finally, in the third step of the analysis, groups were compared on the proximal measures of sensitivity-complimentarity/insensitivity-poor coordination in the mother-infant dyad and on mother-infant and father-infant engagement from the two home observations at 3 months of age. With only three proximal indexes of parent-infant interaction and the need for repeated measures comparisons in the case of the triadic engagement scores, we opted for univariate analyses. The multivariate, discriminant-function approach was restricted to the distal antecedents because there were so many variables under consideration.

LL versus LH. The discriminant-function analysis revealed that the husband and wife prenatal personality and marriage measures along with infant gender could be used to correctly classify 77.1% of the infants with low negative-emotionality scores at 3 months into groups showing low and high levels of negative emotionality 6 months later ($z = 2.83, p < .01$). This is a rate of classification 51% greater than would be expected on the basis of chance alone (Huberty, 1984). In the second step of the analyses, follow-up *t* test to specify important discriminating distal variables revealed that infants who changed from low to high negative emotionality between 3 and 9 months of age, in comparison with those who remained low, had fathers who scored significantly poorer (i.e., had higher scores) on the prenatal measures of interpersonal affect ($Ms = 31.13$ vs. $26.92, t = 3.95, p < .001$) and who were less positive about their marriages before the infant was born ($Ms = 99.94$ vs. $109.80, t = 2.10, p < .05$).

The third step of the analyses of proximal interaction processes revealed that even though the LL and LH groups did not differ with regard to interactions during the mother-infant dyadic observation (i.e., harmony-complimentary), they did differ

---

[5]Discriminant-function analysis is a multivariate-data analytic technique that evaluates the extent to which a series of variables can be used in combination to distinguish subjects' membership in different groups. The method assesses the extent to which subjects assigned to particular groups can be distinguished on the basis of the predictor variables included in the analysis (hit rate). Huberty (1984) provided formulas for determining the extent to which the percent correct classification achieved in the analysis is statistically reliable (*z* score) and the extent to which it proves the rate of accurate prediction of group classification beyond what would be expected by chance.

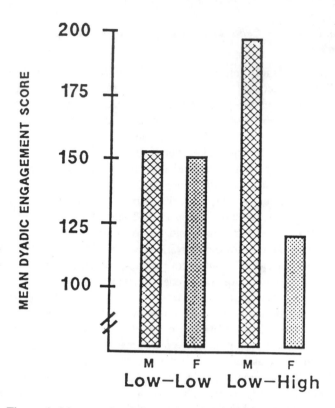

Figure 1. Mean mother-infant (M) and father-infant (F) dyadic engagement scores for negative-emotionality groups that remained low over time (L-L) and changed from low to high (L-H).

in terms of mother-infant and father-infant engagement in the triadic observation. A 2 × 2 (Parent × Group [LL vs. LH]) analysis of variance (ANOVA) indicated that whereas mothers and fathers in the LL group were equally involved with their 3-month-old babies, fathers were less involved than mothers in the LH group, Parent × Group interaction, $F(1,40) = 3.29, p<.08$. This pattern of findings is graphically depicted in Figure 1.

In summary, compared with babies who remained low in negative emotionality, infants who changed from low to high negative emotionality between 3 and 9 months had fathers who were less affectively oriented toward others (interpersonal affect), less positive about their marriages even before their infants were born, and less involved, relative to their wives, with their 3-month-old infants.

HH versus HL. The results of the discriminant-function analysis showed that the prenatal personality and marital measures and infant gender could be used to cor-

TABLE 1

Observed and (Expected) Frequency of Sensitive,
Complementary, Insensitive, and Poorly Coordinated
Mother-Infant Interaction at 3 Months for the High-High
and High-Low Negative-Emotionality Groups

Mother–infant interaction	Negative emotionality group	
	High–high	**High–low**
Sensitive, complementary	1,246 (1,282)	817 (781)
Insensitive, poorly coordinated	1,964 (1,928)	1,138 (1,174)

Note. Values in parentheses represent total observed and expected
15-S sampling epochs (frequency). $\chi^2 (1, N = 52) = 4.48, p < .05$.

rectly classify 78.4% of the infants who had high negative emotionality scores at 3 months into groups with high or low negative emotionality at 9 months ($z = 3.46, p<.001$). This is a rate of classification 52.8% higher than would be expected on the basis of chance alone (Huberty, 1984). Univariate t tests of the prenatal personality and marriage variables revealed that both mothers and fathers of babies who changed from high to low negative emotionality had better self-esteem (i.e., lower scores) than parents of infants who continued to show high negative emotionality (*Ms* of mothers = 26.26 vs. 29.58, $t = 2.30, p<.05$; *Ms* of fathers = 25.53 vs. 27.85, $t = 1.97, p<.05$) and that mothers of these changing infants experienced significantly less conflict and ambivalence in their marriage prenatally than did mothers of infants who remained high in negative emotionality at 3 and 9 months (*Ms* = 26.26 vs. 31.39, $t = 2.43, p<.05$).

Infant characteristics also distinguished these groups. Chi-square analysis indicated that male infants were more likely to remain high in negative emotionality (71.4%), whereas females were marginally more likely to change from high to low (52.9%) between 3 and 9 months, $X^2(1) = 2.93, p<.10$. Furthermore, the total performance score on the NBAS marginally differentiated infants who changed to low negative emotionality from those who stayed high (*Ms* = 2.381 vs. $-1.916, t = 1.96, p<.06$): those who remained high performed more poorly.

Analyses of the proximal measures of parent-infant interaction during the home observations indicated similar patterns of mother and father involvement for the two groups during the triadic observation but significant differences in the mother-infant dyadic observation. Specifically, mother-infant dyads in the group that changed from high to low negative emotionality showed greater than expected frequencies of complementary, responsive, and sensitive interactions and fewer than expected disharmonious, unresponsive, and poorly coordinated exchanges, whereas the reverse was true of dyads with infants who remained highly distressed at both 3 and 9 months, $X^2(1) = 4.48$, $p < .05$. (See Table 1.)

Thus, comparisons of infants who were high in negative emotionality at 3 months and remained high with those who changed from high to low negativity revealed a far more systematic effect of mother and infant factors than those of the LL and LH groups. Specifically, mothers of infants who changed from high to low levels of negative emotionality, relative to those whose infants remained high in negativity from 3 to 9 months, had high self-esteem, experienced less negativity in their marriages before their child's birth, and enjoyed relatively more harmonious, responsive, and complementary interactions with their infants. Infants who changed from high to low negative emotionality were more likely to be female and to evince more behavioral integrity as newborns in comparison to those who remained highly negative over time.

Conditions of Continuity and Discontinuity in Positive Emotionality

Paralleling the analyses performed for negative emotionality, comparisons were made between the LL and LH positive-emotionality groups and between the HH and HL positive-emotionality groups, first using the discriminant-function analysis, which, if successful, was followed by univariate comparisons on distal variables and on the proximal measures of parent-infant interaction.

LL versus LH. Infants who changed from low positive emotionality at 3 months to high positive emotionality at 9 months could be reliably distinguished from those who remained low in positive emotionality using the prenatal parent personality and marriage measures and infant gender in the discriminant-function analysis (76.7% correct classification, $z = 3.23$, $p < .001$, a rate 51.4% greater than that expected by chance; Huberty, 1984). However, univariate tests revealed no significant differences between the LL and LH groups with respect to individual measures of prenatal parent personality or marriage, infant gender, or newborn behavioral performance.

Proximal interaction at the two 3-month observations was found to be different for these two groups of infants. In the case of the triadic observation, a 2 × 2 (Parent × Group [LL vs. LH]) analysis of variance (ANOVA) revealed a significant main effect for group, $F(1, 46) = 5.26$, $p < .05$; parents of infants who changed from low to high positive emotionality were more involved with their babies at 3 months of age than were parents of infants who remained low in positive affect and social responsiveness ($Ms = 159.03$ vs. 126.84). Contrary to expectations, however, interaction in the mother-infant dyad was more complementary, responsive, and harmonious and less unresponsive and poorly coordinated for infants who remained low in positive emotionality in contrast to those who changed from low to high, $\chi^2(1) = 6.17$, $p < .05$. (See Table 2.)

TABLE 2
Observed and (Expected) Frequency of Sensitive,
Complementary, Insensitive, and Poorly Coordinated
Mother-Infant Interaction at 3 Months for the Low-Low and Low-
High Positive-Emotionality Groups

Mother–infant interaction	Positive emotionality group	
	Low–low	Low–high
Sensitive, complementary	860 (825)	485 (520)
Insensitive, poorly coordinated	1,386 (1,421)	932 (897)

Note. Values in parentheses represent total observed and expected 15-S sampling epochs (frequency). χ^2 (1, $N = 48$) = 6.17, $p < .05$.

In sum, although multiple distal factors collectively discriminated LL and LH positive-emotionality groups, no single measure significantly distinguished the groups at a univariate level. Analyses of parent-infant interaction revealed, however, that infants who changed to high positive emotionality at 9 months, relative to those who remained low, experienced more parent involvement during the 3-month triadic observation, but also experienced a lower proportion than expected of responsive, complementary, and harmonious interactions when observed with just their mothers.

HH versus HL. Prenatal parent personality and marital measures and infant gender did not result in a reliable discrimination of infants who remained high in positive emotionality between 3 and 9 months from those who changed from high to low during that time, nor did the measures of parent-infant interaction prove to be different for the HH and HL groups.

Attachment Security and Continuity/Discontinuity in Emotionality

To examine possible consequences of stability and change in both negative and positive emotionality from 3 to 9 months, a series of chi-square analyses were performed. First, separate analyses were conducted to assess relations between continuity and discontinuity in each emotional dimension and attachment security at 12 months. In keeping with the prior analyses of distal and proximal factors, analyses again involved separate comparisons of LL and LH groups and of HH and HL groups. Then the positive- and negative-emotionality groups were combined to test the simultaneous influence of stability or change in both emotional dimensions on infant-mother attachment security.

Negative emotionality. Comparisons of neither LL and LH groups nor HH and HL

TABLE 3
Attachment Security as a Function of Cumulative Risk Associated
With Stability and Change in Negative and Positive Emotionality

Cumulative risk	12-month attachment classification	
	Secure	Insecure
0	15	1
1	21	5
2	8	9

Note. One point given for each of the following conditions: high-high or low-high negative emotionality and low-low or high-low positive emotionality. $\chi^2 (2, N = 59) = 10.42, p < .005$.

groups revealed associations between continuity/discontinuity in negative emotionality and attachment security. Thus, infant-mother attachment security proved to be independent of whether an infant who was low or high in negative emotionality at 3 months remained stable or changed by 9 months.

Positive emotionality. Although the LL and LH groups did not differ significantly in likelihood of being securely attached, the HH and HL positive-emotionality groups did. Infants who changed from high to low positive emotionality between 3 and 9 months were more likely to be classified as insecure at 12 months (57.9%) than infants who remained high in positive emotionality (17.9%), $\chi^2(1) = 8.08$, $p < .004$.

Negative and positive emotionality. To test the hypothesis that stability or change in negative emotionality, although not operating as a significant unique influence on attachment security, might interact with stability/change in positive emotionality to increase or decrease the risk of insecure attachment, a cumulative-risk approach was adopted. More specifically, it was hypothesized that risk for insecurity would be increased if negative emotionality scores remained high (HH) or changed from low to high (LH) or if positive emotionality scores remained low (LL) or changed from high to low (HL). Risk for insecurity was presumed to be decreased if negative emotionality scores remained low (LL) or changed from high to low (HL) or if positive emotionality scores remained high (HH) or changed from low to high (LH). Thus, for purposes of analysis, a risk score of 1 was assigned for group membership in the HH or LH negative-emotionality groups and in the LL or HL positive-emotionality groups, whereas a risk score of 0 was assigned for membership in LL or HL negative-emotionality groups and in the HH or LH positive-emotionality groups. As a result, cumulative-risk scores of 0 (e.g., HL negative and HH positive), 1 (e.g., LH negative and HH positive), or 2 (e.g., LH negative and LL positive) were assigned to each subject with complete data. When security of attachment was examined as a function of cumulative risk, a strong association was discerned, $\chi^2(2) = 10.42$, $p<.005$. As Table 3 indicates, 15/16 (94%) of the infants who had no risk and 21/26 (81%) with a single risk were securely attached to their mothers at 12 months, whereas only 47% of the infants with two risks were so classified.

DISCUSSION

Although several investigations indicate that negative emotionality is significantly stable within the infancy years (Birns, Barten, Bridger, 1969; Gunnar, Mangelsdorf, Larson, & Hertsgaard, 1989; Matheny, Riese, & Wilson, 1985; Miyake, Chen, & Campos, 1985; Riese, 1987), the degree of instability evident in these studies and in the current research raises the possibility that the rank ordering of infants on this dimension of individuality changes a great deal across the first years of life. Indeed, rather than assuming that the limited stability reported in most work is a function of measurement error, the current investigation was based on the presumption, consistent with the theorizing of attachment researchers (e.g., Ainsworth et al., 1978), that such instability reflects, to a significant and important extent, lawful discontinuity (Belsky & Pensky, 1988).

Thus, by examining prenatal family factors and 3-month interactional processes, we sought to illuminate conditions of discontinuity. The fact that this inquiry focused on measurements made prenatally and at 3 months in an effort to account for change in emotionality from 3 to 9 months does not mean that there is something critical about the infant's first 3 months or about the 3- to 9-month period. In fact, given the stability of many family factors and processes studied, all that the findings indicate is that variables measured before any discerned change enabled us to statistically account for change in emotionality. Presumably, processes set in motion before 3 months continue to exert an influence throughout the first year (and probably beyond).

Before considering specific findings of this study, we should note that the decision to restrict our focus to essentially the top and bottom thirds of the sample with respect to the distribution of negative- and positive-emotionality scores was based on two premises. First, we presumed that differences within high and low groups at each point in time could not necessarily be regarded as meaningful, and that an extreme-group approach would reduce the likelihood that subjects would be mistakenly classified as high or low on a particular emotionality dimension. Second, we presumed that extreme-group contrasts would amplify what were expected to be modest effects. Needless to say, such an approach limits the generalizability of the findings, because the full distribution of scores was not subject to investigation.

A variety of the results of our analyses were, in the main, consistent with the limited findings available from the few other pertinent studies that examined correlates of continuity/discontinuity in infant negative emotionality (Engfer, 1986; Matheny, 1986; Washington et al., 1986). The one major exception to this was the unanticipated discovery that harmonious, complementary interactions were disproportionately characteristic of the group that remained low in positive emotionality, whereas the reverse was true in the case of infants who changed from low to high positivity. Why this counterintuitive result emerged remains unclear. Before we try to explain it, we would like to see it replicated. Given the number of analyses run, it may be that it is only a chance finding.

Beyond this single finding, the other significant results repeatedly indicated, as anticipated, that change to lower levels of negative emotionality and to higher levels of positive emotionality was observed when parents (mothers or fathers) were psychologically healthier (higher interpersonal affect or self esteem), marriages were more positive or less negative, mother-infant interaction patterns were more complementary and harmonious, or levels of mother-infant and father-infant engagement were more equal or higher. In contrast, change to higher levels of negative emotionality and to lower levels of positive emotionality was associated with less optimal parent personality, marital characteristics, and interactional processes.

Beyond the general observation that most of the family antecedents of continuity and discontinuity identified in this study were consistent with those anticipated, it should be noted that the distal factors and proximal processes under study proved more successful in accounting for stability and change in negative than positive emotionality. Recall that we had no success in accounting for why some infants who were high in positive emotionality changed by 9 months, whereas others did not; and univariate comparisons of distal factors did not distinguish between the LL and LH positive-emotionality groups. One reason for the limited success in accounting for change in positive emotionality relative to negative emotionality may be that the latter is a more salient characteristic to parents and one that they are more responsive to than positive emotionality. Continuity and discontinuity in positive affect/social responsiveness may result from less deliberate processes, in fact, processes that Malatesta and colleagues' (1989) recent work suggests may be best elucidated through a more microanalytic analysis of interaction than the one used in this investigation, particularly one that emphasizes facial expressions. Perhaps, too, had additional observational data been available, multimeasure compositing could have generated more reliable measures that would have been more sensitive to stability and change in positive emotionality. There is also the possibility that the constructs used in this inquiry as potential conditions of discontinuity, based as they were on prior research on negative emotionality (Engfer, 1986; Matheny, 1986; Washington et al., 1986), may simply have been inappropriate for illuminating factors and processes responsible for stability and change in positive emotionality. Not to be excluded from consideration, also, is the prospect that it is simply easier to measure negative than positive emotionality. In fact, our inability to achieve reliability in observing and recording infant smiles during the 3-month mother-infant observations resulted in this behavior being deleted from the recording form. Whatever the reason why less success was achieved in discriminating between groups that stayed the same and changed with regard to positive emotionality, it is clear that more work on this particular dimension of affectivity is called for.

Perhaps more unexpected than the differential success achieved in accounting for continuity/discontinuity in negative and positive emotionality was the unanticipated discovery that maternal and paternal factors were implicated differentially in accounting for the subsequent emotional functioning of infants who scored high or low in negative affect at 3 months of age. Recall that whereas paternal factors and processes were implicated as important conditions for explaining why babies who scored low in negative emotionality changed to high or remained the same 6 months later, it was maternal factors and processes that emerged as principally responsible for explaining why babies who scored high in negative emotionality at 3 months remained the same or changed over time. Even though these intriguing findings require replication before definitive conclusions can be drawn, the data lead us to tentatively propose that it is mothers who feel good about themselves and their marriages and who participate in disproportionately harmonious exchanges with their young infants who foster sufficient affect regulation to change a highly negative 3-month-old into a not particularly negative 9-month-old, but that it takes an affectively insensitive, maritally dissatisfied, and uninvolved father to turn a not very negative 3-month-old into a highly negative 9-month-old.

Prior research and theory regarding the conditions of discontinuity in negative emotionality and the developmental significance of sensitive mothering make the findings regarding maternal factors and processes easy to assimilate. Presumably, the well-resourced mother capable of initiating and maintaining harmonious interactions with her infant enables the infant to develop skills to regulate his or her own affective distress while at the same time providing care less likely to foster distress and more likely to reduce it when it occurs. Proposing mechanisms that account for the rather systematic set of father characteristics that differentiated infants low in negativity at 3 months who changed and stayed the same 6 months later offers more of a challenge.

One possibility calls attention to the family-system context of the findings. Conceivably, the low level of involvement of men whose infants changed from low to high negativity, coupled with their insensitivity to the emotions of others and dissatisfaction with their marriages, resulted in intrusive, overinvolvement on the part of the mother, which fostered infant distress. Alternatively, mothers' activity may have served to reduce father involvement, which itself reflected marital problems that may also have directly influenced the infant. Certainly consistent with this notion is recent evidence that troubled marriages are often characterized by withdrawn husbands (Gottman & Krokoff, 1989; Markman & Kraft, 1989).

Having discussed findings regarding the antecedent and proximal conditions of continuity and discontinuity in infant emotionality and attachment, consequences need to be considered. Of course, the concept of consequences in this inquiry reflects the temporal ordering of variables rather than any unequivocal pathway of influence. After all, changing patterns of emotionality may as much reflect and be derivative of developing attachment relations as they are the determinants of them. From our perspective, in fact, these potential causes and consequences are reciprocally linked.

It is particularly intriguing, in view of the differential success in forecasting change in positive and negative emotionality, that attachment security was more systematically associated with continuity and discontinuity in positive emotionality than negative emotionality. These results need to be considered in view of two sets of related findings. First, prior work exploring links between infant negative affect and attachment security reveals either no relations (Bates et al., 1985; Belsky & Isabella, 1988; Sroufe, 1985), weak relations (Goldsmith & Alansky, 1987), or relations dependent on social support (Crockenberg, 1981). In contrast, the discovery that infants who change from high to low positive emotionality are disproportionately likely to be subsequently classified as insecure in their attachments to their mothers not only replicates Malatesta and co-workers' (1989) recent findings, but, in so doing, is consistent with the notion that insecurity is associated with the experience of daily life becoming less pleasurable across the first year. The fact that stability and change in negative emotionality contributed to the prediction of attachment security when considered in conjunction with positive emotionality cautions us against concluding that negative affectivity plays no role in the development of attachment security. In fact, the findings suggest that attachment security is associated with developmental processes of affect regulation with regard to both positive and negative emotionality.

In conclusion, the results of this investigation serve to counter the seemingly implicit assumption of much research that instability in infant temperament is primarily a function of measurement error. This study provides substantial evidence that continuity and discontinuity in at least the emotionality aspects of temperament are lawfully related to parental, marital, and infant factors measured before the infant's birth or during the neonatal period, as well as to patterns of parent-infant interaction measured early in the first year and before change in emotionality was discovered. Moreover, the results underscore the emerging recognition that family factors, patterns of infant-affect regulation, and individual differences in infant-mother attachment security are intertwined in a manner likely to affect the future development of the child.

REFERENCES

Ainsworth, M. D. S., Blehar, M. C., Waters, E., & Wall, S. (1978). *Patterns of attachment.* Hillsdale, NJ: Erlbaum.

Ainsworth, M. D. S., & Wittig, B. A. (1969). Attachment and exploratory behavior of one-year-olds in a strange situation. In B. M. Foss (Ed.), *Determinants of infant behavior IV* (pp. 113–136). London: Methuen.

Bates, J. E. (1987). Temperament in infancy. In J. D. Osofsky (Ed.), *Handbook of infant development* (2nd ed., pp. 1101–1149). New York: Wiley.

Bates, J. E., Freeland, C. A. B., & Lounsbury, M. L. (1979). Measurement of infant dif-ficultness. *Child Development, 50,* 794–803.

Bates, J.E., Maslin, C.A., & Frankel, K.A. (1985). Attachment security, mother-child inter-action, and temperament as predictors of behavior problem ratings at age three years. In I. Bretherton & E. Waters (Eds.), Growing points of attachment theory and research. *Monographs of the Society for Research in Child Development, 50*(1–2. Serial No. 209), 167–193.

Belsky, J. (1984). The determinants of parenting: A process model. *Child Development, 55,* 83–96.

Belsky, J., Gilstrap, B., & Rovine, M. (1984). The Pennsylvania Infant and Family Development Project, I: Stability and change in mother-infant and father-infant inter-action in a family setting at one, three, and nine months. *Child Development, 55,* 692–705.

Belsky, J., & Isabella, R. (1988). Maternal, infant, and social-contextual determinants of attachment security. In J. Belsky & T. Nezworski (Eds.), *Clinical implications of attach-ment* (pp. 41–94). Hillsdale, NJ: Erlbaum.

Belsky, J., & Pensky, E. (1988). Developmental history, personality, and family relationship: Toward an emergent family system. In R. Hinde & J. Stevenson-Hinde (Eds.), *Relationships within families* (pp. 193–217). Oxford: Clarendon Press.

Belsky, J., & Rovine, M. (1987). Temperament and attachment security in the strange sit-uation: An empirical rapprochement. *Child Development, 58,* 787–795.

Belsky, J., Rovine, M., & Fish, M. (1989). The developing family system. In M. Gunnar & E. Thelen (Eds.), *Systems and development: Vol. 22. Minnesota Symposia on Child Psychology* (pp. 119–166). Hillsdale, NJ: Erlbaum.

Belsky, J., Rovine, M., & Taylor, D. G. (1984). The Pennsylvania Infant and Family Development Project, III: The origins of individual differences in infant-mother attach-ment: Maternal and infant contributions. *Child Development, 55,* 718–728.

Belsky, J., Taylor, D. G., & Rovine, M. (1984). The Pennsylvania Infant and Family Development Project, II: The development of reciprocal interaction on the mother-infant dyad. *Child Development, 55,* 706–717.

Belsky, J., Youngblade, L., Rovine, M., & Volling, B. (in press). Patterns of marital change and parent-child interaction. *Journal of Marriage and the Family.*

Birns, B., Barten, S. B., & Bridger, W. H. (1969). Individual differences in temperamental characteristics of infants. *Transactions of the New York Academy of Sciences, 31,* 1071–1082.

Braiker, H., & Kelley, H. (1979). Conflict in the development of close relationships. In R. Burgess & T. Huston (Eds.), *Social exchange and developing relationships* (pp. 79–102). San Diego, CA: Academic Press.

Brazelton, T. B. (1973). Neonatal Behavioral Assessment Scale. *Clinics in developmental medicine,* (Vol. 50). London: Heinemann Medical Books.

Buss, A. H., & Plomin, R. (1975). *A temperament theory of personality development.* New York: Wiley-Interscience.

Buss, A. H., & Plomin, R. (1984). *Temperament: Early developing personality traits.* Hillsdale, NJ: Erlbaum.

Campos, J. J., Barrett, K. C., Lamb, M. E., Goldsmith, H. H., & Stenberg, C. (1983). Socioemotional development. In P. H. Mussen (Ed.), *Handbook of child psychology: Vol. 2. Infancy and developmental psychobiology* (pp. 783–915). New York: Wiley.

Campos, J. J., Campos, R. G., & Barrett, K. C. (1989). Emergent themes in the study of emotional development and emotional regulation. *Developmental Psychology, 25,* 394–402.

Cattell, R. B., Eber, H. W., & Tatsuoka, M. M. (1970). *Handbook for the Sixteen Personality Factor Questionnaire (16PF).* Champaign, IL: Institute for Personality and Ability Testing.

Clarke-Stewart, K. A. (1988). Parents' effects on children's development: A decade of progress? *Journal of Applied Developmental Psychology, 9,* 41–84.

Coll, C. G., Zenah, C., Walk, S., Lester, B. M., & Vohr, B. (1989, April). *Early infant temperament: The saliency of positive and negative affect.* Paper presented at the biennial meeting of the Society for Research in Child Development, Kansas City, MO.

Crockenberg, S. (1981). Infant irritability, mother responsiveness, and social support influences on the security of infant-mother attachment. *Child Development, 52,* 857–865.

Crockenberg, S. B. (1986). Are temperamental differences in babies associated with predictable differences in caregiving? In J. V. Lerner & R. M Lerner (Eds.), *Temperament and psychosocial interaction in infancy and childhood: New directions for child development* (pp. 53–73). San Francisco: Jossey-Bass.

Crockenberg, S. B., & Smith, P. (1982). Antecedents of mother-infant interaction and infant irritability in the first three months of life. *Infant Behavior and Development, 5,* 105–119.

Engfer, A. (1986). Antecedents of perceived behavior problems in infancy. In G. A. Kohnstamm (Ed.), *Temperament discussed* (pp. 165–180). Berwyn, PA: Swets North America.

Eysenck, H., & Eysenck, S. (1969). *Personality structure and measurement.* San Diego, CA: Kropp.

Fox, N. A., & Davidson, R. J. (1988). Patterns of brain electrical activity during facial signs of emotion in 10-month-old infants. *Developmental Psychology, 24,* 230–236.

Goldsmith, H. H., & Alansky, J. A. (1987). Maternal and infant temperamental predictors of attachment: A meta-analytic review. *Journal of Consulting and Clinical Psychology, 55,* 805–816.

Goldsmith, H. H., & Campos, J. J. (1986). Fundamental issues in the study of early temperament: The Denver Twin Temperament Study. In M. E. Lamb, A. L. Brown, & B. Rogoff (Eds.), *Advances in developmental psychology* (Vol. 4, pp. 231–283). Hillsdale, NJ: Erlbaum.

Goldsmith, H. H., & Rieser-Danner, L. A. (1986). Variation among temperament theories and validation studies of temperament assessment. In G. A. Kohnstamm (Ed.), *Temperament discussed* (pp. 1–9). Berwyn, PA: Swets North America.

Gottman, J., & Krokoff, L. (1989). Marital interaction and marital satisfaction: A longitudinal view. *Journal of Consulting and Clinical Psychology, 57,* 47–52.

Gunnar, M. R., Mangelsdorf, S., Larson, M., & Hertsgaard, L. (1989). Attachment, temperament, and adrenocortical activity in infancy. A study of psychoendocrine regulation. *Developmental Psychology, 25,* 355–363.

Hubert, N. C., Wachs, T. D., Peters-Martin, P., Gandour, M. J. (1982). The study of early temperament: Measurement and conceptual issues. *Child Development, 53,* 571–600.

Huberty, C. (1984). Issues in the use and interpretation of discriminant analysis. *Psychological Bulletin, 95,* 156–171.

Isabella, R., & Belsky, J. (1985). Marital change during the transition to parenthood and security of infant-parent attachment. *Journal of Family Issues, 6,* 505–522.

Isabella, R., & Belsky, J. (1990). *Interactional origins of infant-mother attachment security: Replication and extension.* Manuscript submitted for publication.

Isabella, R., Belsky, J., & von Eye, A. (1989). Origins of infant-mother attachment: An examination of interactional synchrony during the infant's first year. *Developmental Psychology, 25,* 12–21.

Isabella, R. A., Ward, M. J., & Belsky, J. (1985). Convergence of multiple sources of information on infant individuality: Neonatal behavior, infant behavior, and temperament reports. *Infant Behavior and Development, 8,* 283–291.

Jackson, D. (1976). *Jackson Personality Inventory.* Gaslen, NY: Research Psychologists Press.

Jacobson, J. L., Fein, G. G., Jacobson, S. W., & Schwartz, P. M. (1984). Factors and clusters for the Brazelton scale: An investigation of the dimensions of neonatal behavior. *Developmental Psychology, 20,* 339–353.

Lee, C., & Bates, J. (1985). Mother-child interaction at age two years and perceived difficult temperament. *Child Development, 56,* 1314–1325.

Malatesta, C. Z., Culver, C., Tesman, J., & Shepard, B. (1989). The development of emotion expression during the first two years of life: Normative trends and patterns of individual difference. *Monographs of the Society for Research in Child Development, 54* (1–2, Serial No. 219).

Markman, H., & Kraft, H. (1989). Men and women in marriage: Dealing with gender differences in marital therapy. *The Behavior Therapist, 12,* 51–56.

Matheny, A. P., Jr. (1986). Stability and change of infant temperament: Contributions from the infant, mother, and family environment. In G. Kohnstamm (Ed.), *Temperament discussed* (pp. 49–58). Berwyn, PA: Swets North America.

Matheny, A. P., Jr., Riese, M. L., & Wilson, R. S. (1985). Rudiments of infant temperament: Newborn to 9 months. *Developmental Psychology, 21,* 486–494.

Matheny, A. P., Jr., Wilson, R. S., & Nuss, S. (1984). Toddler temperament: Stability across settings and over ages. *Child Development, 55,* 1200–1211.

McCrae, R., & Costa, P. (1984). *Emerging lives, enduring dispositions: Personality in adulthood.* Boston: Little, Brown.

McNeil, T. F., & Persson-Blennow, I. (1982). Temperament questionnaires in clinical research. In *Temperamental differences in infants and young children* (pp. 20–35). London: Pitman Books Ltd.

Miyake, K., Chen, S., & Campos, J. J. (1985). Infant temperament, mother's mode of interaction and attachment in Japan: An interim report. In I. Bretherton & E. Waters (Eds.), Growing points in attachment theory and research. *Monographs of the Society for Research in Child Development, 50* (1–2, Serial No. 209), 276–297.

Pettit, G. S., & Bates, J. E. (1984). Continuity of individual differences in the mother-infant relationship from six to thirteen months. *Child Development, 55,* 729–739.

Riese, M. L. (1987). Temperament stability between the neonatal period and 24 months. *Developmental Psychology, 23,*216–222.

Smith, P., & Pederson, D. (1988). Material sensitivity and patterns of infant-mother attachment. *Child Development, 59,* 1097–1101.

Sroufe, L. A. (1985). Attachment classification from the perspective of infant-caregiver relationships and infant temperament. *Child Development, 56,* 1–14.

Thomas, A. (1984). Temperament research: Where we are, where we are going. *Merrill-Palmer Quarterly, 30,* 103–109.

Thomas, A., Chess, S., & Birch, H. G. (1968). *Temperament and behavior disorders in children.* New York: New York University Press.

Washington, J., Minde, K., & Goldberg, S. (1986). Temperament in preterm infants: Style and stability. *Journal of the American Academy of Child Psychiatry, 25,* 493–502.

Watson, D., & Clark, L. (1984). Negative affectivity: The disposition to experience aversive emotional states. *Psychological Bulletin, 96,* 465–490.

Watson, D., Clark, L, & Tellegan, A. (1988). Development and validation of brief measures of positive and negative affect: The CANAS Scales. *Journal of Personality and Social Psychology, 54,* 1063–1070.

Watson, D., & Tellegan, A. (1985). Toward a consensual structure of mood. *Psychological Bulletin, 98,* 219–235.

Wille, D. E. (1989, April). *Maternal perception of infant sociability: Impact on mother-infant interaction and quality of attachment.* Paper presented at the biennial meeting of the Society for Research in Child Development, Kansas City, MO.

4

Maternal Representations of Attachment During Pregnancy Predict the Organization of Infant-Mother Attachment at One Year of Age

Peter Fonagy

The Anna Freud Center, London, England

Howard Steele

University College London, England

Miriam Steele

The Anna Freud Center, London, England

While strong restrospective and concurrent associations between maternal and infant patterns of attachment have been noted, this is one of the first reports of a prospective investigation of such associations. The Adult Attachment Interview was administered to 100 mothers expecting their first child, and, at 1-year follow-up, 96 of these were seen with their infants at 12 months in the Strange Situation. Maternal representations of attachment (autonomous vs. dismissing or preoccupied) predicted subsequent infant-mother attachment patterns (secure vs. insecure) 75% of the time. These observed concordances, as well as

Reprinted with permission from *Child Development*, 1991, Vol. 62, 891–905. Copyright 1991 by the Society for Research in Child Development, Inc.

The research was supported by a Commonwealth Scholarship to H. Steele and a Social Sciences and Humanities Research Council of Canada Doctoral Fellowship to M. Steele and grants from the Nuffield Foundation, the Central Research Fund of the University of London, and the Collaborative Research Fund of the Anna Freud Center. The interest of families participating in the research is gratefully acknowledged. Recruitment of subjects was facilitated by H. Brant and A. McMeeking in the Department of Obstetrics and Gynecology, University College Hospital. Mary J. Ward provided training in the coding of the Strange Situation. Karen Pinder, Arabella Kurtz, and Gemma Rocco assisted with data collection and compilation. For comments on earlier drafts and for their support and sustained interest in the work, the authors thank Mary Main, John Bowlby, and George Moran. The authors thank Anna Higgitt for her continued interest and involvement in the research.

*the discordances, are discussed in terms of the uniquely powerful con-
tribution the Adult Attachment Interview makes to the study of representational and intergenerational influences on the development of the
infant-mother attachment.*

There is increasing evidence of an association between the way in which a mother
recalls her own childhood experience and the quality of the relationship existing
between her and her child (Grossmann, Fremmer-Bombik, Rudolph, & Grossmann,
1988; Main & Goldwyn ,1984, in press-a; Main, Kaplan, & Cassidy, 1985; Morris,
1981; Ricks, 1985). The notion of intergenerational concordance in relationship
patterns has a distinguished history in the psychoanalytic literature (Bowlby, 1973,
1988; Emde, 1988; Frailberg, Adelson, & Shapiro, 1975; Freud, 1940/1964) as
well as in epidemiological research (Frommer & O'Shea, 1973; Rutter & Madge,
1976; Rutter, Quinton, & Liddle, 1983). More recently, developmental psychologists, in searching for the roots of individual differences in infant patterns of attachment, have begun to explore the influence of the mother's childhood experience
and personality structure on the child-mother relationship (Belsky & Isabella, 1988;
Grossmann et al., 1988; Haft & Slade, 1989; Main et al., 1985; Ricks, 1985;
Spieker & Booth, 1988; Sroufe, 1985).

John Bowlby's attachment theory provides a plausible explanation for the social
transmission of relationship patterns across generations. Child-caregiver interaction
patterns are internalized early in life and guide the infant's expectations, and evaluations, of relationship experiences. While these internal representations can be
modified by current experience, they are considered resistant to change. They continue to influence relationships throughout childhood, across the lifespan, and even
into the next generation (Bowlby, 1973, 1988). This article addresses the issue of
how expectant mothers' mental representations of attachment may be seen to influence the subsequent quality of the infant-mother relationship.

Attachment research was substantially advanced by the development of a structured interview for classifying an adult's mental representations concerning relationships. The Adult Attachment Interview (George, Kaplan, & Main, 1985)
consists of a series of questions and probes designed to elicit as full a story as possible about the individual's childhood attachment experiences and evaluations of
the effects of those experiences on present functioning. The manner in which these
experiences are conveyed, rather than the nature of the experiences themselves,
yields an overall classification of the adult's current state of mind with respect to
attachment. It has been suggested that these classifications—Dismissing (D),
Preoccupied (E), or Autonomous (F)—bear a systematic association to the Strange
Situation classifications of infant patterns of attachment—Avoidant (A), Resistant
(C), or Secure (B), respectively (Ainsworth & Eichberg, in press; Main & Goldwyn,
in press-a; Main et al., 1985).

Mothers whose interviews are classified Autonomous show objectivity and balance in discussing their childhood experiences, whether favorable or unfavorable, and present a narrative picture that is both coherent and believable. Mothers whose interviews are rated as Dismissing seem cut off from the emotional nature of childhood attachment experiences. Their current state of mind with respect to attachment is variously characterized by idealization, derogation, insistence on the inability to recall, and cognitive formulations divorced from affect. Mothers whose interviews are classified Preoccupied are over involved with their sometimes traumatic childhood experiences at the time of the interview. These experiences appear often to have involved role reversal in which they have assumed the role of parenting the parent(s). Their mind appears overwhelmed and confused by the topic of attachment, evidenced in the interview context by incoherence and preoccupying anger or passivity.

We may understand the relation between mothers' state of mind with respect to attachment and the possible influence of this on maternal behavior and infant security in the following way. Interviews classified Autonomous point to mothers whose minds are not taken up with unresolved concerns regarding their childhood experience and are therefore free to respond to their child's attachment cues. Interviews classified Dismissing indicate a reluctance to acknowledge attachment needs that may make such mothers—who often seem to share a history of rejection by their own mothers—insensitive and unresponsive to their infants' signals. Interviews classified Preoccupied suggest that mothers are likely to provide an inconsistent, confused picture for their infants, giving rise to an anxiously resistant pattern where infants' attempts to deal with their attachment needs are easily frustrated.

Main and Goldwyn (in press-a) report a concordance coefficient of .61 (kappa) between mother and child attachment classification. The figure is particularly impressive since these interviews were conducted with parents of 6-year olds and then correlated with their child's security of attachment as measured 5 years previously (Main et al., 1985). These results have been confirmed by an independent group of investigators (Grossman et al, 1988). However, the retrospective nature of both these studies permits no control for the possibility that mothers' recollections may have been moderated by their evolving relationship with their children. As Sroufe (1985) suggested, a prospective study is the ideal method for assessing the significance of mothers' relationship histories. The attachment theory model of intergenerational concordance predicts that there should be an association between a prenatal assessment of maternal representations of relationships and the subsequent quality of the infant-mother attachment. This article presents findings of a prospective study that examined the association between primiparous mothers' Adult Attachment Interviews, assessed during pregnancy, and Strange Situation assessments of the infant-mother attachment relationship assessed at 1 year.

METHOD

Subjects

One hundred pregnant women were recruited for the London Parent-Child Project. Recruitment for "a study aimed at better understanding how one's own experience of childhood influences the parenting of the next generation" took place during prenatal classes at the obstetrics and gynecology department of University College Hospital. Selection criteria included primiparous status, current cohabitation with the father of the child, fluency in the English language, and age above 20. About 50% of those to whom the study was described agreed to participate. Of the group who declined participation, some did not meet the selection criteria, while others could not obtain agreement from their husbands/partners, despite their interest in participating. A sizable minority were simply not responsive to the idea of participation in the research.

The expectant mothers' ($N = 100$) median age was 31 (range, 22–42). Eighty-two of the women were married to the expectant father at the time of recruitment or married subsequently. At prenatal assessment, median length of residence together was 5 years (range, 1–19). The sample turned out to be a well-educated, white, middle-class group with 70 of the women holding university degrees; all 100 were high school graduates. Twenty-one of the women represented social class I (professional and managerial), 65 social class II (intermediate occupation), nine social class III (skilled occupations), and five social class IV (partly skilled occupations), according to the criteria of the Office of Population Censuses and Surveys (1980). The Registrar General's classification includes a separate 12-point coding of subjects' occupation, allowing for further coding into lower, middle, and upper income groups. Sixty-five of the women were in the middle income group, 21 were in the upper income group, and 14 were in the lower income group. Seventy-five of the expectant mothers were from England, 10 from Scotland or Ireland, and 15 were born outside the United Kingdom. This latter group was primarily Anglo-Saxon or European with only a few from genuinely different cultures.

Between prenatal and 1-year assessments, attrition was low. One mother was excluded from the study because she had twins. Data from one subject were eliminated because she was recently bereaved. Strange Situation data were unavailable for a further two cases because of technical difficulties. Of the 96 children seen in the laboratory, 46 were girls and 50 were boys. No child had a significant auditory or visual handicap. One child (classified secure with mother in the Strange Situation) was born with a cystic hygroma and received considerable medical attention with multiple hospitalizations.

Design

During the last trimester of a first pregnancy, the Adult Attachment Interview (George et al., 1985) was administered to 100 women; 98 were interviewed in their homes, and two were interviewed in the laboratory. While the laboratory setting is normally to be preferred in AAI research, in the present study interviews in the home were favored for the added degree of personal contact involved. To maintain continuity with the sample, all subjects were contacted by telephone and by post at 3 months postpartum. At 12 months postpartum, all the families were invited to the laboratory for the first time, where 96 children were assessed with mother in the Strange Situation.

Adult Attachment Interview Procedure

The interview administered to all subjects closely followed the schedule outlined by George et al. (1985). The Adult Attachment Interview is a structured interview consisting of 18 questions. All interviews were conducted by the same female interviewer and lasted from 30 min to 2 hours, with most lasting approximately 45 min. The interviewer, while trying to put the interviewee at ease, asked only the questions and the relevant probes without looking at the interview text. The interviews were audio-recorded and later transcribed verbatim.

The Adult Attachment Interview is structured entirely around the topic of attachment, principally, the individual's relationship to mother and to father (and/or to alternative caregivers) during childhood. Subjects are asked both to describe their relationship with their parents during childhood and to provide specific biographical episodes to support global evaluations. Ultimate classification depends on the goodness of fit between semantic evaluations and episodic memories.

The interviewer asks directly about childhood experiences of rejection; being upset, ill, and hurt; as well as loss, abuse, and separations. In addition, the subject is asked to offer explanations for the parents' behavior and to describe the current relationship with their parents and the influence they consider their childhood experiences to have on current behavior and, in the present study, future parenting style.

All 100 interviews were independently rated by four judges (Miriam Steele, Howard Steele, and Peter Fonagy, who had received training from Mary Main, and Anna Higgitt, who received training from MS, HS, and PF). The rating procedure followed the established (see Main & Goldwyn, in press-b), and all raters independently studied and rated all interviews. Reliability coefficients were calculated by computing agreements between each possible pair of raters (six estimates) and choosing the median as indicator of reliability. Levels of agreement among the four raters' readings of the interviews were consistently high: On the three-way clas-

sifications, median kappa = .90 (range, .72–.92) as well as on the scales for
Probable Past Experience, median r = .84 (range, .69–.97) and Present State of
Mind, median r = .81 (range, .68–.94).

Each interview was rated on a series of 9-point scales according to criteria specified by Main and Goldwyn (in press-b) where every second point had specific
operational definitions. Three of these scales concerned the adult's probable childhood experience of having been parented in a (1) loving, (2) rejecting, or (3) role-
reversing manner. The adult's probable experience with each parent was rated
separately. A further five scales pertained to subjects' current state of mind with
respect to attachment: (4) idealization, (5) preoccupying anger, (6) derogation, (7)
insistence on the inability to recall, and (8) the overall coherence of the interview.
Notably, preoccupying anger is to be distinguished from derogation. The anger scale
is thought to be most relevant to the Preoccupied classification in its actively resent-
ful (E2) rather than passive form (E1). Derogation, by contrast, is regarded as indicative of the Dismissing classification, derogation of devaluing of attachment being
an attempt to distance oneself from attachment-related feelings including anger.
Furthermore, maternal anger is expected to correlate with infant resistance in its
active, angry form (C1), while maternal derogation is expected to correlate with
infant avoidance.

After assigning Probable Experience and State of Mind scale ratings to an interview transcript, the judge then assigned each interview to one of three categories
reflecting the individual's overall organization of thought concerning attachment:
(1) Dismissing attachment "D," (2) Preoccupied with or entangled by past attachments "E," or (3) Freely valuing, secure, or autonomous with respect to attachment
"F." It is to be noted that in addition to assigning a D/E/F classification, the judge
also decided on the appropriateness of an alternative classification of Unresolved
(U) with respect to past trauma or loss. This is consistent with the observed associations between the U interview status and the recently discovered "disorganized"
pattern of infant attachment (Main & Hesse, in press). In this article we report only
the major D/E/F classifications and not the alternative U classification as this latter
issue is peripheral to the major question under investigation, that is, can the previously reported retrospective patterns be observed prospectively?

The AAI ratings by the four raters were averaged. The associations between the
AAI scales were examined by computing product-moment correlations across the
100 interviews. Table 1 displays these correlations. In light of the relatively high
correlations between scales, a multivariate approach was adopted in all further analyses involving the AAI scale scores.

A discriminant function analysis was performed to identify which of the AAI
scales made the most important contributions to the categorization of the interviews.
Two significant canonical variables were extracted (canonical correlations = .809
and .617, $p \leq$ respectively). The first variable appeared to distinguish the Autonomous

TABLE 1
Product-Moment Correlation Matrix of the Rating-Scale Scores
of 100 Adult Attachment Interviews

	LOVING		REJECTING		ROLE REVERSING	
	Mother	Father	Mother	Father	Mother	Father
Loving^F.............	.67**					
Rejecting^M.......	−.84**	−.57**				
Rejecting^F........	−.43**	−.81**	.48**			
Reversal^M........	−.27*	−.46**	.24	.39**		
Reversal^F.........	−.25	−.13	.23	.11	.42**	
Coherence......	.55**	.49**	−.44**	−.31*	−.32*	−.29*
Poor recall.......	−.38**	−.48**	.21	.35**	.15	.12
Idealization^M...	−.03	−.25	−.02	.23	.07	.15
Idealization^F ...	−.21	.07	.22	−.13	−.20	.18
Anger^M.............	−.54**	−.31*	.62**	.13	.13	.25
Anger^F	−.28*	−.45**	.34**	.45**	.35**	.34**
Derogation^M	−.67**	−.40**	.68**	.28*	.12	.17
Derogation^F.....	−.27*	−.58**	.23	.60**	.23	.17

	Coherence	Inability to Recall	IDEALIZATION		CURRENT ANGER		Dero-gation
			Mother	Father	Mother	Father	
Poor Recall......	−.45**						
Idealization^M...	−.38**	.31*					
Idealization^F ...	−.25	.14	.37**				
Anger^M.............	−.48**	.08	−.11	.19			
Anger^F	−.26	.12	.00	−.13	.58**		
Derogation^M	−.39**	.22	−.16	.20	.48**	.31*	
Derogation^F.....	−.28*	.27*	.19	−.13	.21	.63**	.48**

NOTE.—^M = mother-probable experience with or state of mind concerning; ^F = father-probable experience with or state of mind concerning.
* $p \leq .01$, two-tailed.
** $p \leq .001$, two-tailed.

(F) group from the other two groups (D, E), while the second differentiated between the Preoccupied (E) and Dismissing (D) groups. Correlations between AAI scale scores and canonical variables indicated that coherence of discourse, a loving past relationship with mother and father, and the absence of role reversal contributed highly to the first canonical variable. Present anger, good recall, and the absence of derogation made the most important contribution to the second canonical variable. The complete discriminant function accurately classified 89 of the 100 cases.

Strange Situation Procedure

It is already well established that the Strange Situation is a reliable and valid instrument with which to assess the quality of child-mother attachments (Ainsworth, Blehar, Waters, & Wall, 1978). This 20-min laboratory-based assessment involves two brief separations and two 3-min reunions with the parent. Focus is on the infant's behavior, especially during the reunions, where individual differences are measured in terms of the strategies employed to cope with this stressful situation (i.e., introduction to an unfamiliar place and person, and two brief separations from mother). Of the three major patterns of response, two are thought to reflect an anxious attachment to the parent (either avoidant or resistant) and one is understood to indicate a secure attachment to the parent. Infants whose attachment is coded avoidant tend to appear undistressed during separation and to avoid proximity to the parent upon reunion. Infants whose attachment is coded resistant tend to be distressed by separation and to seek contact during reunion, but rather than being settled by the parent's return, they resist the contact they also seek and are unable to be comforted. Infants whose attachment is coded secure may or may not be distressed by separation, but upon reunion are pleased to see the parent and, if distressed, are easily comforted. Strange Situation assessments, videotaped and audiotaped when the infants were between 12 and 13 months, were subsequently coded by raters blind to the mothers' interview data. Proximity seeking, contact maintenance, resistance, and avoidance during each of the two reunions were coded on the seven-point scales developed by Ainsworth et al. (1978). In addition, all infants were assigned to one of three classifications: secure, avoidant, or resistant. Mary J. Ward coded 35 of the tapes in the context of training three independent coders to high levels of major category agreement, median $r = .88$ (range, .84–.92). On the remaining 61 tapes, median interrater reliability was .91 (range, .88–.94). All Strange Situation tapes were coded by at least two independent coders, both blind to mothers' interview classification, and assigned to one of the three major categories. Disagreements between the two primary raters were conferenced in discussions with a third trained rater, also blind to mothers' interview classification.

Following the Strange Situation procedure, both parents were independently interviewed using a semistructured interview with two major components. The first concerned the presence of major life events or difficulties, including deaths, separations, or changes in employment or financial circumstances. The second aspect of the interview concerned a more detailed inquiry into the individual's experience of the transition to parenthood. Interviews were transcribed; the analysis of the experience of parenthood, however, is not yet complete.

RESULTS

The results are presented in three sections. The first examines the concordance between mothers' Adult Attachment Interview classifications, assessed prenatally, and infants' security of attachment to mother, assessed in the Strange Situation at 12 months. The second examines the particular characteristics of mothers whose interviews were classified secure but whose children were classified insecurely attached in the Strange Situation. The third section considers the distinguishing

TABLE 2

Associations between 96 Mothers' Prenatal Adult Attachment Interview
Classifications and the Strange Situation Classifications of Their
Infants at 12 Months

INFANTS' STRANGE SITUATION CLASSIFICATIONS	MOTHERS' ADULT ATTACHMENT INTERVIEW CLASSIFICATIONS		
	Dismissing (N = 22)	Autonomous (N = 59)	Preoccupied (N = 15)
Avoidant (N = 30) ...	15 (6.9)	8 (18.4)	7 (4.7)
Secure (N = 55)	5 (12.6)	45 (33.8)	5 (8.6)
Resistant (N = 11) ...	2 (2.5)	6 (6.8)	3 (1.7)

	D/E/F → A/C/B Three-Way	F/non-F → B/non-B Two-Way
Observed match ...	66%	75%
Expected match....	44%	52%
Kappa	.38	.48
Chi²	27.6 (df = 4), p ≤ .001	22.54 (df = 1), p ≤ .001

NOTE.—Expected frequencies appear in parentheses. Predicted cells are underscored.

features of mothers whose prenatal interviews were classified insecure but whose children were classified securely attached in the Strange Situation. For all results reported, analyses were repeated excluding those mothers (N = 15) born outside the United Kingdom or Ireland in order to control for the possible influence of cultural factors. Mention is made only where the analyses on the homogeneously U.K./Irish group (N = 81) differ from those attained for the larger London sample (N = 96).

1. The Intergenerational Concordance

Of those adult attachment interviews for which Strange Situation data were available (N = 96), 59 were classified Autonomous, 22 Dismissing, and 15 Preoccupied with respect to attachment. The prediction that a mother's organization of thought concerning relationships, assessed prior to the birth of her child, is associated to her child's security of attachment at 1 year was impressively confirmed. Seventy-five percent of secure mothers had securely attached children; 73% of mothers Dismissing or Preoccupied with respect to attachment had insecurely attached children. The overall two-way (secure-insecure) match between mothers' prenatal interviews and children's security of attachment was 75% (kappa = .48, p ≤ .001, 52% expected by chance alone). The three-way match was 66% (kappa = .38, p ≤ .001, 44% expected). Table 2 shows the observed and expected frequencies for the three-

TABLE 3

Mean Scale-Score Ratings of Mothers' Attachment Interviews Grouped by Infants
Child-Mother Strange Situation Classifications ($N = 96$)

AAI Scales	Avoidant (A) ($N = 30$)	Resistant (C) ($N = 11$)	Secure (B) ($N = 55$)	ANOVA F ($df = 2,93$)	Pair-Wise Comparisons		
					A vs. C	A vs. B	C vs. B
Probable experience:							
Loving/nonrejecting[M]	5.82 (1.64)	7.21 (1.11)	6.54 (1.83)	3.20*	3.26**	2.12*	N.S.
Loving/nonrejecting[F]	5.52 (1.87)	6.60 (1.88)	6.34 (1.61)	2.71	N.S.	N.S.	N.S.
Role reversing[B]	2.06 (1.12)	2.01 (1.01)	1.87 (1.14)	< 1	N.S.	N.S.	N.S.
State of mind:							
Idealization of[B]	3.31 (1.23)	3.57 (1.18)	2.79 (.91)	4.01*	N.S.	2.11*	N.S.
Derogation of[B]	2.21 (1.22)	1.52 (.88)	1.83 (.79)	2.73	N.S.	N.S.	N.S.
Current anger at[B]	2.32 (1.42)	1.84 (1.27)	2.28 (1.30)	< 1	N.S.	N.S.	N.S.
Poor recall[C]	3.90 (1.44)	3.36 (1.26)	3.21 (1.19)	3.10*	N.S.	2.23*	N.S.
Coherence[G]	4.83 (1.34)	5.57 (1.36)	5.96 (1.22)	7.76***	N.S.	3.05***	N.S.

NOTE.—Standard deviations appear in parentheses. Results of pair-wise comparisons by separate variance analysis are expressed as t values with Bonferronized significance levels. M = mother, F = father, B = both parents, C = global state of mind.

* $p \le .05$.
** $p \le .01$.
*** $p \le .001$.

way comparisons between mothers' classification on the Adult Attachment Interview and the infants' Strange Situation classification.

Examination of the observed and expected frequencies in Table 2 clarifies which AAI classifications were found to have particular value for predicting Strange Situation results from prenatal assessments. Autonomous adult classification increases the likelihood of secure infant classification while reducing that of anxious avoidant. Dismissing classification substantially increases the likelihood of anxious avoidant classification while reducing the probability of observing a secure infant pattern of attachment. The Preoccupied classification was of some help in predicting insecure infant status but failed to distinguish anxious-avoidant and anxious-resistant groups. Infants classified insecure resistant could not be predicted on the basis of the classifications of the prenatal AAIs shown in Table 2.

Because of colinearity among the scales, the following transformations were performed. Scores on the loving and the reflexed rejection scales were combined separately with respect to the subject's experience with her mother and father. Reversal, idealization, derogation, and anger scores were combined for the two parents. The means and standard deviations of the AAI scale scores grouped according to the child's Strange Situation classification are shown in Table 3. The eight variables were submitted to one-way multivariate analyses of variance which yielded a significant Wilks's lambda (lambda $= .746$, approximate $F - 1.72$, $df = 16,172$, $p \leqslant .05$). Univariate F tests were performed to examine which of the variables contributed to these group differences. Anxious-resistant and secure children had mothers who recalled their relationship with their mothers as significantly more loving and less rejecting. Idealization was highest among mothers of avoidant and resistant children. Inability to recall was particularly marked among mothers of avoidant children. Coherence was highest among mothers of securely attached infants, significantly distinguishing them from mothers of avoidantly attached infants.

Table 4 portrays the association between prenatal Adult Attachment Interview classification and mean interactive behavior ratings for first and second reunions in the Strange Situation at 1 year. A multivariate analysis of variance was performed which yielded a significant Wilks's lambda (lambda $= .701$, approximate $F = 2.12$, $df = 16,172$, $p \leqslant .01$), indicating that the child's reunion behavior, particularly during the second reunion, was well predicted by the mother's Adult Attachment Interview classification. Univariate ANOVAs performed to explore this association provided strong evidence of the hypothesis that contact maintenance in both Strange Situation reunions would be most marked in infants of mothers whose prenatal interviews were judged Autonomous, while avoidance, as predicted, was most apparent in children of mothers whose interviews were classified Dismissing. Notably, children of mothers whose interviews were classified Preoccupied showed a significantly elevated level of resistance to contact in the second reunion, but not in the first. Similarly, avoidance ratings significantly dis-

TABLE 4

Mean Scores for Reunion Behavior During the Strange Situation at 12 Months by Mothers' Prenatal Adult Attachment Interview Classification

	Dismissing (D) (N = 22)	Preoccupied (E) (N = 15)	Autonomous (F) (N = 59)	Overall F (df = 2,93)	Pair-Wise Comparisons		
					D vs. E	D vs. F	E vs. F
First reunion:							
Proximity and contact seeking ...	1.95 (1.05)	2.74 (2.12)	2.84 (1.62)	2.50	N.S.	N.S.	N.S.
Contact maintenance.......	1.23 (.53)	2.00 (1.56)	2.49 (1.98)	4.40**	1.73	4.38***	N.S.
Resistance to contact..........	1.14 (.35)	1.54 (1.12)	1.62 (1.19)	N.S.	N.S.	N.S.	N.S.
Avoidance of proximity	4.32 (1.43)	3.80 (1.70)	3.22 (1.79)	2.51	N.S.	N.S.	N.S.
Second reunion:							
Proximity and contact seeking ...	2.82 (1.33)	3.17 (1.90)	3.93 (1.69)	2.51	N.S.	N.S.	N.S.
Contact maintenance.......	2.32 (1.91)	3.40 (2.33)	3.91 (2.35)	4.05*	N.S.	3.13**	N.S.
Resistance to contact........	1.96 (1.70)	3.27 (1.94)	1.97 (1.28)	4.83**	1.94	N.S.	2.19*
Avoidance of proximity	4.00 (1.48)	3.13 (1.73)	2.63 (1.72)	5.44**	N.S.	3.50***	N.S.

Note.—Standard deviations appear in parentheses. Pair-wise comparisons are expressed as t values for separate variance with Bonferronized significance levels.

* $p \leq .05$.
** $p \leq .01$.
*** $p \leq .001$.

tinguished Dismissing from Autonomous interviews, but only in the second reunion. This underscores the importance of using two reunions in the assessment of the child's security of attachment.

2. Maternal Attachment Security and Insecurely Attached Children

Fourteen (24%) of the mothers whose interviews were classified Autonomous had insecurely attached infants, eight avoidant and six resistant. Exploration of this difference initially focused on the incidence of major life events over the year intervening between pregnancy and 1-year assessments. One of the 45 and two of the 14, both mothers of avoidantly attached infants, reported having experienced stressful life events (e.g, loss of a loved one, marital strife) during the first year of the child's life. Subsequent analysis of the maternal security/infant insecurity issue were performed with these individuals excluded, as it was felt that the incidence of life events could obscure the picture of the predictive value of the AAI. We also considered the possibility that some of these Autonomous mothers of anxiously attached children may not have been mainstream F's (i.e., F3) in the AAI system of subclassification. Exploration of this possibility led to a counterintuitive findings. Seventy-five percent of Autonomous mothers with anxiously attached children had prototypical Autonomous interviews (F3a or F3b), whereas only 36% of Autonomous mothers with securely attached children had interviews so classified, χ^2 (1) = 4.24.$p \leqslant .05$. Multivariate analysis of variance was then performed to test the hypotheses that the two Autonomous groups could be differentiated on the basis of their AAI scale scores. The analysis yielded a marginally significant Wilks's lambda (lambda = .80, approximate F = 2.53, df = 8,47). Table 5 shows the results of the comparisons between the AAI scale scores assigned to the interviews of each of these interview groups. Individual F tests revealed that the group with insecurely attached infants were consistently rated as somewhat more positive, both in terms of the Probable Experience and the State of Mind scales. They were rated lower in terms of role-reversing experiences with their parents ($p \leqslant .05$). In terms of their present state of mind, this group was also distinguished by their significantly lower rating on the scale for current anger ($p \leqslant .05$).

Of the 11 infants classified anxious resistant in the sample, four were assigned to the passive-resistant (C2) subclass, and all four of these infants belonged to mothers whose prenatal interviews had been classified Autonomous. This is noteworthy because it puts in perspective the significantly lower ratings for preoccupying anger among these mothers. Indeed, *low* maternal anger is an expected correlate of the C2 infant subclassification (Main & Goldwyn, in press-b).

A further comparison was made in order to consider whether these mothers whose interviews were rated so positively and classified Autonomous, but whose infants were observed to be anxiously attached, were more prone to have avoidant

TABLE 5

Mean AAI Scale Scores for Autonomous Mothers with Securely and
Insecurely Attached Children

	Autonomous Mothers with Securely Attached Infants ($N = 44$)	Autonomous Mothers with Insecurely Attached Infants ($N = 12$)	ANOVA F ($df = 1,54$)
Probable experience scales:			
Loving/Nonrejecting[M] ..	6.94 (1.68)	7.16 (1.00)	1.77
Loving/Nonrejecting[F] ...	6.70 (1.42)	6.96 (.94)	2.91
Role reversing[B]	1.68 (.76)	1.31 (.52)·	4.51*
State-of-mind scales:			
Idealization[B]	2.50 (.84)	3.13 (.92)	3.46*
Derogation[B]	1.72 (.82)	1.37 (.34)	2.14
Anger[B]	2.45 (.99)	1.48 (.75)	4.32*
Coherence	6.36 (.94)	6.42 (.57)	< 1
Poor recall	2.95 (.99)	3.04 (.95)	< 1

NOTE.—Standard deviations appear in parentheses. M = mother, F = father, B = both parents.
* $p \leq .05$.

or resistant infants. Here it was revealed that the presence of the resistant infant
patterns was beyond that which would be expected by chance: six, or 55%, of the
11 children classified resistant belonged to this group of Autonomous mothers,
while of the 30 children classified avoidant only six, or 20%, belonged to this group
(Fisher exact $p \leq .05$).

3. Maternal Attachment Insecurity and Securely Attached Children

Of those mothers whose prenatal interviews were classified as Dismissing of
attachment ($N = 22$), five (23%) had securely attached infants. Of the 15 mothers
classified as Preoccupied, five (33%) had securely attached infants. Thus, 27%
of mothers whose interviews were classified as Dismissing or Preoccupied had
securely attached children. In post-hoc exploration of this anomaly, it was noted
that maternal interview classifications appeared to be associated with the country
and culture of upbringing of the mother. While only 27 (33%) of the 81
U.K./Irishborn mothers were classified insecure, 11 (73%) of the 15 subjects born
outside the United Kingdom and Ireland were so classified (Fisher exact $p \leq .01$).
However, this possible overextension of the insecure classification in the case of
non-U.K./Irish subjects could not account for the insecure-mother/secure-child form
of discordance. Of the 27 U.K./Irish mothers who were classified Dismissing or
Preoccupied, 82% had infants coded insecurely attached; of the 11 non-U.K./Irish
mothers in the same group, 55% of the infants were coded insecure (Fisher exact
N.S.).

Consideration was also given to the possibility that the maternal insecurity/infant insecurity type of discordance may have been due to the insecure attachment classification being overextended to those subjects belonging to the lower social classes and/or income groups. There was, however, no association between a mother's demographic characteristics and either her or her infant's attachment classification.

DISCUSSION

Based on prenatal administration of the Adult Attachment Interview to 96 primiparous mothers, we were able, in 75% of the cases, to successfully predict whether an infant would be coded securely or insecurely attached (B/non-B) to mother at 1 year in the Strange Situation. These figures are consistent with those obtained in retrospective (Main & Goldwyn, in press-a, 75% [A/B/C] Grossmann et al., 1988, 77% [B/non-B]) and concurrent (Ainsworth & Eichberg, in press, 80% [A/B/C/D]) administrations of these instruments. Other ongoing research involving prenatal administration of the AAI also suggests that it is possible to predict infant-mother patterns of attachment from pregnancy assessments (e.g., Ward, Botyanski, Plunket, & Carlson, 1991). Unlike past retrospective and concurrent investigations, we did not find the Preoccupied classification to be singularly predictive of the resistant infant classification. The Autonomous and Dismissing interview classifications were powerfully predictive of the secure and avoidant infant classifications, respectively.

The reported accuracy of prediction is impressive when compared with past attempts at identifying determinants of infants' security of attachment in prospective investigations. Previous reports have failed to provide strong evidence of a predictive association between expectant mothers' developmental history and infants' security of attachment (e.g., Belsky & Isabella, 1988). The significance of mothers' developmental history is unlikely to be fully captured unless we are clear about what in an individual's developmental history is of importance for facilitating infants' security of attachment. Predictive power resides, it seems, not in the quality of past experience but in the overall organization of mental structures underlying relationships and attachment-related issues.

The present investigation has additional importance in that it originates in London, where Adult Attachment Interview research has not previously been reported. The frequency distribution of AAI categories as well as Strange Situations, however, matched closely the reports of middle-class samples from North American cities. This reflects the ubiquity of the Bowlby-Ainsworth attachment paradigm and the generalizability of Main's approach to its assessment in adulthood.

Our results indicate that the mother of the securely attached child is able to fluently convey a global representation (whether favorable or unfavorable) of what her relationship to each parent was like during her childhood. At the same time, she is able to provide specific memories that support and elaborate on the global representation of her parents. In presenting to the interviewer her account of her development within her family of origin, she demonstrates an understanding of her own personal development that includes an awareness of the multiple motives (conscious and perhaps unconscious) that guided her parents' behavior toward her. Upon reading the transcript, one is not inclined to derive conclusions different from those being presented by the subject. In other words, there is little idealization of the past, no insistence on an inability to recall, and, overall, there are no significantly distorting mental processes at work. The subject clearly has access to, and is able to express, her feelings without being overwhelmed by them; she is autonomous and freely valuing of attachment—and therefore the prediction, which the present study confirms, that such a woman was substantially more likely to bring to the Strange Situation assessment at 1 year a child who would be classified securely attached to mother. The likely pathways for this effect involve sensitive and responsive patterns of mother-child behavior observed more frequently in women classified as Secure-Autonomous on the Adult Attachment Interview (Crowell & Feldman, 1988; Haft & Slade, 1989). Conversely, mothers classified Dismissing on the Adult Attachment Interview have been shown to manifest a lack of attunement in mother-infant interactions (Haft & Slade, 1989) and restricted patterns of communication between child and parent (Grossmann, 1989).

While mothers of infants who would develop a secure or anxious-avoidant attachment were distinguishable before the child was born, the present study could not easily identify mothers of children who would develop an anxious-resistant attachment. Exploration of the results did, however, reveal two significant associations between infant resistance and maternal interview status. Ratings of infant resistance during the second reunion in the Strange Situation were predictable on the basis of the Preoccupied interview classification. The second observed association between infant resistance and maternal interview status involved the apparent discordance between Autonomous interviews and anxious Strange Situation patterns. The anxious-resistant pattern was significantly associated with a particular type of maternal interview response. This was a response likely to be rated as suggestive of a supportive attachment history, a state of mind typified by low preoccupying anger, some idealization, and an overall impression of security. This was a picture derived from the pregnancy assessment. On the basis of what we subsequently observed in the Strange Situation, we would suggest that there was something fragile about the prenatal interview not detected in our initial ratings of these interviews, which foreshadowed difficulties in adjustment to the caregiving role. This suggestion is consistent with previous findings from prospective longitudinal investigations. Spieker and Booth (1988) found that mothers of resistant infants (unlike mothers of avoidant infants) differed little prenatally from mothers whose infants were classified secure. But a certain fragility, unseen before the child was born, appeared postnatally: they expressed satisfaction with their life and with their infants' temperament despite having higher scores on the Beck Depression Inventory and less confidence in themselves as mothers. This same paradoxical pattern emerged in the present sample where those mothers whose interviews were classified as Autonomous during pregnancy but had insecurely attached children were revealed as presenting a particularly positive picture of their childhood during their prenatal interview. We informally observed in the interview conducted at the time of the Strange Situation, consistent with Spieker and Booth's findings, that these were mothers for whom the maternal experience involved considerable disillusionment, but this requires further systematic investigation. Perhaps the antecedents of the resistant coding are best understood as part of an evolving pattern of a less than successful adaptation to motherhood. This is an accord with the view that mothers of anxiously resistant children have a sensitive set of attachment-related beliefs, but are unable to act consistently on these beliefs (Ainsworth et al., 1978). In other words, it may be worth exploring the hypothesis that there seems to be a certain attachment-related state of mind, perhaps particular to pregnancy, characterized by a somewhat exaggerated secure pattern, which is subsequently associated with infant insecurity. This infant insecurity is perhaps especially prone to take the form of passive resistance and may be mediated by maternal difficulties in adjustment to the caregiving role.

The quality of prediction in any prospective investigation will be moderated by possibilities of change in the mother. The likelihood of change may be substantially increased over the year in which a woman becomes a mother (Benedek, 1959). We cannot be certain at this point in time to what extent the mismatch between apparently heightened security in pregnancy and infants' insecurity at 1 year is due to long-lasting alterations in mental structure (perhaps induced by the transition to motherhood) and to what extent it is due more to transitory shifts (e.g., postpartum depression or lack of support from spouse). A readministration of the Adult Attachment Interview to this group and a matched control group of mothers would yield information as to the extent and nature of possible changes in mental representations of attachment relationships and attachment-related concerns.

Just as the transition to parenthood may occasion disappointment and an inability to consistently employ an appropriate mothering repertoire, so too may entry into the parental role lead to positive alterations in mental structure. This was perhaps operative in those mothers whose prenatal interviews were classified insecure but whose children were later classified as securely attached. We are not proposing that internal working models necessarily change as a function of the initial parenting experience. Yet the accessibility or level of activation of aspects of these mental models may be heightened or attenuated as a function of expectations or events. Particular representations active at any one time exerting control over attachment-related cognitions and behaviors may perhaps be best conceived of as "attachment

stakes." These attachment states are to be distingished from the underlying organization and structure of the internal working model, which may be thought of as
predisposing the individual to particular types of behaviors, analogous to the function of personality traits. Comprehensive models of attachment will need to increasingly focus on the processes by which changes may occur in the representational
processes influencing attachment-related feelings, cognitions and behaviors. There
are a number of clinical service approaches that have begun to incorporate the systematic consideration of these representational processes on the quality of parent-
child relationships (Aber & Baker, 1990; Greenspan & Lieberman, 1988;
Nezworski, Tolan, & Belsky, 1988; Stern-Bruschweiler & Stern, 1989). The further
development and refinement of these clinical/service approaches may be facilitated
by careful use of the Adult Attachment Interview along with the delineation of pertinent situational, person-based, and interactional influences (Sameroff & Chandler,
1975).

In assessing the origins of observed discordances between material working
models of relationships and infants' security of attachment, we need to distinguish
possible errors of measurement from the likelihood of alterations in mental structure. A general, possibly limiting factor that awaits confirmation is the test-retest
reliability of the instrument. Another measurement issue, which emerges from the
current findings, concerns mothers' place of birth. When this does not coincide
with the mainstream culture, it may lead to an underestimation of the extent of
mothers' security/autonomy. Also, certain methodological limitations arise from
pregnancy administrations of the Adult Attachment Interview. In the present study,
the mothers were not probed specifically for fear of loss of the child, an expected
correlate of avoidance in infancy (Main & Goldwyn, in press-b), which when present in significant measure automatically leads the AAI judge to assign the Insecure-
Dismissing classification. One disadvantage, then, of using this measure
prospectively is that attachment states that are activated by the presence of an infant
cannot be assessed and may lead to inaccurate classification.

It is worth noting that the present report does not include consideration of forthcoming pieces of data that may help to eludicate the current portrait of family relationship patterns. It may be that some of the reported discordances will become
more comprehensible when data pertaining to the expected match between maternal
lack of resolution of mourning and infant disorganization are taken into consideration (Main & Hesse, 1990). It is also likely that consideration of the Adult
Attachment classification of the father may provide information pertinent to the
origins of discordance. Past studies have shown that a good marriage with attendant
social support is capable of mitigating the influence of institutional background
on child rearing (Quinton & Rutter, 1988) and to also permit a break from the cycle
of abuse (Egeland, Jacobvitz, & Sroufe, 1988). It may therefore be necessary to
take into account both parents' mental representations not only of their respective

attachment histories but also their representations of one another and of the child (Aber, Slade, Berger, & Kaplan, 1985; Bretherton, Biringen, Ridgeway, Maslin, & Sherman, 1989) if a comprehensive account of the influence of past relationships on present and future relationships is to be provided (Stevenson-Hinde, 1988, 1990).

In summary, the present study provides evidence for lawful continuities in the nature and quality of parent-child relationships across generations. The Adult Attachment interview was shown to be capable of identifying prenatally infants whose attachment to mother is more likely to assume an anxious as opposed to secure form. Many previous studies have shown how these infant patterns of attachment make certain, less than adaptive, developmental pathways more likely (Sroufe, 1988). The availability of an instrument capable of identifying mothers at high risk of evolving such patterns of relationships with their children calls for replication and extension. In addition, it creates new possibilities for preventive work addressed at both attachment-related behaviors and mental representations.

REFERENCES

Aber, J. L., & Baker, A. J. L. (1990). Security of attachment in toddlerhood: Modifying assessment procedures for joint clinical and research purposes. In M. Greenberg, D. Cichetti, & E. M. Cummings (Eds.), *Attachment in the preschool years: Theory, research, and intervention* (pp. 427–460). Chicago: University of Chicago Press.

Aber, J. L., Slade, A., Berger, B., Bresgi, I., & Kaplan, M. (1985). *The parent development interview: Manual and administration procedures.* New York: Barnard College, Department of Psychology.

Ainsworth, M. D. S., Blehar, M. C., Waters, E., & Wall, S. (1978). *Patterns of attachment: A psychological study of the Strange Situation.* Hillsdale, NJ: Erlbaum.

Ainsworth, M. D. S., & Eichberg, C. G. (in press). Effects on infant-mother attachment of mother's unresolved loss of an attachment figure or other traumatic experience. In P. Marris, J. Stevenson-Hinde, & C. Parkes (Eds.), *Attachment across the life cycle.* New York: Routledge.

Belsky, J., & Isabella, R. (1988). Maternal, infant, and social-contextual determinants of attachment security. In J. Belsky & T. Nezworski (Eds.), *Clinical implications of attachment* (pp. 41–94). Hillsdale, NJ: Erlbaum.

Benedek, T. (1959). Parenthood as a developmental phase. *Journal of the American Psychoanalytic Association, 7,* 389–417.

Bowlby, J. (1973). *Attachment and loss: Vol. 2, Separation, anxiety and anger.* New York: Basic.

Bowlby, J. (1988). *A secure base: Clinical applications of attachment theory.* London: Routledge.

Bretherton, I., Biringen, Z., Ridgeway, D., Maslin, C., & Sherman, M. (1989). Attachment: The parental perspective. *Infant Mental Health Journal, 10*(3), 203–221.

Crowell, J. A., & Feldman, S. S. (1988). Mothers' internal models of relationships and children's behavioral and developmental status: A study of mother-child interaction. *Child Development, 59*, 1273–1285.

Egeland, B., Jacobvitz, D., & Sroufe, L. A. (1988). Breaking the cycle of abuse. *Child Development, 59*, 1080–1088.

Emde, R. N. (1988). Development terminable and interminable: I. Innate and motivational factors from infancy. *International Journal of Psychoanalysis, 69*, 23–42.

Fraiberg, S. H., Adelson, E., & Shapiro, V. (1975). Ghosts in the nursery: A psychoanalytic approach to the problem of impaired infant-mother relationships. *Journal of the American Academy of Child Psychiatry, 14*, 387–422.

Freud, S. (1964). An outline of psychoanalysis. In J. Strachey (Ed. and Trans.). *The standard edition of the complete psychological works of Sigmund Freud* (Vol. 23, pp. 137–207). London: Hogarth. (Original work published 1940).

Frommer, E. A., & O'Shea, G. (1973). Antenatal identification of women likely to have problems in managing their infants. *British Journal of Psychiatry, 123*, 149–156.

George, C., Kaplan, N., & Main, M. (1985). *The Adult Attachment Interview.* Unpublished manuscript, University of California at Berkeley, Department of Psychology.

Greenspan, S., & Lieberman, A. (1988). A clinical approach to attachment. In J. Belsky & T. Nezworski (Eds.), *Clinical implications of attachment* (pp. 387–424). Hillsdale, NJ: Erlbaum.

Grossmann, K. (1989, September). *Avoidance as a communicative strategy in attachment relationships.* Paper presented at the Fourth World Congress for Infant Psychiatry and Allied Disciplines, Lugano, Switzerland.

Grossmann, K., Fremmer-Bombik, E., Rudolph, J., & Grossmann, K. E. (1988). Maternal attachment representations as related to patterns of infant-mother attachment and maternal care during the first year,. In R. A. Hinde & J. Stevenson-Hinde (Eds.), *Relationships within families: Mutual influences* (pp. 241–260). Oxford: Clarendon.

Haft, W., & Slade, A. (1989). Affect attunement and maternal attachment: A pilot study. *Infant Mental Health Journal, 10(3)*, 157–172.

Main, M., & Goldwyn, R. (1984). Predicting rejection of her infant form mother's representation of her own experience: Implications for the abused-abusing intergenerational cycle. *Child Abuse and Neglect, 8*, 203–217.

Main, M., & Goldwyn, R. (in press-a). Interview-based adult attachment classifications: Related to infant-mother and infant-father attachment. *Developmental Psychology.*

Main, M., & Goldwyn, R. (in press-b). Adult attachment rating and classification systems. In M. Main (Ed.), *A typology of human attachment organization assessed in discourse, drawings and interviews* (working title). New York: Cambridge University Press.

Main, M., Kaplan, N., & Cassidy, J. (1985). Security in infancy, childhood and adulthood: A move to the level of representation. In I. Bretherton & E. Waters (Eds.), Growing points of attachment theory and research (pp. 66–104), *Monographs of the Society for Research in Child Development, 50*(1–2, Serial No. 209).

Morris, D. (1981). Attachment and intimacy. In G. Stricker & M. Fisher (Eds.), *Intimacy* (pp. 305–323). New York: Plenum.

Nezworski, T., Tolan, W., & Belsky, J. (1988). Intervention in insecure infant attachment.

In J. Belsky & T. Nezworksi (Eds.), *Clinical implications of attachment* (pp. 352–386). Hillsdale, NJ: Erlbaum.

Office of Population Censuses and Surveys (1980). *Classification of occupations and coding index.* London: Her Majesty's Stationery Office.

Quinton, D., & Rutter, M. (1988). *Parenting breakdown: The making and breaking of intergenerational links.* Brookfield, VT: Gower.

Ricks, M. (1985). The social transmission of parental behavior: Attachment across generations. In I. Bretherton & E. Waters (Eds.), Growing points of attachment theory and research (pp. 211–227). *Monographs of the Society for Research in Child Development, 50*(1–2, Serial No. 209).

Rutter, M., & Madge, N. (1976). *Cycles of disadvantage: A review of research.* London: Heinemann.

Rutter, M., Quinton, D., & Liddle, C. (1983). Parenting in two generations: Looking backwards and looking forward. In N. Madge (Ed.), *Families at risk* (pp. 60–98). London: Heinemann.

Sameroff, A. J., & Chandler, M. J. (1975). Reproductive risk and the continuum of caretaking casuality. In F. D. Horowitz (Ed.), *Review of child development research* (Vol. 4, pp. 187–244). Chicago: University of Chicago Press.

Spieker, S., & Booth, C. (1988). Maternal antecedents of attachment quality. In J. Belsky & T. Nezworski (Eds.), *Clinical implications of attachment* (pp. 95–135). Hillsdale, NJ: Erlbaum.

Sroufe, L. A. (1985). Attachment classifications from the perspective of infant-caregiver relationships and infant temperament. *Child Development, 56,* 1–14.

Sroufe, L. A. (1988). The role of infant-caregiver attachment in development. In J. Belsky & T. Nezworski (Eds.), *Clinical implications of attachment* (pp. 18–38). Hillsdale, NJ: Erlbaum.

Stern-Bruschweiler, N., & Stern, D. (1989). A model for conceptualizing the role of the mother's representational world in various mother-infant therapies. *Infant Mental Health Journal, 10*(3), 142–156.

Stevenson-Hinde, J. (1988). Individuals in relationships. In R. A. Hinde & J. Stevenson-Hinde (Eds.), *Relationships within families: Mutual influences* (pp. 68–80). Oxford: Clarendon.

Stevenson-Hinde, J. (1990). Attachment within family systems: An overview. *Infant Mental Health Journal, 11*(3), 218–227.

Ward, M., Botyanski, N., Plunket, S., & Carlson, E. (1991). *The predictive and concurrent validity of the Adult Attachment Interview for adolescent mothers.* Paper presented at the meeting of the Society for Research in Child Development, Seattle.

5

Recent Developments in Attachment Theory and Research

Susan Goldberg

University of Toronto, Ontario

The history and development of attachment theory are reviewed. Research has focused on four major patterns of attachment in infancy: one pattern of secure attachment and three patterns of insecure attachment (avoidant, resistant, and disorganized). These patterns have been shown to reflect different histories of parent-child interaction and affected subsequent development up to age eight. More recently, methods have been developed for identifying similar patterns of attachment in preschoolers, five to seven year olds, and adults. Future research is likely to focus on the development of attachment patterns and their transmission from one generation to another. New data on the relationship between attachment and behavior problems has generated mutual respect and collaboration between clinicians and researchers.

It is widely accepted that the parent-child relationship plays a central role in a child's development, but empirical data to support this hypothesis are very recent and remarkably scant. The most common theoretical approaches to the study of parent-child relationships are psychoanalytic theory (object relations), social learning theory (dependency), and attachment theory. There has been research into each of these, but it is attachment theory that has given rise to a recent wave of empirical studies that has excited both clinicians and researchers. The goal of this article is to review the basic constructs of attachment theory and empirical research.

Reprinted with permission from *Canadian Journal of Psychiatry*, 1991, Vol. 36, 393–400. Copyright 1991 by *Canadian Journal of Psychiatry*.

A CAPSULE VIEW OF ATTACHMENT THEORY

Attachment theory was originally described by Bowlby (1-4), combining ideas from psychoanalysis and ethology. Bowlby argued that affectional ties between children and their caregivers have a biological basis which is best understood in an evolutionary context. Since children's survival depends on the care they receive from adults, there is a genetic bias among infants to behave in ways which maintain and enhance proximity to caregivers and elicit their attention and investment. A complementary evolutionary history biases adults to behave reciprocally. Thus, while psychoanalytic theory emphasizes the caregivers' initial roles in reducing physiological arousal, and social learning theory emphasizes the caregivers as teachers, attachment theory focuses on parents as protectors and providers of security. (All three theories acknowledge that parents play multiple roles, that of teacher, caregiver, playmate, etc.; they differ with respect to which role is considered most influential.) Furthermore, while the psychoanalytic and learning theories view children as initially passive, Bowlby's view credited infants with active participation. Prior theories considered infants to be dependent on caregivers and dependency as a state which must be outgrown. Attachment theory, however, considers it possible for individuals to be reciprocally attached. Attachment is therefore a quality of relationships which lasts one's lifetime. The nature of attachments may be transformed as children develop, but an attachment can endure.

The concept of attachment includes social components (it is a property of social relationships), emotional components (each participant in the relationship feels emotional bonds with the other), cognitive components (each participant forms a cognitive scheme—a "working model" of the relationship and its participants), and behavioral components (participants engage in behaviors that reflect and maintain the relationship). It is the nature and interrelationship of these components that reflect developmental change.

Over the first year, the infant's proximity-promoting behaviors (orienting signals such as cries and vocalizations, and direct actions such as approaching and clinging to the caregiver) become organized into a goal-oriented system focused on a specific caregiver. The mother is usually the first such figure, but others can play this role. When the attachment system is in its goal state (i.e., there is adequate proximity and contact), attachment behaviors subside; when the goal state is threatened, attachment behaviors are activated. Furthermore, because the attachment system operates in the context of other related systems (for example, exploration), the goal is adjusted to fit the context. For a healthy infant in a familiar (safe) environment, the goal may be to remain in the same room with the attachment figure; if the infant is tired or ill or the environment is unfamiliar, the goal becomes greater proximity and contact.

As the child's locomotor, linguistic and social skills develop, the goals of the attachment system are modified to allow for longer separations over greater distances. Cognitive components play a more dominant role and proximity plays a less important role in moderating attachment behavior.

Individuals' working models of a particular relationships include concepts of themselves and others. A more general "working model" of relationships also develops which reflects individuals' experiences in relationships. The quality of both early and later attachments influences self-concepts as well as expectations and attitudes toward social relationships. Individuals whose primary attachment relationships in childhood were satisfying and provided emotional security view themselves as lovable, expect positive interactions with others, and value intimate relationships. Individuals who experienced rejection or harsh treatment as children view themselves as unworthy of love, expect further rejections, and act in ways that elicit rejections. These predictions may not differ radically from those of other theoretical approaches to relationships; however, the evaluation of a theory depends on its ability to be empirically tested.

HISTORY OF RESEARCH INTO ATTACHMENT: AN OVERVIEW

Attachment theory has generated 25 years of productive empirical research. Empirical research was made possible by Ainsworth and her students (5,6), who classified infant-parent attachment between 12 and 18 months of age into three distinct patterns. The first ten to 15 years of research based on this method were devoted to collecting normative data and documenting the precursors and sequelae of different patterns of attachment. Initial efforts to study patterns of attachment in clinical populations followed (for example, maltreated infants, medically ill infants, infants of depressed mothers). These efforts resulted in the addition of a fourth pattern of attachment, which was thought to be potentially more pathological (7,8). However, the inability to examine patterns of attachment beyond infancy soon became a recognized limitation, and more recent work has included the development and validation of methods for assessing attachments in preschoolers (9), five to seven year olds (10), and adults (11). An outline of these schemes is shown in Table I. This conceptual scheme is likely to be completed in the future.

PATTERNS OF ATTACHMENT

Since theories of infant-parent attachment were developed before other age groups were looked at and have been most extensively studied, they will be reviewed in detail as a prelude to introducing the analogues for other age groups. The assessment of infant-mother attachment developed by Ainsworth et al. is based on their hypothesis that the infant's feelings of security are the ontogenetic function of the

TABLE I
Patterns of Attachment at Different Stages of Life

Age	Assessment Method	Patterns of Attachment			
		Secure (B)	Dismissing (A)	Preoccupied (C)	Disorganized (D)
12 to 18 months	Structured observation (Strange Situation)	Secure	Avoidant	Ambivalent/resistant	Disorganized
2¹/₂ to four years	Structured observation (reunions)	Secure	Avoidant	Dependent	Controlling/disorganized
Five to seven years	Structured observation (reunions)	Secure	Avoidant	Dependent	Controlling
Adult	Interview	Autonomous/secure	Dismissing	Preoccupied	Unresolved mourning (loss)

attachment system. Bowlby acknowledged both the phylogenetic goal of protection from predators and external danger and the ontogenetic function of psychologically perceived security. Ainsworth elaborated on the latter in the Strange Situation. The procedure involves observing the infant, caregiver (usually the mother) and a friendly but unfamiliar adult in a series of eight semi-structured episodes in a laboratory playroom (5,6). It relies on the observation of the balance of attachment and exploratory behaviors in response to the manipulations in the eight episodes. The crux of the procedure is a standard sequence of separations and reunions between the infant and each of the two adults. It is felt that over the course of the eight episodes the child experiences increasing distress and a greater need for proximity. The extent to which children cope with these needs and the strategies they use to do so are considered to indicate the quality of attachment.

Scoring depends on a detailed review of videotapes. The infant is rated on behavior directed at the caregiver: seeking contact, maintaining contact, distance interaction, avoidance, and resistance to contact. From this information, the dyad is classified into one of eight subtypes that fall into three broad categories. Although behavior during the entire session is considered, reunion behaviors have been shown to be the most salient feature distinguishing between these patterns (6).

These three patterns reflect strategies used by the infant to manage affective arousal during interactions with, separations from, and reunions with the caregiver. In the secure strategy, the attachment system is activated only when the infant's security is threatened (for example, the caregiver departs and the child is left in an unfamiliar place) and subsides to give the exploratory system free rein when the attachment figure (the secure base) returns. In the avoidant (dismissing) strategy, the attachment system is defensively suppressed so that the child appears to be exploring without concern for security, although he carefully monitors the attachment figure. In the ambivalent/resistant (preoccupied) strategy, the attachment system is continuously activated at the expense of the exploratory system, even when to all outward appearances the child should be safe and comfortable (i.e., the attachment figure is present). Another way of understanding this is to consider the threshold for activating attachment behavior: in the avoidant strategy the threshold is very high, while in the ambivalent/resistant strategy, it is very low. In both insecure strategies, the threshold is set primarily to meet internal needs and is not adapted to the environment. However, in the secure strategy, the threshold is both moderate and sensitive to environmental conditions.

In Ainsworth's original study (5), 65% of the babies exhibited a secure pattern of attachment, 21% an avoidant pattern and 14% an ambivalent/resistant pattern (6). A recent meta-analysis of nearly 2,000 infants from 39 studies conducted in eight different countries showed almost exactly the same distribution, although there were some cultural variations (12). Furthermore, under stable life conditions, patterns of attachment are relatively stable over both the short term (six months)

(13) and the long term (up to five years) (10). These data refer to attachment to the same caregiver assessed on different occasions.

A number of studies have shown that patterns of attachment to the mother and to the father are independent (14–16). This demonstrates that attachment patterns derived from the Strange Situation reflect qualities of distinct relationships rather than a trait of the child. In a recent meta-analysis of 11 studies of attachment to the mother and the father, Fox and his colleagues (17) found a high degree of concordance between patterns of attachment to mother and father, which raises some questions about the trait-versus-relationship interpretation of attachment inferred from the Strange Situation. These findings can be better understood if we consider the relationship between temperament and attachment.

There has been an ongoing discussion in the literature over the extent to which the infant's temperament affects attachment (18–22). It would seem the infants' propensity to become distressed is the primary determinant of behavior during the Strange Situation. However, the most salient behaviors for classification are not the presence or absence of distress, but the infant's style of coping with distress, in particular, use of the attachment figure as a source of comfort. Studies of parent reports of temperament have generally found little association between scores on questionnaires of temperament and security of attachment (22). However, more careful examination of the full classification scheme (including all the subgroups) suggests that there is a temperament dimension inherent in the scheme. Figure 1 illustrates the full classification scheme. Avoidant babies and some secure babies who are slightly avoidant (B_1) are less easily distressed than resistant babies, very secure babies (B_3), and secure babies who are slightly resistant (B_4). If we divide infants according to the degree to which they are likely to become distressed (high/ low distress groups), infants in the high distress group are more likely to be reported as temperamentally "difficult" by parents, and those in the low distress group are more likely to be reported as "easy" (18). Thus, the distress experienced during the Strange Situation is related to the type of security or insecurity, not to security per se.

In the meta-analysis conducted by Fox et al (17), a high degree of concordance was found between the infant's attachment to the mother and father in the high distress (A_1-B_2) and low distress (B_3-C_2) groups. However, within each of these groups, security to the mother and the father were not concordant. Thus, if an infant falls into the A_1-B_2 group with one parent, s/he is likely to fall into the same group with the other parent, but within the A_1-B_2 group, having an A (avoidant) or B (secure) pattern of attachment with one parent does not predict security or insecurity with the other parent. These findings show an association between temperament and behavior on the Strange Situation Test, but they also indicate that security is a characteristic of relationships, rather than an individual trait.

Patterns of attachment behavior during the Strange Situation are related to both

94

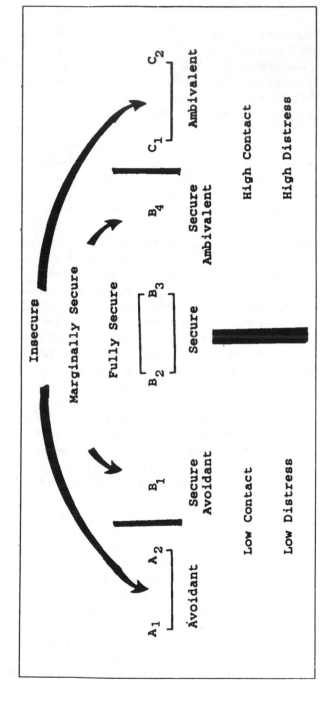

Figure 1. Attachment classifications.

prior and current behavior in the home. Mothers of secure infants have been rated as being more sensitive, responsive, accessible and cooperative during the first year than mothers of insecure infants (23–26). Although there is some evidence that characteristics and/or behaviors of the infant may also predict the quality of attachment, these findings have been less consistent than those on maternal behavior. This suggests that the mother plays a more influential role than the infant in shaping the quality of the relationship.

An increasing number of studies have found that secure infants are more competent than insecure infants in a variety of subsequent cognitive and social skills (27–33). The most ambitious undertaking in this domain is the longitudinal research conducted by Sroufe and his colleagues (31–36) at the Institute for Child Study in Minneapolis. A large sample of children in whom attachment was assessed in infancy are now reaching puberty. Published reports of data up through the early school years consistently document the influences of early attachment on social skills in later life.

Coherent relationships between behavior at home and attachment assessed in the laboratory and between the latter and subsequent development in normative samples have been demonstrated. This has led researchers to use the Strange Situation to explore possible "derailing" of the infant-mother relationship under unusually stressful conditions (for example, premature birth, maltreatment, maternal depression). It was thought that there would be fewer infants with secure attachment relationships with the parent in these populations at-risk. In general, medically ill infants are not more likely to develop insecure patterns of attachment (24,37,38). Some early studies found that maltreated infants are less likely to develop secure attachment relationships (38,39). However, it seems implausible that the majority of maltreated infants or even a substantial minority should be securely attached (7). These studies of "atypical" populations provided the first indication that there might be potential problems in attachment theory or in the assessment methodology. Another intriguing finding was that while there had been a small number of cases that could not be classified into the three pattern scheme, Crittenden's observations of maltreated toddlers (39) and Radke-Yarrow's assessments of preschoolers of depressed mothers (40) uncovered a substantial number of children who seemed to be both avoidant and ambivalent/resistant. In both studies infants with a mixed pattern of attachment were from the most potentially damaging conditions.

Subsequently, Main and Solomon (7,8) reviewed a large number of cases which had not previously been classified or were anomalous (for example, securely attached infants who had been maltreated), by studying video tapes and identified a fourth pattern, which they called "disorganized."

Unlike the previous patterns, which could be described as strategies, the infants in the "disorganized" group did not have a coherent strategy for coping with the separations and reunions during the Strange Situation. In addition, they engaged in unusual and inexplicable behaviors which only made sense if interpreted to reflect confusion or fear of the caregiver. The "mixed" pattern described by Crittenden (39) and Radke-Yarrow (40) was also included in this new disorganized group. Subsequent studies of maltreated children using this new category indicated a high proportion of disorganized attachment (38,41,42). These data lead to the speculation that disorganization is a very insecure pattern of attachment and that some children in previous risk populations who were actually disorganized were initially "misclassified" as secure. This is one area where we can expect further development, and it seems likely that disorganization of attachment may have implications for subsequent psychopathology. However, some observed "disorganization" may also reflect transient responses to events that are normally stressful to a young child (for example, the birth of a sibling). Studies of the disorganized pattern of attachment are needed to provide normative data on the precursors and sequelae of disorganization. Psychiatric populations have not been widely used in studies of attachment. Such studies may make major contributions to both clinical understanding and attachment theory.

BEYOND INFANCY

While a few studies used the Strange Situation on children up to age four (39,41), the absence of methodology for assessing attachment beyond infancy has limited the development of attachment theory. What Bowlby had intended to be a life-span construct became an infancy construct because infancy was the only developmental period in which attachment could be measured. Although it is important to study the sequelae of early attachment in later development, it is equally important to study the development of attachment itself.

The most important new directions concern the development of assessment methods for preschoolers, five to seven year olds, and adults (see Table I). As with the procedures used for infants, those for preschoolers and five to seven year olds rely on videotaped observations of reunions. (The nature and duration of separations are not specified, but typically the child is engaged in a series of tasks with an experimenter.) Adult procedure relies on interviews about the individual's early attachments. A detailed manuscript of the interview is scored. The goal is not to make an objective determination of the nature of these relationships, but rather to assess the individual's current working model of attachment. As shown in Table I, the four patterns previously described for infants can be applied to the other age periods. These classification schemes are relatively new, and research to validate them is only beginning. Nevertheless, these preliminary descriptions provide some sense of the development continuity in attachment patterns which might be possible.

Secure/Autonomous

Secure preschoolers and five to seven year olds, like secure infants, greet a returning parent happily and are able to coordinate attention to the parent and exploration. Separation is less stressful to these children than to infants because their cognitive schemas, which include recognition of parents as independent individuals, are more sophisticated. Older children may engage in enjoyable and absorbing activities during the separation. Thus greeting, while happy, is casual and children usually continue their activities but find a way to involve the parent either by inviting the parent to join the activity or by volunteering information about what they have been doing. Conversation is fluent, and both participants are relaxed. There is comfortable eye contact, and children may initiate physical proximity or contact.

Secure adults (described as autonomous) value attachments and are able to talk coherently and realistically about them. If they had positive relationships with their parents, they can acknowledge and accept their parents' imperfections. If they had a difficult or harsh childhood, they can acknowledge the unhappiness, have come to some understanding of it, and can establish new and important relationships for themselves.

Avoidant/Dismissing

Avoidant preschoolers and five to seven year olds, like avoidant infants, appear to be more interested in other activities than in the parent's return. However, they have learned that social conventions require greetings as well as responses to initiations by the parent. Avoidance in older children is therefore more subtle and is shown by a lack of eye contact, lack of social initiatives and a minimal response to parental overtures. The strategy of avoidance is to maintain neutrality—to do nothing either positive or negative that would draw attention to the relationship.

Avoidant or "dismissing" adults likewise downplay the importance of intimate relationships. They may idealize their childhood experiences without being able to supply supporting details or, in fact, give contradictory examples. Some may speak of negative experiences but do not acknowledge the effects of these experiences. They attempt to limit the influences of attachments on themselves. The reader of the interview transcript can infer a history of lack of closeness or support, or significant rejections.

Dependent/Preoccupied

Among older children, the insecure/ambivalent pattern is labelled "dependent" and, like the infant pattern, its hallmark is preoccupation with the relationship at the expense of other activities. The parent and child may be engaged in a constant struggle for control, the conversation marked by "put-downs" and disagreements. The child is whiny and contentious. Alternatively, the child may emphasize his dependence with extreme coyness (for example, whispering) and feigned helplessness. Even at this age, dependent children are more likely to be visibly upset at the parent's departure than children in other groups.

The adult analogue of this pattern is labelled "preoccupied." These individuals are caught in old struggles with parents, lack a sense of personal identity apart from family or parents, and are unable to evaluate their own role within relationships. They are unable to move beyond details of early memories or current interactions with parents to an objective overview.

Disorganized/Controlling/Unresolved Mourning

This is the least consistent category. Some signs of disorganization similar to those in infants can be seen in preschoolers, especially the youngest preschoolers. However, in older children the disorganized pattern seems to emerge as disorganization in the relationship rather than the individual. The child takes control of the parent in one of two ways. The first is related to caregiving. The child appears to feel responsible for making the parent happy and is overly bright and enthusiastic at reunions. The child works hard to engage the parent. The second is punitive. The child is directly hostile toward the parent in a style that conveys assurance that the parent will comply or meet demands. The child may also ignore the parent when it is clear that such ignoring is a flagrant violation of the social conventions.

The significant feature of adults in the "disorganized" category is unresolved mourning over the loss of an attachment figure. The loss may be a death or loss through divorce or a loss of trust through abuse or neglect. Initial mourning is typically characterized by disorganizing and disorienting experiences. Unresolved mourning is inferred from interview transcripts where signs of continuing cognitive disorganization are shown when the attachment figure is discussed (for example, disbelief in the loss, persisting inappropriate guilt).

At all ages, disorganized individuals are also given an alternative or "forced" classification of one of the other three alternatives (avoidant, secure, ambivalent).

DEVELOPMENT OF ATTACHMENT

We have already noted that a core group of studies on infants found prior observations in the home to be predictors of attachment status based on the Strange Situation. Indeed, behavior during the Strange Situation is a marker or indicator of the relationship history. Since the "disorganized" classification was developed, studies of maltreated children have consistently shown that disorganized attachment is more common in maltreated infants than in controls (38–40, 42). In addition, initial data from an ongoing longitudinal study of the children of clinically depressed mothers document a high rate of "mixed insecure" attachment (A/C, now considered a form of disorganized attachment) among children with mothers who have major bipolar affective disorder (40). These studies support the assertion that secure attachment is the result of appropriately responsive parental care and that inadequate care is the result of very insecure attachment. Furthermore, in the Minnesota longitudinal study (43), it was shown that when infants are tested in the strange situation, at 12 and 18 months, changes in quality of attachment are related to changes in family environment. If the mother's quality of life improved, the infant-mother relationship is more likely to become more secure; if the mother's quality of life deteriorates, infant-mother attachment is likely to become less secure.

Now that methods are available to assess attachment in preschool and early school years, it is possible to evaluate stability and change in attachment relationships over a longer period of time. In the first such study, Main and her associates (10) found that the correlation between security of attachment to the mother at one year and security of attachment to the mother at six years was $r = .76$ ($p < .001$); the analogous correlation for attachment to the father at 18 months and six years was $r = .30$ ($p < .05$). Several other studies of this type are under way. From these we can expect to learn about factors contributing to stability and change in attachment status.

TRANSMISSION OF ATTACHMENT PATTERNS BETWEEN GENERATIONS

With the development of the Adult Attachment Interview (AAI) (11), it is also possible to test whether individuals' experiences of nurturing determine their ability to nurture their own children. Indeed, the first studies of this type show a high degree of concordance between adult "states of mind" regarding attachment and the attachment status of their infants (44–46); parents who are "secure/autonomous" tend to have securely attached infants, those who are "dismissing" tend to have avoidant infants, and those who are preoccupied tend to have ambivalent/resistant infants. While disorganized attachment in infants has been associated with maltreatment and maternal bipolar affective disorder, it also occurs among infants in low risk families. In these circumstances, the initial indications are that disorganized attachment in the infant is associated with unresolved mourning in the parent (46). Although it has not yet been clearly demonstrated, it is possible that parents who maltreat children have experienced traumatic and unresolved loss as a result of inadequate care as children.

The AAI does not purport to provide an accurate picture of childhood. It represents the adult's working model (i.e., present attitudes and feelings) of important relationships during their childhood. Even the preliminary data now available indicate that a significant number of adults with unhappy childhoods are secure/ autonomous adults (10). Likewise, some adults who are insecure were probably securely attached during earlier periods of life. The indications from the current generation of studies are that an adult's cognitions and emotions (i.e., working models) about relationships influence their caregiving, which in turn affects their childrens' attachment status. While those who had secure childhoods clearly have a better chance of becoming secure adults than those whose initial experiences were harsh and rejecting, intervening experiences can change working models of attachment and lead to behavior consistent with the new model. This is good news for clinicians, whose goal is to bring about a positive change through therapeutic intervention. The availability of a method for assessing adult attachment now makes possible the use of pre- and post-therapy assessments to ascertain whether therapy has resulted in changes in working models of attachment.

IMPLICATIONS FOR CHILD PSYCHIATRY

The methods developed by researchers studying attachment can be applied to studies of the relationship between attachment (particularly in infancy) and behavior problems. Most of the existing studies have looked at relatively large cohorts of normally developing children. The number of children likely to have behavior disorders that can be diagnosed would be small in this group. Therefore, the measure of outcome is generally a parent or teacher report checklist (47–49) or a composite score on experimental observation and standardized social competence measures (34–36).

The findings of these studies are equivocal. For example, Sroufe and his colleagues (34–36) have shown that the quality of early attachment is related to later behavior problems in children up to early school age. However, this relationship is stronger in boys than in girls. Lewis and his colleagues (48) reported similar findings, but two other studies (47,49) failed to find such an association.

In our own recent preliminary data, we have found that while there is no consistent relationship between quality of attachment in infancy and scores on the Achenbach's Child Behavior Checklist (CBCL), a different pattern emerges if we consider only children whose parental report scores were high enough to place them in the clinical range. For example, at three years of age, seven percent of children who had had insecure attachment relationships as infants were scored in the clinical range of the CBCL by their mothers, compared with two percent of securely attached infants. Figures based on the fathers' reports were similar: 12% of insecurely attached infants in the clinical range and five percent of securely attached infants. The relative odds of scoring in the clinical range were therefore 2.4 to 3.5 times higher if the child had had an early insecure attachment than if the child had had a secure attachment.

Thus, measures of outcome are important in this type of study. When the actual number of diagnosable cases is expected to be small, a full psychiatric assessment for each child in a large cohort is difficult to justify. Standardized parent and teacher reports, however, do not provide psychiatric diagnoses. It may be that differences in scores below the clinical cutoff are not clinically relevant measures.

An alternative approach, and one that may be of greater use in associating specific diagnoses with particular attachment patterns, is the use of measures of attachment on an experimental basis as part of routine assessment of children referred to clinics for behavior problems. When attachment was measured (using the measure used to assess preschoolers) in 25 children referred for one of the DSM-III-R disruptive behavior disorders and 25 children who were not referred, 84% of the clinic children were classified insecure compared with only 25% of the non clinic group (50). Furthermore, a significantly greater proportion of the children who were referred to the clinic fell into the insecure/controlling category (40% versus 12%). This is the first study to demonstrate an association between clinic status and attachment quality and between a specific diagnosis and a specific form of attachment.

COLLABORATION BETWEEN RESEARCHERS AND CLINICIANS

Much of the work reviewed above has been carried out by psychologists studying child development who communicate with each other and publish their work in journals not routinely read by psychiatrists. Many developmental psychologists remain cautious and skeptical of this work (51). Yet, whenever psychiatrists, particularly child psychiatrists, have been exposed to these ideas, methods and findings, there has been enthusiastic reception. Why is this so?

First, the concepts of attachment theory are familiar to many child psychiatrists. John Bowlby was a psychiatrist and wrote from a psychiatric perspective. However, there is now considerable empirical evidence to support what child psychiatrists already knew: experiences with a primary caregiver influence important aspects of personality. There is the promise in these new findings of a firm scientific basis for some aspects of common belief and practice.

Second, research on attachment combines clinical and experimental techniques. These methods rely on standard manipulations or probes and evaluation of resulting behavior by schemes that can be objectively described and replicated. However, an important component of this evaluation is clinical in nature—reliance on detailed sensitive observations of the patterning and organization of behavior. The training of coders, whether to score reunions from videotape or review interview transcripts, is primarily training in clinical judgment. Detailed descriptions of salient behaviors are provided, but the coder must also learn how to use clinical intuitions. Thus, developmental psychologists working in this field are gaining more appreciation of clinical approaches to human behavior.

Clinicians have been quick to see the possible applications of the methods used in research on attachment to clinical practice. Such efforts could lead to important clinical insights as well as information relevant to attachment theory. However, caution is warranted. These experimental methods are time consuming and costly in clinical practice. Furthermore, the available data are group data, not individual data. We do not know, for example, how frequently classification errors are made or what factors influence them. This is less important for group research data than for the clinical assessment or treatment of individuals. In addition, all but the methods used with infants must be considered to be in a very early stage of development. Nevertheless, a number of projects supported by research funding are using these methods in clinical settings as part of assessment and treatment (50,52), and these projects promise to provide insight into the developmental history of psychopathology.

The result of this research has been a growing collaboration between researchers and clinicians, and between psychologists and psychiatrists. The history of attachment research is short but it has shown early promise. These interdisciplinary collaborations are a necessary step in making that future a reality.

REFERENCES

1. Bowlby J. The nature of the child's tie to his mother. Int J Psychoanal 1958; 39:350–373.
2. Bowlby J. Attachment and loss: attachment. New York: Basic Books, 1969.
3. Bowlby J. Attachment and loss: separation. New York: Basis Books, 1973.
4. Bowlby J. Attachment and loss: loss, sadness and depression. New York: Basic Books, 1980.
5. Ainsworth MDS, Witting BA. Attachment and exploratory behavior of one-year-olds in a strange situation. In: Foss BM, ed. Determinants of infant behavior. London: Methuen, 1969.
6. Ainsworth MDS, Blehar MC, Waters E, et al. Patterns of attachment: a psychological study of the Strange Situation. Hillsdale NJ: Erlbaum, 1978.
7. Main M, Solomon J. Discovery of an insecure-disorganized/disoriented attachment pattern. In: Brazelton TB, Yogman MW, eds. Affective development in infancy. Norwood NJ: Ablex, 1986.
8. Main M, Solomon J. Procedures for identifying infants as disorganized/disoriented during the Ainsworth Strange Situation. In: Greenberg MT, Cicchetti D, Cummings EM, eds. Attachment in the preschool years. Chicago IL: University of Chicago Press, 1990.
9. Cassidy J, Marvin RS. Attachment organization in three- and four-year-olds: coding guidelines (unpublished manual). Charlottesville VA: Department of Psychology, University of Virginia, 1990.
10. Main M, Kaplan N, Cassidy J. Security in infancy, childhood and adulthood: a move to the level of representation. Monogr Soc Res Child Dev 50 1985; (1-2, Serial No. 209):6–104.

11. George C, Kaplan N, Main M. The Berkeley Adult Attachment Interview (unpublished protocol). Berkeley CA: Department of Psychology, University of California, 1985.
12. Van Ijzendoorn MH, Kroonenberg PM. Cross cultural patterns of attachment: a meta-analysis of the strange situation. Child Dev 1988; 59:147–156.
13. Waters E. The stability of individual differences in infant-mother attachment. Child Dev 1978; 49:483–494.
14. Grossmann KE, Grossmann K. Parent-infant relationships in Bielefeld. In: Immelman K, Barlow G, Petrinovich L, et al, eds. Behavioral development: the Bielefeld interdisciplinary project. New York: Cambridge University Press, 1981.
15. Lamb ME. Qualitative aspect of mother-infant and father-infant attachments. Infant Behav Developm 1978; 1:265–275.
16. Main M, Weston DR. The quality of the toddler's relationship to mother and to father: related to conflict behavior and readiness to establish new relationships. Child Dev 1981; 52:932–940.
17. Fox N, Kimmerly NL, Schafer WD. Attachment to mother/attachment to father: a meta-analysis. Child Dev 1991; 62:210–225.
18. Belsky J, Rovine M. Temperament and attachment security in the strange situation: an empirical rapprochement. Child Dev 1987; 8:787–795.
19. Chess S, Thomas A. Infant bonding: mystique and reality. Am J Orthopsychiatry 1982; 52:213–222.
20. Crockenberg SB. Infant irritability, mother responsiveness, and social support influences on security of infant-mother attachment. Child Dev 1981; 52:857–865.
21. Goldsmith HH, Alansky JA. Maternal and infant temperamental predictors of attachment: a meta-analytical review. J Consult Clin Psychol 1987; 55:806–816.
22. Sroufe LA. Attachment classification from the perspective of infant-caregiver relationships and infant temperament. Child Dev 1985; 56:1–14.
23. Belsky J, Rovine M, Taylor DG. The Pennsylvania Infant and Family Development Project. III: the origins of individual differences in infant-mother attachment: maternal and infant contributions. Child Dev 1984; 55:718–728.
24. Goldberg S, Perrotta M, Minde K, et al. Maternal behavior and attachment in low birthweight twins and singletons. Child Dev 1986; 57:34–46.
25. Grossmann K, Grossmann KE. Maternal sensitivity and newborns' orientation responses as related to quality of attachment in northern Germany. Monogr Soc Res Child Dev 1985; 50(1-2, Serial No. 209):233–256.
26. Main M, Tomasini L, Tolan W. Differences among mothers of infants judged to differ in security. Dev Psychol 1979; 15:472–473.
27. Arend R, Gove F, Sroufe LA. Continuity of individual adaptation from infancy to kindergarten: a predictive study of ego resiliency and curiosity in preschoolers. Child Dev 1979; 50:950–959.
28. Bell S. The development of the concept of object as related to infant-mother attachment. Child Dev 1970; 41:291–311.
29. Lieberman A. Preschooler's competence with a peer: relations with attachment and peer experience. Child Dev 1977; 48:1277–1287.

30. Londerville S, Main M. Security of attachment, compliance, and maternal training methods in the second year of life. Dev Psychol 1981; 17:289–299.
31. Matas L, Arend RA, Sroufe LA. Continuity and adaptation in the second year. The relationship between quality of attachment and later competence. Child Dev 1978; 49:549–556.
32. Sroufe LA, Fox N, Pancake V. Attachment and dependency in developmental perspective. Child Dev 1983; 54:1335–1354.
33. Waters E, Wippman J, Sroufe LA. Attachment, positive affect, and competence in the peer group: two studies in construct validation. Child Dev 1979; 50:821–829.
34. Erickson MF, Sroufe LA, Egeland B. The relationship between quality of attachment and behavior problems in a preschool high-risk sample. Monogr Soc Res Child Dev 1985; 50(1-2, Serial No. 209):147–166.
35. Renken B, Egeland B, Marvinney D, et al. Early childhood antecedents of aggression and passive-withdrawal in early elementary school. J Pers 1989; 57:257–281.
36. Sroufe LA, Egeland B, Kreutzer T. The fate of early experience following developmental change: longitudinal approaches to individual adaptation in childhood. Child Dev 1990; 61:1363–1373.
37. Goldberg S. Risk factors in attachment. Can J Psychol 1988; 42:173–188.
38. Spieker SJ, Booth C. Maternal antecedents of attachment quality. In: Belsky J, Nezworski T, eds. Clinical implications of attachment. Hillsdale NJ: Erlbaum, 1988.
39. Crittenden P. Maltreated infants: vulnerability and resilience. J Child Psychol Psychiatry 1985; 26:85–96.
40. Radke-Yarrow M, Cummings EM, Kuczynski L, et al. Patterns of attachment in two- and three-year-olds in normal families and families with paternal depression. Child Dev 1985; 56:591–615.
41. Lyons-Ruth C, Connell D, Zoll D, et al. Infants at social risk: relations among infant maltreatment, maternal behavior, and infant attachment behavior. Dev Psychol 1987; 23:223–232.
42. Carlson V, Cicchetti D, Barnett D, et al. Disorganized/disoriented attachment relationships in maltreated infants. Dev Psychol 1989; 25:525–531.
43. Egeland B, Farber EA. Infant-mother attachment: factors related to its development and changes over time. Child Dev 1984; 55:753–771.
44. Levine L, Ward M, Carlson B. Attachment across three generations: grandmother, mother, and infants. Paper presented at the World Association of Infant Psychiatry and Allied Disciplines, Lugano, Switzerland, 1989.
45. Van Ijzendoorn MH. Intergenerational transmission of parenting: a review of studies in non-clinical populations. Developm Rev (in press).
46. Main M, Hesse E. Parents unresolved traumatic experiences are related to infant disorganized attachment status: is frightened or frightening behavior the linking mechanism? In: Greenberg M, Cicchetti D, Cummings EM, eds. Attachment in the preschool years: theory, research and intervention. Chicago IL: University of Chicago Press, 1990: 161–184.
47. Goldberg S, Corter C, Lojkasek M, et al. Prediction of behavior problems in 4-year-olds born prematurely. Developmental Psychopath 1990; 2:15–30.

48. Lewis M, Feiring C, McGuffog C, et al. Predicting psychopathology in six-year-olds from early social relations. Child Dev 1984; 55:123–136.

49. Bates JE, Bayles K. Attachment and the development of behavior problems. In: Belsky J, Nezworski T, eds. Clinical implications of attachment. Hillsdale NJ: Erlbaum, 1988.

50. Spelz ML. The treatment of preschool conduct problems: an integration of behavioral and attachment concepts. In: Greenberg M, Cicchetti D, Cummings EM, eds. Attachment in the preschool years: theory, research and intervention. Chicago IL: University Press, 1990: 399–426.

51. Lamb ME, Thompson RA, Gardner WP, et al. Security of infantile attachment as assessed in the "strange situation": its study and biological interpretation. Behav Brain Sci 1984; 7:127–147.

52. Lieberman A, Pawl J. Clinical applications of attachment theory. In: Belsky J, Nezworski T, eds. Clinical implications of attachment. Hillsdale NJ: Erlbaum, 1988: 327–351.

6

The Influence of the Family Environment on Personality: Accounting for Sibling Differences

Lois Wladis Hoffman

University of Michigan, Ann Arbor

Findings from behavioral genetics indicate that environment affects personality but that siblings are not alike. This has been interpreted as challenging the idea that child rearing and family events are important. Research from behavioral genetics and developmental psychology is reviewed, suggesting the following: (a) Sibling dissimilarity may be overestimated because of limitations of methodology, measurement, and the outcome variables examined; (b) developmental psychology conceptualizes the family as involving interaction between the person and the environment and personality as multidetermined; thus, sibling dissimilarity is not surprising; (c) objective and subjective family experiences vary for siblings because of birth order, age differences, gender, genetics, and idiosyncratic experiences; (d) sibling differences and similarities may be tied to whether particular outcomes are influenced by specific, varying environments or general family styles.

At the present time there is considerable convergence in the views of researchers in the fields of behavioral genetics and developmental psychology. Developmental psychologists who study the influence of the family environment are aware of genetic influences on intellectual and personality development, and behavioral geneticists are aware of environmental influences. This consensus should enable these two groups of researchers to work together, so that the insights and discoveries

Reprinted with permission from *Psychological Bulletin*, 1991, Vol. 110, No. 2, 187–203. Copyright © 1991 by the American Psychological Association, Inc.

Richard M. Lerner is gratefully acknowledged for his thoughtful suggestions for revising the original manuscript.

of each field can enrich the other and facilitate their mutual quest for understanding human development. Unfortunately, however, the demands of keeping up with research in each area of specialization are so great that it is difficult to stay well informed of the advances in adjacent fields. In addition, even when the quest is the same, the approaches and conceptualizations are so different that there is frequently miscommunication among the different fields of inquiry. This article aims to bridge this gap.

The particular focus here is on the recent publications in behavioral genetics that have concluded that there are environmental influences on personality but that these influences are "nonshared" influences; that is, they are not shared by family members (Loehlin, Willerman, & Horn, 1985; Plomin & Daniels, 1987; Scarr, Webber, Weinberg, & Wittig, 1981). The research that has led to this conclusion indicates that although genetics leaves unexplained a considerable amount of personality variance, family members, and most notably siblings, are not very similar on personality traits. The discovery that children reared in the same family are not very similar with respect to personality has emerged in behavioral genetics as a challenging insight in need of explanation. The conclusion that the environmental influences that affect personality are often different for siblings is one that is shared by the developmental researchers who study the family environment, and some of their research should be helpful in further exploration of the dynamics of nonshared environmental influence or what is better termed *within-family environmental variation* (Loehlin, Willerman, & Horn, 1988). At present, however, differences between the two approaches in how the environment and environmental processes are conceptualized impede cross-fertilization between these two fields. Thus, one specific aim of this article is to clarify how developmental researchers conceptualize environmental influences. The second is to discuss developmental research findings that indicate why environmental influences, even those from within the family, are not the same for different family members.

This article is divided into four sections. The first gives an overview and a critique of the methodology of behavioral genetics that has led to the conclusions that the shared family environment is not important but the nonshared environment is. The second describes how the family is conceptualized currently in developmental psychology. The third section, the main one, discusses some work in developmental psychology that indicates why siblings living in the same family do not share the same environment. It is hoped that this will suggest some possible leads for behavioral geneticists to explore in their own emerging work on why siblings are different from each other. The final section examines sibling similarities and how these can also come about despite the environmental differences.

BEHAVIORAL GENETICS STUDIES

There are four major designs used by behavior geneticists in examining the role of genetics and environment in affecting intelligence and personality. Two of these use samples of twins; two use samples with adopted children.

Twin Studies

One design involves comparing the degree of similarity between monozygotic twins to the degree of similarity between dizygotic twins. Because the former have developed from a single fertilized egg, they have identical genes. The latter have developed from two eggs separately fertilized and thus are simply siblings born at the same time. To the behavioral geneticist, greater similarity in intelligence test or personality scale scores between monozygotic than dizygotic twins indicates a genetic effect. The numerical estimates of heritability and the amount of variance contributed by the shared environment and the unshared environment are computed from these correlations and the difference between them. The size of this difference yields a heritability estimate; it is double the difference between the two correlations. The nonshared environment is the difference between the monozygotic twin correlation and 1 (or 100%). That is, their similarity, reflected in the size of the correlation, represents shared genetics and shared environment; their dissimilarity represents the nonshared environment. The residue, that is, the estimated heritability plus the estimate of the nonshared environment subtracted from 1, yields the estimated shared environment.[1]

This design has been criticized for various reasons, such as the assumption of additive gene factors, but to the developmental psychologist the major problem has to do with the assumption that monozygotic and dizygotic twins have equally similar environments (Lewontin, Rose, & Kamin, 1984). Not only do parents treat monozygotic twins more similarly than dizygotic twins, as research has indicated (Lytton, 1977; Scarr & Carter-Saltzman, 1979), but the sheer fact that monozygotic twins look exactly alike, whereas dizygotics do not, ensures that they will have more similar environments. There is abundant evidence that adults and peers, parents and siblings, respond differently to different appearances (Hartup, 1983; Langlois, 1986; Sorell & Nowak, 1981). And, indeed, dizygotic twins who are very similar in appearance and mistakenly identified as monozygotic are more similar on personality traits than other pairs of dizygotic twins (Scarr & Carter-Saltzman, 1979; L.W. Hoffman, 1985). Thus, from the physical appearance dimension alone, same-sex dizygotic twins

---

[1]This is an adequate description for present purposes but it is slightly oversimplified because it does not take into account the estimate of error variance.

cannot have as similar an environment as do monozygotic twins. However, a big thrust in developmental psychology today has to do with the child as elicitor of parental behavior and also as interpreter of the environment. Much of how a parent behaves is a response to the child, and in addition, much of what the child experiences is his or her interpretation of events (Scarr & McCartney, 1983). Thus, the genetically identical twins would experience more similar environments because of other genetically shared traits besides physical appearance. The possibility that monozygotic twins have more similar environments than dizygotic twins throws off the assumptions of this twin design and raises questions about the very, specific *numerical* estimate of variances due to heritability, unshared environment, and shared environment.

Behavioral geneticists have argued and presented evidence that it is the genetic similarity between monozygotic twins that drives the greater environmental similarity (Lytton, 1977). This has been used as a defense of the twin design. However, a greater similarity in environment induced by greater similarity in genetics still means that monozygotic twins have more similar, or shared, environments than dizygotic twins. Although similar behaviors in children will elicit similar responses in one mother, these responses are different than would be elicited in a different mother (Crockenberg, 1986). Thus, the higher correlations in personality test scores shown by monozygotic twins is partly because their environments are more similar. The difference in the size of the two correlations is inflated by that portion of the personality trait similarity between monozygotics that stems from their greater shared environment. This method overestimates the heritability factor and underestimates the contribution of the shared environment. As one might expect, the heritability estimates yielded by the twin studies are considerably higher than those yielded by the adoption studies—particularly with respect to personality variables (Scarr et al., 1981).

A different twin design involves comparing the correlations between scores of monozygotic twins who have been reared apart and monozygotic twins reared together and sometimes also to dizygotic twins reared together and sometimes also to dizygotic twins reared apart and together. This design can have the advantage of examining the contribution of the shared family environment. It has a disadvantage, however, introduced by the peculiarities of the samples of separated twins. The occurrence of twins who are reared separately is rare, and it is difficult to locate an appropriate unbiased sample; thus, studies using this technique have often been severely criticized by both behavioral geneticists and developmental psychologists (Farber, 1981; R.M. Lerner, 1986; Scarr & Kidd, 1983). Furthermore, the separated twins in these studies have rarely been separated since birth and have often been reared in similar environments.[2] As Bronfenbrenner (1986) has shown, the degree

---

[2]In a recent study of separated twins by Bouchard, Lykken, McGue, Segal, and Tellegen (1990) very

of similarity among twins is considerably reduced when they are reared, not only in different families, but also in different community environments.

The results from the separated twin studies, like the simple comparisons of monozygotic and dizygotic twins reared in their family of birth, support the hypothesis of a genetic influence on personality traits and a greater effect of the nonshared than the shared environment. Note, however, that this pattern does not always prevail. With both designs, the shared family environment has sometimes shown a major influence. For example, a recent analysis by Tellegen and his colleagues (Tellegen et al., 1988) that compared monozygotic and dizygotic twins reared separately and together found that the shared environment showed a considerable effect on the traits of "social closeness" and "positive emotionality." Plomin, Foch, and Rowe (1981) concluded from a study of nonseparated twins that the family environment, and not genetics, was the major source of individual differences in aggression, as measured with Bobo clown laboratory procedures. And, as another example, Coon and Carey (1989) found in a study of nonseparated twins that the effects of the shared environment were greater than heredity in determining musical ability. Thus, although the focus of this review is on the general absence of environmentally produced sibling similarity, it should be clear that this does not describe all personality variables (Rose & Kaprio, 1987). This point is taken up again in the fourth section.

Adoption Studies

A more powerful research design used by behavioral geneticists involves obtaining measures from children, adopted at or shortly after birth, and comparing their scores with those of biological parents, who did not interact with them, and those of adoptive parents who reared them. Similarity in scores between biological parents and the offspring they did not rear demonstrates a genetic effect. Similarity between the adoptive parent and the child would indicate an environmental effect. The most impressive of the adoption studies is the Texas adoption project (Horn, 1983). The data set includes both IQ scores and personality test scores for the biological mothers, the adoptive parents, the adopted child, and the siblings of the adopted child—both other adopted children and those born to the adoptive parents. Furthermore, data have been collected from the adoptive families at two points—when the children were elementary school age and 10 years later. This study provides an excellent test of the genetic hypothesis. A significant correlation between the scores of biological parents and children who were given up for adoption within

---

high estimates of genetic influence and low estimates of influence from the shared family environment were reported. However, in this study, the age at separation varied, and some monozygotic twins had maintained contact during childhood. Furthermore, some had been together for 20 years before assessment.

2 weeks of their birth clearly demonstrates a genetic effect. In the case of IQ scores, the results are impressive, and the genetic influence is clearly demonstrated (Horn, 1983; Horn, Loehlin, & Willerman, 1979). In the case of the personality scores, the results have been more modest. The childhood scores yielded few significant relationships (Scarr & Kidd, 1983). The data collected in the second wave yielded a relationship accounting for about 20%–25% of the variance (Loehlin, 1989; Loehlin, Willerman, & Horn, 1987).

Although this design is appropriate for testing a genetic hypothesis, there has been criticism of the other side of the design—the test for environmental influences (Bronfenbrenner, 1985; L.W. Hoffman, 1985). This test involves examining the correlation between adoptive parent IQ scores and the IQ scores of the adopted child for the test of environmental influences on intelligence and examining the correlations between adoptive parent personality test scores and the adopted child's personality test scores for a test of environmental influences on personality. Both sets of correlations were close to zero. These results are seen as showing no effect of the family environment. However, although looking for similarity in scores between biological and adopted-away children is appropriate for a test of genetic influence, neither the adoptive mother's IQ scores nor her personality test scores seem appropriate as measures of the relevant environment.

Researchers in developmental psychology have identified various aspects of family life that appear to affect the child's cognitive development. These include the amount of parent-child interaction, the kind of interaction the variety of stimulation provided, the degree of independence training, and a host of other variables (Bradley & Caldwell, 1984; Hess & Holloway, 1984; Wachs & Gruen, 1982). Maternal IQ scores, particularly within the narrow range represented in adoption studies, would not be expected to tap such differences in parental behavior. Furthermore, in a longitudinal study of adopted families by Leon Yarrow and his colleagues (Yarrow, Goodwin, Manheimer, & Milowe, 1973) behavioral observations of mother-infant interaction obtained when the children were 6 months old did predict the adopted child's IQ scores at 10 years of age. Measures of the mother's level of stimulation and responsivitiy to the infant showed significant correlations with the 10-year-olds' IQs that ranged in the middle 50s.

Turning to the personality evidence, again, similarity between biological parents and offspring they have not reared provides irrefutable evidence of genetic influence. However, the test of the environmental influence, examining personality similarity between the rearing parents and the adopted offspring, is questionable. Before discussing this issue, another adoption design is described because similar methodological problems are involved.

Another adoption design that has been used in drawing the conclusion that the shared family environment does not contribute to the child's personality development involves comparing families with adopted children to a sample of families with nonadopted children (Scarr & Weinberg, 1983). In this case, there are no data on the birth parents of the adopted children, and the two samples, the adoptive families and the nonadoptive families, are independent. The most widely cited study using this design is the Minnesota study of adolescents conducted by Sandra Scarr and her colleagues (Scarr & Weinberg, 1983; Scarr et al., 1981). The heritability estimate for the personality variables examined in this study is similar to that in the Texas study, about .22, both studies yielding lower estimates than are found in most twin studies (Scarr & Kidd, 1983). Like the Texas study, they found only a modest relationship between the biological parents' personality test scores and their adolescent children's scores even though in the Minnesota study they were also the rearing parents. The correlation between rearing parents and their *adopted* children was also like the Texas study—close to zero.

The question is, however, is a correlation between the personality traits of adoptive parents and their adopted children an appropriate test of environmental influence? Developmental psychologists, when looking for a family environment effect on personality, do not seek trait similarity between parents and children but look instead at child-rearing patterns, or parent-child interaction, or sometime parental attitudes toward children and expectations (Baumrind, 1971; Sigel, 1985). Environmental influences do not produce clones of the parent. To explain dependency in a child, one would not expect to find a dependent parent but rather an overprotective one. Anxiety might develop from having an anxious parent, but it might also result because the parent creates a frightening world. A sense of powerlessness may be more likely to develop in a child when the parents are all-powerful and domineering than when they also feel powerless (Strodtbeck, 1958). Having an extremely competent and self-assured parent may make a child feel inadequate in contrast. The model that works well for showing genetic influence is not the lack of similarity in traits between parents and children does not seem convincing evidence of the absence of a family effect.

A set of analyses that seems more relevant for many of these environmental issues is the comparison of siblings, because siblings have been reared in the same family with the same parents. Both of these adoption studies, as well as others (Loehlin et al., 1985), have compared the personality traits of children reared in the same family. By and large, they show that biologically related siblings are more similar than siblings who are not biologically related, but siblings are *not* very similar (Scarr et al., 1981).

What do these sibling results indicate? To the behavioral geneticists, the greater sibling similarity in nonadoptive families than in adoptive families shows some effects of genetics, but the correlations are so low even in the biological families that genetics does not seem to explain much of the personality variance, and thus they are more interested than before in environmental influences. However, the relative absence of sibling similarity in the adoptive family has also reinforced their view that the environment siblings share contributes little to personality development. They have therefore turned their attention toward understanding what environmental factors make siblings different, that is, toward understanding within-family environmental variation (Loehlin et al., 1988; Plomin & Daniels, 1987).

To an environmentally oriented developmental psychologist, the difference between the biological sibling similarity and the adopted sibling similarity may reflect genetic factors, as behavioral geneticists conclude, but it may also reflect differences in the dynamics of the adoptive family. It is possible that parents treat adopted children differently than they treat nonadopted children, and that knowing one is an adopted child is itself an environmental variable affecting the impact of the parent's influence, thus diminishing similarity among adopted children. In a previous publication (L.W. Hoffman, 1985), it was even suggested that the family dynamics are different in a family in which all the children are adopted than where some are adopted and some are born to their parents. Data from the Minnesota Transracial-Adoption Study (Scarr & Kidd, 1983) show that IQ scores are as similar for adopted siblings as for biological siblings but significantly more similar than for mixed-sibling pairs. It is not only genetic relatedness that differentiates adopted and nonadoptive families is not as compelling to those who study the family environment as it is to the behavioral geneticists.

Nevertheless, the lack of personality trait similarity among siblings that is revealed in this research is one that environmentally oriented developmental psychologists can easily accept (Lamb, 1987; Wachs, 1987). It is important to point out, however, that for the adoption studies, as for the twin studies, this pattern cannot be generalized to all personality traits. Most of the personality tests used in this research are those that tap dimensions for which there was some previous evidence of a genetic effect (Scarr et al., 1981), such as the Eysenck Personality Inventory. Sibling similarity is somewhat higher on other tests, such as the Holland Interest Styles, for both adoptive and nonadoptive families, and this is particularly true when there is similarity between mothers' and fathers' scores (Grotevant, 1979; L.W. Hoffman, 1985). Furthermore, the general pattern of greater sibling similarity in the nonadoptive families than in the adoptive families does not prevail across all personality variables, even on the Eysenck Personality Inventory (Scarr et al., 1981). Nevertheless, the data indicate that on most of the traits examined in this research, siblings are not very similar, and this is a conclusion about which both groups of researchers concur (Lamb, 1987; Wachs, 1987).

At this point, an overview has been presented of the behavioral genetics research that has led to the conclusion that although environment plays a role in personality development, it is not an environment that siblings share. Some of the evidence that demonstrates the absence of a shared-family environment has been criticized, from the viewpoint of a researcher of the family environment—either because the measures do not adequately tap the relevant environment, as with the mother's IQ as a measure of the quality of the home environment, or because the model does not reflect environmental influence patterns, as with seeking personality trait similarity between parents and children.

There are also differences among the various researchers within both fields. Many behavioral geneticists who rely on the twin studies might estimate that the environmental variance to be accounted for is less than that suggested by the adoption studies. Developmental psychologists may have reservations about how far the conclusions about the absence of sibling similarity can be generalized (Lamb, 1987; Wachs, 1987). For example, the case seems better established for the personality variables than for IQ because some of the studies of IQ have shown similarity among nonrelated adopted siblings (L.W. Hoffman, 1985) and for some personality traits more than others. In addition, it is important to emphasize that any conclusions are limited to the populations studied, that is, populations that are relatively advantaged, not those that are economically deprived (Scarr-Salapatek, 1971). Despite these differences, there is basic consensus across behavioral genetics and developmental psychology that both genetics and environment play a role in personality development and that environmental influences do not result in sibling similarity.

Paradoxically, this consensus has revealed basic misunderstandings between these two groups of researchers. In several publications by behavioral geneticists, the discovery that siblings are not alike on personality traits is announced with considerable excitement and with the statement that this is counter to the prevailing view in developmental psychology. In addition, it is asserted that if siblings are not alike in personality, the aspects of the family environment that are typically studied, such as child rearing patterns and parental divorce, cannot play an important part in affecting personality development (Loehlin et al., 1987; Plomin & Daniels, 1987; Rowe, 1987; Tellegen et al., 1988). The behavioral geneticists assume that such variables, if operating, would make siblings alike in personality. Environmentally oriented developmental psychologists, on the other hand, hold that these influences operate differently for different children, and thus the absence of sibling similarity does not mean these variables are not having an effect (Lamb, 1987; Wachs, 1987).

DEVELOPMENTAL CONCEPTION OF THE FAMILY ENVIRONMENT

To developmental psychologists today who study the family environment, it is conceptualized as dynamic and transactional in nature. Thus siblings do not typically experience the same objective environment. In addition, its effects are moderated by the individual and thus even the effects of the same objective environment are not the same for each child in the family because each is different in terms of genetics and environmental history (Wachs, 1983). Because siblings are born at different points in the family cycle, are different ages at any particular point, may be different genders, and have different temperaments and physical appearance, their objective environment may be different and their subjective experience may be different.

In addition, the family environment is not a global variable; rather it is multidimensional, and the effects on personality outcomes depend on combinations of variables, some of which may be objectively the same for siblings, some of which may be different. Furthermore, researchers of the family environment today are aware that nonfamily experiences contribute to personality development, in an interactive fashion, and that personality is not set in childhood but can be affected by subsequent life experiences.

Objective Environmental Differences

With respect to their objective environment, whether one is considering parental behavior, family events, or social setting impacts, the objective environment is likely to be somewhat different for each child. A second-born child, for example, cannot receive as much attention as a firstborn in early infancy because the mother has two children to care for (Lasko, 1954). The fact that a firstborn has a mother who is a novice and each later born has an experienced mother has significance for the mother's behavior toward the child and her developmental expectations (Baskett, 1985; Lewis & Kreitzberg, 1979). Any family event, such as divorce or unemployment, is presented differently to different age children. Thus, divorce may make the mother more of a peer to a teenaged daughter but more of an erratic disciplinarian to a preschool son (Hetherington & Camara, 1984; Weiss, 1979). When economic adversity hit during the depression of the 1930s, adolescent sons were expected to take on outside employment and contribute to the family income but younger sons and daughters were not (Elder, 1974). There is abundant evidence, to be described more fully in the next section of this review, that parents treat sons differently from daughters (Huston, 1983) and they behave differently in the presence of each—for example, they are more likely to fight in the presence of sons than of daughters (Hetherington & Camara, 1984).

As already noted, different physical appearance can elicit different parental behavior (Langlois, 1986). Parental behavior is affected also by the child's temperament, and thus a child's genetics and previous experiences may evoke different parental treatment (Crockenberg, 1986; J.V. Lerner & Galambos, 1986; Thompson, 1986). For example, early predispositions in the child set off parent reactions that, in turn, affect the child, and even minor differences can be augmented by this interactive process. Differences as subtle as the sound of the neonate's cry have been shown to evoke different responses in both parents and unrelated adults (Lamb & Bornstein, 1986; Malatesta, Culver, Tesman, & Shepard, 1989; Wiesenfeld & Malatesta, 1982). Experimental studies have also shown that parental responses to the same stimuli, such as recorded infant cries, are not homogeneous. They can be affected, for example, by whether the parent is an experienced parent or a new parent (Lounsbury & Bates, 1982). Because the point is often missed, it is important to reiterate, however, that temperament, even in early infancy, is not necessarily a manifestation of genetics. Research by Plomin and Defries (1985) found no relationship between the temperaments of adopted infants and their biological parents' personalities but did find similarities to their adoptive parents' personalities (Loehlin et al., 1988).

Thus, within-family environmental variance may come from different environmental stimuli that children encounter because they are treated differently by their parents and they are born at different times into different family constellations and circumstances. This does not mean that there may not also be aspects of the family environment that are the same for siblings, but, if one conceives of personality as a result of multiple interacting influences (Mischel, 1973), then these environmental variations can be important in accounting for differences among siblings in personality.

Subjective Environmental Differences

In addition, however, unless siblings are monozygotic twins, each is different genetically and, because of both genetic differences and environmental differences such as those just described, each reacts differently even to the same environmental stimuli. Thus, for example, Patterson (1976) has shown that aggressive children may respond differently to punitive discipline than nonaggressive children, and Dodge (Dodge & Somberg, 1987) has shown that the interpretation of ambiguous intent mediates aggressive response. Some evidence suggests that boys may be more vulnerable than girls to environmental influence (L.W. Hoffman, 1975) and that infants' responses are mediated by temperament (Thompson, 1986).

Particularly pertinent to the idea of different interpretations of environmental stimuli is the recent emphasis in socialization research on the role of cognition. Because siblings are different ages, they interpret events differently. The egocentric preschool child, for example, interprets the father's departure at the time of divorce as a response to his own behavior, an error an older child in the family would not ordinarily make (Wallerstein & Kelly, 1979). The same family event can thus be interpreted differently, producing a different emotional response and self-attribution, and can have a different impact on personality development. This approach views children as endlessly coding and interpreting their surroundings and contrasting themselves to others.

The emphasis on the child as an interpreter of his or her environment, and also the research on the child as an elicitor of parent behavior, are both part of the new emphasis in socialization research on the child as an active agent in his or her own socialization. This is not a new idea. It is an approach that was suggested by Bell (1968) 23 years ago and by Lewin (1935) 56 years ago, but it is now the dominant thrust in developmental psychology (Clarke-Stewart & Friedman, 1987; Hetherington & Parke, 1986; Hoffman, Paris, Hall, & Schell, 1988; R.M. Lerner, 1986; Shaffer, 1987). Different children evoke different interpersonal responses, attend to different aspects of their environment, and process environmental influences differently. This process has been described from a genetic standpoint in a classic article by Scarr and McCartney (1983). To the environmentally oriented developmental psychologist, however, the active child is shaped by the environment and his or her developmental level as well as by genetics.

Thus, the current conceptualization of the family environment in developmental psychology is that environment is not the same for all children in the family, and also that the impact of the environment on personality is mediated by the child's interpretation and response.

Multidimensionality

The family environment includes many different aspects that operate in interaction, and different combinations of family variables may have different effects (Baumrind, 1971; Bronfenbrenner, 1989; Eisenberg, 1988). The terms used by behavioral geneticists, *shared and nonshared environments*, are operationally defined as environmental influences that have resulted in sibling similarity or dissimilarity; they are inferred from the outcome. Yet to the developmental psychologist, a common environmental experience that affected each child might not result in the same personality trait if other inputs were not the same. Thus, it is possible that there is an aspect of the family environment that has affected all of the children, but that it is expressed in different ways. For example, research has shown that in a family with a very domineering father, a child with whom the father has a warm and compassionate relationship is likely to model his dominance, but a child who experiences his dominance without this moderating relationship is likely to feel impotent through his or her reciprocal role in relations to the dominant father and to be submissive (Eron, Walder, & Lefkowitz, 1971; L.W. Hoffman, 1961). Thus, two brothers with a dominant father, one of whom shares a warm relationship and the other who does not, will become very different on the trait of dominance. Their difference would lead the behavioral geneticist to say their environment is unshared. Nevertheless, both children have responded to the same quantity of dominance in the father.

Research in developmental psychology typically examines combinations of "environment" and "person" variables that are directly measured and controls on other variables in predicting to child outcomes. The focus is more on the process of influence than the outcome. An outcome, such as a personality trait, cannot tell one the environmental influences. Different scores on a personality inventory for a trait do not mean that common environmental experiences did not go into that outcome, but only that the total environmental package was not the same. Because there are so many aspects of the environment that interact in affecting personality, it is not likely that even a common experience that marks all of the children in some way will result in the same outcome (Hetherington, 1989).

Nonfamily Experiences

The childhood years in the family ware still seen by environmental researchers as particularly important influences on personality development (Lamb & Bornstein, 1986). These are important both because of the special vulnerability to influence of this period and because each subsequent influence builds on the preceding. Thus these early influences affect the person who then elicits and inter- prets subsequent environmental experiences.

However, the subsequent experiences also affect the person. Developmental researchers today do not see personality as set in childhood, nor as set in the family, but as subject to change throughout the life span through interactions in a variety of settings (Brim & Kagan, 1980; Hartup, 1989; Rutter, 1979).

In summary, the current conceptualization of the family environment in devel- opmental psychology is that it is not the same for all children in the family and also that the impact of the environment on personality is mediated by the child's interpretation and response. It is conceived of as multidimensional with effects on personality depending on combinations of interacting units. Although the family environment of childhood is particularly important in affecting personality, other environments and subsequent experiences also have an effect.

A considerable amount of research in developmental psychology has examined sources of environmental variation within families. Some of this research is reviewed in the following section. This should provide both some answers to the question behavioral geneticists are currently asking, "What environmental influences make siblings different?", and some leads for future research. In the final section of this article, the question considered is "What environmental influences make siblings similar?" In view of the way environment is conceptualized by developmental psy- chologists today, the latter question seems the more challenging.

WHY ARE CHILDREN IN THE SAME FAMILY DIFFERENT?

The question addressed in this section is the title of a recent article by Plomin and Daniels (1987): Why are children in the same family so different from one another? The answer they proposed invokes the principle of what social psychol- ogists call *relative deprivation*; that is, it's not what you have but what you have relative to the others around you. This theory is usually attributed to Stouffer, Suchman, DeVinney, Star, and Williams (1949). In the 1940s, they investigated the soldiers' morale during World War II. They found that in the branches of the service in which there were the most promotions, the Air Force notably, there was the most dissatisfaction with rank. They proposed that it is one's relative deprivation rather than one's absolute deprivation that leads to discontent. One compares oneself to the people at hand. In a very loving family, then, a child who feels she receives less love than her sister may feel unloved. If the comparison group is one's siblings, then Plomin and Daniels suggested that within-family differences may be more important than between-families differences in their effects on personality.

The evidence presented is meager. Plomin and Daniels (1987; Daniels, Dunn, Furstenberg, & Plomin, 1985) relied on subject reports off differential treatment and found that perceiving oneself as less favored in the family, such as experiencing less maternal closeness or less influence in the family decisions than siblings, is related to dissatisfaction with oneself. It is quite possible that both perception of self and the perception of one's family role are measuring the same general personality trait. Nevertheless, the process they described is certainly relevant. Furthermore, it can be extended beyond the idea of interpretations of parental treatment to other areas—such as the development of self-concept. A familiar example is the very intelligent child in a highly accomplished family who perceives himself as intellectually inadequate. The tallest child in a short family may think of herself as tall even through the school years when social comparison would indicate otherwise. Contrast with siblings can be very important in affecting one's self-concept, and these contrasts are often highlighted by parents, even when the differences are small in comparison to the population range.

There are, however, many other sources of sibling differences, many of which have been demonstrated in developmental psychology research. Five sources of sibling differences are discussed: (a) ordinal position, (b) the age of the child when an event occurs, (c) gender, (d) the child's physical appearance,[3] and (3) idiosyncratic experiences.

Ordinal Position

First, family roles and sibling interactions are very much affected by ordinal positions. Firstborn children are treated differently by parents throughout life than are subsequent children (Cushna, 1966; Hilton, 1967; Rothbart, 1971). In addition,

---

[3]Attractiveness rather than temperament is discussed as an eliciting variable because the empirical evidence is more solid. Research on temperament has been hampered by the problem of distinguishing whether the temperament is a response to the mother's behavior or a cause of the mother's behavior. When measures use mother's reports of infant temperament, the problem is compounded because the mother's report may reflect her attitude as well as the child's characteristics (Crockenberg, 1986).

it is a different experience to be an older sibling than it is to have an older sibling (Abramowitz, Corter, Pepler & Stanhope, 1986; Brim, 1958; Lamb, 1977). The firstborn child enters the family at a very different point in the family's development. This child is the greatest disruptions to the couple's relationship, and at each stage in the firstborn's life, he or she is dealing with inexperienced parents (R.M. Lerner & Spanier, 1978; W. Miller & Newman, 1978). In the United States today, for many new parents this is the first child they have ever cared for or had much experience with at all (Alpert & Richardson, 1980). Parents are more likely to have inappropriate developmental expectations for the firstborn. Everything the first child does is done as a pioneer. He or she is the first to enter school; the younger siblings have already heard his or her firsthand accounts when they enter, and they have a sibling in the school that first day. The firstborn, at adolescence, presents the parents for the first time with the new teenage patterns in dress, dating, and curfew hours. By the time the next child is an adolescent, the parents are more knowledgeable about the current peer culture.

One of the best studies demonstrating different parental treatment of first- and second-born siblings is one from the 1950s. It was conducted by Lasko (1954) and was part of the Fels Longitudinal study that followed the children from birth through adulthood. The study obtained frequent home observations of parent-child interaction for all the children in the family. Lasko compared the mother's behavior toward the firstborn, second born, and third born, measured when each child was the same age. For example, she compared the mother's behavior toward the firstborn at 1 year of age with the same mother's behavior toward the second born when that child was 1 and each with the third child at age 1. There were striking differences through the first 6 years with greater convergence for the variables examined after that age. The variables examined included child centeredness, acceptance, intensity of contact, affection, acceleration, readiness of explanation, and several other measures. Her findings revealed that the firstborn starts from a more favorable position than any subsequent child ever experiences, particularly with respect to more attention. At the birth of the second child, however, the first child drops to a point lower than the second child experiences at the same age. By the time the first child is 3 or 4, the firstborn is treated less warmly and more restrictively and coercively than the second child is at the same age. For the second child, if a third is born at age 3, the mother's behavior toward the child is altered, in a similar but less extreme way, with a loss of warmth and attentiveness. But if the third child is born when the second is 4, change is minor. Despite these differences in the siblings' experiences there were consistencies in mothers' methods of handling children and in their policies of child rearing across their children.

These findings seem different from data reported recently by Dunn and her colleagues (Dunn, Plomin, & Daniels, 1986; Dunn, Plomin, & Nettles, 1985). Dunn also examined mother-child interaction with firstborn children when they were 1 year old and compared it with the same mother's interaction with the second child when that child was 1, and repeated the comparisons for age 2. Her comparisons reported *similarity* in the mother's behavior toward the first- and second-born child. The different results, however, can be explained by differences in the design. Dunn observed mother-child interaction when the mother was alone with the child. Lasko (1954) observed mother-child interaction in the natural home setting. In the home situation, the mothers were rarely alone with either child once the second was born, and it is in the context of the increased responsibilities for the mother that the second child brings, as well as the need to control the first child's behavior toward the second, that the mother's behaviors change.

There are many other studies that have found differences in parental treatment of firstborn children, some looking at differences between firstborn and second born within a family, some contrasting parents interacting with a firstborn child with other parents interacting with a second-born child (Parke & Sawin, 1975; Thoman, Leiderman, & Olson, 1972). Findings include the following: Fathers talk to and touch firstborn sons as infants more than any subsequent child (Parke & Sawin, 1975). They are also more likely to discipline firstborn children than later ones. A special involvement with the firstborn by both parents is manifested throughout childhood (Baskett, 1985; Jacobs & Moss, 1976; Lewis & Kreitzberg, 1979). Conversations at the family dinner table are pitched to the level of the firstborn. In a laboratory puzzle-solving task, mothers with firstborns were more involved in getting the child to complete the task successfully (Hilton, 1967). Parents interfere with more activities of the firstborn, and the firstborn are given more responsibilities than the later born (Cushna, 1966; Hilton, 1967; Rothbart, 1971).

There are also studies that have examined sibling interaction. Although some of this research has noted the imitation of the older by the younger, leading to shared mannerisms and speech styles (Abramovitch, Corter, & Lando, 1979; Brim, 1958; Lamb, 1977, 1978; Pepler, Corter & Abramovitch, 1982; Samuels, 1977), others have focused on the reciprocality of sibling roles that can lead to differentiation (Abramovitch, Pepler, & Corter, 1982; Cicirelli, 1976, 1982). For example, older children are often given the responsibility for younger ones, which can be generalized to other peer relationships, whereas younger ones may be more likely to develop an expectation that they will be cared for.

Most of the research on ordinal position effects focuses on how the *objective* environment is affected. Thus, the studies reviewed have indicated objective differences between firstborn and later-born children in parental treatment and family ecology (Lasko, 1954; Lewis & Kreitzberg, 1979; Parke & Sawin, 1975). Some of the research has also examined differences in the children's interactions with the environment, such as the tendency of the younger to observe and imitate the older (Brim, 1958; Lamb, 1978; Pepler et al., 1982). This is an example of when one child selectively seeks out or attends to specific aspects of the environment, a pattern that has been called *niche picking* (Scarr & McCartney, 1983). However, there has been very little research into how ordinal position might affect the subjective environment, although it seems possible that the differences in objective environments would have an impact on children that would, in turn, lead to different interpretations of common environments.[4]

On the other hand, ordinal position has been related to various child outcome measures, most often to levels of achievement and IQ scores (S. Schacter, 1963; Zajonc, 1983), but also to personality variables such as anxiety level and peer popularity. Firstborn children are generally found to attain higher professional status (S. Schacter, 1963), have higher IQ scores (Zajonc, 1983), higher anxiety (Lahey, Hammer, Crumrine, & Forehand, 1980), and less peer popularity (N. Miller & Maruyama, 1976) than later-born children. These relationships are consistent with the ordinal position effects on environmental differences. For example, more early parental attention, family conversation pitched at the firstborn's level, and high parental expectations are all likely to lead to higher achievement and higher IQ scores. However the actual step-by-step empirical links have not been made.

Behavioral geneticists have often noted that the amount of variance in personality traits that ordinal position accounts for is small, and thus they have dismissed it as unimportant (Plomin & Daniels, 1987). This ignores two aspects of the relationship: (a) The relationship is indirect—ordinal position affects environment, which in turn affects outcome; and (b) personality outcomes are affected by a multiplicity of interacting environmental influences, and any given one is unlikely to explain much variance.

Child's Age at Time of Event

A second source of different experience is the child's age when a family event occurs. In contrast to the ordinal-position research, investigations of the child's age as a source of sibling differences focus mainly on the subjective environment. Because the child's cognitive understandings and affective needs vary with age, the objectively same event has very different significance for different age siblings. This is true for both major and minor events. A hospitalization of the mother may be a significant event for the 9-month-old but not for the 5-year-old sibling (Yarrow, 1964). The age of the child when the mother returns to employment seems to make

---

[4] A study by Daniels et al. (1985) did analyze the relationship between ordinal position and siblings' perceptions of the family environment, but the results were not reported. Birth order, age, and gender were all examined, and it was reported that "several of these correlations" were statistically significant but none accounted for more than "4% of the variance of sibling difference scores" (Daniels et al., 1985, p. 770). However, which relationships were significant was not indicated.

a difference in its effects (Weinraub & Jaeger, 1990). Because nontwin siblings are different ages, the same event may be a different experience.

Divorce is used here as an example because divorce has been cited by behavioral geneticists as a shared family experience that has been ruled out as an important environmental variable by the absence of sibling similarity across personality traits (Rowe, 1987). Yet, the developmental research has indicated that the event is experienced differently depending on the age of the child when the divorce occurs. There are several studies that have explicitly examined the different effects of divorce when it occurs at different stages in the child's life, such as the research of Kalter and his associates (Kalter & Rembar, 1981), the more recent investigation by Allison and Furstenberg (1989), or the clinical studies of Wallerstein and Kelly (Kelly & Wallerstein, 1975; Wallerstein & Kelly, 1979).

For the young child, the sheer loss of routines in the family that accompanies the initial stages of divorce is disturbing. In addition, the young child's egocentrism can lead to interpreting the father's departure as a response to him or her with a resulting guilt and sense of abandonment that lasts beyond the early years. There is also a misinterpretation of the mother's moods, with the young child interpreting the mother's distress as rejection or anger toward the child.

The child who is older when the divorce occurs has a more accurate interpretation of the events and the parents' emotions. The school-aged child also has more supports outside the family and more opportunity to escape the emotional upset of the custodial parent (Kelly & Wallerstein, 1975). For the child who is closer to adolescence, there is often embarrassment, and anxiety about the sexuality of the parent that comes to the fore, particularly when there is a new partner for one or both parents (Hetherington & Camara, 1984). At the same time, the older child, particularly a daughter, can take on new roles, new responsibilities, and sometimes new companionship with the mother. This can have positive aspects, such as a new sense of competence and value, but it has also been described as "growing up too fast" (Weiss, 1979).

In short, the studies show that each child experiences the divorce through his or her level of understanding and the needs and anxieties that are ascendant at the particular age. In this sense, then, the same divorce may be experienced by siblings of different ages as a different environmental influence. Divorce may seem like an experience that is shared by siblings, but its interpretation and impact are not shared.

Although most of the research that examines how the child's age moderates environmental effects has focused on the child's interpretations, differences in the objective environment for children of different ages when a family event occurs have also been observed. New role assignments, for example, often depend on the ages of the children. Some of the divorce research just described (Weiss, 1979) shows this: another example is Elder's (1974) classic study of children growing up during the economic depression of the 1930s, which also shows this. Economic adversity had a very different effect on the environments of different-aged children and important consequences for personality differences in adulthood. Adolescent sons who had experienced prosperity in childhood, but whose families were particularly hit with economic reversals during the depression, were called on to supplement the family income. This experience appeared to facilitate long-term ego development, resulting in a pattern of occupational achievement and stability in adulthood. Younger boys whose families were heavily hit experienced the income loss as children and did not have a role in the family's coping efforts. Their development followed a very different pattern. As adults, they were less self-directed and occupationally effective than their age cohorts whose families had escaped economic reversals. Thus, the same family event, heavy economic loss during the depression, had different effects on different age sons because their age moderated their family roles and objective experiences when adversity hit.

Gender

The third source of sibling differences to be discussed is the child's gender. Fifteen years ago, a widely read book by Maccoby and Jacklin (1974) appeared that summarized a considerable range of research and concluded that there was little solid evidence for gender differences in children's behavior or performance, nor in their parental treatment. The book led to several severe critiques (Block, 1976; 1978) and a flurry of research. At this point there are abundant data demonstrating that parents do treat boys and girls differently (Huston, 1983, 1985). Research with toddlers and preschoolers has shown, for example, that girls are given help more quickly when performing a task, that their bids for dependency—such as clinging to the mother's skirt or seeking body contact as she works in the kitchen—are more often reacted to positively, whereas boys' similar attempts are discouraged (Fagot, 1978, 1985). Boys are given earlier autonomy and less restricted opportunities for play outside the home (Fagot, Hagan, Leinbach, & Kronsberg, 1985; L.W. Hoffman, 1977; Saegert & Hart, 1976). The physical environment and the toys provided are different for each sex (Eccles & Hoffman, 1984; Rheingold & Cook, 1975). For older children, expectations for achievement and evaluations of competence are different (Eccles & Hoffman, 1984). As previously mentioned, there are even data indicating that parents are more likely to fight with each other in front of a male child (Hetherington & Camara, 1984). Parents often report that they do not or would not treat sons differently from daughters, but behavioral observations or child-specific reports reveal differently (Fagot, 1982; L.W. Hoffman, 1977). Sons who display behavior seen as atypical for males ar particularly pressured by parents and peers to change their ways.

Thus, males and females do experience objectively different family environments.

That much of this difference is due to parents' sex role beliefs and not to characteristics of the child has been demonstrated by the studies that have used the same children as the stimulus but changed the information about whether they were male or female and then observed the responses of adult subjects. A diapered infant left in the care of adult subjects elicited sex role stereotyped behavior to match whatever sex the infant was assigned by the researchers (Seavey, Katz, & Zalk, 1975). In another study, the cries of an infant were interpreted as anger by subjects when told the infant was a boy and as fear when told the infant was a girl (Condry & Condry, 1976). As a third example, the aggressiveness of children's play, viewed on a videotape, was judged differently when subjects were told the children were boys than when they were told they were girls (Condry & Ross, 1985).

In addition, some of the differences in parental behavior are consistent with sex stereotypes, but inconsistent with actual gender differences. For example, female infants are perceived and handled as though they were more fragile and vulnerable, but in fact the male neonate is less mature at birth than the female and more vulnerable to disease and infant mortality (Minton, Kagan, & Levine, 1971; Moss, 1967). Male children are allowed to cross the street by themselves at a younger age, but differences in maturity level and impulsivity would seem to suggest that females are ready earlier (L.W. Hoffman, 1975; 1977).

Nevertheless, some of the differences in parental behavior are no doubt elicited by gender differences in children's behavior. One interesting example comes from the longitudinal work of Moss (1967). Moss found that by 3 months, mothers of female infants were more responsive to the infants' cries than mothers of male infants. It was proposed that this pattern developed because of differences in maturity levels of males and females at birth (L.W. Hoffman, 1975). Because females are more mature at birth, their early crying is more often a response to hunger or environmental stimuli rather than to internal body states. As a result, the mother's responses to female infant cries with feeding, changing, or covering are more often rewarded with the cessation of crying. Because mothers of males are less often rewarded in this way, their responsively declines. Thus, even a small gender difference may affect parent behavior and set off a chain of interaction.

It is likely that gender differences in aggressiveness (Macoby & Jacklin, 1974) evoke different parental response, and differences in aggressiveness within male samples have been shown to affect parental reaction (Elder, Caspi, & Nguyen, 1986; Elder, Nguyen, & Caspi, 1985; Patterson & Dishion, 1988). In Hetherington's work (Hetherington & Camara, 1984), a particular accompaniment of divorce for 4-year-old sons was a cycle of angry exchanges with the mother and aggression in the peer group. This pattern still marked the sons' behavior 2 years after the divorce and, even 6 years after, was reflected to the views of the child by his peers, even though his actual aggression by then had subsided. This response to divorce was not found for daughters. It is not possible to say precisely that the hostile interchanges with the mother, and the pattern of erratic discipline of sons that was observed, resulted because of gender differences in response patterns per se because the environmental conditions themselves were not the same for boys and girls, but it is an interpretation consistent with the results (Hetherington & Camara, 1984).

Gender is also seen as affecting the processing of the environment. According to the cognitive developmental theory of Kohlberg (1966), once children attain *gender constancy*, the understanding both of what their gender is and that it will never change, they seek to acquire gender-ascribed traits and behaviors. This sets off a self-socializing process that includes selectively attending to the environment— watching and modeling, for example, gender-appropriate models.

Kohlberg's (1966) theory of sex role development had not been empirically tested, but there is other evidence of gender-based niche picking. For example, whether the origin of the pattern lies in socialization experiences or genetics is unknown, but research has shown that gender is related to self-selected play activities and that young children self-select same-sex companions (Connor & Serbin, 1977; Maccoby, 1989; Masters & Furman, 1981). Because different play patterns have also been shown to have an effect on personality and cognitive development, in both experimental and natural observation studies, this process may be an important link to personality differences (Connor & Serbin, 1977; Eccles & Hoffman, 1984; L.W. Hoffman, 1977).

Physical Appearance

The fourth factor that has been shown to lead to different sibling experiences is a genetic one, physical appearance. Many studies demonstrate that more attractive children elicit more positive responses and evaluation from parents, other adults, and peers (Hartup, 1983; Langlois, 1986; Lenerz, Kucher, East, Lerner, & Lerner, 1987; R.M. Lerner, 1987; Sorell & Nowak, 1981). This work has used laboratory research designs and natural observations—in homes and in schools. One study involved 150 families in which infants' attractiveness was assessed by an independent panel of judges (Langlois, 1986; Langlois & Casey, 1984). Mother-infant interactions were systematically observed from the child's birth through 9 months. Mothers of attractive babies were more involved with the baby and less involved with others. More attractive infants, particularly daughters, were more often kissed, cooed to, smiled at, and cuddled. These relationships increased over the 9-month period. The attractiveness of firstborn infants was also correlated (at -.43) with maternal attitudes, which measured disappointments in the infant. These same patterns were revealed in studies that looked at fathers' as well as mothers' behavior (Parke & Sawin, 1975), in studies that used filmstrips or pictures of infants or children, and in studies with unrelated adults who judged the personality of the baby or the seriousness of a reported transgression by an older child (Berkowtiz & Frodi, 1979; Dion, 1972, 1974; Langlois, 1986; Stephan & Langlois, 1984).

It is interesting that in studies that have measured the child's attractiveness, behavior, and the attributions of peers about their behavior or competence, attractiveness and attributions are related across the years, but attractiveness and behavior do not show a relationship in early childhood (Adams & Crane, 1980; Clifford & Walster, 1973; Dion & Stein, 1978; Hartup, 1983; Langlois, 1986; Langlois & Downs, 1979; Styczynski, 1976; Styczynski & Langlois, 1980). That relationship emerges only in older children. Thus studies have found that young children rated by judges as unattractive are seen as more aggressive and less competent, but their behavior does not support that judgment. Among older children, however, behavioral measures of aggression and competence do relate to attractiveness (Langlois & Downs, 1979; Styczynski, 1976). It has been suggested that this reflects a self-fulfilling prophecy: Less attractive children are reacted to more negatively by others, and their subsequent behavior patterns are a response to these attributions and interactions (Hartup, 1983; Langlois, 1986).

In most of the research, physical attractiveness is a potent elicitor of parent, peer, and teacher response for both boys and girls (Lenerz et al., 1987), although the effect is sometimes stronger when the child is female (Langlois & Casey, 1984). In one interesting case, however, the effect was found only for girls. Research by Elder and his colleagues (Elder et al., 1986; Elder et al., 1985) showed that during economic hardship and unemployment, fathers were more punitive and less supportive of daughters, but only if they were unattractive. If they were attractive, in some cases economic hardship actually increased supportiveness and lessened punitiveness. In this research, boys' attractiveness made no difference in the parenting outcomes of economic hardship.

There are other aspects of physical appearance that have been investigated. For example, the child's closer resemblance to one parent rather than the other brings forth different responses from each parent and may influence the child's identification with each. The size of the child is also important. Being tall for age, for example, evokes higher developmental expectations. Being chubby or thin is associated with more peer rejection and with being given more "personal space" by peers in interactions (R.M. Lerner, 1987). All of these can be differences among siblings and lead to different environmental experiences.

Idiosyncratic Experiences

A fifth source of differential sibling effects is the obvious one that some children have different experiences from their siblings because of random events—an illness, witnessing a parental interaction unseen by the other children, or an accident. In addition, there is a whole set of events that occur outside the family and affect personality. Interactions with peers have been particularly examined.

The impact of chance encounters and random events on personality development can be considerable, as indicated in personal histories and clinical studies (Bandura, 1982), but they are difficult to study empirically. They can be one-time occurrences that have particular significance, such as overhearing a conversation between one's parents that leads the child to believe he or she was an unwanted child or a less valued one, or there can be a continuous experience such as having a widowed grandmother move into the household and share one child's bedroom. Such family experiences that are not shared by siblings are very likely to occur, and their significance for personality differences lies in their ability to affect the child's other environmental interactions and interpretations.

Only a few of these child-specific experiences, however, have been studied empirically: those that occur with sufficient frequency that a sample can be assembled. For example, there are studies exploring the effects of hospitalization during childhood and the effects of various specific chronic illnesses such as diabetes, cystic fibrosis, and cancer (Hagen, Myers, & Alswede, in press; Pless, 1984). These studies point up both the direct effects of the illness on the child's personality development, particularly the self-concept, and the effects on the parents' differential treatment of their children. The research indicates that chronic illness is likely to affect the developmental path of both the ill child and the siblings, but the direction of the effects is different (Freeman & Hagen, 1990; Hagen, Anderson, & Barclay, 1986; Lobato, 1983). Among the findings are that the illness may involve a shift in sibling hierarchies with the ill child treated as the younger and the healthy as the older, despite actual ordinal position; and that the ill child may be overprotected and unnecessarily encouraged in dependency patterns (Hagen et al., in press).

In addition to child-specific family experiences, however, there are many experiences outside the family that are not shared by siblings and are important in affecting personality development. As noted earlier, although developmental psychologists see the early years and the family environment as particularly important, environmental influences operate throughout the life span (Brim & Kagan, 1980; Rutterr, 1979). Thus, as siblings move beyond the family, it is inevitable that they will have unshared experiences, and these will contribute to the lack of personality similarity.

For example, siblings have different peer groups and different experiences with them. The peer group provides the child with his or her first opportunity for comparison with age mates, and a considerable amount of research has examined the effects of children's peer groups on their self-concepts and social behavior. Studies has indicated that by 8 years of age, children engage in social comparison: they evaluate themselves in terms of how their performance contrasts with that of their immediate peers (Hartup, 1983; Rubble, Boggiano,

Feldman, & Loebl, 1980). Although the degree of self-confidence obtaining earlier may buffer this process, new information and discrepancies can lead to change. This can change again at different developmental stages, such as adolescence, when new peer group standards and different individual talents and attributes may emerge (Hartup, 1989).

WHY WOULD SIBLINGS BE ALIKE?

Evidence has been presented that the objective environment of siblings is not the same. Parents' behavior changes with subsequent children as their experience and the stress in their lives change, and it is different in response to the different stimuli that each child presents. The whole family dynamics are altered to each additional child. There are different expectations and different roles assigned, often based on the child's ordinal position, gender, and individual qualities. In addition, different children interpret experiences differently—because of their age and gender, and also because of interpersonal differences that can develop from both genetic and environmental influences. If one adds to that the evidence that personality result from multiple influences from within the family and from outside, then the discovery that siblings are not alike on personality traits is not surprising.

Are Siblings Different?

But is it true that siblings are not alike? Despite the accumulation of evidence from behavioral genetics that environmental influence accounts for a considerable amount of sibling difference, there is also evidence even from these data for sibling similarity. Thus, although Plomin and Daniels asserted that "environmental influences make two children in the same family as different from one another as are pairs of children selected randomly" (1987, p.1), Lykken (1987) has pointed out that this is not all the case: The average intraclass correlation for siblings on personality traits is greater than zero. It is often a statistically significant correlation; it is simply not a high one. Furthermore, for some traits, as noted earlier, there is considerable sibling similarity that cannot be attributed to genetics.

It is unfortunate that more attention has not been given by either behavioral geneticists or developmental psychologists to exploring which traits and which measures show environmentally produced similarity among siblings because this might suggest hypotheses about the different processes involved. When the developmental psychologist examines the effects of the family environment on the child, the research is always child specific. Thus, in studies of child rearing, the researcher measures how the parent behaves toward the particular child for whom the outcome measures are obtained. Because of awareness of other influences, the developmental researcher controls on as many of these variables as possible. The child's ordinal position, gender, and age are almost always controlled by either statistics or the research design. The parents' education is also controlled lest that be the variable carrying the relationship. Furthermore, behavioral observations rather than self-reports are typically used. Because of the complexities and expense of this design, siblings are rarely included (Wachs, 1983), and sibling similarity is rarely examined in developmental research.

Behavioral genetics data, on the other hand, consist primarily of comparisons of siblings' scores on self-report personality inventories to see the relative importance of genetics, environmental influences that result in sibling differences, and the environmental influences that result in sibling similarity. The relatively low overall influence of what is called the shared family environment is commonly noted, but little attention is given to which variables do or do not show this influence either within individual studies or across different investigations.

Some of the behavioral genetics research, however, seems to indicate that what might be considered attitudes shows more sibling similarity than the more typical personality measures (Loehlin et al., 1988). Conservatism and religiosity, for example, have been found to be particularly affected by the shared family environment (Loehlin, 1987). Interest areas also seem to show sibling similarity. For example, scores from the Holland Interest Styles, as noted earlier, show marked sibling similarity when the parents are similar to each other (Grotevant, 1979). Interest and involvement in music show clear sibling similarity, with the common family environment more important than genetic factors (Coon & Carey, 1989).

The outcomes examined in developmental psychology research on the family environment are rarely personality traits, they are more often coping skills, competency, and moral internalization, and these are not the variables examined in the behavioral genetics work. Furthermore, the self-report personality inventories such as the California Psychological Inventory, the Minnesota Multiphasic Personality Inventory, and the Eysenck Personality Inventory, which are used in behavioral genetics, are rarely used in developmental research. If self-report measures are used, they are usually concept-specific instruments, such as the Nowicki-Strickland Children's Locus of Control Scale (Nowicki & Strickland, 1973) as a measure of personal effectiveness, but more often measurement relies on behavioral observation. It seems possible, therefore, that the prevalence of sibling differences in the behavioral genetics research is a function of the particular concepts studied and the instruments used to tap them.

For example, aggression, when measured by behavior in a laboratory setting, showed a marked effect of the shared environment (Plomin et al., 1981), as indicated earlier. This is a measure frequently used in developmental psychology. However, in the behavioral genetics research that uses self-report personality measures, aggression shows very little nongenetic sibling similarity (Loehlin et al., 1988). It may be that self-report measures bring out siblings' tendency to focus on differences from the siblings (F.F. Schacter, 1982). This tendency may be augmented by the subjects' knowledge that their siblings were also being tested. Behavioral observations, on the other hand, which are not based on an intrafamily frame of reference, may show that they are actually quite similar compared with the population range. Thus, at this point, it is not really known that siblings are not similar. They may be similar in some respects, but not in others.

Different Environment–Outcome Links

In views of the evidence cited earlier for differences in siblings' experiences and processing of the environment, how might sibling similarity be explained? Why might siblings be similar on some characteristics but dissimilar on others?

For different behavior patterns, different aspects of the environment are important (Wachs, 1983). Furthermore, some aspects of the environment are more subject to intrafamily variation that others. It seems likely, then, that some outcomes would be less likely to show siblings similarity. An example might be dependency. In the preceding section of this review, data were cited showing that daughters were more likely to be rewarded for dependency, whereas sons were more likely to be punished (Fagot, 1978). In sibling relationships, later-born children are more likely to expect help fro firstborn children than the reverse (Abramovitch et al., 1982). Idiosyncratic experience such as chronic illness are likely to bring forth parental overprotection (Hagen et al., in press). All of these environmental variables have been linked to the development of dependency (Maccoby & Masters, 1970). Therefore, dependency may be a characteristic that is particularly likely to show sibling variability. Social competence and moral internalization, on the other hand, have been related to more general parenting styles, such as the tendency for parents to give explanations for their influence attempts, relying on inductive discipline rather than power assertion or love withdrawal, the tendency to allow the child a more active role in decisions, and the general warmth and involvement of the parents (Baumrind, 1967; M.L. Hoffman, 1986). Sibling similarity might be expected, then, for these characteristics because the antecedent environmental variables are general parenting styles that are not likely to vary greatly across siblings.[5]

In addition, some outcomes measures are more vulnerable to influence at specific developmental stages, others throughout the life span. Some are shaped by multiple environmental inputs, whereas others have more specific environmental ties

---

[5]The concept of *dominance* is measured by the California Psychological Inventory and the Thurstone Temperament Schedule and did not show sibling similarity for adopted or nonadopted sibling pairs (Loehlin et al., 1985). This label may seem similar to the concept of dependency, but it is actually tapping a different dimension (Maccoby & Masters, 1970). Similarly, "altruism" and "empathy," as measured by personality inventories, do not show sibling similarity (Loehlin et al., 1988), but these are quite different from the prevailing concepts and measures of moral internalization used in developmental research (M.L. Hoffman, 1986).

(Erikson, 1963; Rutter, 1979; Wachs, 1983). These differences would affect whether the outcomes would show sibling similarity.

What is assumed here is that even though there are differences in a parent's behavior toward different children, there is also a similarity of style across children that differentiates one parent from another. This general consistency is shown in both the Lasko (1954) study and the Dunn et al. (1985) study discussed in the previous section. Although the Lasko study showed that firstborn children experienced different environments than later-born children, like Dunn and her colleagues, she found a commonalty of style across children that differentiated one mother from another. It seems likely that some personality traits, attitudes, and behavior patterns are more affected by general family patterns and by commonalties of style, whereas others are more influenced by individual environmental encounters that vary across siblings.

Thus, there is evidence of sibling similarity, as well as sibling differences, but most of the variables that have been shown to be affected by the family environment in the developmental studies have not been examined in the behavioral genetics research. Existing studies of sibling similarity rely heavily on self-report personality inventories. Whether behavioral measures, or measures of broader range of outcome variables, would show the same patterns is open to question. A fuller picture of sibling similarities and differences would be helpful in forming hypotheses about the socialization processes involved.

However, a reasonable hypothesis is that siblings may not be similar on those characteristics that are particularly affected by the kinds of environmental experiences that are likely to vary across siblings, but they may be more similar on characteristics that are responsive to more general family patterns. This hypothesis assumes that certain child characteristics are more likely to show sibling similarity than others and that this reflects different kinds of environmental influences that determine each set. It is consistent with the prevailing approach in developmental psychology, but incorporates the work in behavioral genetics that has been concerned with comparing siblings across families to identify characteristics in which they are similar.

Salience as a Determinant of Sibling Similarity

A quite different hypothesis is that the characteristics that show sibling similarity will vary from family to family depending on what environmental influences are most salient or most uniformly present. This might be particularly important in the transmission of values or interests. Thus, in some families certain values are strongly and unambivalently endorsed and encouraged by word and by example. It might be sociopolitical involvement, as in the family of Joseph and Rose Kennedy. It might be a concern for others—an emphasis on role taking and empathy that comes through in verbal input and in the parents' behavior toward the children, each other, and nonfamily members. It might be an emphasis on making money or academic achievement, family centeredness, or an interest area such as sports. If salience is the major determinant of sibling similarity, this might not be revealed in the customary research because the dimension would be different across families. However, salience might also be a moderating variable that increases sibling similarity effects.

Another factor that may influence sibling similarity is uniformity between parents. Sibling similarity on the Holland Interest Styles was only slightly higher than for personality measures except when parental agreement was introduced. When the parents' scores were similar, however, sibling similarity increased significantly for both biological and adopted siblings (Grotevant, 1979).

This pattern of similarity between parents leading to increased uniformity in the children should operate in other areas. For example, the family environment is an important learning place for values, attitudes, coping styles, work orientations, and even styles of parenting. When parents differ, the children may model one or the other, or neither because the difference weakens the effect of each. But when the parents present the same pattern, the chances are increased that each child will adopt it, thus increasing sibling similarity. Uniformity between family influences and the broader social milieu should also have this effect. Thus, the neighborhood or community setting can also affect sibling similarity (Bronfenbrenner, 1989).

This second hypothesis that salience or uniformity might increase sibling similarity is not an alternative to the first but an additional one that might be particularly applicable to values or interest areas. It might also be a supplementary one, for salience or uniformity could increase the impact of environmental influence that was common across siblings. Thus, what is suggested here is that although the research shows that the family environment is not the same across siblings either objectivity or subjectively, some outcome variables may be tied to aspects of the family environment that show less intrafamily variability. For these, similarity between sibling would be more likely, and salience and uniformity could increase the effect.

CONCLUSION

This review has addressed issues raised by research from behavioral genetics that shows that, for many personality traits, environmental influence is important but siblings are not alike. These results are provocative and important in their potential influence. Recent publications in behavioral genetics have suggested that these findings challenge the basic assumptions of the research in developmental psychology that examines the effects of the family environment on personality development. To behavioral geneticists, these data raise questions as to whether child rearing patterns, or family events such as divorce, can be seen as important in explaining individual differences in personality. If they were important, would not the effects be the same for all children in the family? Would not siblings be alike?

Research from both behavioral genetics and developmental psychology have been reviewed here to make two major points. First, the absence of sibling similarity may be less general than is asserted because of limitations in the methodology and in the range and measurement of the outcome variables. If, for example, the genetic influence is being overestimated by the methodologies used, as suggested here, then the degree of environmentally produced sibling similarity is being underestimated. If the heavy reliance on self-report personality inventories is showing more sibling difference than would a broader range of outcome variables and behavior-based measures, then again, sibling similarity is being underestimated.

Second, personality results from complex interacting influences that include objective and subjective factors. There is always a person interacting with the environment, and this affects the objective experience and the interpretation. It is a cumulative, transactional process. Although some aspects of the family environment may be the same across siblings, other aspects are not the same. Research shows that children within the same family have different environmental experiences and different reactions to these experiences because of their order of birth, different ages when any particular event occurs, their gender, genetic differences, and idiosyncratic encounters. Thus, finding that siblings are not the same on personality traits is not surprising from the viewpoint of developmental psychology.

It seems likely from the research reviewed here that siblings are different in some respects and similar in others. However, questions of what environmental conditions might lead to sibling similarity or dissimilarity have not been investigated. It is possible that certain outcome variables are more likely to show similarity than others depending on the kinds of environmental influences involved. It is also possible that some family environments are more conducive to sibling similarity than others. Research on the environmental processes that lead to sibling similarities and differences can be an important new direction for unraveling the complexities of social development. The real value of this recent research from behavioral genetics does not lie in implications for reinterpreting existing research in developmental psychology, but rather in its impetus to research on the environmental precursors of sibling similarities and differences.

REFERENCES

Abramovitch, R., Corter, C., & Lando, B. (1979). Sibling interaction in the home. *Child Development*, 50, 997–1003.

Abramovitch, R., Corter, C., Pepler, D.J., & Stanhope, L. (1986). Sibling and peer interaction. *Child Development, 57*, 217–229.

Abramovitch, R., Pepler, D., & Corter, C. (1982). Patterns of sibling interaction among preschool-age children. In M.E. Lamb & B. Sutton-Smith (Eds.), *Sibling relationship* (pp. 61–86). Hillsdale, NJ: Erlbaum.

Adams, G.R., & Crane, P. (1980). An assessment of parents' and teachers' expectations of preschool children's social preference for attractive or unattractive children and adults. *Child Development, 51*, 224–231.

Allison, P.D., & Furstenberg, F.F., Jr. (1989). How marital dissolution affects children: Variations by age and sex. *Developmental Psychology, 25*, 540–549.

Alpert, J.L., & Richardson, M.S. (1980) Parenting. In L.W. Poon (Ed.), *Aging in the 1980s* (pp. 441–454). Washington, DC: American Psychological Association.

Bandura, A. (1982), The psychology of chance encounters and life paths. *American Psychologist, 37*, 747–755.

Baskett, L.M. (1985), Sibling status effects: Adult expectations. *Developmental Psychology, 21*, 441–445.

Baumrind, D. (1967). Childcare practices anteceding three patterns of preschool behavior. *Genetic Psychology Monograph, 4*(1, Pt.2).

Baumrind, D. (1971). Current patterns of parental authority. *Developmental Psychology Monograph, 4*(Pt. 2).

Bell, R.Q. (1968). A reinterpretation of the direction of effects in studies of socialization. *Psychological Review, 75*, 81–95.

Berkowitz, L., & Frodi, A. (1979). Reactions to a child's mistakes as affected by her/his looks and speech. *Social Psychology Quarterly, 42*, 420–425.

Block, J.H. (1976). Issues, problems, and pitfalls in assessing sex differences. *Merrill-Palmer Quarterly, 22*, 283–308.

Block, J.H. (1978). Another look at sex differentiation in the socialization behaviors of mothers and fathers. In J. Sherman & F. Denmark (Eds.), *Psychology of women: Future directions of research* (pp. 29–87). New York: Psychological Directions.

Blum, H. (1983). Adoptive parents: Generative conflict and generational continuity. In A.J. Solnit, R.S. Eister, & P.B. Neubauer (Eds.), *The psychoanalytic study of the child* (Vol 38, pp. 141–163), New Haven, CT: Yale University Press.

Bouchard, T.J., Jr., Lykken, D.T., McGue, M., Segal, N.L., & Tellegen, A. (1990). Sources of human psychological differences: The Minnesota Study of Twins Reared Apart. *Science, 250*, 223–250.

Bradley, R.H., & Caldwell, B.M. (1984), The relation of infants' home environments to achievement test performance in the first grade: A follow-up study. *Child Development, 55*, 803–809.

Brim, O.G., Jr. (1958). Family structure and sex role learning by children: A further analysis of Helen Koch's data. *Sociometry, 21*, 1–16.

Bronfenbrenner, U. (1985, April). *Organism-environment interaction from an ecological perspective.* Paper presented at the biennial meeting of the Society for Research in Child Development. Toronto, Ontario, Canada.

Bronfenbrenner, U. (1986). Ecology of the family as a context for human development: Research perspectives. *Developmental Psychology, 22* (6), 723–742.

Bronfenbrenner, U. (1989). Ecological systems theory. In R. Vasta (Ed.), *Six theories of child development* (pp. 185–246). Greenwich, CT: JAI Press.

Cicirelli, V.G. (1976). Siblings helping siblings. In V.L. Allen (Ed.), *Children as tutors* (pp. 138–149). San Diego, CA: Academic Press.

Cicirelli, V.G. (1982). Sibling influence throughout the lifespan. In M.E. Lamb & B. Sutten-Smith (Eds.), *Sibling relationships: Their nature and significance across the lifespan* (pp. 267–284). Hillsdale, NJ: Erlbaum.

Clarke-Stewart, A., & Friedman, S. (1987). *Child development: Infancy through adolescence.* New York: Wiley.

Clifford, M.M., & Walster, E. (1973). The effects of physical attractiveness on teacher expectations. *Sociology of Education, 46*, 248–258.

Condry, J.C., & Condry, S. (1976). Sex and aggression. *Child Development, 56*, 225–233.

Connor, J. & Serbin, L.A. (1977). Behaviorally based masculine and feminine activity preference scales for preschoolers: Correlates with other classroom behaviors and cognitive tests. *Child Development, 48*, 1411–1416.

Coon, H., & Carey, G. (1989). Genetic and environmental determinants of musical ability in twins. *Behavioral Genetics, 19*, 183–193.

Crockenberg, S.B. (1986). Are temperamental differences in babies associated with predictable differences in care-giving? In J.V. Lerner & R.M. Lerner (Eds.), *Temperament and social interaction in infants and children. New directions for child development* (pp. 53–74). San Francisco: Jossey-Bass.

Cushna, B. (1966, September). *Agency and birth order differences in very early childhood.* Paper presented at the 74th Annual Convention of the American Psychological Association, New York.

Daniels, D., Dunn, J., Furstenberg, F.F., & Plomin, R. (1985). Environmental differences within the family and adjustment differences within pairs of adolescent siblings. *Child Development, 56*, 764–774.

Dion, K.K. (1972). Physical attractiveness and evaluations of children's transgression. *Journal of Personality and Social Psychology, 24*, 207–213.

Dion, K.K. (1974). Children's physical attractiveness and sex as determinants of adult punitiveness. *Developmental Psychology, 10*, 772–778.

Dion, K.K., & Stein, S. (1978). Physical attractiveness and interpersonal influence. *Journal of Experimental Social Psychology, 14*, 97–108.

Dodge, K.A., & Somberg, D.R. (1987). Hostile attributional biases among aggressive boys are exacerbated under conditions of threat to the self. *Child Development, 58*, 213–224.

Dunn, J.F., Plomin, R., & Daniels, D. (1986). Consistency and change in mothers' behavior towards young siblings. *Child Development, 57*, 348–356.

Dunn, J.F., Plomin, R., & Nettles, M. (1985). Consistency of mothers' behavior toward infant siblings. *Developmental Psychology, 21*, 1188–1195.

Eccles, J.S., & Hoffman, L.W. (1984). Sex roles, socialization, and occupational behavior. In H.W. Stevenson & A.E. Siegel (Eds.), *Child development research and social policy* (pp. 367–420). Hillsdale, NJ: Erlbaum.

Elder, G.H., Jr. (1974). *Children of the Great Depression.* Chicago: University of Chicago Press.

Elder, G., Caspi, A., & Nyguyen, T. (1986). Resourceful and vulnerable children: Family influence in hard times. In R.K. Silbereisen, K. Eyferth, & G. Rudinger (Eds.), *Development as action in context* (pp. 167–186). New York: Springer-Verlag.

Elder, G., Nyguyen, T., & Caspi, A. (1985), Linking family hardship to children's lives. *Child Development, 56,* 361–375.

Erikson, E.H. (1963). *Childhood and society* (2nd ed.). New York: Norton.

Eron, L.D., Walder, L.O., & Lefkowitz, M.M. (1971). *Learning of aggression,* Boston: Little, Brown.

Fagot, B.I. (1978). The influence of sex of child on parental reactions to toddler children. *Child Development, 49,* 459–465.

Fagot, B.I. (1982). Adults as socializing agents. In T.M. Field, A. Huston, H.C. Quay, L. Troll, & G.E. Finley (Eds.), *Review of human development* (pp. 304–315). New York: Wiley.

Fagot, B.I. (1985) Beyond the reinforcement principle. *Developmental Psychology, 21,* 1097–1104.

Fagot, B.I., Hagan, R., Leinbach, M.D., & Kronsberg, S. (1985). Differential reactions to assertive and communicative acts of toddler boys and girls. *Child Development, 56,* 1499–1505.

Farber, S.L. (1981). *Identical twins reared apart: A reanalysis.* New York: Basic Books.

Feeman, D.J., & Hagen, J.W. (1990). Effects of childhood chronic illness on families. *Social Work in Health Care, 14,* 37–53.

Grotevant, H.D. (1979). Environmental influences on vocational interest development in adolescents from adoptive and biological families. *Child Development, 50,* 854–860.

Grotevant, H.D. (1984, August). *Exploration and negotiation of differences within families during adolescence.* Invited address at the 92nd Annual Convention of the American Psychological Association, Toronto, Ontario, Canada.

Hagen, J.W., Anderson, B., & Barclay, C.R. (1986). Issues in research on the young chronically ill child. *Topics in Early Childhood Special Education,* 5(4), 49–57.

Hagen, J.W., Myers, J.T., & Allswede, J.S. (in press). The psychological impact of children's chronic illness. In D.L. Featherman, R.M. Lerner, & M. Perlmutter (Eds.), *Life span development and behavior* (Vol. 11). Hillsdale, NJ: Erlbaum.

Hartup, W.W. (1983). Peer relations. In P.H. Mussen (Ed.), *Handbook of child psychology: Socialization, personality and social development* (4th ed., pp. 102–196). New York: Wiley.

Hartup, W.W. (1989). Social relationships and their developmental significance. *American Psychologist, 44,* 120–126.

Hess, R.D., & Holloway, S.D. (1984). Family and school as educational institutions. In R.D. Parke (Ed.), *Review of child development research: Vol. V. The family* (pp. 179–222). Chicago: University of Chicago Press.

Hetherington, E.M. (1989). Coping with family transitions: Winners, losers, and survivors. *Child Development, 60,* 1–14.

Hetherington, E.M., & Camara, K.A. (1984). Families in transition. In R.D. Parke (Ed.), *Review of child development research* (Vol. 7, pp. 398–439). Chicago: University of Chicago Press.

Hethering, E.M., & Parke, R. (1986). *Child development: A contemporary viewpoint*. New York: McGraw-Hill.

Hilton, I. (1967). Differences in the behavior of mothers toward first- and later-born children. *Journal of Personality and Social Psychology, 7*, 282–290.

Hoffman, L.W. (1961). The father's role in the family and the child's peer group adjustment. *Merrill-Palmer Quarterly, 7*, 97–105.

Hoffman, L.W. (1977). Changes in family roles, socialization, and sex differences. *American Psychologist, 32*, 644–657.

Hoffman, L.W. (1985). The changing genetics/socialization balance. *Journal of Social Issues, 41*, 1, 127–148.

Hoffman, L.W., Paris, S., Hall, E., & Schell, R. (1988). *Developmental psychology today*. New York: Random House.

Hoffman, M.L. (1986). Moral development. In M.H. Bornstein & M.E. Lamb (Eds.), *Developmental psychology* (2nd ed., pp. 309–366). Hillsdale, NJ: Erlbaum.

Horn, J.M. (1983). The Texas adoption project: Adopted children and their intellectual resemblance to biological and adoptive parents. *Child Development, 54*, 268–275.

Horn, J.M., Loehlin, J.C., & Willerman, L. (1979). Intellectual resemblance among adoptive and biological relatives: The Texas adoption project. *Behavior Genetics, 9*, 177–207.

Huston, A.C. (1983). Sex-typing. In P.H. Mussen (Ed.), *Handbook of child psychology* (4th ed., Vol. 4, pp. 387–467). New York: Wiley.

Huston, A.C. (1985). The development of sex-typing. *Developmental Review, 5*, 1–17.

Jacobs, B.S., & Moss, H.A. (1976). Birth order and sex of sibling as determinants of mother-infant interaction. *Child Development, 47*, 315–322.

Kalter, N., & Rembar, J. (1981). The significance of a child's age at the time of parental divorce. *American Journal of Orthopsychiatry, 51*, 85–100.

Kelly, J.B., & Wallerstein, J.S. (1975). The effects of parental divorce. *American Journal of Orthopsychiatry, 45*, 253–254.

Kohlberg, L.K. (1966). A cognitive-developmental analysis of children's sex-role concepts and attitudes. In E.E. Maccoby (Ed.), *The development of sex differences* (pp. 82–172). Stanford, CA: Stanford University Press.

Lahey, B.B., Hammer, D., Crumrine, P.L., & Forehand, R.L. (1980). Birth Order × Sex interactions in child behavior problems. *Developmental Psychology, 16*, 608–615.

Lamb, M.E. (1977, July). *The relationships between mothers, fathers, infants and siblings in the first two years of life*. Paper presented at the biennial conference of the International Society for the Study of Behavioral Development, Pavia, Italy.

Lamb, M.E. (1978). Interactions between 18-month-olds and their pre-school-aged siblings. *Child Development, 49*, 51–59.

Lamb, M.E. (1987). Niche picking by siblings and scientists. *Behavioral and Brain Sciences, 10*, 30.

Lamb, M.E., & Bornstein, M.H. (1986). *Development in infancy* (2nd ed.) New York: Random House.

Langlois, J.H. (1986). From the eye of the beholder to behavioral reality: Development of social behaviors and social relations as a function of physical attractiveness. In C.P. Herman, M.P. Zanna, & E.T. Higgins (Eds.), *Ontario symposium on personality and social psychology* (Vol. 3, pp. 23–51). Hillsdale, NJ: Erlbaum.

Langlois, J.H., & Casey, R.C. (1984, March). *Baby beautiful: The relationship between infant physical attractiveness and maternal behavior.* Paper presented at the fourth biennial International Conference on Infant Studies, New York.

Langlois, J.H., & Downs, A.C. (1979). Peer relations as a function of physical attractiveness: The eye of the beholder or behavioral reality? *Child Development, 50*, 409–418.

Lasko, J.K. (1954). Parent behavior toward first and second children. *Genetic Psychology Monographs, 49*, 97–137.

Lenerz, K., Kucher, J.S., East, P.L., Lerner, J.V., & Lerner, R.M. (1987). Early adolescents' physical organismic characteristics and psychosocial functioning: Findings from the Pennsylvania early adolescent transition study (PEATS). In R.M. Lerner & T.T. Foch (Eds.), *Biological-psychosocial interactions in early adolescence* (pp. 225–248). Hillsdale, NJ: Erlbaum.

Lerner, J.V., & Galambos, N.J. (1986). Temperament and maternal employment. In J.V. Lerner & R.M. Lerner (Eds.), *Temperament and social interaction in infants and children: New directions for child development* (pp. 75–88). San Francisco: Jossey-Bass.

Lerner, R.M. (1986). *Concepts and theories of human development* (2nd ed.) New York: Random House.

Lerner, R.M. (1987). A life-span perspective for early adolescence. In R.M. Lerner & T.T. Foch (Eds.), *Biological-psychosocial interactions in early adolescence* (pp. 9–34). Hillsdale, NJ: Erlbaum.

Lerner, R.M., & Spanier, G.D. (Eds.). (1978). *Contributions of the child to marital quality and family interaction through the life span.* San Diego, CA: Academic Press.

Lewin, KA. (1935). *A dynamic theory of personality.* New York: McGraw-Hill.

Lewis, M., & Kreitzberg, V.S. (1979). Effects of birth order and spacing on mother-infant interactions. *Developmental Psychology, 15*, 617–625.

Lewontin, R.C., Rose, S., & Kamin, K.J. (1984). *Not in our genes.* New York: Pantheon Books.

Lobato, D. (1983). Siblings of handicapped children: A review. *Journal of Autism and Developmental Disorders, 13*, 347–364.

Loehlin, J.C. (1987). Twin studies, environment differences, age changes. *Behavioral and Brain Sciences, 10*, 30–31.

Loehlin, J.C. (1989, May), *Personality resemblance and personality change in adoptive families: Evidence from the Texas Adoption Project.* Paper presented at the Society of Biological Psychiatry Annual Meeting, San Francisco.

Loehlin, J.C., Willerman, L., & Horn, J.M. (1985). Personality resemblances in adoptive families when children are late-adolescent or adult. *Journal of Personality and Social Psychology, 39*, 101–133.

Lounsbury, M.L., & Bates, J.E. (1982). The cries of infants of differing levels of perceived temperamental difficulties: Acoustic properties and effects on listeners. *Child Development, 53*, 677–686.

Lykken, D.T. (1987). An alternative explanation for low or zero sib correlations. *Behavioral and Brain Sciences, 10*, 31.

Lytton, H. (1977). Do parents create, or respond to, differences in twins? *Developmental Psychology, 13*, 456–459.

Maccoby, E.E. (1989, August). *Gender and relationships: A developmental account.* Invited address presented at the 97th Annual Convention of the American Psychological Association, New Orleans, LA.

Maccoby, E.E., & Jacklin, C.N. (1974). *The psychology of sex differences.* Stanford, CA: Stanford University Press.

Maccoby, E.E., & Masters, J.C. (1970). Attachment and dependency. In P.H. Mussen (Ed.), *Charmichael's manual of child psychology* (Vol. 2, pp. 73–158). New York: Wiley.

Malatesta, C.Z., Culver, C., Tesman, J.R., & Shepard, B. (1989). The development of emotion expression during the first two years of life. *Monographs of the Society for Research in Child Development 54*(1–2, Serial No. 219).

Masters, J.C., & Furman, W. (1981). Popularity, individual friendship selection, and specific peer interactions among children. *Developmental Psychology, 17*, 344–370.

Miller, N., & Maruyama, G. (1976). Ordinal position and peer popularity. *Journal of Personality and Social Psychology, 33*, 123–131.

Miller, W., & Newman, L. (Eds.). (1978). *The first child and family formation.* Chapel Hill NC,: University of North Carolina Press.

Minton, C., Kagan, J., & Levine, J.A. (1971). Maternal control and obedience in the two-year old. *Child Development, 42*, 1873–1894.

Mischel, W. (1973). Toward a cognitive social learning reconceptualization of personality. *Psychological Review, 80*, 252–283.

Moss, H.A. (1967). Sex, age, and state as determinants of mother-infant interaction. *Merrill-Palmer Quarterly, 13*, 19–36.

Nowicki, S., & Strickland, B.R. (1973). A locus of control scale for children. *Journal of Consulting and Clinical Psychology, 40*, 148–154.

Parke, R.D., & Sawin, D. (1975, April). *Infant characteristics and behavior as elicitors of maternal and paternal responsibility in the newborn period.* Paper presented at the biennial meeting of Society for Research in Child Development, Denver, CO.

Patterson, G.R. (1976). The aggressive child: Victim and architect of a coercive system. In E.J. Mash, L.A. Hamerlyncck, & L.C. Handy (Eds.), *Behavior modification and families: Vol. 1. Theory and research* (pp. 218–239). New York: Brunner/Mazel.

Patterson, G.R., & Dishion, T.J. (1988). Multilevel family process models: Traits, interactions, and relationships. In R. Hinde & J. Stevenson-Hinde (Eds.), *Relationships within families: Mutual influences* (pp. 283–310). Oxford, England: Clarendon Press.

Pepler, D., Corter, C., & Abramovitch, R. (1982) Social relations among children: Siblings and peers. In K. Rubin & H. Ross (Eds.), *Peer relationships and social skills in childhood* (pp. 209–227). New York: Springer-Verlag.

Pless, I.B. (1984). Clinical assessment: Physical and psychological functioning. *Pediatric Clinics of North America, 31*, 33–45.

Plomin, R., & Daniels, D. (1987). Why are children in the same family so different from one another? *Behavioral and Brain Sciences, 10*, 1–22.

Plomin, R., & Defrieds, J.C. (1985). *Origins of individual differences in infancy: The Colorado adoption project.* San Diego, CA: Academic Press.

Plomin, R., Foch, T.T., & Rowe, D.C. (1981). Bobo clown aggression in childhood: Environment not genes. *Journal of Research in Personality, 15*, 331–342.

Rheingold, H.L., & Cook, K.V. (1975). The contents of boys' and girls' rooms as an index of parents' behavior. *Child Development, 46*, 459–463.

Rose, R.J., & Kaprio, J. (1987). Shared experience and similarity of personality: Positive data from Finnish and American twins. *Behavioral and Brain Sciences, 10*, 35–36.

Rothbard, M.K. (1971). Birth order and mother-child interaction in an achievement situation. *Journal of Personality and Social Psychology, 17*, 113–120.

Rowe, D.C. (1987). The puzzle of nonshared environmental influences. *Behavioral and Brain Sciences, 10*, 37–38.

Ruble, D.N., Boggiano, A.K., Feldman, N.S., & Loebl, J.H. (1980). Developmental analysis of the role of social comparison in self-evaluation. *Developmental Psychology, 16*, 105–115.

Rutter, M. (1979). Maternal deprivation 1972–1978: New findings, new concepts, new approaches. *Child Development, 50*, 283–305.

Saegert, S., & Hart, R. (1976). The development of sex differences in the environmental competence of children. In P. Burnett (Ed.), *Women in society* (pp. 87–116). Chicago: Maaroufa Press.

Samuels, H.R. (1977, April). *The role of the sibling in the infant's social environment.* Paper presented at the biennial meeting of the Society for Research in Child Development, New Orleans, LA.

Scarr, S., & Carter-Saltzman, L. (1979). Twin method: Defense of a critical assumption. *Behavior Genetics, 9*, 527–542.

Scarr, S., & Kidd, K.K. (1983). Developmental behavior genetics. In P.H. Mussen (Ed.), *Handbook of child psychology: Vol. II. Infancy and developmental psychobiology* (4th ed., pp. 345–433). New York: Wiley.

Scarr, S., & McCartney, K. (1983). How people make their own environments. *Child Development, 54*, 425–435.

Scarr, S., Webber, P.L., Weinberg, R.A., & Wittig, M.A. (1981). Personality resemblance among adolescents and their parents in biologically related and adoptive families. *Journal of Personality and Social Psychology, 40*, 885–898.

Scarr, S., & Weinberg, R.A. (1983). The Minnesota adoption studies: Genetic differences and malleability. *Child Development, 54*, 260–267.

Scarr-Salapatek, S. (1971). Race, social class, and IQ. *Science, 174*, 1285–1295.

Schacter, F.F. (1982). Sibling deidentification and split-parent identification: A family tetrad. In M.E. Lamb & B. Sutton-Smith (Eds.), *Sibling relationships: Their nature and significance across the life-span* (pp. 123–152). Hillsdale, NJ: Erlbaum.

Schacter, S. (1963). Birth order, eminence, and higher education. *American Sociological Review, 2,* 757–767.

Seavey, C.A., Katz, P.A., & Zalk, S.R. (1975). Baby X: The effects of gender labels on adult responses to infants. *Sex Roles, 1,* 103–110.

Shaffer, D.R. (1987). *Social and personality development.* Pacific Grove, CA: Brooks/Cole.

Sigel, I. (Ed.). (1985). *Parental belief systems: The psychological consequences for children.* Hillsdale, NJ: Erlbaum.

Sorell, G.T., & Nowak, C.A. (1981). The role of physical attractiveness as a contributor to individual development. In R.M. Lerner & N.A. Bush-Rossnagel (Ed.), *Individuals as producers of their development* (pp. 389–446). San Diego, CA: Academic Press.

Stephan, C., & Langlois, J.H. (1984). Baby beautiful: Adult attributions of infant competence as a function of infant attractiveness. *Child Development, 55,* 576–585.

Strodtbeck, F.L. (1958). Family interaction, values, and achievement. In D.C. McClelland, A.L. Baldwin, U. Bronfenbrenner, & F.L. Strodtbeck (Eds.), *Talent and society* (pp. 135–194). Princeton, NJ: Van Nostrand Reinhold.

Stouffer, S.A., Suchman, E.A., DeVinney, L.C., Star, S.A., & Williams, R.M., Jr. (1949). *The American soldier, studies in social psychology in World War II* (Vol. 1). Princeton, NJ: Princeton University Press.

Styzynski, L.E. (1976). *Effects of physical characteristics on the social, emotional, and intellectual development of early school age children.* Unpublished doctoral dissertation, University of Texas at Austin.

Styczynski, L.E., & Langlois, J.H. (1980). *Judging the book by its cover: Children's attractiveness and achievement.* Unpublished manuscript, University of Texas at Austin.

Tellegen, A., Lykken, D.T., Bouchard, T.J., Wilcox, K.J., Segal, N.L., & Rich. S. (1988). Personality similarity in twins reared apart and together. *Journal of Personality and Social Psychology, 54,* 1031–1039.

Thoman, E.B., Leiderman, P.H., & Olson, J.P. (1972). Neonate-mother interactions during breast feeding. *Developmental Psychology, 6,* 110–118.

Thompson, R.A. (1986). Temperament, emotionality and infant social cognition. In J.V. Lerner & R.M. Lerner (Eds.), *Temperament and social interaction in infants and children. New directions for child development* (pp. 35–52). San Francisco: Jossey-Bass.

Wachs, T.D. (1983). The use and abuse of environment in behavior-genetic research. *Child Development, 54,* 396–407.

Wachs, T.D. (1987). The relevance of the concept of unshared environment to the study of environmental influences: A paradigmatic shift or just some gears slipping? *Behavioral and Brain Sciences, 10,* 41–42.

Wachs, T.D., & Gruen, C.E. (1982). *Early experience and human development.* New York: Plenum Press.

Wallerstein, J.S., & Kelly, J.B. (1979). Children and divorce: A review. *Social Work, 13,* 468–475.

Weinraub, M., & Jaeger, E. (1990). The timing of the mother's return to the work place: Effects on the developing mother-infant relationship. In J.S. Hyde & M.J. Essex (Eds.),

Parental leave and child care: Setting a research and policy agenda (pp. 28–37). Philadelphia: Temple University Press.

Weiss, R.S. (1979). Growin up a little faster. *Journal of Social Issues, 35*, 97–111.

Wiesenfeld, A.R., & Malatesta, C.Z. (1982). Infant distress. In L.W. Hoffman, R.J. Gandelman, & H.R. Shiffman (Eds.), *Parenting, its causes and consequences* (pp. 123–139). Hillsdale, NJ: Erlbaum.

Yarrow, L.J. (1964). Separation from parents during early childhood. In M.L. Hoffman & L.W. Hoffman (Eds.), *Review of child development research* (Vol. 1, pp. 89–136). New York: Russell Sage Foundation.

Yarrow, L.J., Goodwin, M.S., Manheimer, H., & Milowe, I.D. (1973). Infancy experiences and cognitive and personality development at ten years. In L.J. Stone, H.T. Smith, & L.B. Murphy (Eds.), *The competent infant: Research and commentary* (pp. 1274–1281). New York: Basic Books.

Zajonc, R.B. (1983). Validating the confluence model. *Psychological Bulletin, 93*, 457–480.

7

The Development of the Subconcepts of Death in Young Children: A Short-Term Longitudinal Study

Alice Lazar

Montgomery County Public Schools, Rockville, Maryland

Judith Torney-Purta

University of Maryland, College Park

A short-term longitudinal design and the probabilistic latent class method of analysis were used to study the development of young children's understanding of death, 99 first and second graders were interviewed individually in the fall and spring. The results support the notion that the subconcepts of death—irreversibility, cessation, causality, and inevitability—need to be studied separately and in relation to one another. Children first understand the subconcepts of irreversibility and inevitability. Development of these subconcepts does not seem to be conditional on each other. However, at least one of these subconcepts must be understood before the child understands the subconcepts of cessation or causality. The pattern of development of these subconcepts is different when the referent object is human versus animal. The overall methodology offers promise in understanding the development of these concepts in young children.

In the last 25 years, death has become a more acceptable topic of study. The relevance of the child's conceptualization of death became even more timely as hun-

Reprinted with permission from *Child Development*, 1991, Vol. 62, 1321–1333. Copyright ©1991 by the Society for Research in Child Development, Inc.

This study is based on a portion of the first author's doctoral dissertation, conducted under the supervision of the second author. The participation of the parents and children at the Charles E. Smith Jewish Day School, Blessed Sacrament, and Our Lady of Lourdes Elementary schools is acknowledged with gratitude. Thanks are also expressed to Kathleen Galdi and Esther Starobin for their help in collecting and analyzing the data.

dreds of thousands of schoolchildren witnessed the death of the astronauts, including a teacher, in the *Challenger* space shuttle. Parents and teachers alike were unsure of what the children understood in regard to this tragedy, and how to discuss it with them. Those who are concerned with helping children adjust to bereavement have emphasized the child's cognitive understanding of death as affecting his or her adjustment (e.g., Furman, 1974; Smilansky, 1981a). Others say that accidents, a major cause of death of children, may be more frequent if the child does not comprehend the finality of death (e.g., McIntire, Angle, & Struempler, 1972). Also, suicide gestures may be used for getting attention when the child does not see death as irreversible (Orbach & Glaubman, 1978, 1979).

The findings of research on children's understanding of death have suffered from flaws in design. First, because of the sensitivity of the topic, many of the studies use more highly selective samples than are used in other research areas. For example, Lazar (1985) and Townley and Thornburg (1980) received permission to conduct interviews with children from less than 25% of the parent populations polled. Koocher (1974) and Yalom (1980) point out the difficulties of obtaining clearance from human-subjects research committees and school boards for doing studies involving explicit questioning of young children about death.

A second factor contributing to the limitations of the data is methodology. Many researchers in this area have attempted to integrate the concept of death into a Piagetian framework, without considering other aspects. Stambrook and Parker (1987) reviewed the relevant literature and suggested that the variability of findings may be related to sociocultural factors, further confounded by the use of cross-sectional data.

In addition, some studies suggest that a child's understanding of death appears to be affected by the type of object being referred to, and other task requirements are also influential (Candy-Gibbs, Sharp, & Petrun, 1985; Richards & Siegler, 1984). The child may use different structures and processes when responding to animals and humans (Gelman & Spelke, 1981). Orbach, Talmon, Kedem, and Har-Even (1987) found different basic sequential patterns of development of five subconcepts depending on the referent object—humans or animals. Also, children understand a great deal more than they can express verbally, and therefore there is the need for an inquiry that will draw out meaningful information (Yalom, 1980).

A third factor contributing to the lack of understanding in this area is that most investigations have examined only one or two aspects of the concept of death. A review of the literature by Speece and Brent (1984) identified three subconcepts to be included in a definition of a "mature" understanding of death. They omitted a component, "causality," found to be significant by others, suggesting at least four subconcepts to be studied. The way they are measured is frequently not similar from study to study. The following are definitions of the four subconcepts, with some examples of methodology and related findings.

Irreversibility —This involves the child's ability to conceptualize that the dead never can come back to life. Studies show discrepant results. White, Elsom, and Prawat (1978) found that less than half of their fourth graders understood irreversibility when responding to questions about a character in a story read to them. In contrast, Swain (1979) found that almost every child after the age of 4 said that death was irreversible. She interviewed children using a semi-structured format that allowed the subjects to explain their responses. In one study, children were asked questions like, "How can you make dead things come back to life?" which appeared to confuse many children (Koocher, 1973).

Cessation —This involves the child's ability to conceptualize that all biological, sensational, emotional, and cognitive functions have ceased. When answering questions in a structured interview (McIntire et al., 1972), about two-thirds of subjects aged 5 to 10 years understood this completely. However, only about one-half of White, Elsom, and Prawat's 9- and 10-year-olds were classified as understanding this concept. Most Israeli 4-year-olds found it easier to grasp cessation of processes such as sight, hearing, and motion but had difficulty verbalizing cessation in regard to feeling, thought, and consciousness. Most children of 5, in response to a standardized interview (Smilansky, 1987), showed a mature understanding of the subconcept of cessation. Results of other individual interviews found a developmental sequence of cessation: Children first realize that the dead cannot eat or speak. As they grow older, they understand the less obvious dysfunctions, that is, that the dead cannot drink or hear. Older children said the dead cannot feel cold or smell flowers, and still older ones said that the dead cannot dream or know they are dead (Kane, 1979).

Causality —This involves the child's ability to understand the objective causes of death. Some studies found that young children use immanent-justice notions to explain death (Gartley & Bernasconi, 1967). It has also been suggested that younger children give more external causes (e.g., "They get shot," "They have an accident"), while older ones give more internal causes (e.g., "They have heart attacks or cancer," "They get old")(Wass, 1984).

Inevitability —This involves the child's ability to conceptualize the idea that death is universal and inevitable, including the fact that he or she too will die. Most studies (e.g., Childers & Wimmer, 1971; Gartley & Bernasconi, 1967; Swain, 1979) found that more than half of children from 6 to 7 years of age and above understand that subconcept.

There are just a few studies that examined all of these concepts. Smilansky's (1987) extensive, but cross-sectional, research with Israeli 4–10-year-olds showed an earlier understanding of death concepts by this sample than would be predicted from many of the studies in the literature. A recent study (Schonfeld & Smilansky, 1989) compared her data from the lower socioeconomic class with a similar

American sample. The findings suggest that Israeli children understand the subconcepts of irreversibility and cessation before American children do. These studies thus support the hypothesis that the subconcepts are learned differentially, and suggest a developmental progression of the subconcepts. However, they did not interpret the evidence as indicating a structural interrelation of the subconcepts. Smilansky's data suggest that for Israeli children, irreversibility is understood first, cessation next, inevitability after that, and causality last.

Walco (1982) also examined the component attributes of the concept of death. The subconcepts were defined similarly to Smilansky's. He also found that the subconcepts develop independently without evidence of a specific structural interrelation. Orbach et al. (1987) used Smilansky's questionnaire and cross-sectional data in an attempt to identify sequential patterns of development of the subconcepts. Their findings suggest that the order appears to be irreversibility, inevitability, cessation, and causality. When a fifth concept, old age, was considered, referent-object differences were found. That is, children seemed to understand this concept first when asked about human death, but later (between cessation and causality) in regard to animal death.

Hoffman and Strauss's (1985) data suggest that universality (i.e., inevitability, as defined here) is understood first, followed by cessation, irreversibility, and causality. They say that understanding the inevitability of the biological act of death is a separate subconcept, and that this develops last.

To fully understand the development of the concept of death in children, one needs to look at each of the subconcepts both separately and in relation to each other. Investigation of the development of the understanding of the subconcepts of death should also attempt to determine whether there is a consistent pattern of development for the majority of children. Previous studies used cross-sectional samples, which did not allow for such analysis (Stambrook & Parker, 1987).

This short-term longitudinal study studied the development of each subconcept both over time and in relation to the other subconcepts. It investigated the development of the child's conceptualization of death by looking at the subconcepts of irreversibility, cessation, causality, and inevitability to answer the following question: What developmental changes take place in the understanding and organization of the subconcepts of death in first and second graders during a 7-month period? This age range was chosen as previous research suggested that there is a consolidation of the understanding of these subconcepts in 6- and 7-year-old children (Speece & Brent, 1984).

Specifically, what are the patterns of change when the same children's responses are evaluated at two different times? Is there a consistent hierarchial structure in the development of the subconcepts, such that certain subconcepts tend to develop before or are prerequisite to others?

METHOD

Subjects

Introductory letters were sent to the principles of a conservative Jewish elementary school and two Roman Catholic elementary schools serving the same upper-middle-class populations in the suburbs of Washington, DC. Approximately 97% of the children were white.

Letters and parent surveys were sent to parents of all of the first and second graders. Parents were asked to complete a parent survey, but only those children for whom parents also gave written consent were interviewed. As an incentive to respond, parents were told that a donation to the Christa McAuliffe Scholarship Fund would be made in the name of the class at each school returning the most surveys (without reference to whether permission was given or withheld). The first set of data was collected in October of 1986; the second, in May of 1987.

The parent survey was designed to furnish demographic information regarding the population as a whole and to identify variables that discriminated between those parents who gave permission for the child's participation in the study and those who did not. Included on the permission form was a request that parents not prime their children for the interview.

Slightly over 40% of the total group responded by returning the parent survey; approximately 30% of the total group of parents gave permission for their children to be interviewed. Of the 141 respondents, eight did not complete the parent survey. Although permission was given to interview 103 children, two were not fluent in English, and for two, the parent surveys were received after the first interviews were completed. Therefore, 99 children were interviewed. At the time of collection of the second set of data, one subject had moved, thus reducing the Time 2 sample to 98. In no case had a child in the sample suffered the death of a parent or a sibling.

The mean educational level for the parents was between completion of a college degree and postgraduate studies. The PPVT-R, form M (Dunn & Dunn, 1981a) was also administered to each child participating in the first interview. This test yields an age-equivalent, receptive-language score (Dunn & Dunn, 1981b). The child sample as a whole had a receptive-language score of 8 1/2 years, that is, 1 to 2 years higher than their chronological ages (i.e., mean age equivalent, in months, of 102.60; standard deviation of 19.25).

A comparison of those children for whom parents gave permission to participate in the interview with those who did not indicated that there were no differences between the groups on religion, degree of religiosity, parents' education level, grade, gender, experience with human or animal death, or the number of situations where death was discussed. Responses to the second parent survey, after the Time 2 interview, revealed that very few children mentioned having been interviewed at either time. The only two parents who said that they remembered their children talking about their reaction to the interview reported that the children had remarked that the questions reminded them of the death of their pets.

Child Interview

The research instrument used with the children was the Questionnaire for Examination of Development of the Concept of Death, by Smilansky (1981b), which had been translated into English. It offers a positive methodological alternative to much other research, as its mode of inquiry is structured while still seeking and basing the scoring on the reasoning underlying "yes/no" responses. This interview also looks at the various aspects of the overall concept of death while controlling for the referent object; the same questions were asked regarding human and animal death.

The questionnaire explored the children's understanding of the four subconcepts of death, with the following questions: (1) *irreversibility* (no. 4)—"If a person/dog dies and has been buried in his grave for a long time, can he become a living person/dog again? Why?" (no. 5)—"If a person/dog dies and has not been buried yet, can he be a living person/dog again? Why?" (2) *cessation* (nos. 2, 3, 6, 7, 8)—"Can a dead person/dog see [hear, move, know, feel]? Why?" (3) *causality* (no. 1)—"What kinds of things do people/dogs die of? What are some reasons [causes] that people/dogs die of?" and (4) *inevitability* (no. 9)—"Does everyone/every dog die? Why? Will you/your pet die?"

Each subconcept was scored 0 to 3, according to Smilansky's criteria. For example, a score of 3 points for irreversibility requires two correct answers and two correct explanations. A score of 2 points is given where there are two correct answers (i.e., "no") and only one correct explanation; the second explanation was either omitted or insufficient. A score of 1 point is where there is one correct response with a correct explanation, or two correct answers, but neither explanation is correct. A score of zero is given when the child answered two wrong or gave no response. To receive a score of 3 for the subconcept of cessation, the child must say "no" to all the related questions and give all correct explanations. Two points are given when either one of the answers is wrong or one of the explanations shows a lack of understanding. Each wrong explanation voids a correct response. One point is given if two of the answers are not correct or the explanations are wrong. A zero is given when there are three or less correct answers. For the subconcept of causality, the child must respond "old age" and one other cause to receive 3 points. A score of 2 points is given where the only response is "old age." One point is given for one or more correct answers without "old age." A score of zero is given for no correct response. For 3 points on the subconcept of inevitability, the child must show understanding of the universality of death—that all people/animals die, without exception. Two points are given when the child says that everybody/every animal is going to die but him or her, only old people die, or only old people die and he or she will die when he or she gets old. A score of 2 points is also given for a response that all people/animals die, without a correct explanation. One point is given when the child gives other general ideas of groups dying for reasons other than old age (e.g., "No, just sick people") and when the child generalizes to others beyond himself/herself (e.g., "Yes, except for me and my parents/pet"). A score of zero is given when the child responds, "No one has to die."

For purposes of the scaling involved in this study, each response was then scored as "concept mastered" (i.e., a perfect score of 3) or "concept not mastered" (i.e., a score of less than 3).

Smilansky, using large Israeli samples, found test-retest reliability based on a 6-week interval to be .84. Also, an analysis of interitem consistency yielded a Cronbach alpha of .77. Factor analysis demonstrated that the four factors corresponding to these subconcepts together accounted for 67% of the variance.

Procedure

Each subject was interviewed individually in a room near the respective classrooms, with Smilansky's questionnaire, for approximately 15 min. The interviewer was a school psychologist with extensive experience relating to children. Questions were asked in a low-key manner, and responses were written down by the interviewer as they were given. Half the students answered the questions about animal death first; half answered the questions about human death first. Another school psychologist administered the PPVT-R, using the standardized instructions. This general procedure, without the PPVT-R, was repeated after 7 months.

Interrater Agreement

Using Smilansky's criteria, six independent judges were asked to score responses of 10 randomly chosen subjects. Percent agreement was 94%.

Analysis

The data analyzed here were eight scores (i.e., the four subconcepts related to human death and to animal death). To identify the developmental sequence of acquisition of the subconcepts, the probabilistic latent class model, as proposed by Dayton and Macready (1976), was used. This method involves a deterministic, model-fitting strategy rather than a hypothesis-testing strategy. As such, it provides a statistical assessment of fit of hypothesized hierarchies from which one can infer the order of acquisition of the various components. Model 5 (Dayton & Macready,

1978), which assumes that the error probabilities are constant across all items, was used to assess goodness of fit of several hypothesized hierarchical structures for Time 1 (October) data. Subsequently, the method was used to see if such pattern sequences were stable. That is, goodness of fit was then assessed for Time 2 (May) data for both referent objects (i.e., human and animal death). Specifically, the model requires that frequencies of possible response patterns "mastered/not mastered" for each subconcept he obtaining and then tested for viable fit to a hypothesized latent hierarchical structure. This model does not depend on the assumption of task equivalence (Dayton & Macready, 1976).

RESULTS

The Questionnaire

The internal consistency of the questionnaire measured by coefficient alpha appears to be adequate for three or the four subconcepts (alpha was .73, .81, .70 for irreversibility, cessation, and inevitability, respectively). This measure of reliability was low for the subconcept causality (alpha = .44). A coefficient of interitem reliability for the entire questionnaire was .68.

A statistical analysis to determine the impact of the order of presentation of human versus animal death questions on the overall scores resulted in F values of 1.32 and .26 comparing the means of total human and total animal scores, which were not significant ($p > .05$). Therefore, the rest of the analyses were conducted without regard to this variable. The order of questions within the animal/human set was not varied. It is important to note that although the order of questions within category was not randomized, the order of referent object (human and animal) was counterbalanced. This means, for example, that the question about causality of human death, was the first question asked for half the children but the eleventh question asked for the other half.

Results of the Analyses of Development

The study examined the development of children's understanding of death by analyzing the hierarchy of responses to the questions at the two interviews, held 7 months apart. The subconcepts of irreversibility, cessation, causality, and inevitability were analyzed individually and in relation to one another.

Table 1 presents the mean scores of the children for each of the subconcepts as they pertain to human and animal death at Time 1 and Time 2. There was no statistically significant difference between human and animal responses (i.e., t tests) in understanding of irreversibility and cessation. At Time 1, however, more children understood the subconcepts of causality an inevitability when the questions were

Table 1

Means and Standard Deviations of Subconcept Scores Related to
Human and Animal Death

	Mean Scores (Time 1)	t Values (H vs. A)	Mean Scores (Time 2)	t Values (T1 vs. T2)
Irreversibility:				
Human	2.50 (.85)	.67	2.58 (.77)	.94
Animal	2.55 (.78)		2.58 (.72)	.34
Cessation:				
Human	1.73 (1.20)	.63	2.09 (1.06)	2.78*
Animal	1.81 (1.20)		2.27 (1.05)	3.70*
Causality:				
Human	2.01 (.98)	4.87*	2.00 (1.00)	.09
Animal	1.45 (.92)		1.93 (1.03)	3.74*
Inevitability:				
Human	2.57 (.69)	3.54*	2.79 (.58)	3.13*
Animal	2.31 (.90)		2.76 (.54)	4.61*

NOTE.—Raw scores range from 0 to 3; *t* values of human vs. animals at Time 1 and differences between means Time 1 and Time 2; Time 1 n = 99 and Time 2 n = 98.
* $p < .05$.

asked pertaining to humans. They had relative difficulty understanding and/or explaining their understanding of these subconcepts when they were asked in regard to animal death. At Time 2, the gap appears to have closed between the referent objects for both causality and inevitability. However, at Time 2, the children's responses to questions regarding the cessation of different functions at death differed significantly for the two referent objects, with the higher score for the questions related to animal death.

Comparisons of mean subconcept scores at Time 1 and Time 2, related to both human and animal death, revealed that most of the scores improved significantly over time (see Table 1). Only understanding of irreversibility related to both referent objects, and causality as related to human death, did not improve over time. However, development during the 7-month time interval of this study made a difference in the child's understanding of cessation and inevitability related to human and animal death, and of causality related to animal death.

A summary of the results related to the individual subconcepts indicates that for the subconcept *irreversibility*, some children gave relatively sophisticated answers. For example, when asked if the dead person who is not buried can become a live person again, one child responded, "No, because still if he is not buried, it's the same thing. He can't experience himself." Some children gave more concrete responses. In response to whether the dead animal that was put in the trash can could come alive again, one child said, "He wouldn't want to be alive again because he would have to smell the trash can." However, most 6- and 7-year-old children understood this concept (consistent with a pilot study of Lazar, 1985; and Smilansky, 1987). The children's scores did not change significantly over the 7-month period (see Table 1), nor was there any difference associated with the referent object. Even at the time of the first interview, a majority of the children demonstrated mastery of the subconcept of irreversibility for both referent objects.

Cessation is a more complex subconcept. Five aspects of cessation were assessed: hearing, moving, seeing, knowing, and feeling. At Time 1, the children had difficulty with this concept as it relates both to humans and animals. Seven months later, the subjects had a significantly better understanding of this concept. At that time, 60% of the children had mastery of this subconcept when asked in regard to animal death, but only 47% demonstrated mastery for this subconcept as related to human death.

The subconcept of *causality* is measured by asking the child for reasons why people die. According to Smilansky, to show that one completely understands this subconcept, the child must give "old age" plus another cause of death. At Time 1, the children scored significantly lower on causality as related to animal death than for human-related death. At Time 2, the percentage of children demonstrating mastery of this subconcept in relation to human death remained just below 50%. However, scores for the animal-related data increased significantly from Time 1 to Time 2. These differences are probably what is contributing to the relatively low internal consistency of this variable in regard to animal death. The results have to be interpreted cautiously. The problem may be a function of Smilansky's definition of mastery of this subconcept: The child must indicate that one of the causes of death is "old age." Relatively few children at Time 1 gave "old age" as a cause of animal death.

In addition to "old age" the causes of death given by these 6- and 7-year-olds included AIDS, drugs, cancer, heart attacks, shooting, and poisoning. Some unusual responses were, "They fall off the Empire State Building; from the snow; from eating soap."

The subconcept of *inevitability* is measured by the child's ability to understand that everyone will die. There was significant improvement from Time 1 to Time 2 (see Table 1) in the children's understanding of this subconcept for both referent objects. Even at Time 1, a majority of the children demonstrated mastery of this subconcept. When asked why he thought everyone will die, one boy said, "Because if everyone lived to 555 there would be too many people on this planet and also they would get too big like a giant." Another child said everyone has to die because otherwise "the world would get filled up . . . and be squished." A more religious interpretation was that everyone dies because "Adam and Eve ate the apple. If they hadn't, everyone would live forever and there would be no guns or knives or old."

Developmental hierarchy of subconcepts The development of the subconcepts has rarely been studied in regard to their relation to one another. It is therefore difficult

Table 2
Percentage of Subjects Responding According to a Specific
Response Pattern of Four Subconcepts, Related to Human and
Animal Death, at Time 1 and Time 2

	HUMAN		ANIMAL	
PATTERN	Time 1	Time 2	Time 1	Time 2
---	10	4	11	7
R—	7	4	18	2
-S-......................	1	0	1	1
RS—......................	5	2	8	3
--C-......................	2	1	1	2
R-C-......................	5	0	3	0
-SC-......................	0	0	0	1
RSC-	4	4	5	0
---N......................	5	11	13	5
R--N	12	12	8	8
-S-N......................	3	1	2	5
RS-N	10	15	15	21
--CN	6	5	1*	5
R-CN......................	16	15	5	10
-SCN......................	3	4	1	4
RSCN......................	10	20	7	24

NOTE.—"-" = not mastered; R, S, C, or N = mastery of that sub-concept, where R = irreversibility, S = cessation, C = causality, and N = inevitability. The sequences are in backward binomial order. Time 1 $n = 99$, Time 2 $n = 98$.

to hypothesize an underlying developmental pattern or latent hierarchy with much certainty.

The hierarchies suggested by the literature and from the data were tested for fit using the probabilistic method for identifying latent developmental hierarchies. Table 2 presents the 16 possible response patterns, in backward binomial order, for the four subconcepts, related to humans and animals, at Time 1 and 2, and the percentage of subjects responding accordingly. The respective positions (following the questionnaire, and not necessarily related to any hypothesized developmental order) are: irreversibility (R), cessation (S), causality (C), and inevitability (N).

Table 3 indicates four hierarchies tested for viable fit of the data. The observed frequencies of the patterns were compared to hypothesized estimated probabilities. Then the Time 1 pattern goodness of fit was compared to the Time 2 data and/or the data of the other referent object to assess stability. The method used here is a deterministic one, and therefore the obtained probability values are guides by which one can assign a range of fit. Thus, a chi-square with a probability value of .20 or greater indicates good fit of the model to the data, a probability value

Table 3
Possible Latent Subconcept Hierarchies Tested for Viable Fit, Chi-Squares,
Degrees of Freedom, and Goodness of Fit

1 (Lit.)[a]	2 (Lit.)	3 (Hum. Data)	4 (Ani. Data)
----	----	----	----
R---	---N	R--N	R---
R--N	R--N	RS-N	---N
RS-N	RS-N	R-CN	RS-N
R-CN	S-CN	RSCN	RSCN
RSCN	RSCN		

Data Analyzed	Chi-Square	df	Goodness of Fit[c]
1 (literature based):[a]			
Time 1 human	2.33	8	Good
Time 2 human	20.40	8	Poor
Time 1 animal	19.64	8	Poor
Time 2 animal	15.63	8	Poor
2 (literature based):			
Time 1 human	3.31	8	Good
Time 2 human	8.33	8	Good
Time 1 animal	[b]		Indeterminant
Time 2 animal	7.85	8	Good
3 (Time 1 human data based):			
[Time 1 human	3.31	9	Good]
Time 2 human	21.26	9	Poor
Time 1 animal	71.72	9	Poor
Time 2 animal	13.67	9	Fair
4 (Time 1 animal data based):			
Time 1 human	[b]		Indeterminant
Time 2 human	37.34	9	Poor
[Time 1 animal	10.48	9	Good]
Time 2 animal	16.45	9	Fair

NOTE.—Time 1 n = 99, Time 2 n = 98.
[a] Criterion for hierarchy.
[b] Data did not fit within the boundaries of the model.
[c] Good, $p > .20$; fair, $p = .20$ to $.05$; poor, $p < .05$.

of .20 to .05 is indicative of fair fit, and a probability value of less then .05 is indicative of poor fit. In some cases the model did not determine any fit with the data (Dayton & Macready, 1976).

The first hypothesized subconcept sequence was suggested by the literature. It hypothesizes that irreversibility (R) is understood first, followed by comprehension of inevitability (N). After these two concepts are understood, the child then develops understanding of cessation (S) and/or causality (C). The Time 1 human-related data fit this pattern. Thus, the understanding of both irreversibility and inevitability appears to be a prerequisite for understanding of either of the other two. However, when this hierarchy was tested for stability with the Time 2 human-related data and both sets of animal-related data, poor fit was found. The criterion for the second hierarchical pattern was also suggested from the literature. Here, however, understanding of inevitability is thought to be first, and then irreversibility. This model also proposes that understanding of both cessation and causality develop later. Comprehension of the latter two subconcepts is not conditional on each other. As can be seen from Table 3, the Time 1 human-related data fit the model well. The good fit of the Time 2 human-related data suggests that the model is stable over time. What is also apparent is that the Time 1 animal-related data again did not fit the model at all, yet the Time 2 animal data fit well. These results suggest that development of the understanding of the subconcepts is referent-object dependent at first. However, once the child starts to generalize his or her understanding of these subconcepts, comprehension of the subconcepts related to animal death follows the same pattern as does the development of the understanding of the subconcepts as pertains to human death.

The criterion for the third set of sequential patterns is the Time 1 human-related data. It represents the sequences in which 12% or more of the subjects responded. The latent hierarchy proposed here is that understanding of irreversibility and inevitability occurs first. Understanding of both of them is necessary for either cessation or causality to be understood. It is similar to the first two proposed models, except that it does not hypothesize which subconcept is understood first. As this model was generated by the Time 1 human-related data, the fit to these data is an artifact. However, when tested with data from the later time period, this particular model is not stable. Also, as with the first two models, the Time 1 animal-related data do not fit the model. However, the Time 2 data for this referent object have fair fit with this model, again, supporting the idea that development of the understanding of the subconcepts is, at least at first, referent-object dependent.

The criterion for the last hierarchy tested for viable fit was the Time 1 animal-related data. It represents those sequences to which 13% or more of the subjects responded. This model suggests that either irreversibility or inevitability is understood first, and their understanding is not conditional on one another. However, this model says that understanding of cessation is conditional on the comprehension of both irreversibility and inevitability, and that understanding of cessation precedes understanding of causality. The results (see Table 3) are as expected based on the above findings. The human-related data did not fit the model at either time. The Time 2 animal data appear to fit only fairly well. The use of this analysis with the data-generated hierarchy tends to demonstrate again that, at first, understanding of the subconcepts is related to the referent object.

Although the model that best describes the pattern of development of the understanding of the subconcepts of death cannot be definitively specified, the results do suggest that studying the development of children's understanding of death as a global concept is inappropriate. Further, the referent object must be specified.

Table 4
Frequencies of Subjects Demonstrating Mastery of Cessation, According to
Whether They Had Mastered Inevitability and/or Irreversibility

	With Inevitability and/or Irreversibility		Without Inevitability and/or Irreversibility	
	Time 1	Time 2	Time 1	Time 2
Human:				
Cessation not mastered	51	47	12	5
Mastered	35	46	1	0
Animal:				
Cessation not mastered	48	30	12	9
Mastered	38	57	1	2

NOTE.—Time 1 n = 99, Time 2 n = 98.

The best-fitting hierarchical sequence appears to be that based on previous literature: Understanding of inevitability develops first, followed by irreversibility. Comprehension of cessation and causality develop later, and understanding of these two subconcepts is not conditional on each other. The data seem to confirm that understanding cessation and causality is dependent on understanding of irreversibility and/or inevitability.

Table 4 illustrates this in a different way. It presents the number of subjects demonstrating mastery of cessation according to whether they had mastered inevitability and/or irreversibility at Time 1 and Time 2 for each referent object. For the human data, only one subject demonstrated mastery of cessation without receiving a perfect scores on irreversibility and/or inevitability. The animal-related data yielded similar results.

Table 5 presents a similar frequency table regarding mastery of the subconcept causality. Only three subjects demonstrated mastery of causality, without mastery of either irreversibility or inevitability, related to human- or animal-related data, at Time 1 and Time 2.

Thus, the data support part of the developmental pattern: The understanding of cessation and causality is not dependent on each other but is dependent on the understanding of irreversibility and/or inevitability.

DISCUSSION

Children's understanding of death remains a topic that adults are reluctant to have broached with children. Although approximately 40% of the parent population polled responded to a mailed survey, less than one-third of all the parents permitted their children to participate in the interview. This is significantly below that for

Table 5
Frequencies of Subjects Demonstrating Mastery of Causality, According
to Whether They Had Mastered Inevitability and/or Irreversibility

	With Inevitability and/or Irreversibility		Without Inevitability and/or Irreversibility	
	Time 1	Time 2	Time 1	Time 2
Human:				
Causality not mastered	42	45	11	4
Mastered................................	43	48	3	1
Animal:				
Causality not mastered	63	44	10	8
Mastered................................	24	43	2	3

NOTE.—Time 1 n = 99, Time 2 n = 98.

other topics studied with young children (e.g., Perrin & Gerrity, 1981). Adults are reluctant to have children talk about death. However, when asked, "Do you ever think about death?" 83% of the children said that they do.

Ninety-nine 6- and 7-year-olds attending parochial schools were interviewed individually in the fall (Time 1) and spring (Time 2). The data were the responses to a structured interview that assessed children's understanding of four previously identified subconcepts of death (irreversibility, cessation, causality, and inevitability) in regard to both human and animal death. The questionnaire therefore met the criteria of an appropriate task requirement, while affording an opportunity to see if responses were a function of a referent object. Internal consistency was found to be adequate for all the subconcepts when measured for the questionnaire as a whole. Only the reliability of the subconcept of causality in regard to animal death appeared to be somewhat dubious.

Three of the four subconcepts were understood better when related to human death. It has previously been assumed that the child will begin to understand the concept in relation to animals and then later generalize it to humans. These data seem to support the opposite ordering. The only subconcept that seems to be understood better in regard to animal death is cessation. Perhaps this is because children have more actual visual experiences with death of an animal. For example, when a child sees a dead bird or squirrel in the street, he or she soon learns that the dead animal does not move. Few children have actually seen a dead person. This finding is consistent with McIntire et al.'s (1972) finding that children gave more realistic responses regarding what happens to the dead body of a pet than of a human.

The short-term longitudinal study allowed the examination of patterns of development of the subconcepts of death. Significant changes were noted within only

7 months, with many children showing mastery of most of the subconcepts at Time 2. Whether the Time 1 interview served to spur the child to seek some of the answers to the questions is not known. Almost all of the children said that they remembered the first interview. However, parents reported that they recalled hearing very little, if anything, about it. If the interview motivated the children to seek explanations or confirmation of their ideas, they apparently did not seek such help from their parents. Perhaps the initial interview was the catalyst for the modification and organization of vague ideas already part of the children's repertoire.

The responses to the questions related to the specific subconcepts indicated that a significant number of children understood causality related to animal death better at Time 2. Similarly, scores for cessation and inevitability related to both referent objects improved significantly over the 7 months. At Time 1, slightly more than half of the children understood inevitability, while at Time 2, almost every child understood this concept. However, even at Time 2, less than half the children were able to fully define causality related to human death. Although understanding of irreversibility did not significantly change over the 7-month period, it is important to note that 70% of the children understood this subconcept at Time 1.

Cessation appears to be a complex subconcept. The literature (e.g., Kane, 1979; Smilansky, 1987) suggests that some aspects of cessation are understood earlier than others. Differential development may have contributed to the initial low percentage of mastery, and merits further investigation. Also, it is interesting that although some children could correctly explain why a dead person cannot move or hear, when asked why they cannot see, they gave a more concrete response: "Because their eyes are closed." A higher level of language ability may be necessary to explain all the aspects of cessation.

Many previous studies attempted to get at what children understood about the subconcepts via indirect methods (e.g., drawings, confusing questions) and/or incomplete question sets (e.g., dealing with a subset of subconcepts). Smilansky's study was, at the time this study was designed, the most carefully piloted measure of questions devised to be clear to children, and it was also the one that represented the best possibility for reliability of scoring. Smilansky and others (e.g., Hoffman & Strauss, 1985) have used a format that helps elicit from young children the most relevant understanding of the subconcepts. Questions measuring the four subconcepts were interspersed in the interview. A different number of questions was necessary to maximize measurement of the children's understanding of the subconcepts. Because task equivalence of the questions has not been investigated, an analytic technique that did not make this assumption was employed.

A probabilistic model was used to identify a possible underlying structure to the development of the subconcepts of death. It appears that children first understand the subconcepts of irreversibility and inevitability, and that their development does not seem to be conditional on one another. However, one or both of these subconcepts need to be understood before the child understands the subconcepts of cessation and/or causality.

One alternative explanation is that these results are an artifact of the order in which the questions were presented. However, the order of each group of questions (i.e., for human and animal death) was counterbalanced, and a comparison of scores showed no difference related to that order of presentation. Further, the most viable developmental sequence of subconcepts suggested by the analysis does not correspond to the orders of questions in the interview. A future study might more fully rule out a priming hypotheses by further counterbalancing order within referent category.

At first, the rate of development of the subconcepts seems to be different, depending on whether the referent object is human or animal. As the child starts to generalize his or her understanding of the subconcepts, hierarchies of response related to animal death begin to follow the same pattern as does the development of the understanding of the subconcepts pertaining to human death. Statements about the identified developmental patterns are tentative. There were 16 possible patterns for these data, and a relatively large number of children understood most of the subconcepts at Time 2. Future research data from children somewhat younger would provide a better picture of the development of the subconcepts.

Alternatively, using 6- and 7-year-old subjects who are more representative, intellectually and socioeconomically, of the population as a whole would confirm whether these results were generalizable to most children at this age.

The scoring criteria established by Smilansky should also be reconsidered. She defined understanding of causality as being able to tell that the cause of death is "old age" and at least one other cause. The criterion of "old age" may be thought of as an attempt to construct a continuum matching other things known about children's developing cognition, progressing from external, concrete, and visible causes (e.g., accidents) to integrate internal causes involving biological processes (such as aging). However, the signs typically identified with old age, such as graying or wrinkles, are not readily recognized in animals. To children, frailty may be associated with illness rather than old age. Size also may be considered as a variable related to age or growth. However, this dimension may not be readily recognized by a young child in relation to a pet. Further, "old age," in and of itself, may not be a cause of death but rather be correlated with factors that cause death. Carey (1985) suggests that the types of responses given by most 6- and 7-year-olds are things that happen to people (e.g., "get shot") or disease that people contract. She suggests that at this age, the child does not conceptualize death in regard to what happens within the body as a result of these external events or as a result of aging. If the questions/scoring were modified accordingly, it might be that the subconcept of causality develops last. This is clearly a field in which better measures are needed. Such measures might well be based on the kind of analysis presented here, retaining the questions from Smilansky that appear valuable and developing new questions and scoring criteria for other subconcepts. The issue of differences in performance demands of the subconcept tasks should also be addressed in further measurement development.

The results support the hypothesis that studying the development of the concept of death, as a global concept, is inappropriate. The subconcepts do develop differentially, and an investigation of their development must study them separately and in relation to one another. The results also reinforce the need to examine children's response to questions related to different referent objects when attempting to understand the development of such subconcepts in young children. This investigation indicates that the short-term longitudinal design, together with the probabilistic method, offers a viable model for future research.

It appears that although children have limited direct experience with death, they are integrating ideas and experiences and are developing an understanding of related subconcepts. The best way to measure such understanding is to ask direct questions that will elicit such information from young children. Although many adults continue to be reluctant to broach the topic of death with children, most children are thinking about death and developing an understanding of the subconcepts associated with it.

REFERENCES

Candy-Gibbs, S.E., Sharp, K.C., & Petrun, C.J. (1985). The effects of age, object, and cultural/religious background on children's concepts of death. *Omega*, 15, 329–346.

Carey, S. (1985). *Conceptual change in childhood*. Cambridge, MA: MIT Press.

Childers, P., & Wimmer, M. (1971). The concept of death in early childhood. *Child Development*, 42, 1299–1301.

Dayton, D.M., & Macready, G.B. (1976). A probabilistic model for validation of behavioral hierarchies. *Psychometrika*, 41, 189–204.

Dunn, L.M., & Dunn, L.M. (1981a). *Peabody Picture Vocabulary Test—revised: Form M*. Circle Pines, MN: American Guidance Service.

Dunn, L.M., & Dunn, L.M. (1981b). *Peabody Picture Vocabulary Test—revised: Manual for Forms L and M*. Circle Pines, MN: American Guidance Service.

Furman, E. (1974). *A child's parent dies: Studies in childhood bereavement*. New Haven, CT: Yale University Press.

Gartley, W., & Bernasconi, M. (1967). The concept of death in children. *Journal of Genetic Psychology*, 110, 71–85.

Gelman, R., & Spelke, E. (1981). The development of thought about animate and inanimate objects: Implications for research on social cognition. In J. Flavell & L. Ross (Eds.) *Social cognitive development* (pp. 43–66). New York: Cambridge University Press.

Hoffman, S.I., & Strauss, S. (1985). The development of children's concepts of death. *Death Studies*, 9, 469–482.

Kane, B. (1979). Children's concepts of death. *Journal of Genetic Psychology*, 134, 141–153.

Koocher, G.P. (1973). Childhood, death, and cognitive development. *Developmental Psychology*, 9, 369–375.

Koocher, G.P. (1974). Conversations with children about death—ethical considerations in research. *Journal of Clinical Child Psychology*, 3, 19–21.

Lazar, A. (1985). *Preschoolers, first, and third-grade children's understanding of the sub-concepts of death—a comparative study.* Unpublished manuscript, available from author.

McIntire, M.S., Angle, C.R., & Struempler, L.J. (1972). The concept of death in Midwestern children and youth. *American Journal of Diseases of Children*, 123, 527–532.

Orbach, I., & Glaubman, H. (1978). Suicidal aggressive and normal children's perception of personal and interpersonal death. *Journal of CLinical Psychology*, 34, 850–857.

Orbach, I., & Glaubman, H. (1979). Children's perception of death as a defensive process. *Journal of Abnormal Psychology*, 88, 671–674.

Orbach, I., Talmon, O., Kedem, P., & Har-Even, D. (1987). Sequential patterns of five sub-concepts of human and animal death in children. *Journal of the American Academy of Child and Adolescent Psychiatry*, 26, 578–582.

Perrin, E.C., & Gerrity, P.S. (1981). There's a demon in your belly: Children's understanding of illness. *Pediatrics*, 67, 841–849.

Richards, D.D., & Siegler, R.S. (1984). The effects of task requirements on children's life judgments. *Child Development*, 55, 1687–1696.

Schonfeld, D.J., & Smilansky, S. (1989). A cross-cultural comparison of Israeli and American children's death concepts. *Death Studies*, 13, 593–604.

Smilansky, S. (1981a). Different mourning patterns and the orphan's utilization of his intellectual ability to understand the concept of death. *Advances in Thanatology*, 5, 39–55.

Smilansky, S. (1981b). *Manual for questionnaire of the development of death conceptualization.* Unpublished manuscript, Tel Aviv University, Department of Psychology, Tel Aviv.

Smilansky, S. (1987). *On death: Helping children understand and cope.* New York: Peter Lang.

Speece, M.W., & Brent, S.B. (1984). Children's understanding of death: A review of three components of a death concept. *Child Development*, 55, 1671–1686.

Stambrook, M., & Parker, K.C.H. (1987). The development of the concept of death in childhood: A review of the literature. *Merrill-Palmer Quarterly*, 33, 133–157.

Swain, H. (1979). Childhood views of death. *Death Education*, 2, 341–358.

Townley, K. & Thronburg, K.R. (1980). Maturation of the concept of death in elementary school children. *Educational Research Quarterly*, 5, 17–24.

Walco, G. (1982). *Children's concepts of death: A cognitive training study.* Paper presented at the 90th annual convention of APA, Washington, DC.

Wass, H. (1984). Concepts of death: A developmental perspective. In H. Wass & C.A. Corr (Eds.), *Childhood and death* (pp. 3–24). Washington, DC: Hemisphere.

White, E., Elsom, B., & Prawat, R. (1978). Children's conceptions of death. *Child Development*, 49, 307–310.

Yalom, I.D. (1980). *Existential psychotherapy.* New York: Basic.

Part II
VULNERABILITY AND COMPETENCE

The articles in this section represent the increasing literature on stress and resilience. They deal with stressors that place children at risk for poor outcomes, resilience, and with ways of promoting positive adaptations.

In the first article, Terr theorizes about the stress of psychic trauma and the characteristics that the majority of children display. Childhood trauma is defined as one sudden external blow to the psyche (Type I) or a series of blows (Type II) that are beyond the child's capacity for coping. Clinical cases studied include the traumas of sexual abuse, kidnapping, and witness to murder. Four common symptoms observed are visualized or otherwise repeatedly perceived memories, repetitive behaviors, trauma-specific fears, and changed attitudes about people and the future. Additional features characteristic of Type I and Type II traumas and the implications of trauma for subsequent psychiatric diagnosis, including multiple personality, are described.

The next paper represents an innovative collaborative effort that focuses on one specific stress—physical child abuse. By combining across two studies, using similar measures but demographically different samples, Trickett, Aber, Carlson, and Cicchetti are able to describe the interaction of SES with parenting style, abuse, and developmental outcomes. Data on a total of 132 4- to 8-year-old abused and comparison children and their mothers were available. There were two measures of child-rearing context. The developmental outcomes assessed were receptive vocabulary and behavioral problems. Results indicate that the effects of maltreatment are distinguishable from those of low socioeconomic class. However, abuse-comparison differences were greater for the working class than for the low-income group. The findings have implications for programs tailored to groups at risk for child abuse.

Focusing on multiple contextual risk factors, Barocas, Seifer, Sameroff, Andrews, Croft, and Ostrow examine attentional and cognitive outcomes among preschoolers. The data were derived from a longitudinal study of mothers with varying degrees of mental illness and their children. Overall, the greater the level of environmental risk, the lower will be the intellectual performance of the child. Of importance in this study was the inclusion of mediating factors. Maternal teaching style, specifically affective quality, influenced children's intellectual performance through their self-regulatory skills and attentional capacity. The authors also address important methodological issues, including the validity of laboratory assessments of parent–child behavior.

The next article is a review of the developmental psychopathology literature on children's adaptation to life stressors. Luthar and Zigler define the main constructs associated with risk research, specifically stress and competence, and the methodological problems associated with their measurement. The authors review theoretical models of stress resistance and factors that moderate the effects of stress. This article is an excellent summary of the issues involved in risk research.

We conclude this section with an article on competence. Weissberg, Caplan, and Harwood review the literature on prevention programs. Prevention is often a neglected area in the training of child psychiatrists and psychologists. The authors describe the need for primary prevention and the different types of programs, including family support, early childhood education, and school-based programs. A few of the successful prevention programs in each area are reviewed. This article emphasizes the need for professionals to expand beyond treating specific mental disorders to treating the whole child.

8

Childhood Traumas: An Outline and Overview

Lenore C. Terr

University of California, San Francisco

Childhood psychic trauma appears to be a crucial etiological factor in the development of a number of serious disorders both in childhood and in adulthood. Like childhood rheumatic fever, psychic trauma sets a number of different problems into motion, any of which may lead to a definable mental condition. The author suggests four characteristics related to childhood trauma that appear to last for long periods of life, no matter what diagnosis the patient eventually receives. These are visualized or otherwise repeatedly perceived memories of the traumatic event, repetitive behaviors, trauma-specific fears, and changed attitudes about people, life, and the future. She divides childhood trauma into two basic types and defines the findings that can be used to characterize each of these types. Type I trauma includes full, detailed memories, "omens," and misperceptions. Type II trauma includes denial and numbing, self-hypnosis and dissociation, and rage. Crossover conditions often occur after sudden, shocking deaths or accidents that leave children handicapped. In these instances, characteristics of both type I and type II childhood traumas exist side by side. There may be considerable sadness. Each finding of childhood trauma discussed by the author is illustrated with one or two case examples.

Mental conditions brought on by horrible external events in childhood present a wide range of findings. If one looks only at the clinical manifestations of trauma in a given day in the life of the traumatized child, one could diagnose conduct disorder, borderline personality, major affective disorder, attention deficit hyperactivity, phobic disorder, dissociative disorder, obsessive-compulsive

Reprinted with permission from *American Journal of Psychiatry*, 1991, Vol. 148, No. 1 (10–20). Copyright © 1991 by the American Psychiatric Association.

disorder, panic disorder, adjustment disorder, and even such conditions, as yet unofficial in the nomenclature, as precursors of multiple personality or acute dissociative disorder, and not be wrong. If one projects this multiplicity of technically correct diagnoses onto a traumatized child's adulthood, one finds even more diagnostic leeway.

We must organize our thinking about childhood trauma, however, or we run the risk of never seeing the condition at all. Like the young photographer in Cortázar's short story and Antonioni's film, "Blow Up," we may enlarge the diagnostic fine points of trauma into such prominence that we altogether lose the central point—that external forces created the internal changes in the first place. We must not let ourselves forget childhood trauma just because the problem is so vast.

Studies of adults in mental hospitals[1], adults suffering from multiple personalities[2], adults who are borderline [3], and adolescents who go on to commit murder[4] show that these adults and adolescents very often were abused or shocked in their own childhoods. Studies of adult rape victims demonstrate that they often were raped or incestuously abused as children and that they are quite prone to being raped again—and again—in their adult lives[5]. Those who harm children have often been harmed themselves as children[6]. And some of those who indulge in self-mutilation or who make repeated suicide attempts give vivid past histories of long-standing childhood horrors[7].

One could say that childhood trauma is so ubiquitous to the psychiatric disorders of adolescence and adulthood that we should forget it, that it cancels itself out. We know, however, that not every child is directly shocked or personally subjected to terror from the outside. Most children come from relatively kind, nonabusive families. Most youngsters are never enrolled in a pedophilic day-care center or happen upon a satanic cult. The chances of experiencing a frightening flood, hurricane, or earthquake are not that great. The chances of witnessing a murder or of being kidnapped are not overwhelmingly high. Numbers of children should be able to get through their childhoods without any direct exposure to a traumatic event or series of terrible events. And they apparently do so.[8,9]

Even if we were to broaden the diagnosis of childhood trauma, as I will propose in this paper, to allow in any child mentally harmed enough by a single external event or a long-standing series of such events to qualify for a trauma-related diagnosis, we could not possibly cover everything that we see in adults as a result of these early traumas—the borderline patients, the patients with multiple personality disorder, and the chronic victims or victimizers, for instance. We will still need our adult diagnostic schemes and our adult treatment plans. But perhaps, if we looked in a more organized fashion at childhood psychic trauma and at what it does, we would recognize it as the important etiologic determinant that it actually is. We could begin to see how childhood trauma works. And we could study it better.

Like childhood rheumatic fever, which causes a number of conditions in adulthood ranging from mitral stenosis to subacute bacterial endocarditis to massive heart failure, childhood psychic trauma leads to a number of mental changes that eventually account for some adult character problems, certain kinds of psychotic thinking, considerable violence, much dissociation, extremes of passivity, self-mutilative episodes, and a variety of anxiety disturbances. Even though heart failure and subacute bacterial endocarditis in adulthood look very different from one another and demand specific treatments, their original cause—the childhood rheumatic fever—gives an organizing pattern to the physician's entire approach. Every good internist knows how to obtain and assess a history of rheumatic fever, even though it was the pediatrician who originally diagnosed and treated the sick child.

In this paper, I will define childhood trauma and point to four features that characterize almost all of the conditions resulting from extreme fright in childhood. These four features are seen in children suffering the results of events that were single, sudden, and unexpected, the classical Freudian traumas[10,11], and in children responding to long-standing and anticipated blows, those resulting in the various child abuse syndromes[12,13], survivor syndromes[14-16]. These four features appear to last for years in the course of the condition. They are often seen in adults who were traumatized as children, even though the adults now carry other diagnoses. Only one or two of these four features may be evident in an individual traumatized as a child; but from the history it is often evident that the other features played an important part in the person's life.

I will divide all of the trauma-stress conditions of childhood into two rough categories and call them type I and type II childhood traumas. I will propose that children suffering from type I traumas, the results of one sudden blow, differ in certain ways from children suffering from type II traumas, the results of long-standing or repeated ordeals. I will conclude with a note on the crossover conditions, childhood traumas that appear to settle between the two major types that I propose.

This paper is largely theoretical, although each point will be illustrated with a clinical example. It is based, in part, upon three studies: the Chowchilla kidnaping study [8,17,18], a retrospective study of 20 preschoolers suffering from a wide range of traumas that were documented by third parties[19], and a study of normal latency-aged children's and adolescents' responses to the Challenger space shuttle explosion[9]. The paper is primarily based, however, upon my clinical notes taken from more than 150 individual children who came for evaluation or treatment after a variety of externally generated horrors. The paper is an attempt to organize and to provide a scheme of thinking about childhood psychic trauma. It is not meant in any way as a last-minute addition to the *DSM-IV* process or as a proposal for a new and revisionary *DSM-V*. Instead, it is an outline and overview of a group of phenomena that may go their various ways into the adult diagnostic groups but that should still hold together in our thinking because of their association with the earliest traumas.

I will define childhood trauma as the mental results of one sudden, external blow or a series of blows, rendering the young person temporarily helpless and breaking past ordinary coping and defensive operations. As the reader will note, I have broadened the concept of traumas to include not only those conditions marked by intense surprise but also those marked by prolonged and sickening anticipation. All childhood traumas, according to my definition, originate from the outside. None is generated solely within the child's own mind. Childhood trauma may be accompanied by as yet unknown biological changes that are stimulated by the external events. The trauma begins with events outside the child. Once the events take place, a number of internal changes occur in the child. These changes last. As in the case of rheumatic fever, the changes stay active for years—often to the detriment of the young victim.

FOUR CHARACTERISTICS COMMON TO MOST CASES OF CHILDHOOD TRAUMA

There are several well-known characteristics that distinguish the traumas of childhood. Thought suppression, sleep problems, exaggerated startle responses, developmental regressions, fears of the mundane, deliberate avoidances, panic, irritability, and hypervigilance are prominent among these.

I consider four characteristics, however, particularly important in traumatized children no matter when in the course of the illness one observes the child and no matter what age the child is at the time. They are: 1) strongly visualized or otherwise repeatedly perceived memories, 2) repetitive behaviors, 3) trauma-specific fears, and 4) changed attitudes about people, aspects of life, and the future.

One note on traumatic dreams, the classic Freudian sign of trauma that I have not included in my list of four: the repetitive dream is a hallmark of trauma, but it is not always seen in childhood trauma, especially in children under age 5. Dreaming appears to be something that develops into what we recognize as dreaming by about age 3 or 4[20]. Before that, infants physically demonstrate that they are dreaming by making mouthing movements or little sounds in their sleep. Toddlers may scream from sleep without awakening, but this kind of dreaming is often too primitive and inexpressive to establish that traumatic dreams are actually taking place[21]. In a study of 20 children with documented traumas that occurred before the age of 5, only four of them verbalized the contents of their dreams[19]. The repeated dream apparently is very difficult to find in most traumas before the age of 5. Furthermore, these dreams often take deeply disguised forms as time progresses after the traumatic event. In those children old enough to dream and to remember their dreams, traumatic dreaming may occur at intervals several years apart or in such deeply disguised forms that the process becomes extremely difficult to distinguish from other forms of dreaming.

Visualized or Otherwise Repeatedly Perceived Memories

The ability to re-see or, occasionally but less frequently, to re-feel a terrible event or a series of events is an important common characteristic of almost all externally generated disorders of childhood[22]. Re-seeing is so important that it sometimes occurs even when the original experience was not at all visual[22]. Tactile, positional, or smell memories may also follow from long-standing terrors or single shocks. But the tendency to revisualize appears to be the strongest of all of these re-perceptions in childhood trauma. Visualizations are most strongly stimulated by remainders of the traumatic event, but they occasionally come up entirely unbidden.

The vivid and unwelcome nature of returning traumatic visualizations marks them as special to these externally generated conditions. Children tend to see their traumas and old ordeals at leisure—during times when they are bored with classes, at night before falling asleep, and when they are at rest listening to the radio or watching television. As opposed to those traumatized as adults, traumatized children rarely find themselves abruptly interrupted by sudden, dysphoric visualizations.

Even those who were infants or toddlers at the time of their ordeals and thus were unable to lay down, store, or retrieve full verbal memories of their traumas tend to play out, to draw, or to re-see highly visualized elements from their old experiences[19]. In cases in which the facts of a sexual abuse are not known, for instance, children may indicate their internalized visions of the abuse by sketching what they see in their mind or acting it out almost like a movie picture. Such children may use their visual and positional senses, senses that may outlast the verbal memory itself, to draw pictures of themselves "at the most scary moments of [their] life." Of course, other posttraumatic features should be present too, if the child actually was a trauma victim.

> Three and a half years after experiencing a series of traumatic events, a 5-year-old child was discovered (through pornographic photographs confiscated by U.S. Customs agents) to have been sexually misused in a day-care home between the ages of 15 and 18 months. The girl's parents did not dare speak to her about what they had learned from the investigators. They, in retrospect, realized that she had been sketching hundreds of nude adults beginning from the time when she had first begun to draw.
>
> While playing in my office, this child told me that a baby she had just drawn was "all naked" and "a bad girl." Unknowingly, she had

just depicted herself. Despite the fact that the little girl's only verbal memory of the events was "I think there was grave danger at a lady—MaryBeth's—house," her volumes of drawings represented strongly visualized elements that she had retained and had needed to recreate from these very early, nonverbal experiences.

A 40-year-old mental health professional began working at a facility for male juvenile delinquents. On his long rides home he began seeing himself as a toddler—attacked in a shack by a group of older children. The man drove to the town where he had lived until he was 4 years old, and he found the shack that he had "pictured." The shack stood catercornered to his old house.

Repetitive Behaviors

Play and behavioral reenactments are frequent manifestations of both the single blow and the long-standing terrors of childhood. Psycholphysiologic repetitions are less frequently observed in ordinary practice, but they gain particular importance in certain cultures[23]. Posttraumatic play, defined by the players as "fun," is a grim, long-lasting, and particularly contagious form of childhood repetitive behavior[24]. Although reenactments lack the element of "fun," they also repeat aspects of the terrible events. Reenactments can occur as single behaviors, repeated behaviors, or bodily responses. Repetitive behaviors may even be seen in children who were exposed to traumatic events before the age of 12 months[19]. In other words, children who have no verbal memory whatsoever of their traumas may be seen to feel physical sensations or play or act in a manner that evokes what they originally experienced at the time of the event. The 5-year-old girl described in the previous case vignette, for instance, experienced "funny feelings" in her "tummy" every time she saw a finger pointed at her. The pornographic pictures confiscated by the customs authorities showed an erect penis jabbing the very spot on the 15–18-month-old child's belly that she had indicated when, at age 5, she spoke of the "funny feelings."

The childhood survivors of single shocks and of long-standing terrors are usually entirely unaware that their behaviors and physical responses repeat something of the original set of thoughts or emergency responses. Thus, the presence or absence of behavioral reenactments may at times be better determined from interviews with third parties.

Behavioral reenactments may recur so frequently as to become distinct personality traits. These may eventually gather into the personality disorders of adulthood, or they may recur so physiologically as to represent what seems to be physical disease. Long after most repeated nightmares have disappeared into deeply disguised form, reenactments continue to characterize the behaviors of traumatically stressed children. Recent psychiatric investigation into the lives and works of important artists—Edgar Allen Poe, Edith Wharton, René Magritte, Alfred Hitchcock, and Ingmar Bergman[25], Stephen King[26], and Virginia Woolf[27]—show that these artists reenacted childhood traumas behaviorally throughout their lifetimes and also played out their traumas in artistic works spanning their entire careers. If one could live a thousand years, one might completely work through a childhood trauma by playing out the terrifying scenario until it no longer terrified. The lifetime allotted to the ordinary person, however, does not appear to be enough.

> A 6-year-old girl walked into a circus tent and was suddenly attacked by a runaway lion. The animal tore open her scalp and bit into her face. The girl had to undergo several surgical procedures to repair what happened within a few seconds' time. She was left with an uneven hairline and a large bald spot. After the extraordinary experience, the little girl preferred "Beauty Parlor" to all other games of pretend. She combed her younger sister's hair repeatedly, often bringing the younger child to tears over the roughness of the combing. The little girl's dolls developed bald spots and uneven hairlines without anyone ever observing exactly how these anomalies came into being. The child, previously outgoing and friendly, stuck close to home and rarely ventured out into her neighborhood. At age 6, her main hopes for the future were to grow up, and become a runway model or a "beauty parlor lady."

Trauma-Specific Fears

Some of the specific fears related to the shocks and long-standing extreme external stresses of childhood can be avoided by moving out of town or by changing houses or neighborhoods. Fears can be conditioned away by repeatedly facing the feared object. Most extremely stressed or psychically traumatized children continue to harbor one or two trauma-related fears, however, well into adulthood. Fears of specific things that are related to experiences precipitated by traumatic events are fairly easy to spot, once one knows what the trauma might have been. This type of literal, specific fear is pathognomonic of the childhood traumas. Whereas neurotically or developmentally phobic children may fear *all* dogs, the dog-bitten youngster will fear the German shepherds, the Dobermans, or whatever species actually created the traumatic state. Whereas neurotically anxious children fear growing up or getting married, traumatized youngsters fear (and re-create) oral sex, anal intercourse, or whatever particular sexual abuse they originally experienced.

Traumatized children tend also to fear mundane items—the dark, strangers, looming objects, being alone, being outside, food, animals, and vehicles, for instance. In fact, fears of the dark and of being alone are strongly connected with sudden shocks in the early years[9]. But these mundane fears may also be connected with a number of other emotional disorders and developmental stages of childhood. The panic and extreme avoidances observed following terrifying events, in connection with this mundane group of fears, *do* make them important to childhood trauma. But the specific, literal kinds of fear noted in the preceding paragraph almost "label" the traumatic condition. When one sees this literal kind of fear lasting throughout the years despite the natural tendencies toward spontaneous desensitization, childhood trauma is the most likely cause.

> A girl was sexually misused by her father from age 5 to age 15, at which time she ran away from home, never to return. As a married adult of 38, she feared sex with her husband unless she initiated the act herself. She responded to the female-on-top or side-to-side positions, positions that had not originally been taken by her father. Any sexual positioning that was evocative of the incestuous set of sexual postures stimulated fear, pain, and revulsion.

Changed Attitudes About People, Life, and the Future

The sense of a severely limited future, along with changed attitudes about people and life, appears to be important in the trauma and extreme stress disorders originating in childhood. The limitation of future perspective is particularly striking in traumatized children because ordinary youngsters exhibit almost limitless ideas about the future. Truisms, such as "I live one day at a time" or "I can't guess what will happen in my lifetime," come from the rethinkings that occur in the years after traumatic events. Ideas such as "You can't trust the police" or "You can't count on anything or anyone to protect you" also follow from single and long-standing, repeated traumas. Sexually traumatized girls may shrink away from men or accost them with overfriendly advances. Part of this behavior is reenactment, but part reflects attitudinal changes. Limitations in scope and future perspective in childhood trauma victims seem to reflect the ongoing belief that more traumas are bound to follow. Traumatized children recognize profound vulnerability in all human beings, especially themselves. This shattering of what Lifton and Olson call "the shield of invincibility"[28] and what Erikson terms "basic trust" and "autonomy"[29] appears to characterize almost all event-engendered disorders of childhood. The feeling of futurelessness of the traumatized child is quite different from that of the depressed youngster. For the traumatized, the future is a landscape filled with crags, pits, and monsters. For the depressed, the future is a bleak, featureless landscape stretched out to infinity.

> A 17-year-old boy, searching for a freeway shoulder on which to stop

his disabled car, was hit from the rear by a speeder. The boy's automobile exploded. He flew out completely unscathed but watched helplessly as his best friend burned to death in the passenger seat.

For months after the event the boy could not work and spent most of his days moping. He was plagued with bad dreams and fears of further disaster. He began psychotherapy; and when I said to him at the end of an early session, "See you next week," he asked, "How do you know it will be next week? Who knows? I may die on my way out of your office. I may be killed out there on the sidewalk. I don't count on seeing you next week. I live day to day—day to day."

A 15-year-old girl came for psychiatric treatment because, since she was attacked at age 8, she had failed to volunteer or speak up in class. Since her acceptance in an academic high school, she could achieve no more than Bs because she was too quiet.

The girl had experienced significant changes in her attitudes about life and people while she was lying in a hospital room for 3 months, following repairs to her vagina, anus, and peritoneum. A man had grabbed her from a Chinatown sidewalk on her way home from school. He had taken her into an abandoned garage and attacked her vagina with a pair of chopsticks. The girl had decided after her ordeal that she was "chosen" by the deranged man because she had "showed too much." Never again, she had vowed to herself, would she ever "show." People could not be trusted, she believed. Life must be endured, not savored.

FEATURES CHARACTERISTIC OF THE SINGLE-BLOW TRAUMAS, TYPE I DISORDERS

The type I traumatic conditions of childhood follow from unanticipated single events. These are classical childhood traumas by Anna Freud's definition[30]. These are also the most typical posttraumatic stress disorders that one finds in childhood, usually meeting the criteria of repetition, avoidance, and hyperalertness that represent the major divisions in our diagnostic manual, *DSM-III-R*. Those children who suffer the results of single blows appear to exhibit certain symptoms and signs that differentiate their conditions from those resulting from the more complicated events. The findings special to single, shocking, intense terrors are 1) full, detailed, etched-in memories, 2) "omens" (retrospective reworkings, cognitive reappraisals reasons, and turning points), and 3) misperceptions and mistimings. Type I traumas do not appear to breed the massive denials, psychic numbings, self-anesthesias, or personality problems that characterize the type II disorders of childhood.

Full, Detailed Memories

With the exception of youngsters below the approximate age of 28 to 36 months, almost every previously untraumatized child who is fully conscious at the time that he or she experiences or witnesses one terrible event demonstrates the ability to retrieve detailed and full memories afterward[19]. Verbal recollections of single shocks in an otherwise trauma-free childhood are delivered in an amazingly clear and detailed fashion. Children sometimes sound like robots as they strive to tell every detail as efficiently as possible. As a matter of fact, children are sometimes able to remember more from a single event than are the adults who observed the same event[24]. A few details from a traumatic event of childhood may be factually wrong because the child initially misperceived or mistimed the sequence of what happened. But children with type I disorders seem to remember the event and to give impressively clear, detailed accounts of their experiences.

This remarkable retrieval of full, precise, verbal memories of almost all single-blow traumas makes one conclude that these memories stay alive in a very special way, no matter how much conscious suppression the traumatized child is attempting. Memories of prolonged or variably repeated childhood abuses, on the other hand, appear to be retained in spots, rather than as clear, complete wholes[19]. Amnesias, as a matter of fact, are often reported in children who seem to be heading for the multiple personality disorders of adulthood[31]. Children who have been repeatedly physically or sexually abused may waver in their accusations of abusers and waver in the completeness and the detail of their memories. But children who have been traumatized a single time do not often forget. As Malle says at the conclusion of his autobiographical film, *Au Revoir Les Enfants* (1987), a tale of single, terrible event from his boyhood in occupied France, "Over forty years have passed, but I will remember every second of that January morning until the day I die."

> The first time that he visited the psychiatrist, a 5-year-old boy minutely described his stepfather's murder of his baby brother. The incident had occurred 2 weeks earlier. The boy knew just where under the television table in a motel room he had been hiding. He reported exactly where he had been sitting and lying before taking cover. He described the types of blows that fell upon his younger sibling and meticulously repeated the attacker's phrases and threats. He said that he had been trying to forget all of this but could not. The boy's teacher had been reprimanding him for repeatedly hiding under the desks and tables at school, but neither teacher nor student recognized the significance of this "bad behavior."

Omens

During and after single-blow shocks, children tend frequently to ask themselves "Why?" and "Why me?" In this way they attempt to gain retrospective mastery over the randomness, the lack of control, and the "less-than-humaneness" of the trauma that they endured. When children traumatized by a single event belatedly develop a reason why everything happened, a purpose to the entire affair, or a way that the disaster could have been averted, considerable mental energy goes into these reworkings of the past. I have termed these belated reshiftings, reasons, and warnings "omens"[17], while Pynoos et al. call them "cognitive reappraisals"[11]. I believe that we are describing the same phenomenon. This kind of rethinking and reworking occurs much more often after one sudden external shock than it does after a prolonged series of terrible experiences. Children who have found omens or reasons to explain why they suffer often feel intensely guilty. Although victims of type II childhood trauma also experience profound guilt, the sense of guilt does not often consciously align itself to the "Why me?" question. The repetitions and long-standing nature of the type II stressors make the inquiry "How could I have avoided it?" far less pressing than the question "How will I avoid it the next time?"

The omen or cognitive reappraisal is a belated way in which the singly traumatized child tries to deal retroactively with what had been entirely unexpected—a sudden, surprising psychological blow. Because repeated horrors encourage a sense of anticipation and expectation, different means of coping come to be employed. These means of coping eventually create the defining characteristics of the type II disorders, characteristics that are unmatched in the type I disorders.

> An 8-year-old boy's mother bought him a fancy skateboard, admonishing him to ride only on the sidewalk. The first Saturday morning the boy rode his skateboard on the sidewalk, he was run over by a car backing out of a neighbor's driveway. The boy commented a year later, "I can't help thinking many, many times about what Mom said about riding skateboards on sidewalks."

> A 16-year-old girl received a slice of pizza from her best friend as a birthday present. Biting into the pizza, she was poisoned by a corrosive toxin. The girl suffered from internal injuries for more than 6 weeks. Even though the real source of the poison was found by health officials at the pizza parlor, the injured girl thought again and again about the nature of her relationship with the friend who had purchased the pizza. In minutest detail she tried to figure out at what point her friend had decided to kill her.

Misperceptions

Misidentifications, visual hallucinations, and peculiar time distortions often occur to children who have experienced single, intense, unexpected shocks[22,32]. In contrast to this, the long-standing, extreme external stresses that affect children are often engineered by perpetrators known to them—caretakers, teachers, or family members, for instance. Because of a child's familiarity with such perpetrators, the chances of early misperceptions become slim. Two important exceptions to this general rule are when a type II victim thinks that he or she "sees" a once-familiar abuser years after losing track of the person and when a known, long-standing perpetrator was never perceived correctly by the child because of a disguise that he or she was wearing (as in satanism and cults).

Many of the type I childhood traumas include visual misperceptions and hallucinations. These perceptual distortions may seem to indicate organic mental conditions or psychoses, but a few bizarre sightings do not "make" a brain disorder or a schizophrenic episode. Visual hallucinations and illusions are observed in children shortly after traumatic events and, at times, long after sudden, unanticipated shocks. Massive releases of neurotransmitters in the brain at the time of the terror may account for these problems with perception. But the types of substances and mechanisms are, as yet, unknown.

> A 7-year-old girl rode in a station wagon alongside her sister and two cousins on a family outing to the mountains. A loose boulder from an adjacent hillside smashed into the roof of the girl's car, killing one cousin and the girl's older sister, while sparing the girl and her other young cousin. For the ensuing year, the surviving girl "saw" her sister at her bedside almost every night. The dead sister visited the living child dressed in pink, green, and orange outfits. She appeared fully fleshed, as she was in life. The vision said nothing. The young survivor felt upset by a sense of menace emanating from her sister's "ghost," yet, at the same time, she felt oddly comforted by the sight.

FEATURES CHARACTERISTIC OF VARIABLE, MULTIPLE, OR LONG-STANDING TRAUMAS, TYPE II DISORDERS

Type II disorders follow from long-standing or repeated exposure to extreme external events. The fist such event, of course, creates surprise. But the subsequent unfolding of horrors creates a sense of anticipation. Massive attempts to protect the psyche and to preserve the self are put into gear. The defenses and coping operations used in the type II disorders of childhood—massive denial, repression, dissociation, self-anesthesia, self-hypnosis, identification with the aggressor, and aggression turned against the self—often lead to profound character changes in the youngster. Even though a repeatedly abused youngster may not settle into a recognizable form of adult character disorder until the late teens or early twenties, extreme personality problems may emerge even before the age of 5.

The emotions stirred up by type II traumas are 1) an absence of feeling, 2) a sense of rage, or 3) unremitting sadness. These emotions exist side by side with the fear that is ubiquitous to the childhood traumas. Type II disorders, under the scrutiny of able mental health professionals, may come to be diagnosed in childhood as conduct disorders, attention deficit disorders, depression, or dissociative disorders. Recognition of the expanded group of traumas that I am suggesting here may help to define a common etiology and range of findings for many of these childhood conditions. Of course, if a child originally was traumatized, one would expect to find vestiges of the repeated visualizations, repeated behaviors and physiologic sensations, specific fears, and revised ideas about people, life, and the future that appear to characterize the childhood traumas.

Denial and Psychic Numbing

Denial and psychic numbing have long been considered classic findings of the posttraumatic stress disorders. Diagnostic problems often arise, however, because massive denial and emotional shutdown are so often evanescent or absent in children who have gone through single shocks[17]. Although conscious suppression of thoughts will take place in any kind of trauma, and although brief, limited denial and numbing may last from moments to hours after a shocking event, massive denial and psychic numbing are primarily associated with the long-standing horrors of childhood, what I would call the type II traumas. Children who experience this type of stress may employ such extreme numbing and denial that they look extremely withdrawn or inhuman. When very young, they may assume the guise of Spitz's "hospitalism" babies[33] or of "hail fellow well met" superficiality[34], both of which are signs of failure of attachment and of personality organization.

Children who experience type II traumas do not complain of going "numb." The sense of going dead is one that depends upon years of subjectively knowing what it was to feel alive. On the other hand, children who have been repeatedly brutalized or terrorized *do* exhibit massive denial to the eyes of the trained observer. Such children avoid talking about themselves. They often go for years without saying a thing about their ordeals. They valiantly try to look normal at school, in the neighborhood, and on the playground. They may tell their stories once or twice and entirely deny them later. (This is quite different from some children who have experienced type I traumas, who may tell their stories even at kindergarten Show and Tell.)

Children who experience type II traumas often forget. They may forget whole segments of childhood—from birth to age 9, for instance. Where one sees the difference between these "forgetful" children and ordinary youngsters is in the multiply traumatized child's relative indifference to pain, lack of empathy, failure to define or to acknowledge feelings, and absolute avoidance of psychological intimacy. Repeatedly brutalized, benumbed children employ massive denial—and when their denial-related behaviors cluster together, the resultant childhood personality disorder (one that cuts across adult narcissistic, antisocial, borderline, and avoidant categories) is massive.

Profound psychic numbing in children occurs as an accommodation to the most extreme, long-standing, or repeated traumatic situations. Childhood physical and sexual abuse represent two of these extremes. What still makes the underlying idea of "trauma" the correct etiology and pathogenesis here is the fact that the specific fears, the repeated play, the behavioral and physiologic reenactments, the tendencies toward visualizations, and the revised ideas about life, people, and the future seem to persist in so many of these children for years after the last abuse stops.

> Suzanna was 6 years old when her teenaged brother began sexually molesting her. (It turned out that he, in turn, had been sexually molested by a junior high school teacher before he began abusing Suzanna.) Suzanna once tried to tell her mother, "Nobody's supposed to touch you in your—" (she pointed at her genitals). But after that she said nothing further to her parents, teachers, or friends until the school nurse discovered what was happening 2 ½ years after it began.
>
> On psychiatric examination when she was age 9, Suzanna spent much of the first hour pushing her index finger back and forth through a small hole she had made with the rest of her fingers. She repeatedly rubbed the loose couch pillows over one another. She said of her experiences with her brother, "He put his penis where I pooped. It hurt. I told him it hurt, but he said nuttin' back. I didn't like that at all. It didn't really frighten me. Not really. I just made up my mind to think about other things."
>
> When Suzanna was asked how she was able to do this mind trick, "to think about other things," she replied, "I say 'I don't know' over and over to myself. When I say my prayers I keep saying the last word of the prayer. Sometimes I do it a hundred times. I say 'I don't know' a lot of times in my mind each day . . . . Sometimes now I find myself not feeling things. I don't feel sad or mad when I should be. The people at my school think I'm funny because of it."

Self-Hypnosis and Dissociation

Spontaneous self-hypnosis, depersonalization, and dissociation are important outcomes of repeated, long-standing terrors (the type II traumas). Children who have been the victims of extended periods of terror come to learn that the stressful events will be repeated. Some of these children, the ones, perhaps, who have an innate ease of hypnotizability, spontaneously fall upon the technique of self-hypnosis. This mechanism enables a child mentally to escape. Suzanna, the child described in the previous paragraph, used the repetition of a single word, the last word of her prayers, to accomplish this escape from pain and worry. She also lulled herself into minitrances by saying, "I don't know" in her mind. The children at school recognized her affect to be unusual. But nobody but the child herself could recognize the self-hypnosis.

Traumatized children who use a great deal of self-hypnosis may, in fact, go on to develop adult multiple personality disorders[35]. This is probably a rare condition. Spontaneous dissociation, however, accounts for a number of more commonly observed findings in abused children—bodily anesthesias, feelings of invisibility, and amnesias for certain periods of childhood life.

Multiple personality disorder, a syndrome in search of its own place in our diagnostic manuals, belongs here, at least in terms of etiology—the repeated, extreme, long-standing traumas of childhood. In children, periods of time that cannot be accounted for, problem behaviors, visual and auditory hallucinations, and headaches appear to indicate that the child is suffering from multiple personality precursors[36]. Most self-hypnotizing children who are type II trauma victims fall short of the multiple personality or precursors diagnoses, however, They develop, instead, anesthesias to bodily pain, sexual anesthesia, and extreme emotional distancings. Children who come to expect the repetition of terrors remove themselves in any way that they can. These emotional removals are not possible for the ordinary type I trauma victim.

> Frederick was 7 years old when he was sent to live with his aunt because his mother found out, through a tape recording set up to catch her husband at infidelity, that Frederick's stepfather had been throwing him against walls while she worked the evening shift. Frederick did not tell anyone his year-long story, despite two visits to the emergency room and one neighbor-instigated protective service investigation.
>
> While in his aunt's custody, Frederick glanced down at the playground pavement one day and saw blood. After several seconds of searching for a wounded companion, Frederick realized that it was *he* who was bleeding. The boy realized he could feel no pain.
>
> In a psychotherapy session I asked Frederick how he could make this sort of thing happen. "It jus' happens now," he said. "I used to pretend I was at a picnic with my head on Mommy's lap. The first time

my stepdaddy hit me, it hurt a lot. But then I found out that I could make myself go on Mommy's lap [in imagination], and Winston couldn't hurt me that way. I kept goin' on Mommy's lap—I didn't have to cry or scream or anything. I could *be* someplace else and not get hurt. I don't know how many times Winston punched me out. I wasn't always payin' attention. Like I told you, first I'd be at a picnic on Mom's lap. Later I didn't have to think of no picnic—jus' her lap. Now if somethin' makes me bleed, I don't think of no lap at all. I jus' don't feel no pain."

Jamie was repeatedly abused by his alcoholic father. He had also repeatedly observed his father beat his mother. At age 8, he witnessed his mother shoot his father to death. When he was 9, the child was psychologically evaluated. At that time he told me, "I started some planets. I made my planets up as a game. But it's real now. It's no game anymore." Jamie described a safe planet he had invented long ago, his own planet. He also had invented a number of very unsafe planets where people "got killed." He said that he had come to achieve invisibility by repeatedly visiting his own safe planet and avoiding the unsafe ones. "Starting when I was 6," he said, "I began to feel invisible. When my Mom pointed a gun at my Dad . . . I was thinking like 'I didn't see it,' like 'This didn't happen.' I blinked to see if I was dreaming . . . . I remember at first pretending I wasn't there—that I didn't see it—that I was on my own planet. I had gone there a lot before. When Mom and Dad would fight, I would try not to hear, not to see. I'd try to go to sleep. Normally, I couldn't. I'd try to get out of the room where they were. I'd try to visit my planet. But now my mind, yes, it just goes blank. Mostly it happens at home. A few minutes at a time."

Jamie repeatedly dreamed by night about his father's death. And he visualized the killing by day. But from the moment that his dad was shot, Jamie wondered if he himself could turn invisible. "I know I can," he said. "I do it here on earth. I do it all the time on my planet. You're just going to have to believe me. My friends believe it . . . . When my father was being shot I felt invisible. But if I turned invisible in front of everybody, they'd take away my powers."

Rage

Rage, including anger turned against the self, is a striking finding in those post-traumatic disorders that are brought on by repeated or long-standing abuses, the type II disorders. One observes rage and its negative, extreme passivity, in those type II disorders originating in places where trust originally resided. Dorothy Otnow Lewis and her group reported that among adolescent delinquents who go on to commit murder, chronic physical abuse is a key findings within a cluster of several other key findings[36]. The rage of the repeatedly abused child cannot safely be underestimated.

Reenactments of anger may come so frequently in the type II trauma disorders that habitual patterns of aggressiveness are established. The rage may become so fearsome to the child as to crate extremes of passivity. Wild fluctuations of both active anger and extreme passivity may so dominate the clinical picture that the young person is eventually given a diagnosis of borderline personality. Defenses against rage such as passive into active and identification with the aggressor also put their own peculiar stamps on the type II child. Type II children have been known to attack their own bodies. Self-mutilations or physically damaging suicide attempts occur. The festering anger of the repeatedly abused child is probably as damaging a part of the condition as is the chronic numbing. Both of these, in fact, the numbing and rage, probably figure later in the antisocial, borderline, narcissistic, and multiple personality diagnoses that are so often part of the picture of the type II traumatized child grown up.

> A 5-year-old boy whose new stepmother had been tying him with ropes and leaving him locked up in closets behaved well at kindergarten. At home, however, he took scissors to his stepmother's best lingerie. He sprinkled India ink twice into the family wash. He consistently managed not to eat the food his stepmother prepared for him. The boy's stepmother said he was asking for the punishments she gave him. And so the abuses escalated.

> A 45-year-old woman had been a teenager in summer camp when the atomic bomb destroyed her home in Hiroshima. (Her immediate family was spared; all were out of town on Aug. 6, 1945.) As an adult, the woman could not get along well with her American-born husband, alternately accusing him of laziness, ineptitude at work, and infidelity. From the time her daughter turned 13, the woman began believing the girl to be promiscuous, a liar, a drug addict, and a thief. The woman could not get along with her co-workers at the international law office where she worked. She was able, she said, to relate only to customers from Japan. They reminded her "of the people [she] used to know at home when [she] was a girl." I invited the woman to come to my office to talk about her experiences with the bomb. She made two appointments for this purpose but failed to appear for either. Obviously, too much time had elapsed to prove any cause-and-effect hypothesis here.

It is interesting, however, that the woman's anger and suspiciousness rested only with American and American-influenced people. Native Japanese persons, the victims, not the perpetrators of the atomic bomb, were entirely spared her wrath.

CROSSOVER TYPE I-TYPE II TRAUMATIC CONDITIONS OF CHILDHOOD

When a single psychological shock takes a child's parent's life, leaves a child homeless, handicapped, or disfigured, or causes a child to undergo prolonged hospitalization and pain, the ongoing stresses tend to push the changes in the child toward those characteristics of the type II childhood traumas. In these cases one often finds features of both the type I and the type II conditions. Those children with permanent handicaps, longstanding pain, or loss of significant objects are often forced into making significant character changes or using numbing tricks to minimize their pain. They may still retain, however, the characteristics typical of responses to single events—clear memory, perceptual distortions, and omens.

Perpetual Mourning and Depression

Psychic shock interferes with childhood bereavement and vice versa[37]. The combined psychological effects of shock and grief continue to drag on throughout childhood. As time goes by, and the childhood mourning does not proceed through its ordinary stages[38], the young trauma victim is reinjured—from the inside this time—through prolonged exposure to sadness and loss. The psychological condition of mixed mourning and trauma in youth may take the guise of major affective disorder and may have to be treated as such, at least at first. There is a high rate of depression in refugee children from brutal regimes[15,16]. An explanation for this finding may be the unresolved trauma that potentiates and extends the unresolved grief, the grief that furthers the trauma, or both.

A 4-year-old boy watched his older sister's evisceration in a freak accident in a children's swimming pool. Before the disaster she had asked him to play, but he had refused. The little girl then sat down on an exposed drain pipe. The boy spent a couple of years after the accident using wooden blocks to build his own perfect pool. He blamed himself for not agreeing to play with his sister, an act, he felt, that caused his sister's injury. The boy retained a clear memory of all of the events. He showed symptoms typical of type I trauma.

Following his sister's death in transplantation surgery 2 years after the accident, the boy began to retreat from his friends, avoid participating in class, and stay silent much of the time. His teachers complained about his extreme passivity and said he was losing ground in subjects in which he had already proved himself. He lost some weight and stopped sleeping through the night. He lost his playfulness and began losing his friends. His 2 years of mourning had introduced type II characteristics into a previously pure type I disorder.

Childhood Disfigurement, Disability, and Pain

Children who are physically injured in psychically traumatic accidents tend perpetually to mourn old selves, personas that were previously intact and perfect. Even when perpetual grief is not the problem, posttraumatic physical handicaps frequently demand considerable personality reorganization in order that the child can live with a new, limited self. In children, character rearrangements may become massive. To deal with the pain and procedures accompanying traumatic accidents, children may employ self-hypnosis. They may experience self-revulsion, unremitting guilt and shame, impotent rage at their peers who shun and tease them, and sadness. Suicide attempts are not infrequent in this group. Robert Stoller suggested in a recent paper that some extremes of adult sadomasochistic behavior may originate in painful illnesses, injuries, and procedures during childhood. Rather than self-hypnotizing, these children may divert themselves from the pain by self-stimulating—and thus perpetually associate their pain with sexuality[39]. Childhood syndromes of injury and shock do not consistently qualify, under *DSM-III-R* criteria, as posttraumatic stress disorders[40]. But these mixed syndromes of depression, numbing, rage, and fright often carry many of the four characteristics that I associate with childhood traumas. Adjustment to a sudden surprise, coupled with a prolonged ordeal, often lies at the origin of the problem.

A kindergartner climbed onto a large department store display table, causing it to fall over onto her face as her grandmother paid the clerk for a purchase.. The child's facial bones were smashed, and although they were beautifully reconstructed, she looked quite different than she had before the accident. Old friends did not recognize her, and other kindergartners told the child that she must be pretending to be Belinda—she could not actually *be* Belinda.

The little girl, previously outgoing, mischievous, and vivacious, took on a quiet, remote, and perfectly well-behaved mode of behavior. Two years after the accident she said, "I was a devil before, but I was punished for it. Now I'm good." Despite the fact that she experienced bad dreams, liked to play alone under chairs, and tended to mutilate her

dolls' faces, Belinda's character change dominated all other posttraumatic findings.

SUMMARY

There appears to be a group of problems brought on in childhood by the experience of extreme fright generated by outside events. Some of these childhood problems are created by one external shock, and others are created by a multiplicity
of blows. Untreated, all but the mildest of the childhood traumas last for years.
The child's responses, in fact, may create a number of different kinds of problems
in adult life. There are four characteristics, however, that seem to affect almost
everyone subjected to extreme terrors in childhood. These findings seem to last
and can be retrieved in histories. They include repeated visualizations or other
returning perceptions, repeated behaviors and bodily response, trauma-specific
fears, and revised ideas about people, life, and the future. These four findings appear
to remain clustered together in childhood trauma victims even when other diagnoses
seem more appropriate. Like rheumatic fever, childhood trauma creates changes
that may eventually lead to a number of different diagnoses. But also like rheumatic
fever, childhood trauma must always be kept in mind as a possible underlying mechanism when these various conditions appear.

If one takes all of the disorders of childhood brought on by extreme external
events and puts them into the general category of trauma, they can be roughly subdivided into two groupings: type I, which is brought on by one sudden shock, and
type II, which is precipitated by a series of external blows. Crossover conditions
are quite common and develop when one blow creates a long-standing series of
childhood adversities.

REFERENCES

1. Carmen E (H), Rieker PP, Mills T: Victims of violence and psychiatric illness. Am J
   Psychiatry 1984; 141:378–383
2. Bliss E: Multiple Personality, Allied Disorders, and Hypnosis. New York, Oxford
   University Press, 1986
3. Walsh R: The family of the borderline patient, in The Borderline Patient. Edited by
   Grinker F, Werble B. New York, Jason Aronson, 1977
4. Lewis DO, Lovely R, Yaeger C, et al: Toward a theory of the genesis of violence. J
   Am Accad Child Psychiatry 1989; 28:431–436
5. Russell D: The Secret Trauma. New York, Basic Books, 1986
6. Silver LB, Dublin CC, Lourie RS: Does violence breed violence? Contributions from
   a study of the child abuse syndrome. Am J Psychiatry 1969; 126:404–407
7. Herman J, Van Der Kolk B. Traumatic antecedents of borderline personality, in

Psychological Trauma. Edited by Van Der Kolk B. Washington, DC, American Psychiatric Press, 1987

8. Terr L: Life attitudes, dreams, and psychic trauma in a group of "normal" children. J Am Acad Child Psychiatry 1983; 22:221–230

9. Terr L: Children's responses to the Challenger disaster, in New Research Program and Abstracts, American Psychiatric Association 143rd Annual Meeting, Washington, DC, APA, 1990

10. Frued S: Beyond the pleasure principle (1920), in Complete Psychological Works, standard ed, vol 18. London, Hogarth Press, 1955

11. Pynoos R, Frederick C, Nader K, et al: Life threat and posttraumatic stress in school age children. Arch Gen Psychiatry 1987; 44:1057–1063

12. Green A: Dimensions of psychological trauma in abused children. J Am Acad Child Psychiatry 1983; 22:231–237

13. McLeer S, Deblinger E, Atkins M, et al: Post-traumatic stress disorder in sexually abused children. J Am Acad Child Adolesc Psychiatry 1988; 27:650–659

14. Kinzie JD, Sack W, Angell R, et al: The psychiatric effects of massive trauma on Cambodian children. J Am Acad Child Adolesc Psychiatry 1986; 25:370–383

15. Kinzie JD, Sack W, Angell R, et al: A three-year follow-up of Cambodian young people traumatized as children. J Am Acad Child Adolesc Psychiatry 1989; 28:501–504

16. Kestenberg J: Child survivors of the Holocaust—40 years later. J Am Acad Child Psychiatry 1985; 24:408–412

17. Terr L: Children of Chowchilla. Psychoanal Study Child 1979; 34:547–623

18. Terr LC: Chowchilla revisited: the effects of psychic trauma four years after a school-bus kidnapping. Am J Psychiatry 1983; 140:1543–1550

19. Terr L: What happens to the memories of early childhood trauma? J Am Acad Child Adolesc Psychiatry 1988; 27:96–104

20. Mack J: Nightmares and the Human Conflict. Boston, Little, Brown, 1970

21. Terr L: Children's nightmares, in Sleep and Its Disorders in Children. Edited by Guilleminault C. New York, Raven Press, 1987

22. Terr L: Remembered images in psychic trauma. Psychoanal Study Child 1985; 40:493–533

23. Kinzie JD: Severe posttraumatic stress syndrome among Cambodian refugees, in Disaster Stress Studies. Edited by Shore J. Washington, DC, American Psychiatric Press, 1986

24. Terr L: "Forbidden games." J Am Acad Child Psychiatry 1981; 20:740–759

25. Terr L: Childhood trauma and the creative product. Psychoanal Study Child 1987; 42:545–572

26. Terr L: Terror writing by the formerly terrified. Psychoanal Study Child 1989; 44:369–390

27. Terr L: Who's afraid in Virginia Woolf? Psychoanal Study Child 1990; 45:531–544

28. Lifton R, Olson E: The human meaning of total disaster. Psychiatry 1976; 39:1–18

29. Erikson E: Childhood and Society. New York, Norton, 1950

30. Frued A: Comments on trauma, in The Writings of Anna Freud, vol V, 1956–1965:

Research at the Hampstead Child Therapy Clinic and Other Papers. New York, International Universities Press, 1969

31. Kluft R: Childhood multiple personality disorder, in Childhood Antecedents of Multiple Personality. Edited by Kluft R. Washington, DC, American Psychiatric Press, 1985

32. Terr L: Too Scared to Cry. New York, Harper & Row, 1990

33. Spitz R: Hospitalism, Psychoanal Study Child 1945; 1:64–72

34. Terr LC: A family study of child abuse. Am J Psychiatry 1970; 127:665–671

35. Spiegel D: Multiple personality as a posttraumatic stress disorder. Psychiatr Clin North Am 1984; 7:101–110

36. Lewis DO, Moy E, Jackson LD, et al: Biopsychosocial characteristics of children who later murder: a prospective study. Am J Psychiatry 1985; 142:1161–1167

37. Eth S, Pynoos R: Interaction of trauma and grief in childhood, in Post-traumatic Stress Disorder in Children. Edited by Eth S, Pynoos P. Washington, DC, American Psychiatry Press, 1985

38. Osterweis M, Solomon F, Green M (eds): Bereavement. Washington, DC, National Academy Press, 1984

39. Stoller R: Consensual sadomasochistic perversions, in the Psychoanalytic Core. Edited by Blum H, Weinshel EM, Rodman FR. New York, International Universities Press, 1989

40. Stoddard FJ, Norman DK, Murphy JM: A diagnostic outcome study of children and adolescents with severe burns. J Trauma 1989; 29:471–477

9

Relationship of Socioeconomic Status to the Etiology and Developmental Sequelae of Physical Child Abuse

Penelope K. Trickett
National Institute of Mental Health, Bethesda, Maryland

J. Lawrence Aber
Columbia University, New York City

Vicki Carlson
Washington University, St. Louis, Missouri

Dante Cicchetti
University of Rochester, New York

This article studies how socioeconomic status (SES) may be related to the etiology of physical child abuse and to the consequences of abuse for child development. It reports a collaboration of two independent child abuse research projects. The general perspective and design of these two projects overlapped, which made possible the assessment of the generalizability of findings across samples from two geographical locations that differ in ethnic and socioeconomic composition. The total sample consisted of 132 4- to 8-year-old physically abused and comparison children and their mothers. Measures of child-rearing context and child development common to both projects were examined. Results indicated robust effects of abuse and similar patterns in both projects. In some instances, interactive effects of SES with abuse status were

Reprinted with permission from *Developmental Psychology*, 1991, Vol. 27, No. 1, 148–158. Copyright © 1991 by the American Psychological Association, Inc.

This article was supported in part by the W. T. Grant Foundation. The original research studies were supported by the National Institute of Mental Health, the National Center for Child Abuse and Neglect, the W. T. Grant Foundation, and the Spencer Foundation. We are grateful to Marianne Celano for her assistance with the statistical analyses. We would especially like to thank Edward F. Zigler, whose formative influence on our development as researchers indirectly made possible this collaborative effort.

found, suggesting different relationships between SES and certain child-rearing approaches in abusive and nonabusive families.

In the past decade, there has been an increasing recognition of the complex multiple determinants of child abuse and its sequelae and of the need for well-designed, developmentally oriented research if progress is to be made in understanding this phenomenon (e.g., Belsky, 1980; Cicchetti & Rizley, 1981; Zigler, 1980). Early research tended to have a narrow focus, to be poorly grounded in the knowledge of normal child development, and, frequently, to use inadequate control groups, which resulted in conflicting, unreplicable findings (Aber & Cicchetti, 1984). The call for improved research has been heeded by a number of developmental psychologists, and the results of these studies are beginning to appear in the literature and other public forums (see, e.g., Aber & Allen, 1987; Crittenden, 1988; Kaufman & Cicchetti, 1989; Reid, 1986; Schneider-Rosen, Braunwald, Carlson, & Cicchetti, 1985; Trickett & Kuczynski, 1986; Trickett & Susman, 1988). This permits some optimism that there will soon exist a significant increase in solid knowledge about abusive families, with important implications for both prevention of abuse and intervention.

However, a very important issue is not being addressed by this new wave of research studies. This is the question of the influence of socioeconomic status (SES) both on etiological factors and on the consequences of abuse for children's development. An early and long-lasting controversy in the child abuse field has been whether differences in SES affect the etiology and prevalence of abuse and, if so, why or how (see, e.g., Gelles, 1973; Light, 1973; Parke & Collmer, 1975). There is currently a moderate consensus about whether the prevalence of abuse is higher in lower-SES families: Recent studies have indicated that although there may be a reporting bias such that lower-SES abusive families are proportionately more likely to be reported to the authorities than are middle-class abusive families, it is likely that abuse in fact occurs more frequently among lower-SES families (Garbarino, 1977; National Center for Child Abuse and Neglect, 1988; Pelton, 1978; Straus & Gelles, 1986; Straus, Steinmetz, & Gelles, 1980). However, no research has focused on the processes that could account for this relationship between SES and abuse rates. One possibility is provided by the large literature on the relationship between SES and certain child-rearing practices and attitudes. This literature has demonstrated a relationship between lower SES and greater use of authoritarian punishment, lower parental involvement and nurturance, and lower emphasis on independence (see Gecas, 1979, for a thorough and integrative review). So far, no empirical investigations have focused on child-rearing practices and SES in samples of abusive families.

Similarly, the question of how SES might mediate the consequences of abuse for children's development has long been a matter of speculation. Elmer (1977), for example, found no differences in social and emotional developmental sequelae between abused children and a matched lower-SES control group and so concluded that lower SES has a more important effect on children's development than does abuse history. That is, Elmer suggested that the impact of poverty on children's development is so deleterious that any additional impact of abuse or maltreatment is not discernible. This conclusion runs counter to additive theories of risk (see, e.g., Rutter, 1979; Sameroff & Seifer, 1983), which posit that the number of risk factors, including both those associated with poverty and those associated with maladaptive parenting, combine additively to increase the likelihood and degree of developmental problems in children. Several recent research studies (e.g., Aber & Allen, 1987; Carlson, Cicchetti, Barnett, & Braunwald, 1989; Coster, Gersten, Beeghly, & Cicchetti, 1989; Hoffman-Plotkin & Twentyman, 1984; Kaufman & Cicchetti, 1989) have shown that in some domains of development, maltreatment has demonstrable, deleterious effects even in welfare-dependent samples. However, the issue of how low SES may mediate these effects has been ignored.

These issues of the relation of SES to the processes involved in the etiology of abuse and to the developmental consequences of abuse were addressed by the collaboration of two research projects, the Harvard Child Maltreatment Project (HCMP; Cicchetti, Carlson, Braunwald, & Aber, 1987) and the NIMH (National Institute of Mental Health) Child Abuse Project (Trickett, Susman, & Lourie, 1980), which were both concerned with the etiology of abuse and with its consequences for the social and emotional development of the children involved. Fortuitously, the general perspective and design of these two projects were quite similar, which made possible an unusual opportunity to assess the generalizability of patterns of findings across samples from two geographical locations that differed in ethnic and social class composition.

Both of these studies used a multimethod approach to assess the child-rearing environment or context of the abusive homes and the social and emotional development of abused children. Not only were the constructs being measured similar, but in a number of instances, the specific measures used were the same. On the basis of ecological theories of the etiology of child abuse, both projects assessed features of the child's environment at the microsystem level (specifically, the parent's child-rearing practices and values) and at the mesosystem level (specifically, family climate; Aber, Allen, Carlson, & Cicchetti, 1989; Belsky, 1980; Garbarino, 1977; Parke & Collmer, 1975). We reasoned that abusive families would score higher on certain child-rearing factors (such as authoritarian control and lack of encouragement of autonomy) and family-climate factors (such as conflict and lack of cohesion) than would demographically matched nonmaltreating families (see Trickett & Susman, 1988).

On the basis of developmental theories of psychopathology (Cicchetti, 1984, 1987; Kohlberg, Ricks, & Snarey, 1983; Sroufe & Rutter, 1984), both projects also assessed identical features of the child's development in the cognitive domain (specifically, relative cognitive maturity) and the behavioral domain (specifically, behavioral symptomatology such as depression and aggression). Again, we reasoned that abused children would score lower on cognitive maturity and higher on behavioral symptomatology than would demographically matched nonmaltreated children (Aber et al., 1989). Finally, each study had rich data about the demographic characteristics of the sample that made it possible to obtain several identical indices of SES.

Although these two research projects were quite similar in many respects, they differed considerably in two important respects: (a) the sample selection strategy and, consequently, (b) the SES and family structure of the participating children and parents. The differences are described in detail in the Method section. In brief, one project was a large-scale study whose subjects were 1- to 8-year-old, lower-SES, predominantly welfare-dependent children who were victims of various types of maltreatment. The other was a smaller project with 4- to 11-year-old, predominantly working-class physical abuse victims. Because of the differences in the age ranges of the subjects and in the type of maltreatment experienced by the children, we decided to select similarly defined subsamples of physically abused 4- to 8-year-old children from each project for this collaborative effort.

Thus, the purpose of the present collaborative study was to ask two general sets of questions. The first set, framed in a "cross-cultural," comparative fashion, concerned the generalizability of patterns of findings across different samples of maltreated children and their families, with one sample consisting of primarily single-parent families living in poverty and the other of primarily two-parent working-class families. The second set of questions concerned the association between the effects of maltreatment and etiological and developmental factors over and above the effects of SES. More specifically, we asked the following questions: What are the patterns of differences in child-rearing contexts of physically abusive and nonabusive families from two geographically and demographically different samples? What are the patterns of differences in behavioral symptomatology and cognitive maturity in physically abused and nonabused children from two geographically and demographically different samples? After controlling the variations in key demographic characteristics such as race and marital status, what are the unique contributions of SES, maltreatment status, and their interactions in statistically predicting variation in etiological factors and developmental sequelae?

METHOD

Subjects

The subjects in the present study were subsamples drawn from the two larger child maltreatment research projects. The HCMP is a large-scale cross-sectional and longitudinal study with a total sample of over 400 maltreated and comparison children between the ages of 1 and 8. The maltreatment group included the full range of types of maltreatment found in the state and private protective service systems from which the families were recruited. The children had experienced a variety of physical and sexual abuse, neglect, emotional maltreatment, and other conditions of inadequate child rearing and came from predominantly urban, lower-SES, welfare-dependent, single-parent families. This project also had a demographically similar nonmaltreated comparison group. The NIMH Child Abuse Study, on the other hand, was a smaller scale study with 28 abusive families (with a child between 4 and 11 years old) and 28 comparison families matched on a number of demographic variables; these subjects were predominantly suburban, working-class, two-parent families. In this study, abusive families, referred from local protective service agencies in the Washington, DC, metropolitan area, were selected on the basis of the presence of physical abuse perpetrated by a parent but with no evidence of sexual abuse. Abuse group subsamples were selected from both projects by choosing all families with a child between the ages of 4 and 8 who had been physically but not sexually abused. It should be noted that the criteria used for evidence of physical abuse were somewhat different for the two projects: For the HCMP, all forms of maltreatment originally qualified for selection into the sample; later, physical abuse status (not necessarily perpetrated by a resident parent) was determined by a caseworker. (In fact, in 91% of the cases, the perpetrator was identified as a resident parent.) For the NIMH project, the criterion for selection into the sample was evidence of a physical injury perpetrated by a resident parent.

For the HCMP sample, 37 families met the selection criteria; for the NIMH sample, the number was 21 families. Families from the two original comparison groups were selected on the basis of age of child (4–8 years). Additionally, for the HCMP sample, randomly selected girls were dropped from the comparison group until it had the same gender proportion as the abuse group. (Because the NIMH abuse and comparison groups had been matched on gender, this procedure was not necessary for these groups.) The HCMP comparison group consisted of 53 families; the NIMH comparison group consisted of 21 families.

Table 1 summarizes the demographic characteristics of the abuse and comparison groups from these two samples. As can be seen, the four groups did not differ in the mean age of the child, in the proportion of boys in the sample, or in the number of children in the families. The two samples did differ in the proportion of non-Whites, in the proportion of single-parent families, and in social class as measured by the Hollingshead Four-Factor Scale of Socioeconomic Status (Hollingshead, 1975; see also Carlson & Celano, 1987). The Hollingshead Scale is a measure of SES that is derived fro each family from a formula that combines weighted scores for parents' educational level and occupational type. Figure 1 shows the distribution of scores for the two samples. Scores can range from 8 (elementary school edu-

TABLE 1
Demographic Characteristics of the Two Samples

| | HCMP | | NIMH | |
| | Abuse | Comparison | Abuse | Comparison |
Measure	($n = 37$)	($n = 53$)	($n = 21$)	($n = 21$)
Mean age of child	5.84	5.68	6.20	6.13
% male child	62	62	67	67
% White	89	87	60	67
% single-parent families	68	72	33	30
Mean number of children in family	3.11	2.50	2.43	2.23
Mean Hollingshead score[a]	22.60	23.66	31.45	34.86

Note. HCMP = Harvard Child Maltreatment Project; NIMH = National Institute of Mental Health. Signficant sample differences were as follows: For percent White, χ^2 (3, $N = 131$) = 10.87, $p < .01$; for percent single-parent families, χ^2 (3, $N = 131$) = 17.16, $p < .001$; and for mean Hollingshead score, $F(3, 128) = 10.10$, $p < .001$.
[a] Hollingshead (1975).

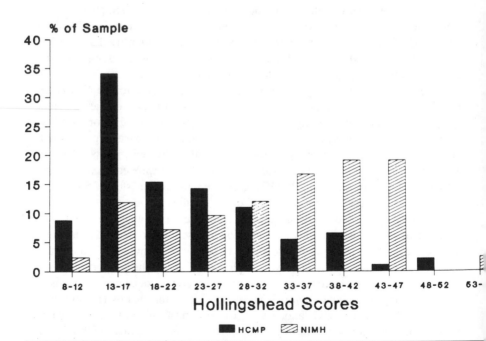

Figure 1. Distributions of Hollingshead scores (Hollingshead, 1975) for the Harvard Maltreatment Project (HCMP) and National Institute of Mental Health (NIMH) samples.

cation, chronically unemployed) to 66 (graduate degree, large business owner or professional). For the HCMP sample, the scores ranged from 8 to 50; for the NIMH sample, from 11 to 53. As Figure 1 illustrates, scores for the HCMP sample are positively skewed, whereas scores for the NIMH sample are negatively skewed. Thus, it is important to note that despite a significant difference in the mean score, there is considerable overlap in the distributions.

The HCMP sample can generally be characterized as lower SES, with a high proportion of single-parent families and a relatively low proportion of minorities. The NIMH sample is of a significantly higher SES, with a high proportion of two-parent families and a higher proportion of minority families and with most parents having a high school degree and a skilled blue-collar job. Although heterogeneous, the NIMH sample is probably best described as working class. There were no significant differences in demographic characteristics between the abuse and comparison groups overall or for either sample and no significant interaction effects of group and sample on demographic characteristics.

Measures

Four measures common to both original studies were selected for analysis. Of these, two measured child-rearing context and two measured child developmental status. For the HCMP, the child-rearing measures were collected in the child's home and the developmental measures were collected in a laboratory set up like a family room or playroom as part of over 20 hr of data collection. For the NIMH study, these measures were administered to children and mothers in a home-like research laboratory as part of about 7 hr of data collection.

Child-rearing context. The Family Environment Scale (FES; Moos & Moos, 1981) is a 90-item true-false measure of various aspects of the family psychosocial environment that yields 10 subscale scores. As conceptualized by Moos (1984), these subscales fall into one of three overarching "mesosystem" domains of the family's psychosocial environment: interpersonal relationships, personal growth, and system maintenance (see Appendix for subscale definitions; the manual [Moos & Moos, 1981] provides detailed information about reliability, validity, and norms). The subscale scores reported here are standard scores based on the test's norms (Moos & Moos, 1981).

The Child-Rearing Practices Q-Sort (CRPQ; Block, 1981) consists of 91 items about child-rearing practices and beliefs that are sorted into seven categories according to how descriptive each statement is of the mother's child rearing. These 91 items are then combined into 21 subscales. (For a listing of the items on each of these subscales, see Block, 1981.) There is considerable evidence for the test-retest reliability and validity of the CRPQ (e.g., Block, 1981; Block, Block, & Morrison, 1982). On a conceptual basis, 13 of the 21 subscales were selected for analysis and grouped into three general child-rearing dimensions: enjoyment of the child and parental role, parental authoritarian control, and parental encouragement of autonomy (see Table 3). These three "microsystem" categories are very similar to the primary dimensions of child rearing identified by Baumrind (1967, 1971), Maccoby and Martin (1983), and others. Dimensions similar to these have also been identified repeatedly as being related to SES (Gecas, 1979).

Developmental status. The Peabody Picture Vocabulary Test—Revised (PPVT, Dunn & Dunn, 1981) is a measure of receptive language abilities that correlates approximately .70 with full-scale IQ scores. The PPVT has been found to be highly related to motivational factors associated with school performance (Aber & Allen, 1987) and to be especially sensitive to specific test-taking influences (see, e.g., Zigler, Abelson, & Seitz, 1973) and is thus regarded in the present study as a measure of cognitive maturity rather than cognitive ability per se. (Information about reliability, validity, and the standardization sample is available in the manual; Dunn & Dunn, 1981.) The PPVT was administered to all children in the standard fashion.

The Child Behavior Checklist (CBC) is a measure of behavior problems that was filled out by the child's mother. (See Achenbach & Edelbrock, 1983, for extensive information on reliability, validity, and standardization.) For the present analyses, the total behavior-problem raw score was examined, as were four age- and gender-specific subscale scores (social withdrawal, depression, somatic complaints, and aggression). These four subscales were chosen both because of their conceptual relevance and because they are common to the preschool and school-age versions of the CBC for both boys and girls (see Aber et al., 1989, for a detailed discussion). Because these scales are constructed somewhat differently for different age-gender groupings, raw scores from these scales were normalized within each of the four age-gender groups (i.e., boys vs. girls, 4 and 5 years old vs. 6 years old and above).

RESULTS

Examining Group Differences

The general analytic strategy for examining group differences and assessing the patterns across samples was to conduct Status (abuse, comparison) × Sample (HCMP, NIMH) multivariate or univariate analyses of variance on each of the dependent measures. Because of our interest in examining patterns of findings in an area not yet examined empirically, we decided that, whenever the alpha level was less than .10 for multivariate Fs, univariate effects where p was less than .05 would be examined. Scheffé tests were used for post hoc analyses.

Child-rearing context. For the FES, a Status × Sample multivariate analysis of variance (MANOVA) was conducted on the 10 subscales. Significant multivariate *F*s were found for status, sample, and the interaction term. Univariate *F*s were then examined for each of the 10 subscales; these findings are summarized in Table 2. As can be seen, status effects predominated. The usual pattern of these findings was that the means for the two NIMH groups were at the extremes (i.e., the highest and lowest of the four groups), with the means for the two HCMP groups being in similar relationship to one another but not so extreme. Thus, the abuse groups scored highest on the negative factors (e.g., Conflict), whereas the comparison groups scored highest on the positive factors (e.g., Cohesion). There were significant sample effects for only two of the subscales, Conflict and Moral Religious Emphasis, with the NIMH sample lower on the former and higher on the latter than the HCMP sample. The two significant Status × Sample interaction terms were for Conflict and Active Recreational Orientation. For Conflict, post hoc analyses showed that the NIMH comparison group was significantly lower than the other three groups, which were quite similar to one another. For the Active Recreational Orientation subscale, the NIMH abuse group was significantly lower than the other three groups, which did not differ from one another.

For the CRPQ, Status × Sample MANOVAs were run on each of the three groups of subscales described earlier (see Table 3). A significant multivariate *F* for status was found for the group of subscales concerning enjoyment of child and parental role. A trend for status for the subscales concerning encouragement of autonomy also was found. In the enjoyment of child and parental role category, all three subscales were significantly different: Abusive mothers were lower on Enjoyment of Parental Role and Emotional Expressiveness and higher on Negative Affect Toward Child than were comparison mothers. A trend for the Status × Sample interaction term for this category was also found. Post hoc analyses indicated that the more negative scores on the two of these three subscales for which there were significant univariate *F*s were primarily due to the NIMH abuse group. For the encouragement of autonomy category, inspection of univariate *F*s revealed that abuse-group mothers were lower on Encouraging Independence and Openness to Experience and higher on Suppression of Sexual Curiosity than were comparison mothers.

These same MANOVAs revealed a significant multivariate *F* for sample for the group of subscales concerning authoritarian control and a trend for those concerning encouragement of autonomy. Univariate *F*s indicated that the NIMH sample was higher on Control by Guilt, Emphasis on Early Training, and Overprotectiveness and lower on Rational Guidance of the Child than the HCMP sample. A significant Status × Sample interaction term was also found for this dimension. Post hoc analyses indicated that the NIMH abuse group was significantly lower on Rational Guidance of the Child than were the other three groups.

Developmental status. For the PPVT, a Status × Sample analysis of variance (ANOVA) revealed a borderline effect for status ($p < .10$), with the abused children

TABLE 2
Ten Subscales of the Family Environment Scale for the Two Samples

| | HCMP | | | | NIMH | | | | Significant F ratios | | |
| | Abuse | | Comparison | | Abuse | | Comparison | | | | |
Subscale	M	SD	M	SD	M	SD	M	SD	Status	Sample	Interaction
Cohesion	51.68	15.75	57.36	10.59	47.86	12.28	56.95	6.84	9.10**		
Expressiveness	48.18	11.61	52.96	15.49	47.33	11.46	56.62	11.19	7.13**		
Conflict	55.96	13.24	55.41	8.08	53.57	8.59	42.19	10.06	7.65***	13.03***	6.03*
Independence	45.96	11.16	45.59	13.53	39.95	14.62	45.52	11.63			
Achievement orientation	51.14	10.36	50.55	7.95	53.14	11.32	45.14	8.55	4.45*		
Intellectual–cultural orientation	43.37	10.37	50.36	11.82	43.05	8.46	51.62	7.52	12.70***		
Active–recreational orientation	50.14	9.53	50.96	10.56	40.71	13.75	53.86	10.33	8.49**		
Moral–religious emphasis	50.91	7.03	54.46	9.01	56.52	6.59	60.67	7.84	5.78*	13.43***	6.87**
Organization	52.23	10.60	51.96	10.24	51.86	9.48	58.48	10.21			
Control	59.95	8.40	55.46	9.50	58.09	6.56	56.33	6.26	3.21*		
Multivariate F									2.70**	4.71***	2.38*

Note. HCMP = Harvard Child Maltreatment Project; NIMH = National Institute of Mental Health.
* $p < .05$. ** $p < .01$. *** $p < .001$.

TABLE 3
Three Categories of the Child Rearing Practices Q-Sort for the Two Samples

Category/subscale	HCMP Abuse M	HCMP Abuse SD	HCMP Comparison M	HCMP Comparison SD	NIMH Abuse M	NIMH Abuse SD	NIMH Comparison M	NIMH Comparison SD	Status	Sample	Interaction
	HCMP				NIMH				Significant F ratios		
	Abuse		Comparison		Abuse		Comparison		Status	Sample	Interaction
	M	SD	M	SD	M	SD	M	SD			
Enjoyment of child and parental role									7.93****		2.33*
Enjoyment of Parental Role	4.50	1.07	4.48	1.17	3.95	1.15	4.81	0.95	3.38**		
Emotional Expressiveness	5.56	0.68	5.98	0.52	5.32	0.77	6.01	0.65	20.37****		4.23**
Negative Affect Toward Child (reversed)	5.27	1.46	5.57	1.29	4.51	1.47	5.92	0.72	11.75****	2.54**	4.96**
Authoritarian control											2.41**
Authoritarian Control	2.91	0.71	2.56	0.55	3.03	0.74	2.82	0.78			
Control by Guilt	3.47	1.07	3.36	1.07	4.38	1.11	3.59	1.17		7.30***	
Control by Anxiety	3.67	1.38	3.43	1.24	3.98	1.10	3.95	1.45			
Emphasis on Early Training	2.32	0.92	2.24	1.10	3.25	1.28	2.54	1.79		6.58**	
Rational Guidance (reversed)	2.20	0.99	2.26	0.93	2.98	1.00	2.24	0.78		4.51**	5.03**
Encouragement of autonomy									2.01*	2.16*	
Encouraging Independence	4.35	0.95	4.48	0.81	3.78	1.16	4.59	0.74	7.19***		
Openness to Experience	5.50	0.80	5.66	0.91	4.94	1.25	5.77	0.96	7.21***		
Supression of Sexual Curiosity (reversed)	5.01	0.98	5.28	1.24	5.06	1.13	5.69	1.02	4.34**		
Overprotectiveness (reversed)	5.05	0.81	5.23	0.84	4.64	0.66	4.99	0.72		4.60**	
Parental Worry (reversed)	3.09	1.34	3.00	1.24	2.67	1.37	3.62	1.43			

Note: HCMP = Harvard Child Maltreatment Project; NIMH = National Institute of Mental Health.
*$p < .10$. **$p < .05$. ***$p < .01$. ****$p < .001$.

showing lower cognitive maturity than the comparison children (see Table 4). There were no other significant effects for this measure.

For the CBC, a Status × Sample ANOVA was run on the total behavior-problem score, and a MANOVA was conducted on the four behavior-problem subscale scores. Means, standard deviations, and significance levels are listed in Table 4. A significant status effect was found for the total behavior-problem score. There was also a significant F for the Status × Sample interaction. As can be seen in Table 4, both abuse groups have higher behavior-problem mean scores than both comparison groups, with the NIMH abuse group having the highest score and the NIMH comparison group the lowest score. Post hoc analyses indicated that the NIMH abuse group mean is significantly higher than that of both comparison groups. For the four behavior-problem subscale scores, there was a significant multivariate F for status. The univariate Fs for status were significant for all but the Somatic Complaints subscale. In all cases, the pattern was similar to that found for the total behavior-problems score, with NIMH scores at the extremes and HCMP scores falling between these extremes.

Demographic Characteristics as Predictors of Child-Rearing Context and Child Development

To examine more specifically the function of the demographic differences of the two samples in producing the sample and Sample × Abuse Status effects of the analyses described above, a series of hierarchical multiple regressions were conducted in which race, marital status, SES, abuse status, and the SES × Abuse Status interaction term were entered, in that order, as predictors of child-rearing context and child development. Race and marital status were entered first to control for any variance due to these two variables (which significantly differentiated the two samples) before entering the variables of primary interest: SES, abuse status, and their interaction. The 10 FES subscales and the 13 CRPQ subscales were reduced to five composite scores for ease of interpretation. For the FES, one composite score, family relationships index, consisted of the Cohesion, Expressiveness, and Conflict (reversed) subscales; a second composite score, community resources index, was the average of the Active Recreational Orientation, Intellectual-Cultural Orientation, and Moral Religious Emphasis subscales (see Corse, Schmid, & Trickett, 1990; Holahan & Moos, 1981, for more details about the rationale and construction of these composite scores and for information on adequate internal consistency). For the CRPQ, the three categories of subscales were converted into composite scores by averaging the subscale scores within each category. The alphas for these composites were .63 for enjoyment of child and parental role, .66 for authoritarian control, and .72 for encouragement of autonomy. The intercorrelations

TABLE 4
Development Sequelae for the Two Samples

Measure	HCMP				NIMH				Significant F ratios	
	Abuse		Comparison		Abuse		Comparison		Status	Interaction
	M	SD	M	SD	M	SD	M	SD		
Peabody Picture Vocabulary Test	90.81	17.86	98.26	15.58	91.30	19.50	95.62	15.73	3.35*	—
Child Behavior Checklist										
Total behavior problems	54.64	22.66	45.19	20.66	67.90	28.06	34.76	16.67	24.42***	7.55**
Social Withdrawal[a]	0.10	0.94	-.06	0.99	0.49	0.84	-0.45	0.79	8.38**	—
Depression[a]	0.11	0.85	-.01	0.96	0.46	1.30	-0.56	0.60	8.98**	—
Somatic Complaints[a]	0.12	1.03	-.05	1.10	-0.01	0.80	-0.27	0.81	—	—
Aggression[a]	0.16	1.06	-.14	0.84	0.62	1.14	-0.47	0.74	13.66***	—

Note: HCMP = Harvard Child Maltreatment Project; NIMH = National Institute of Mental Health.
[a] In z scores.
* $p < .10$. ** $p < .01$. *** $p < .001$.

TABLE 5
Predictors of Ecological Context: Results of Hierarchical Multiple
Regression Analyses

Measure	FES Composite Scores		CRPQ Composite Scores		
	FRI	CRI	ECPR	AC	EA
Race					
R^2	.01	.01	.00	.03	.00
F	0.58	0.65	0.08	3.34	0.02
` Beta	.082	-.087	.026	.168	-.012
Marital status					
R^2	.01	.01	.02	.03	.01
F	0.20	0.00	2.70	0.47	1.20
Beta	.048	.000	-.153	.064	.103
SES					
R^2	.04	.04	.02	.05	.16
F	3.05	2.71	0.29	2.08	20.42***
Beta	.215	.204	.058	-.153	.449
Abuse status					
R^2	.15	.17	.13	.10	.20
F	9.90**	12.74***	13.64**	6.13*	5.85*
Beta	.322	.363	.328	-.224	.206
Interaction of SES and status					
R^2	.15	.18	.17	.15	.21
F	0.33	0.86	5.21*	7.24**	0.77
Beta	.259	.413	.870	-1.04	.326

Note. FES = Family Environment Scale; CRPQ = Child-Rearing Practices Q-Sort; FRI = Family Relationships Index; CRI = Community Resources Index; ECPR = Enjoyment of Child and Parental Role; AC = Authoritarian Control; EA = Encouragement of Autonomy; SES = Socioeconomic Status.
* $p < .05$.   ** $p < .01$.   *** $p < .001$.

of all five child-rearing context composite variables ranged from .17 to .64 (absolute value), with a median of .42 and only one coefficient above .54.

Table 5 presents the results of these multiple regressions. As can be seen, despite significant within-group variability, neither race nor marital status were ever significant predictors of child-rearing context. SES significantly predicted only one index of child-rearing context, encouragement of autonomy. Families who were higher in SES reported more encouragement of autonomy and more independence in the child. Most important, after we controlled for the effects of SES and the other demographic variables, abuse status was a significant predictor of all five child-rearing context variables. Abuse-group status was related to lower scores on the family relationship and community resources indices, enjoyment of the child and parental role, and encouragement of autonomy and to higher scores on authoritarian control. There were two child-rearing context variables for which the SES-status interaction term was a significant predictor: enjoyment of child and parental role and authoritarian control. Figure 2 illustrates these interactions; the relationship between SES and the residualized scores for the child-rearing context variables (partialing out the variance accounted for by race and marital status) is plotted. For enjoyment of child and parental role, this score increases with increasing SES for the comparison group, whereas no such relationship holds for the abuse group. For authoritarian control, there is a negative relationship with SES for the comparison group but no association between these two variables for the abuse group.

Identical multiple regressions were conducted for the two child development scores, cognitive maturity (as measured by the PPVT) and total behavior problems (see Table 6). As with the ecological variables, marital status was never a significant predictor. Race was significant only for cognitive maturity, with minority children scoring lower than White children. SES also was a significant predictor of cognitive maturity, with higher SES being associated with higher cognitive maturity. After we controlled for both race and SES, abuse status was also a significant predictor of cognitive maturity, with abused children scoring lower than comparison children. Abuse status was also a significant predictor of total behavior problems. Furthermore, the SES-status interaction term also was significant: For the comparison group, there was no relationship between number of problems and SES, whereas for the abuse group, these two variables were positively associated (see Figure 2; again, behavior-problem scores were residualized, controlling for race and marital status).

DISCUSSION

Two limitations of this study should be mentioned at the outset. First, the data presented are cross-sectional and do not give definitive evidence of the direction of causality. Although the findings are consistent with decades of child-rearing research and theory concerning the impact of the child-rearing environment and other experiences on child development (see, e.g., Maccoby & Martin, 1983), what is really needed to provide more conclusive evidence is that extremely rare and difficult phenomenon, a prospective, longitudinal study. Second, this research was based on just two samples that differed in SES and other demographic characteristics in multiple and somewhat idiosyncratic ways, as mentioned earlier. The results say nothing about, for example, the relationship between child-rearing context and abuse among the rural poor or the upper-middle class. Further research needs to be done to extend the present findings.

Nonetheless, the results of this collaborative study represent one of the most rigorous attempts to date to investigate the relationship between SES and child abuse

202

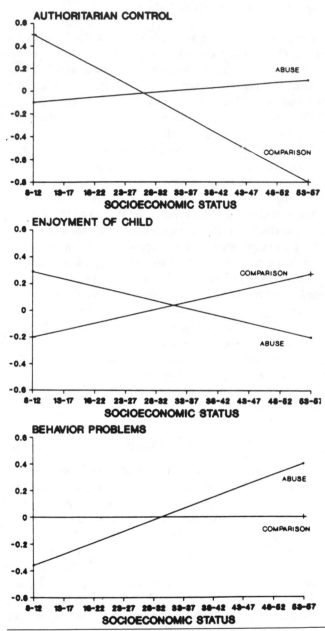

Figure 2. The interaction of abuse status and socioeconomic status for authoritarian control, enjoyment of child and parental role, and total behavior problems after partialing out the effects of race and marital status.

TABLE 6

Predictors of Development Sequelae: Results of Hierarchical
Multiple Regressions

Measure	Cognitive maturity			Total behavior problems		
	R^2	F	Beta	R^2	F	Beta
Race	.09	12.42**	.297	.00	0.00	−.002
Marital status	.09	0.11	−.028	.00	0.23	.046
SES	.16	10.63**	.307	.00	0.00	.006
Abuse status	.19	5.31*	.187	.14	17.83**	−.376
Interaction of SES and status	.20	0.19	.160	.18	5.50*	−.896

Note Fs are for the change in R^2 from the previous step. SES = socio-economic status.
* $p < .05$. ** $p < .001$.

in terms of both etiological factors and consequences for child development. The consistency of the patterns that emerge from the group difference analyses, along with the regression results, provides strong support for the notion that there are differences in the developmental ecologies of abusive homes beside those attributable to low SES. Although these differences include the expected heightened conflict, control, and punitive discipline techniques (Parke & Collmer, 1975; Trickett & Kuczynski, 1986; Wolfe, 1985), of perhaps greater importance are the differences in the emotional climates of the homes and in expectations for and satisfaction with the child. For the abusive families, a picture emerges of worried parents with little enjoyment of parenting and little satisfaction with and expressed affection for the child, of isolation from the wider community, and of lack of encouragement for the development of autonomy and independence in the child while nonetheless holding high standards of achievement for the child. Much research has suggested that such an environment has deleterious consequences for children across many domains including social, emotional, and cognitive development (Aber & Allen, 1987; Maccoby & Martin, 1983).

Also of importance is the fact that the abuse-comparison difference in authoritarian control is apparent only in the regression analyses. Considerable research has shown that this variable, or ones similar to it such as the use of harsh physical punishment, is negatively correlated with SES (see, e.g., Gecas, 1979; Hess, 1970; Kohn, 1959). In the present study, with SES controlled for, the difference between the abuse and comparison groups emerges. As Figure 2 shows, the comparison group showed the expected relationship between these variables: The higher the SES, the lower the espousal of belief in authoritarian control techniques. For the abusive families, on the other hand, this relationship does not exist. The significant SES-status interaction for the variable indexing enjoyment of child and parental role can be interpreted similarly: As the stresses associated with poverty decrease, expressed enjoyment of parenting increases for the comparison group. This expected relationship does not hold for the abuse group.

We also found robust maltreatment effects on child development, thus further challenging Elmer's (1977) notion that maltreatment effects cannot be distinguished from the deleterious effects of low social class (see also Aber & Allen, 1987; Cicchetti & Carlson, 1989). This was especially clear for parent-reported child behavior problems for which strong abuse-comparison differences were found with no sample or SES main effects in any of the analyses. The picture for cognitive maturity is more complicated. As is true for authoritarian control, the abuse-comparison difference for cognitive maturity is clearer in the regression analyses. In these analyses, an effect of race was found. This is a common finding in the research literature, and the PPVT in particular has been found to be especially prone to test-administration effects that tend to put minorities at a disadvantage (see Zigler, Abelson, & Seitz, 1973; Zigler & Butterfield, 1968; see also Moore, 1986, for a recent investigation of socialization practices in minority families and children's test-taking styles affecting IQ test performance). More important here is the fact that after race and marital status are controlled for, SES is a significant predictor of cognitive maturity. As with authoritarian control, this is a frequent research finding (Hess, 1970) and, in a parallel fashion, it is only after SES is controlled for that the significant abuse-comparison difference emerges (see also Aber & Allen, 1987; Trickett, 1988).

However, the general conclusion of robust differences in both ecological context and child development for abusive and nonabusive families must be qualified by acknowledging that there are patterns that differentiate the two samples examined, as is clearly shown in the group-difference analyses. That is, the abuse-comparison differences found in this study for both the child-rearing context variables and the child development variables tend to be much greater for the NIMH sample (primarily working class) than for the HCMP sample (primarily lower class). The significant SES-status interaction found in the regression analyses for total behavior problems probably reflects this phenomenon as well (that is, for abused children but not comparison children, higher SES was associated with more behavior problems). Although one could attribute the generally enhanced environments and better child development of the NIMH comparison group to the advantages of higher social class, how can one explain the more severe impairment of the NIMH abuse group?

There are several possible explanations for this phenomenon, including the following. First, there are demographic differences in the samples, including the higher proportion of single-parent families in the HCMP sample and the higher average

SES status of the NIMH sample, which may reflect differential protective service referral patterns. That is, we speculate that children from higher-class, two-parent families may need to pass a higher threshold of severity of abuse to be referred (Aber, 1980; Gelles, 1973). Second, the manner in which the samples were originally selected might have brought more instances of severe abuse into the NIMH sample, where criteria specifically included a visible injury by a resident parent. These differences across samples may illustrate the implications of recruiting a more diverse sample of protective service cases from state caseloads (HCMP) versus targeting a research-defined abuse group (NIMH) even when also obtained from protective services. It would have been valuable to have had independent ratings on a common metric of the severity of abuse to test this hypothesis of class differences in the severity of abuse necessary for referral, but no such metric presently exists. Indeed, the field needs a way to operationalize severity of maltreatment if progress on these and related issues is to be made (see Cicchetti & Barnett, in press, for an elaboration).

The "cross-cultural," group-difference approach to the examination of sample differences demonstrates that how clearly one can see the impact of child maltreatment over and above the effects of social class depends considerably on the characteristics of the samples in question. Scientists need to spend more time and effort measuring and describing the demographic characteristics of their samples if we are going to understand fully these relationships (Mueller & Parcel, 1981). It seems that the lower the SES, the harder it is to separate the effects of SES and abuse; this is especially true for those factors that are often correlated with SES (such as, in the present study, authoritarian disciplinary techniques and cognitive maturity). In fact, the interactions illustrated in Figure 2 suggest that among the lowest SES families in this study, the differences between abusive and nonabusive families are essentially nondiscernible. For higher-SES children, the experiences in abusive and nonabusive homes may be more different, leading, concomitantly, to greater differences in development.

We need more research studies that focus on the mediators of the relationships between SES and child-rearing context and child development in both abusive and nonabusive samples. Such studies are necessary if we are to understand more clearly the dynamic processes that link lower SES and physical abuse. Only then will it be possible to develop the prevention and intervention programs tailored to specific high-risk groups that are needed to reduce this enormous social problem.

REFERENCES

Aber, J. L. (1980). The involuntary child placement decision: Solomon's dilemma revisited. In G. Gerbner, C. Ross, & E. F. Zigler (Eds.), *Child abuse: An agenda for action* (pp. 156–182). New York: Oxford University Press.

Aber, J. L., & Allen, J. P. (1987). The effects of maltreatment on young children's socioemotional development: An attachment theory perspective. *Developmental Psychology, 23*, 406–414.

Aber, J. L., Allen, J. P., Carlson, V., & Cicchetti, D. (1989). The effects of maltreatment on development during early childhood: Recent studies and their theoretical, clinical and policy implications. In D. Cicchetti & V. Carlson (Eds.), *Child maltreatment: Theory and research on the causes and consequences of child abuse and neglect* (pp. 579–619). Cambridge, England: Cambridge University Press.

Aber, J. L., & Cicchetti, D. (1984). The socio-emotional development of maltreated children: An empirical and theoretical analysis. In H. Fitzgerald, B. Lester, & M. Yogman (Eds.), *Theory and research in behavioral pediatrics* (Vol. 2, pp. 147–205). New York: Plenum Press.

Achenbach, T. M., & Edelbrock, C. S. (1983). *Manual for the Child Behavior Checklist and Revised Child Behavior Profile.* Burlington, VT: Queen City Printers.

Baumrind, D. (1967). Child care practices anteceding 3 patterns of preschool behavior. *Genetic Psychology Monographs, 78*, 43–88.

Baumrind, D. (1971). Current patterns of parental authority. *Developmental Psychology Monographs, 4*(1, Pt. 2).

Belsky, J. (1980). Child maltreatment: An ecological integration. *American Psychologist, 55*, 83–96.

Block, J. H. (1981). *The child-rearing practices report (CRPR): A set of Q items for the description of parental socialization attitudes and values.* Unpublished manuscript, University of California, Berkeley.

Block, J. H., Block, J., & Morrison, A. (1982). Parental agreement-disagreement on child-rearing orientations and gender-related personality correlates in children. *Child Development, 52*, 965–974.

Carlson, V., & Celano, M. (1987, August). *Comparison of three SES measures in two high-risk samples.* Paper presented at the 95th Annual Convention of the American Psychological Association, New York.

Carlson, V., Cicchetti, D., Barnett, D., & Braunwald, K. (1989). Disorganized/disoriented attachment relationships in maltreated infants. *Developmental Psychology, 25*, 525–531.

Cicchetti, D. (1984). The emergence of developmental psychopathology. *Child Development, 55*, 1–7.

Cicchetti, D. (1987). Developmental psychopathology in infancy: Illustration from the study of maltreated youngsters. *Journal of Consulting and Clinical Psychology, 55*, 837–845.

Cicchetti, D., & Barnett, D. (in press). Toward the development of a scientific nosology of child maltreatment. In D. Cicchetti & W. Grove (Eds.), *Thinking clearly about psychology: Essays in honor of Paul Meehl.* Cambridge, England: Cambridge University Press.

Cicchetti, D., & Carlson, V. (Eds.). (1989). *Child maltreatment: Theory and research on the causes and consequences of child abuse and neglect.* Cambridge, England: Cambridge University Press.

Cicchetti, D., Carlson, V., Braunwald, K., & Aber, J. L. (1987). The sequelae of child maltreatment. In R. Gelles & J. Lancaster (Eds.), *Research in child abuse: Biosocial perspectives* (pp. 277–298). Chicago: Aldine.

Cicchetti, D., & Rizley, R. (1981). Developmental perspectives on the etiology, intergenerational transmission and sequelae of child maltreatment. *New Directions for Child Development, 11*, 32–59.

Corse, S. A., Schmid, K. D., & Trickett, P. K. (1990). Social network characteristics of abusing and non-abusing mothers and their relationships to parenting beliefs. *Journal of Community Psychology, 18*, 44–59.

Coster, W. J., Gersten, M. S., Beeghly, M., & Cicchetti, D. (1989). Communicative functioning in maltreated toddlers. *Developmental Psychology, 25*, 1020–1029.

Crittenden, P. M. (1988). Relationships at risk. In J. Belsky & T. Nezworski (Eds.), *Clinical implications of attachment* (pp. 136–174). Hillsdale, NJ: Erlbaum.

Dunn, L., & Dunn, L. (1981). *Manual for the Peabody Picture Vocabulary Test—Revised.* Circle Pines, MN: American Guidance Service.

Elmer, E. (1977). *Fragile families, troubled children.* Pittsburgh, PA: University of Pittsburgh Press.

Garbarino, J. (1977). The human ecology of child maltreatment: A conceptual model for research. *Journal of Marriage and the Family, 39*, 721–732.

Gecas, V. (1979). The influence of social class on socialization. In W. Burr (Ed.), *Contemporary theories about the family* (Vol. 1, pp. 365–401). New York: Free Press.

Gelles, R. J. (1973). Child abuse and psychopathology: A sociological critique and reformulation. *American Journal of Orthopsychiatry, 43*, 611–621.

Hess, R. D. (1970). Social class and ethnic influences on socialization. In P. H. Mussen (Ed.), *Manual of child psychology* (3rd ed.). New York: Wiley.

Hoffman-Plotkin, D., & Twentyman, C. (1984). A multimodal assessment of behavioral and cognitive deficits in abused and neglected preschoolers. *Child Development, 55*, 794–802.

Holahan, C., & Moos, R. (1981). Social support and psychological distress: A longitudinal analysis. *Journal of Abnormal Psychology, 90*, 365–370.

Hollingshead, A. F. (1975). *Four-Factor Index of Social Status.* Unpublished manuscript, Yale University, Department of Sociology, New Haven, CT.

Kaufman, J., & Cicchetti, D. (1989). The effects of maltreatment on school-aged children's socioemotional development: Assessments in a day-camp setting. *Developmental Psychology, 25*, 516–524.

Kohlberg, L., Ricks, D., & Snarey, J. (1983). Childhood developments as a predictor of adaptation in adulthood. In L. Kohlberg (Ed.), *Developmental psychology and early education* (pp. 91–172). New York: Longman.

Kohn, M. L. (1959). Social class and the exercise of parental authority. *American Sociological Review, 24*, 352–366.

Light, R. J. (1973). Abused and neglected children in America: A study of alternative policies. *Harvard Educational Review, 43*, 556–598.

Maccoby, E. E., & Martin, J. A. (1983). Socialization in the context of the family: Parent-child interaction. In P. H. Mussen (Series Ed.) & E. M. Hetherington (Vol. Ed.),

Handbook of child psychology: Vol. 4. Socialization, personality, and social development (4th ed., pp. 1–101). New York: Wiley.

Moore, E. G. J. (1986). Family socialization and the IQ test performance of traditionally and transracially adopted black children. *Child Development, 22,* 317–326.

Moos, R. H. (1984). Context and coping: Toward a unifying conceptual framework. *American Journal of Community Psychology, 12*(1), 5–36.

Moos, R. H., & Moos, B. S. (1981). *Manual for the Family Environment Scale.* Palo Alto, CA: Consulting Psychologists Press.

Mueller, N., & Parcel, T. L. (1981). Measures of socioeconomic status: Alternatives and recommendations. *Child Development, 52,* 13–30.

National Center for Child Abuse and Neglect. (1988). *Study of national incidence and prevalence of child abuse and neglect.* Washington, DC: U. S. Department of Health and Human Services.

Parke, R. D., & Collmer, C. W. (1975). Child abuse: An interdisciplinary analysis. In E. M. Hetherington (Ed.), *Review of child development research* (Vol. 5, pp. 509–590). Chicago: University of Chicago Press.

Pelton, L. (1978). Child abuse and neglect: The myth of classlessness. *American Journal of Orthopsychiatry, 48,* 608–617.

Reid, J. B. (1986). Social-interaction patterns in families of abused and nonabused children. In C. Zahn-Waxler, E. M. Cummings, & R. Iannotti (Eds.), *Altruism and aggression: Social and biological origins* (pp. 238–255). Cambridge, England: Cambridge University Press.

Rutter, M. (1979). Protective factors in children's responses to stress and disadvantage. In M. W. Kent & J. E. Rolf (Eds.), *Primary prevention of psychopathology; Vol. 3. Social competence in children* (pp. 49–74). Hanover, NH: University Press of New England.

Sameroff, A., & Seifer, R. (1983). Sources of continuity in parent-child relations. In M. Lewis (Chair), *Sociability and change in parent-child interaction in normal and at-risk children.* Symposium conducted at the meeting of the Society for Research in Child Development, Detroit, MI.

Schneider-Rosen, K., Braunwald, K., Carlson, V., & Cicchetti, D. (1985). Current perspectives in attachment theory: Illustrations from the study of maltreated infants. In I. Bretherton & E. Waters (Eds.), *Growing points in attachment theory and research: Monographs of the Society for Research in Child Development* (pp. 194–210). Chicago: University of Chicago Press.

Sroufe, L. A., & Rutter, M. (1984). The domain of developmental psychopathology. *Child Development, 55,* 17–29.

Straus, M. A., & Gelles, R. J. (1986). Societal change and change in family violence from 1975 to 1985 as revealed in two national surveys. *Journal of Marriage and the Family, 48,* 465–479.

Straus, M. A., Steinmetz, S., & Gelles, R. (1980). *Behind closed doors: Violence in the American family.* New York: Doubleday/Anchor.

Trickett, P. K. (1988, August). *The social and emotional development of physically abused children: Relationships with child-rearing beliefs and practices.* Paper presented at the Fifth Australian Developmental Psychology Conference, Sydney, Australia.

Trickett, P. K., & Kuczynski, L. (1986). Children's misbehaviors and parental discipline strategies in abusive and nonabusive families. *Developmental Psychology, 22*, 115–123.

Trickett, P. K., & Susman, E. J. (1988). Parental perceptions of child-rearing practices in physically abusive and nonabusive parents. *Development Psychology, 24*, 270–276.

Trickett, P. K., Susman, E. J., & Lourie, I. (1980). *The impact of the child-rearing environment on the abused child's social and emotional development* (Protocol No. 80-M-112). Bethesda, MD: National Institute of Mental Health.

Wolfe, D. A. (1985). Child-abusive parents: An empirical review and analysis. *Psychological Bulletin, 97*, 462–482.

Zigler, E. F. (1980). Controlling child abuse: Do we have the knowledge and/or the will? In G. Gerbner, C. J. Ross, & E. F. Zigler (Eds.), *Child abuse: An agenda for action* (pp. 3–34). New York: Oxford University Press.

Zigler, E. F., Abelson, W. D., & Seitz, V. (1973). Motivational factors in the performance of economically disadvantaged children on the Peabody Picture Vocabulary Test. *Child Development, 44*, 293–303.

Zigler, E. F., & Butterfield, E. (1968). Motivational aspects of changes in IQ performance of culturally deprived nursery school children. *Child Development, 39*, 1–14.

APPENDIX

Family Environment Subscales

Relationship Dimensions

1. Cohesion: the degree of commitment, help, and support family members provide for one another.
2. Expressiveness: the extent to which family members are encouraged to act openly and to express their feelings directly.
3. Conflict: the amount of openly expressed anger, aggression, and conflict among family members.

Personal Growth Dimensions

4. Independence: the extent to which family members are assertive and self-sufficient and make their own decisions.
5. Achievement Orientation: the extent to which activities (such as school and work) are cast into an achievement-oriented or competitive framework.
6. Intellectual-Cultural Orientation: the degree of interest in political, social, intellectual, and cultural activities.
7. Active-Recreational Orientation: the extent of participation in social and recreational activities.
8. Moral-Religious Emphasis: the degree of emphasis on ethical and religious issues and values.

System Maintenance Dimensions

9. Organization: the degree of importance of clear organization and structure in planning family activities and responsibilities.
10. Control: the extent to which set rules and procedures are used to run family life.

10

Social and Interpersonal Determinants of Developmental Risk

Ralph Barocas

George Mason University, Fairfax, Virginia

Ronald Seifer and Arnold J. Sameroff

Brown University, Providence, Rhode Island

Thomas A. Andrews

Rochester, New York

Roxanne T. Croft

New Brunswick, New Jersey

Ellen Ostrow

Silver Spring, Maryland

It was hypothesized that maternal teaching style (MTS) and a child's attentional performance mediate the relation between contextual risk factors and intelligence quotient (IQ). One hundred fifty-nine 4-year-old children and their mothers in a longitudinal study of children at risk for mental disorder participated in a maternal teaching task, a Luria bulb-squeeze procedure, and a delayed-match-to-sample (DMS) task in the laboratory. Maternal teaching, Luria, and DMS performance added significant variance to the risk-IQ prediction equation. The influence of MTS and attentional performance was examined through regression and structural equation-model analyses. Contextual risk was strongly related to a child's preschool IQ, but this connection may be mediated by maternal interaction and child attentional performance.

Reprinted with permission from *Developmental Psychology*, 1991, Vol. 27, No. 3, 479–488. Copyright 1991 by the American Psychological Association, Inc. The research reported here was supported by the National Institute of Mental Health and the W. T. Grant Foundation. This article was completed while Ralph Barocas was a visiting professor at the Department of Psychiatry and Human Behavior, Brown University.

211

The role that social context plays in defining the limits of the child's cognitive growth is discussed.

The study of environmental risk factors in the development of cognitive and social difficulties in children benefits from the simultaneous examination of multiple contextual risk factors. A child's social and intellectual competence is related to a group of factors that, in addition to biological factors, include the socioeconomic status (SES) of the family, stressful life events within a family, family size, and parental mental-health status. As the number of risk factors increases, children's intellectual and social performance decreases (Barocas, Seifer, & Sameroff, 1985; Morisset, Barnard, Greenberg, Spieker, & Booth, 1989; Rutter, 1979; Sameroff, Seifer, Barocas, Zax, & Greenspan, 1987; Werner & Smith, 1982).

This report extends previous work where a cumulative multiple-risk index of maternal, family, and social-status variables predicted intelligence quotient (IQ) and social adjustment in 4-year-old children (Barocas et al., 1985; Sameroff, Seifer, Barocas et al., 1987; Sameroff, Seifer, Zax, & Barocas, 1987). One important result was that different combinations of risk factors yielded similar IQ outcomes even when the total numbers of risk factors were equal, permitting a conclusion that no single risk factor was dominant. Despite these promising results, relatively little is known of the processes that transform social, family, and individual risk events into individual differences in psychological functioning.

Vygotsky's (1978, 1986) sociocultural approach provides a framework in which the role of selected social and maternal factors in the development of self-regulatory skills central to higher order intellectual functioning may be examined. On the basis of Vygotsky's perspective, we developed a model in which the connection between risk and IQ is evaluated with regard to the mediating influences of maternal teaching style (MTS) and the 4-year-old child's self-regulatory performance. This model posits that (a) young children develop cognitive capacities in the context of adult-mediated experience, (b) self-regulation is an important achievement of this developmental period and leads to general cognitive competence, and (c) the increasing presence of contextual risk factors has a cumulative adverse impact on intellectual performance, mediated by the mother's teaching style and the child's self-regulation ability.

THE CONTEXT OF ADULT GUIDANCE

Vygotsky (1978) assigned a central role to adult guidance in the evolution of the child's behavior (Luria, 1976; Vygotsky, 1978; Wertsch, 1985). Piaget (1926) and others (e.g., Werner & Kaplan, 1963) identified the internalization of social activity as a mechanism of development, but it was Vygotsky and Luria who elaborated this theme and identified the shared problem-solving activity of child and adult as defining the primary framework for cognitive growth (see also Freund, 1990; Rogoff, 1987).

Vygotsky (1978) used his concept of the zone of proximal development to describe how individual mental development originates in social interaction. He suggested that a basis for prediction of a child's future independent performance is found in the child's current performance with adult guidance. Adult guidance that fosters cognitive growth is bracketed at one end by redundancy of information that offers no new material to the child and at the other end with information beyond the comprehension of the child. Effective adult guidance must fall within this bracketed range (see also Fogel & Thelen, 1987).

Variation in how adults may guide children has been studied. For example, Sigel and his colleagues (Sigel, 1972; Sigel, McGilicuddy-DeLisa, Flaugher, & Rock, 1982) examined parental instruction in terms of the distancing required in the mental operational demands placed on children. Demands that require less distancing are tied to the here and now of immediate stimulation (e.g., labeling or demonstration). They do not encourage independent representation by the child. High-distancing instructions are less connected to the specific task and encourage active representations by the child (e.g., planning or evaluation of outcome). Although Sigel's work implies that the highest distancing strategies would be most effective, Vygotsky's (1978) work suggests that these high-distancing teaching strategies must be within the child's zone of proximal development to effectively encourage development of representational competence. It may be that intermediate distancing demands, those that are just slightly removed from immediate activity, are best at promoting cognitive growth in preschool-aged children.

Sigel's (1972; Sigel et al., 1982) approach is consonant with other schemes for studying parental teaching style in its emphasis on scoring the interactions with regard to how variations in parent behavior impact on child behavior (e.g., Hess & Shipman, 1965; Price, 1984; Wood, Bruner, & Ross, 1976). The quality of Sigel's system that is attractive for the current research is its emphasis on explicitly scoring parental behavior for its representational demands on the children in contrast to other systems that are more classificatory in terms of specific child behaviors.

Historically, studies of teaching style grew out of an interest in the promotion of cognitive skills (Hess & Shipman, 1965). As a result, examination of parental behavior in terms of its cognitive content has received the strongest emphasis. However, it is increasingly apparent that the affective quality of the parental behavior is also important in promoting cognitive as well as emotional growth in young children (e.g., Estrada, Arsenio, Hess, & Halloway, 1987).

MEASUREMENT OF SELF-REGULATION

Self-regulation is central to intellectual functioning and may be an important by-product of adult guidance. Directing attention and exerting semantic control over voluntary motor responses are evolving abilities in preschool children and are fundamental to the higher intellectual functions of planning and problem solving, which involve self-regulation of motor and cognitive activity. Vygotsky (1978, 1986) and Luria (1961) each developed methods to study different aspects of the early maturation of regulatory behavior mediated by adult guidance, particularly by means of the speech-language system. Although neither established a relation between a child's performance in these situations and social context, they believed that individual differences in cognitive functioning included reflections of the child's social world.

Luria (1961) used a simple task to document the developmental course of the ascendance of word meaning over other motor activity. Children were instructed to squeeze a bulb in one hand in response to a light signal. On different trials, he paired the stimulus onset with an appropriate verbal instruction ("squeeze") or an inappropriate one ("don't squeeze"). Younger children squeezed the bulb even when told not to do so; the verbal instruction, supplied by Luria or self-supplied by the child, had no inhibitory or semantic value for these younger children. Their motor responses were also inefficient and imprecise, resulting in perseveration errors (extra squeezes), squeezes with the wrong hand or with both hands, and squeezes during the interstimulus interval. Only later in development, when the child was able to inhibit the response in a complete and efficient manner, was semantic control of behavior said to be evident (Balamore & Wozniak, 1984; Tinsley & Waters, 1982).

Vygotsky (1986) emphasized the functional self-guiding aspect of spontaneous private speech, which he believed was central to understanding relations among thought, language, and action. Murray (1979) used a delayed match-to-sample (DMS) procedure to assess the functional significance of spontaneous speech-for-self. He found that this laboratory situation, which requires a discrimination and a delay in response, was useful in eliciting spontaneous speech during the delay period. Furthermore, the speech was positively correlated with the child's successful performance.

RISK ADULT GUIDANCE, SELF-REGULATION, AND IQ

Family and social-context factors are useful in the prediction of children's intellectual and social adjustment (Barocas et al., 1985; Rutter, 1979; Sameroff, Seifer, Barocas et al., 1987). Vygotsky (1978, 1986) identified adult guidance as an intervening psychological mechanism between contextual factors and individual development. He argued that all of the child's higher mental functions, which include attention, memory, and concept formation, originate in human interaction (Vygotsky, 1978). Consequently, to the extent that risk factors influence parental interactive styles, they also promote individual differences in basic self-regulatory skills that become manifest in intellectual functioning.

Saxe, Guberman, and Gearhart (1987) presented data from several studies of early number development in support of this perspective. They analyzed sociocultural factors, parent-child interaction, and the individual development of children, and found that social class was related to parental expectations of children, number activities in the home, degree of simplification in teaching interactions, and differences in the unassisted performance of the children. Their main conclusion was that number concepts evolve from everyday number activities that are embedded in adult-guided social practices.

Although there has been little research in SES from the Vygotskian perspective, the work of Saxe and co-workers (1987) and others show that lower status is associated with cognitive aspects of maternal teaching strategies that may discourage optimal representational competence in children (e.g., Bee, Van Egeren, Streissguth, Nyman, & Leckie, 1969; Hess & Shipman, 1965). Affective aspects of these adult-child interactions have also been related to risk and outcome. Warm and supportive approaches to children may operate to enhance healthy adjustments as has been reported in connection with mother-infant attachment, teaching styles, and environmental risk (Bretherton, 1985; Estrada et al., 1987; Patterson, Cohn, & Kao, 1989; Rutter, 1979, 1987).

The processes described previously are examined in this report. Parent-child teaching interactions, children's self-regulatory performance, and IQ were measured in 4-year-old children whose families were described in terms of a variety of risk factors. Specifically, we evaluate the hypothesis that mother-child interaction in a teaching situation and child self-regulated attentional abilities are useful as mediators in the explanation of the relation between risk and IQ.

METHOD

Subjects

The participants in this study were 159 families enrolled in the Rochester Longitudinal Study, which examined mothers with varying degrees of mental-health problems and their children (Sameroff, Seifer, & Zax, 1982). These families were seen previously during the prenatal period and when the child was newborn, 4 months, 12 months, and 30 months of age. Assessments on the attention and IQ procedures described later were performed when the child was 4 years of age (mean age = 49.0 months; SD = 1.37).

The families in this study were heterogenous on demographic and mental-health status. Hollingshead SES ranged from 1 to 5 ($M = 3.76$, $SD = 1.14$); education ranged from 3 to 18 years ($M = 11.73$, $SD = 2.58$); 58 (36%) of the families were Black; 26 (16%) of the mothers were unwed when their child was born; 62 (39%) were diagnosed as having mental illness of varying levels of severity. There were more boys than girls in the sample (94 vs. 65), and 48 (30%) of the children were firstborn.

The 159 children in this study were from families who had complete protocols on all of the measures. The original prenatal sample was 337 families. Of these, 198 completed a majority of the 4-year assessment, but 39 were lost for this study because of equipment failures on the Luria or DMS tasks (described later), leaving the final sample of 159. When compared with either the total prenatal attrition sample or the untested 4-year sample, the study group did not differ or approach significance on any of the demographic factors described previously here. In the total prenatal attrition sample, SES was 3.68, mother education was 12 years, 31% were Black families, 16% of parents were single mothers, 40% of mothers had mental illness, 52% of children were boys, and 29% of children were firstborn.

Multiple-Risk Index

An environmental multiple-risk index derived from earlier assessments was used in the analyses to summarize the demographic and mental-health status of the families, and is described in detail elsewhere (Sameroff, Seifer, Barocas et al., 1987). Assessments were made during the first year unless otherwise indicated. The risk index is a sum of ten 0–1 scores for the following (numbers in parentheses are the percentage assigned to the risk category for each measure): presence of mental illness (39%) determined by structures psychiatric interview prenatally and at 30 months; high anxiety (27%) determined through the first 4 years by the IPAT Anxiety Scale questionnaire (Cattell & Scheier, 1963), the Eysenck and Eysenck (1969) Neuroticism scale, and the Rutter (1979) Malaise scale; rigid parental perspectives (25%) determined at 4 years by the Kohn (1977) Parental Values and the Sameroff and Feil (1985) Concepts of Development Questionnaire; low spontaneous interaction (24%) during home observations at 1 year of age; less than high-school education (40%); low occupational level (19%); minority status (36%); no father in household (40%); many stressful life events (27%) determined by social-medical histories during the first 4 years; and 4 or more children in the family (18%). Scores ranged from 0 to 8 ($M = 2.88$, $SD = 2.16$). There were 51 families with low risk (scores of 0 or 1), 47 families with medium risk (scores of 2 or 3), and 61 families with high risk (scores of 4 or greater). Again, there was no evidence of selective attrition on this multiple-risk measure; the average of multiple-risk scores for the families not considered in this report was 2.82.

Laboratory Procedure at 4 Years

MTS procedure. After a brief introduction, the mother and child were brought into a room, and the mother was instructed to teach her child to fold a boat from a square piece of paper. On the table at which they were seated was a model that detailed the five steps necessary to complete the paper boat. Mothers were instructed to give their child whatever help was necessary but not to touch the paper the child was folding or do the task for the child. The procedure was videotaped (Croft, 1977).

The tapes were scored in two ways. First was the mental operational demand (MOD) of the mother's verbal statements to the child (Flaugher & Sigel, 1980; Sigel, 1972). These MODs are classified in three mutually exclusive and exhaustive categories: high, medium, and low. The high-level MODs require more distancing from the immediate task by the child and are presumed to promote cognitive representation (e.g., "See what we have to do here, make these folds to make a boat"). Low MODs are not distanced from the task and require little representation by the child (e.g., "Fold the paper in half"). The medium MODs are intermediate, requiring some distancing and representation (e.g., "Let's see what the next fold is"). The proportion of each type of MOD to the total number of MODs was calculated. Because the three scores are linearly related, only two (low and medium MOD) were used in analyses. The average proportion of low MODs was .83 ($SD = .13$); medium MODs, .06 ($SD = .05$); and high MODs, .11 ($SD = .10$). This indicates that the medium and high MODs were not the routine means by which the teaching occurred but were intermittent statements that aided the child in gaining a broader understanding of the task at hand.

The second scoring was of the affective tone of the mother during the interaction. Four 5-point rating scales were used: positive, negative, flattened, and involved. Positive and negative were defined as the expression in words, voice, or body movement; flattened was defined as evidence of diminished expression of affect or body movement; involved was defined as the degree to which the parent was engaged and enthusiastic about the task.

Kappa coefficients for both MOD scoring and affect ratings among raters for 20 protocols was between .85 and .90 in all cases. Ratings were performed by trained students and Ronald Seifer.

DMS procedure. After the teaching task was completed, the mother left the room to complete an interview, and the DMS procedure was initiated (Cumming & Berryman, 1965; Ferraro, Francis, & Perkins, 1971; Murray, 1979). The child was seated in front of a panel with three .65-cm light sources horizontally positioned 3 cm apart at eye level (currently available as Lafayette Instrument Pigeon Key with Three Color Display, Model 80123). The center light was a standard stimulus, and the matching lights were on either side, which were translucent disk-shaped response switches (illuminated from the rear) that the child could press. Each light could be either red or green (Ostrow, 1980).

In simultaneous-match training, the child was instructed to press the button that was the same color as the center stimulus light (no statements about speed or accuracy were made, but the child was encouraged to do the best he or she could, and the speed of the task was indicated by the nature of the training stimuli). The stimulus light appeared for 2 s, and then the two matching lights lit up for 2 s, during which time the child could respond. The interstimulus interval was 5 s. During training, the stimulus light remained on through the entire trial. As soon as the child had four successive correct simultaneous matches, the delay trials were begun. A second examiner, controlling the apparatus behind a one-way mirror, signaled the examiner who was in the room with the child when the training criterion was reached. If the child went 40 trials without attaining this criterion, no delay trials were conducted. At each correct match, one M&M candy was deposited in a chute with a Plexiglas cover so that it was visible to the child (pilot testing indicated that without the cover children would hold the candy in their hand and make a mess).

If the child successfully completed training, the examiner repeated the instructions and left the room, and the delay trials were begun. Each block of 10 trials consisted of five red and five green stimulus lights arranged by computer so that no color appeared three times in succession, and the presence of the red and green lights in the response buttons was arranged so that no color appeared in a position more than twice in succession. The delay periods for the blocks were 1, 2, 5, and 10 s, respectively.

While the task was ongoing, the child's speech was audiotaped, and the stimulus color and child's response noted. Unfortunately, the speech samples were too few to permit an analysis of the relationship between speech and successful mediation. Consequently, this report is limited to only the behavioral description of the DMS performance.

The data were reduced by forming four groups of children: Nonlearners were those who did not achieve the criterion of four correct simultaneous-match training trials (39%); learners were those who met the training criterion but whose performance did not achieve 70% correct matches in the first 1-s delay block (31%); decrementers were those who achieved 70% correct on the 1-s delay block but whose performance dropped below this criterion by the 10-s delay (11%); nondecrementers were those who maintained a minimum of 70% correct through the 10-s delay trial (19%). Children were assigned a score of 1 if they were nonlearners, 2 if they were learners, 3 if they were decrementers, and 4 if they were nondecrementers. This summary measure is referred to as DMS group.

Luria bulb-squeeze task. After the DMS task was completed, the panel in front of the child was changed to one that had a 4.5-cm light source at the child's eye level. The child held a 3.5 × 5-cm rubber bulb in each hand that was connected to the center of the panel (hemline markers purchased from Singer Sewing Co.). The examiner sat next to the child during this procedure. Children first demonstrated that they could correctly understand the words *red* and *green* as well as the ability to squeeze the bulb one time in their preferred hand. They were then given the instruction that when a green light appeared, they should squeeze the bulb in their (preferred) hand one time, and not to squeeze either bulb when a red light came on. They were then asked to demonstrate what they would do when a green light came on and when a red light came on. When the children correctly squeezed one time ("What will you do when the green light comes on?") and no times ("What will you do when the red light comes on?"), the task was begun. No children had difficulty with this instructional set. As with the DMS, no explicit speed or accuracy instructions were given; it was stipulated only that the children should do their best.

The first block consisted of eight green- and eight red-light trials, arranged randomly by computer so that no color appeared three times in succession. The light remained on for 2 s and the interstimulus interval was 2 or 3 s (arranged randomly by computer so that no interval occurred more than three times in succession). If the child was not looking at the panel, the examiner said "Look at the light now" before the next trial.

The second block was similar to the first, except that the examiner said "go" once when the green light appeared and "don't go" when the red light appeared. On the third block, the child was instructed to say "go" one time and squeeze the bulb one time when the green light appeared; and "don't go" one time and not squeeze when the red light appeared. The fourth block was identical to the first block. For each block, there were eight green and eight red stimuli, with the same on-time and interstimulus interval as the first block. There was a pause of about 1 min between blocks while the relevant instructions were repeated.

The child's responses from each bulb (by means of a pressure transducer), the presence of speech (by means of a voice-activated switch), and the on-off status of each light color was recorded on a Grass Model 79 polygraph. These paper records were later scored for the following criteria for each trial: hit (one squeeze by the preferred hand in response to the green light), miss (no squeeze in response to the green light), wrong (a squeeze in response to the red light), extra hit (a second squeeze in response to the red light), interval squeeze (a squeeze in the interstimulus interval), overflow (a non-preferred-hand squeeze in the presence of a preferred-hand squeeze), nonpreferred overflow (a non-preferred-hand squeeze in the absence of a preferred-hand squeeze). This scoring was highly reliable; rater agreement was over .90 in 20 protocols.

A summary score of all of the errors of commission was computed, which will be referred to as Luria errors. This included mistakes (wrongs plus interval squeezes), overflows (overflow plus nonpreferred overflow), and perseveration (extra hit plus extra wrong). The mistakes, overflows, and perseverations for each block were converted to z scores, and these 12 z scores were summed. The Cronbach alpha for this scale was .87. The misses, an error of omission, were not included in this summary score.

IQ assessment. After the attention tasks were completed, four verbal scales of the Wechsler Primary and Preschool Scale of Intelligence (WPPSI), similarities, comprehension, information, and vocabulary, were used (Wechsler, 1967). The total prorated verbal IQ score (M = 103.5; SD = 17.5; range = 62–156) was used in analyses. The use of IQ tests in a study with Black and White children and the problems in interpretation of group differences are noted. However, this study was not concerned with group differences in outcome, but with patterns of correlations with the IQ outcome. Group differences have typically not been found for these types of relations (Jensen, 1980).

To summarize the data reduction, final variables from the teaching procedure were mother's positive affect, negative affect, flattened affect, involvement, low MOD, medium MOD, and high MOD; from the Luria bulb-squeeze procedure was child Luria errors; from the DMS was child DMS group; and from the WPPSI exam was the child verbal IQ. The multiple-risk score described previously here was also used in analyses.

RESULTS

This study took as its departure an earlier report that established that risk factors associated with the family and mother predict a child's intellectual functioning. This relation was again evaluated but with the addition and elaboration of other predictive measures selected to illuminate the vehicles of transmission, which may intervene between family characteristics and individual intellectual performance.

Table 1 shows the correlations among maternal and family risk factors, ratings for MTS, child attention and self-regulatory behavior, and child intellectual performance. Maternal and family risk factors have a clear and important impact on intellectual functioning (Sameroff, Seifer, Barocas et al., 1987), indicated by the obtained correlation of -.61. The greater the risk, the lower the intellectual performance of the child. It is useful to recall that these risk factors are not attributes of the child, but rather attributes of the context within which the child is developing.

Second, the risk factors and maternal teaching ratings are also significantly related. Highest risk scores are associated with less expression of positive emotion, more expression of negative emotion, and less expressiveness and involvement with the child during the teaching situation. Also, these parents are less likely to use teaching strategies believed to foster the use of abstraction by their children.

Third, maternal- and family-risk scores are significantly related to each of the attention/self-regulating measures. The greater the risk, the less likely the child was to negotiate the DMS situation successfully, and the more likely the child was

TABLE 1
Correlations Among Risk, Maternal Teaching, Attention, and Outcome Measures

Factor	Factor									
	1	2	3	4	5	6	7	8	9	10
1. WPPSI verbal IQ	—									
2. Contextual risk	-.61	—								
3. MTS positive	.54	-.57	—							
4. MTS negative	-.45	.41	-.58	—						
5. MTS flattened	-.46	.46	-.63	.61	—					
6. MTS involved	.44	-.46	.52	-.40	-.51	—				
7. MTS low MOD	-.15	.19	-.07	-.10	-.00	-.02	—			
8. MTS med MOD	.39	-.45	.34	-.19	-.27	.19	-.43	—		
9. MTS high MOD	.19	-.22	.21	-.06	-.09	.10	-.70	.32	—	
10. Luria errors	-.29	.28	-.28	.24	.18	-.22	.08	-.10	-.19	—
11. DMS group	.51	-.36	.38	-.35	-.33	.23	.00	.08	.00	-.23

Note. Correlations of .16 or greater are significant at $p < .05$; correlations of .21 or greater are significant at $p < .01$. The number of cases is 159. WPPSI = Wechsler Primary and Preschool Scale of Intelligence; MTS = maternal teaching style; MOD = mental operational demand; med = medium; DMS = delayed-match-to-sample task.

to fail to inhibit unnecessary motor activity in the Luria bulb-squeeze situation. Although these tasks were related, and both assess attentional and mediational skills, the DMS situation emerged as the superior predictor of IQ: $r = .51$ for DMS and $-.29$ for Luria ($t = 2.57$, $p < .05$).

Fourth, the relation of each of the teaching and child measures to IQ shows much the same pattern they had with regard to risk. Uninvolved parents who display negative emotion and little enthusiasm in the teaching situation have children with lower IQs. Additionally, teaching styles that support the child's dependence on abstraction and generalization positively covary with IQ.

Table 2 shows the hierarchical multiple-regression analysis in which maternal- and family-risk factors are entered into the prediction equation first, followed by the maternal teaching measures and by the child's laboratory-attention measures (Cohen & Cohen, 1983). When maternal teaching is added, a significant increase of 9% in variance explained is achieved; when the attention measures are entered, an additional significant increase of 7% is obtained. Taken together, these measures of maternal and family risk, MTS (particularly the affective aspects), and the child's attention and self-regulation as assessed in the DMS and Luria situations account for more than half the variance in IQ.

Subgroup Differences

The patterns of relations among variables detailed in Tables 1 and 2 were examined in three sets of subgroups: boys versus girls, Whites versus non-Whites, and

TABLE 2
Summary of Hierarchical Multiple-Regression Analysis With
Verbal IQ as Criterion

Predictor variables	R^2	R^2 change	F (change)
Step 1			
Contextual risk	.376	.376	94.43*
Step 2			
MTS positive			
MTS negative			
MTS flattened			
MTS involved			
MTS low MOD			
MTS medium MOD	.468	.092	4.35*
Step 3			
Luria errors			
DMS group	.538	.071	11.38*

Note. MTS = maternal teaching style; MOD = mental operational demand; DMS = delayed-match-to-sample task; IQ = intelligence quotient.
* $p < .01$.

ill mothers versus healthy mothers. The matrix in Table 1 contains 45 correlations, and there was no evidence for substantial subgroup effects beyond those expected by chance given the number of correlations compared; at most 6.67% of the correlations compared were significantly different. For boys versus girls, 1 of the 45 correlations was significantly different; for Whites versus non-Whites, 3 of 45 were different; for mentally ill versus nonmentally ill mothers, 0 of 45 were different. Also, within all six subgroups, the hierarchical regression relations held. That is, the proportion of variance explained by Steps 2 and 3 (the effects of maternal teaching and child attention after risk was partialed) was about the same as reported in Table 2 for the entire sample.

Structural Modeling

The regression analyses described previously here are consistent with hypotheses stated at the outset. However, because several analyses would be necessary to examine different aspects of the model, there is no single test of whether our data are consistent with the proposed theoretical explanation. To address this problem, we used a structural-equations-model approach to our data. Such models allow for the examination of complex hypotheses (particularly those with multiple criterion variables and indirect paths) as well as direct comparison of the adequacy of competing models. The major hypothesis examined was whether the indirect path from contextual risk to child IQ, by means of maternal teaching and child attention, was necessary to explain the risk by IQ correlation.

Models were evaluated by using BMD EQS/PC2.10 (Bentler, 1986). The measurement model included three latent variables. The first was indicated by the four MTS affect ratings and is referred to as MTS-affect. The second latent variable was indicated and medium MOD and is called MTS-MOD. The third latent variable was indicated by the Luria composite score and the DMS group and is called attention. The contextual risk and child IQ are each defined by a single measured variable. The structural portion of the model in its most general form included a direct path from risk to IQ and indirect paths from risk to IQ by means of either MTS-affect or MTS-MOD and then attention (see Figure 1).[1] The sample size for these analyses is adequate. Including the measurement model, structural model, and relevant error terms, a maximum of 26 parameters were estimated. Through the use of Bentler's (1986) guideline of 5 cases for each parameter estimated, 130 cases would be the minimum necessary.

This general model provided a satisfactory fit to the obtained data, $\chi^2(30, N = 159) = 41.53, p = .08$; Bentler-Bonet fit index $= .961$. However, the parameter associated with the direct path from risk to IQ was not significant, and the Wald test for dropping parameters suggested that this parameter could be dropped.[2] Indeed, when this path was eliminated from the model, a similar degree of fit was observed, $\chi^2(31, N = 159) = 41.54, p = .10$; Bentler-Bonnet fit index $= .966$, and the Lagrange multiplier tests for adding parameters (see Footnote 2) did not suggest any additions. The difference in chi-square between these nested models is .01 (with 1 df), which does not approach significance. A third model was examined where the direct path between risk and IQ was kept and the indirect paths were eliminated (by dropping the parameter from attention to IQ). This model showed a significant decrease in goodness of fit, $\chi^2(31, N = 159) = 78.99, p < .001$;

---

[1]The model in Figure 1 has been slightly simplified for ease of presentation. In fact, there are three additional paths: from risk to maternal teaching negative, from risk to maternal teaching flat, and from risk to maternal teaching medium MOD. These paths were included because preliminary analysis indicated they were necessary to achieve adequate fit. They are not related to the main hypotheses examined, but are related to measurement aspects of the model. They indicate that there is a relation between risk and some of the maternal teaching variables not accounted for by the MTS latent variable. Note that none of these three paths are relevant to the prediction of 4-year IQ. If these paths are not used in the analyses, the conclusions about relative merits of the models is exactly the same. The only difference is that all of the models have slightly elevated chi-square levels; the best $\chi^2 (34, N = 159) = 64.04$ $p < .01$, although the *relative* chi-square difference among the models is unchanged.

[2]Bentler (1986) described two tests relevant to decisions about adding or dropping parameters in structural-equation models. The Wald test examines whether parameters in a particular model may be dropped without significantly affecting goodness of fit. The Lagrange multiplier tests examine whether parameters not included in a particular model would significantly increase the goodness of fit. Both of these approaches are exploratory in nature; they examine all possible parameters and do not adjust nominal alpha rates. They are presented here to note that these exploratory, computer-generated suggestions fit precisely with the hypothesis-driven comparisons among models that were made.

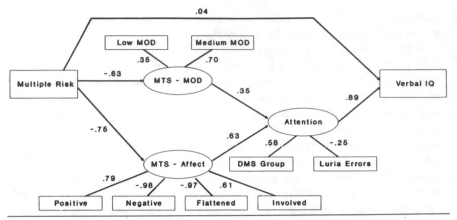

Figure 1. Structural model for prediction of child verbal intelligence quotient (IQ). (MOD = mental operational demand; MTS = maternal teaching style; DMS = delayed-match-to-sample task.)

Bentler-Bonnet fit index = .853. Note also that the difference in chi-square from either of the previous models is about 38, far greater than the significance level for a 1 degree-of-freedom test. The Lagrange multiplier test suggested adding a path from attention to IQ, precisely the indirect path that was eliminated.

It should be noted that the path from MTS-MOD to attention did not reach significance ($z = 1.38$). When removed from the model, there was not a significant decrease in chi-square, a difference of 1.46 with 1 degree of freedom. The mediated effect appears stronger with respect to maternal affect than with cognitive teaching strategy.

In sum, two competing explanations of the data were examined, each of which implied different predictive paths. The best fitting and most parsimonious model included a direct path from risk to IQ mediated first by MTS (particularly affect) and then by child attention, but no direct path from risk to IQ. The addition of the direct path did not provide an increase in explanatory power given the observed data. This finding is stronger than the original hypothesis, which merely posited the necessity of the indirect path but not the elimination of the direct path. However, firm attributions about causality are premature without replication, longitudinal study designs, or experimental manipulations of relevant behaviors.

DISCUSSION

This study examined one model of how a group of social, family, and individual risk factors were related to a child's intellectual functioning. It was generally guided by the suggestion that there is a direct relation between the development of intrapersonal mental activity and the interpersonal context provided the child during the developmental period (Vygotsky, 1978). The child's independent behavior is considered partly a product of the internalization of events that occur in interpersonal exchange. Thus, the opportunities and limits for much of the child's cognitive growth are defined by the world within which the child lives. If the child receives guidance from adults whose lives are diminished by circumstance, then that child may suffer a corresponding loss of opportunity to internalize growth-enhancing experiences. Simultaneous examination of measures selected from the different levels of social, family, and individual organization may offer the best understanding of the determinants of a child's functioning (Bronfenbrenner, 1979; Saxe et al., 1987). Here these included social factors such as SES, family factors such as number of children in the family, and individual factors such as performance on self-regulatory attention tasks.

Analysis indicated that a model hypothesizing indirect effects of cumulative risk on child IQ by means of maternal teaching and child self-regulated attention fit the observed data. In particular, the affective components of the mothers' teaching were related to child self-regulation and attention. When these indirect paths were included in the model, it was no longer necessary to posit a direct relation between cumulative risk and child IQ. There were no meaningful subgroup effects. No evidence pointed to differences among boys and girls, among White versus non-White, or among mentally ill versus nonmentally ill mothers in terms of patterns of relations among variables.

Although the results demonstrate support for the importance of adult guidance and self-regulation in understanding risk-competence relations, there were many other domains not assessed in this study. For example, issues of social support, sensitivity during interactions, peer influences, preschool or daycare experiences, to name a few, were not considered. These and other factors are good candidates for adding to our understanding of how broadly defined contextual risk becomes manifested in individual differences in cognitive competence.

Laboratory Versus Contextual Assessment

The assessments in this study were performed in the laboratory and raise the question of generalizability to everyday contexts. The maternal teaching task used here, as well as those used by others, are attempts to standardize everyday parent-child activity. Some investigators who have addressed this issue of ecological validity more directly through the observation of children engaged in teaching tasks, both at home and in the laboratory, report no differences as a result of setting (Borduin & Henggler, 1981). Additional research also supports the view that the relation of teaching style to either demographic characteristics or child behavior does not appear to vary as a function of setting (e.g., Bee et al., 1969; Laosa, 1980;

Price, 1984). Despite the minimal amount of empirical evidence, some credence may be extended to the use of laboratory assessments of mother-child teaching interactions.

The Luria and DMS procedures are less amenable to home administration or observational analogues. However, the major component of each task, executing an adult instruction sometimes with a discrimination involved, is an event that occurs many times during each day in the life of the 4-year-old child.

Contextual Versus Maturational Effects

The examination of self-regulation as described here is dependent on developmental maturity and prompts the question of what limits biological inevitabilities might place on the contributions of social factors. Although control of a response such as a bulb squeeze or the recall of a color after a few seconds delay is ultimately achieved in all healthy children, there are individual differences in its accomplishment. These differences, like those measured on scales of intelligence, provide the opportunity to enrich our understanding of the context of development. The disentanglement of maturational and contextual influences and the assignment of causal roles is difficult. However, differences in rates of acquisition of self-regulation, attention, and other cognitive behaviors that may be fundamentally maturational in nature have been associated with later important adjustment behaviors. For example, Mischel, Shoda, and Rodriguez (1989) showed that individual differences in the voluntary delay of gratification in 4-year-olds, a behavior mastered by all children within another year or 2, is predictive of adolescent cognitive and social competence.

General Measurement Issues

Precise determination of individual differences in specific behavior domains such as attention is always difficult in pre-school-age children. Our original intent was to examine carefully how the language system serves attentional capabilities by means of individual self-regulation in the children studied. As noted previously here, the DMS procedure yielded too few speech samples to perform such analyses. Also when composite measures of both attention protocols were computed, we relied on a relatively modest relation between the Luria and DMS results (which was sufficient for the structural-equation-modeling procedures). There is clearly a need for better measures to accurately assess qualities of attention and self-regulation in these young children.

In the MTS assessments, the behavior of interest with respect to MODs made up only 17% of those sampled, and may have contributed to the marginal utility of MODs in the overall model. In contrast, the ratings of affect, which were more useful in the overall model, relied on behavior observed throughout the entire procedure. Such discrepancies prompt questions as to whether different results are due to differences in the phenomena or to artifacts of the sampling and assessment systems. Low-frequency responses, such as higher level MODs, may require more sampling over longer time periods to reduce variability resulting from measurement error and thereby increase predictive power.

Theoretical Implications of Results

The data here enlarge the understanding of the development of individual differences because they comment on the relation between risk and intellectual performance. The results suggest that risk may be mediated by aspects of maternal teaching, particularly the emotional climate established by the mother. Moreover, these affective qualities of the mothers were relatively independent of their teaching strategies. Maternal teaching climates rated as aversive or indifferent to the child, and to a lesser extent those that did not foster the elaboration of representation skills, were associated with poorer self-regulatory performance. These children showed an excess of activity that interfered with successful execution of a simple voluntary task and more difficulty in the mastery of a mediational attentional task. These same children also earned lower IQ scores. Overall, the data are consistent with the hypothesis that one way in which maternal teaching might influence IQ is through its relation to the acquisition of efficient self-regulatory behavior.

Two issues related to speculation about causality merit discussion: maternal IQ and direction of influence in the teaching situation. One measure not included in this study was maternal IQ. Some have suggested that this is an important determinant of children's IQ independent of environmental characteristics (e.g., Scarr, 1985). Yet others indicate that context is the primary determinant (e.g., Gottfried & Gottfried, 1984). If IQ is largely inherited and only subject to minor environmental influences, then one could observe a correlation between maternal teaching and child outcome, even when the maternal teaching does not truly mediate child intelligence; the same factor (i.e., high maternal IQ) could produce both the teaching strategies and the child performance. Our data indicate that the affective rather than cognitive strategies predicted the children's IQ. It is less likely that maternal IQ would mediate the mother's affective style more than their cognitive strategies. This study was not designed to examine issues of inheritance and cannot be conclusive about specific causal mechanisms, but this important and enduring issue should be addressed in future work.

A related issue is the direction of effects in parent-child interactions. The model evaluated in this study suggests that maternal teaching promotes individual differences in cognitive function. However, the probability that child functioning affects maternal teaching must also be considered, as the findings of Saxe and associates

(1987) suggest. We believe that research designs will continue to become more complex, enabling the demonstration of bidirectional influences, which is consistent with transactional models of development (Sameroff, 1983).

Determining direction of effect is often motivated by the desire to ascertain causal relationships. A straightforward approach involves comparing variables measured at one point in time with those measured at a later point in time. Those temporally prior are sometimes interpreted as causal in nature. In this longitudinal study, we measured many child variables during the first year of life. However, there were no meaningful patterns of relations in the child measures from earlier to later years. Those relations that were present were with family and context variables and were aggregated in the multiple-risk index (Sameroff, Seifer, Baldwin, & Baldwin, 1989). Even if there were such relations among child variables, a more rigorous research design and analysis strategy would be necessary to account for autocorrelation effects that may produce spurious conclusions about causality. This study was not designed with such considerations in mind and is not well suited to make definitive statements about causal relations.

From a more practical perspective, this study suggests that impaired development might be the outcome of the accumulation of risk factors operating concomitantly at differing levels of social, family, and individual organization. Unfortunately, interventions with multiproblem families that address all aspects of their risk for developmental problems are costly and difficult to implement. However, if the observation regarding cumulative impact of risk is correct, then intervention at any one level or organization (which could address a meaningful subset of the risk factors) may have significant impact through the reduction of the overall risk burden. Future studies might examine whether this hypothesis is correct.

In summary, mothers who were poor, had four or more children, suffered from a mental disorder, or did not benefit from the presence of another adult in the household had children with lower intelligence. These same mothers were less likely to receive positive affective ratings, and their children were more likely to encounter difficulties on the self-regulatory tasks. Among the models examined, the one that best fit the data suggested that the maternal teaching approach, partly determined by social and family-risk factors, acted to influence intellectual performance by affecting the child's self-regulatory skills.

REFERENCES

Balamore, U., & Wozniak, R. H. (1984). Speech-action coordination in young children. *Developmental Psychology, 20,* 850–858.

Barocas, R., Seifer, R., & Sameroff, A. J. (1985). Defining environmental risk: Multiple dimensions of psychological vulnerability. *American Journal of Community Psychology, 13,* 429–443.

Bee, H. L., Van Egeren, L. F., Streissguth, A. P., Nyman, B. A., & Leckie, M. S. (1969). Social class differences in maternal teaching strategies and speech patterns. *Developmental Psychology, 5*, 726–734.

Bentler, P. (1986). *Lagrange multiplier and Wald tests for EQS and EQS/PC*. Los Angeles: BMDP Statistical Software.

Borduin, C. M., & Henggler, S. W. (1981). Social class, experimental setting, and task characteristics of mother-child interaction. *Developmental Psychology, 17*, 209–214.

Bretherton, I. (1985). Attachment theory: Retrospect and prospect. In I. Bretherton & E. Waters (Eds.), Growing points of attachment theory and research. *Monographs of the Society for Research in Child Development, 50*(1-2, Serial No. 209), 3–38.

Bronfenbrenner, U. (1979). Contexts of child rearing: Problems and prospects. *American Psychologist, 34*, 844–850.

Cattell, R. B., & Scheier, I. H. (1963). *Handbook for the IPAT anxiety scale questionnaire* (2nd ed.). Champaign, IL: Institute for Personality and Ability Testing.

Cohen, J., & Cohen, P. (1983). *Applied multiple regression/correlation analysis for the behavioral sciences* (2nd ed.). Hillsdale, NJ: Erlbaum.

Croft, R. G. F. (1977). *The relationship of maternal teaching style and socioeconomic status to four-year-old children's locus of control orientation*. Unpublished doctoral dissertation, University of Rochester, New York.

Cumming, W. W., & Berryman, R. (1965). The complex discriminated operant: Studies of matching and related problems. In D. I. Mostofsky (Ed.), *Stimulus generalization* (pp. 284–330). Stanford, CA: Stanford University Press.

Estrada, P., Arsenio, W. F., Hess, R. D., & Halloway, S. D. (1987). Affective quality of the mother-child relationship: Longitudinal consequences of children's school relevant cognitive functioning. *Developmental Psychology, 23*, 210–215.

Eysenck, H. J., & Eysenck, S. B. G. (1969). *Personality structure and measurement*. San Diego, CA: Knapp.

Ferraro, D. P., Francis, E. W., & Perkins, J. J. (1971). Titrating delayed matching to sample in children. *Developmental Psychology, 7*, 488–493.

Flaugher, J., & Sigel, I (1980). *Parent-child interaction observation schedule (PCI)*. Princeton, NJ: Educational Testing Service.

Fogel, A., & Thelen, E. (1987). Development of early expressive and communicative action: Reinterpreting the evidence from a dynamic systems perspective. *Developmental Psychology, 23*, 747–761.

Freund, L. S. (1990). Maternal regulation of children's problem-solving behavior and its impact on children's performance. *Child Development, 61*, 113–126.

Gottfried, A. W., & Gottfried, A. E. (1984). Home environment and cognitive development in young children of middle socioeconomic status families. In A. W. Gottfried (Ed.), *Home environment and early cognitive development: Longitudinal research* (pp. 57–115). San Diego, CA: Academic Press.

Hess, R. D., & Shipman, V. C. (1965). Early experience and the socialization of cognitive modes in children. *Child Development, 36*, 869–886.

Jensen, A. R. (1980). *Bias in mental testing*. New York: Free Press.

Kohn, M. L. (1977). *Class and conformity* (2nd ed.). Chicago: University of Chicago Press.

Laosa, L. M. (1980). Maternal teaching strategies and cognitive styles in Chicano families. *Journal of Educational Psychology, 72*, 45–54.

Luria, A. R. (1961). *The role of speech in the regulation of normal and abnormal behavior.* New York: Liveiryut.

Luria, A. R. (1976). *Cognitive development, its cultural and social foundation.* Cambridge, MA: Harvard University Press.

Mischel, W., Shoda, Y., & Rodriguez, M. L. (1989). Delay of gratification in children. *Science, 244*, 933–938.

Morisset, C. E., Barnard, K. E., Greenberg, M. T., Spieker, S. J., & Booth, C. L. (1989, March). *Environmental influences on early language development: The context of social risk.* Paper presented at the meeting of the Society for Research in Child Development meeting, Kansas City, MO.

Murray, D. J. (1979). Spontaneous private speech and performance on a delayed match-to-sample task. *Journal of Experimental Child Psychology, 27*, 286–302.

Ostrow, E. (1980). *Maternal teaching style and delayed match-to-sample performance in four-year-old children.* Unpublished doctoral dissertation, University of Rochester, New York.

Patterson, C. J., Cohn, D. A., & Kao, B. T. (1989). Maternal warmth as a protective factor against risks associated with peer rejection in children. *Development and Psychopathology, 1*, 21–38.

Piaget, J. (1926). *The language and thought of the child.* New York: Harcourt, Brace.

Price, G. G. (1984). Mnemonic support and curriculum selection in teaching by mothers: A conjoint effect. *Child Development, 55*, 659–668.

Rogoff, B. (1987). Specifying the development of a cognitive skill in its interactional and social context: Commentary. *Monographs of the Society for Research in Child Development, 52*(2, Serial No. 216), 153–159.

Rutter, M. (1979). Protective factors in children's responses to stress and disadvantage. In W. Kent & J. E. Rolf (Eds.), *Primary prevention of psychopathology (Vol. 3): Social competence in children* (pp. 49–74). Hanover, NH: University Press of New England.

Rutter, M. (1987). Psychosocial resilience and protective mechanisms. *American Journal of Orthopsychiatry, 57*, 316–331.

Sameroff, A. J. (1983). Developmental systems: contexts and evolution. In W. Kessen (Ed.), *Handbook of child psychology: Vol. 1. History, theories, and methods*(4th ed., pp. 237–294). New York: Wiley.

Sameroff, A. J., & Feil, L. (1985). Parental concepts of development. In I. E. Sigel (Ed.), *Parental belief systems: The psychological consequences for children* (pp. 84–104). Hillsdale, NJ: Erlbaum.

Sameroff, A. J., Seifer, R., Baldwin, C., & Baldwin, A. (1989, March). Continuity of risk from early childhood to adolescence. In R. Barocas (Chair), *Development and risk from early childhood to adolescence: The Rochester Longitudinal Study.* Symposium presented at the meeting of the Society for Research in Child Development meeting, Kansas City, MO.

Sameroff, A. J., Seifer, R., Barocas, R., Zax, M., & Greenspan, S. (1987). Intelligence quotient scores of 4-year-old children: Social environmental risk factors. *Pediatrics, 79,* 343–350.

Sameroff, A. J., Seifer, R., & Zax, M. (1982). Early development of children at risk for emotional disorder. *Monographs of the Society for Research in Child Development, 47*(7, Serial No. 199).

Sameroff, A. J., Seifer, R., Zax, M., & Barocas, R. (1987). Early indicators of developmental risk: Rochester Longitudinal Study. *Schizophrenia Bulletin, 13,* 383–394.

Saxe, G. B., Guberman, S. R., & Gearhart, M. (1987). Social processes in early number development. *Monographs of the Society for Research in Child Development, 52*(2, Serial No. 216).

Scarr, S. (1985). Constructing psychology: Making facts and fables for our times. *American Psychologist, 40,* 499–512.

Sigel, I. E. (1972). The distancing hypothesis revisited: An elaboration of a neo-Piagetian view of the development of representational thought. In M. E. Meyer (Ed.), *Cognitive learning* (pp. 33–46). Bellingham, WA: Western Washington State College Press.

Sigel, I. E., McGillicuddy-DeLisa, A. V., Flaugher, J., & Rock, D. A. (1982). *Parents as teachers of their own learning disabled children.* Princeton, NJ: Educational Testing Service.

Tinsley, V. S., & Waters, H. S. (1982). The development of verbal control over motor behavior: A replication and extension of Luria's findings. *Child Development, 53,* 746–753.

Vygotsky, L. S. (1978). *Mind in society: The development of higher psychological processes.* Cambridge, MA: Harvard University Press.

Vygotsky, L. S. (1986). *Thought and language.* Cambridge, MA: MIT Press.

Wechsler, D. (1967). *The Wechsler Preschool and Primary Scale of Intelligence.* New York: Psychological Corporation.

Werner, E. E., & Smith, R. S. (1982). *Vulnerable but invincible: A longitudinal study of resilient children and youth.* New York: McGraw-Hill.

Werner, H., & Kaplan, B. (1963). *Symbol formation.* New York: Wiley.

Wertsch, J. V. (1985). *Culture, communication, and cognition: Vygotskian perspectives.* Cambridge, England: Cambridge University Press.

Wood, D., Bruner, J., & Ross, G. (1976). The role of tutoring in problem solving. *Journal of Child Psychology and Psychiatry, 17,* 89–100.

11

Vulnerability and Competence
A Review of Research on Resilience
in Childhood

Suniya S. Luthar

Yale University, New Haven, Connecticut

Edward Zigler

Yale University, New Haven, Connecticut

The developmental psychopathology literature addressing issues of children's resilience and vulnerability in dealing with life stresses is reviewed. The contribution and methodological limitations of research on stress and competence are examined, theoretical concepts of resilience are discussed, and findings with respect to protective mechanisms, as well as data from longitudinal studies, are presented. Directions for further research are outlined.

In the face of life stresses, many children develop behavioral and psychological difficulties. Other children, referred to as "resilient" or "stress-resistant," defy expectation by developing into well-adapted individuals in spite of serious stressors in their lives. In recent years, a great deal of empirical work has focused on resilience and vulnerability. This paper reviews the literature on resilience within the field of developmental psychopathology. In the first of the paper's five sections, approaches to defining the two central constructs in resilience research—stress and competence—are examined. Methodological issues associated with the various operational definitions are considered in some detail. Theoretical models of stress-resistance are outlined in the second section of the paper. The third and fourth sections of the paper contain, respectively, empirical findings on factors that moderate

Reprinted with permission from *American Journal of Orthopsychiatry*, 1991, Vol. 61, No. 1, 6–22. Copyright © 1991 American Orthopsychiatric Association.

Research was supported by funds from the National Institute of Child Health and Human Development (Grant No. PO1-HD03008) and from the Smith Richardson Foundation.

the effects of stress, and data obtained from longitudinal studies. Implications for future research on resilience are discussed in the concluding part of the paper.

CENTRAL CONSTRUCTS IN RISK RESEARCH

Definitions of Stressors

Horowitz (1989) has delineated five types of risk literature: the high-risk infant literature, which includes research on infants born prematurely or following prenatal complications; the conduct disorder literature, focusing on behavioral disorders and the conditions that dispose toward them; "behavioral teratogenesis," in which the focus is on infancy and the exposure to environmental agents such as lead and alcohol; research on sensitive or critical periods, conducted largely with nonhuman animals; and developmental psychopathology, focusing on emotional/social maladjustment and competence, and on factors that are ameliorative against stress. This review is confined to studies within the developmental psychopathology literature.

Life events research. In studies on childhood stress resistance, a commonly used approach to operationalizing stress is the life events method. This technique uses self-report measures to obtain a count of stressful life events encountered by respondents. Typically, such measures (Coddington, 1972; Johnson & McCutcheon, 1980; Swearingen & Cohen, 1985) consist of a list of items judged to be experienced frequently by children and adolescents, and respondents are asked to indicate events experienced in the recent past. There is a large literature on the methodological issues associated with measures of life events (Cohen, 1988; Johnson, 1986; Johnson & Bradlyn, 1988; Monroe, 1982; Tausig, 1982; Thoits, 1983; Zimmerman, 1983). A brief overview of salient issues is presented here.

Many of the early life events measures (e.g., Coddington, 1972; Holmes & Rahe, 1967) contained a heterogeneous mix of events ranging from trivial to severe, desirable to undesirable, and subjectively judgmental to objectively descriptive (Dohrenwend & Dohrenwend, 1978; Garmezy & Rutter, 1985). Scales developed in recent years have addressed some of these limitations. In measures such as the Life Events Checklist (Johnson & McCutcheon, 1980), the Junior High Life Experiences Survey (Swearingen & Cohen, 1985), and the Adolescent Perceived Events Scale (Compas, Davis, Forsythe, & Wagner, 1987), respondents are asked not just whether they have experienced a particular event, but also whether they perceived that event as being desirable or undesirable, and the extent to which it has affected their lives.

The life events measures cited above have been found to have acceptable psychometric properties in terms of both reliability and validity (Cohen, 1988; Johnson & Bradlyn, 1988). Research employing measures such as these can be strictly empirical, controlled, and precise (Anthony, 1987). Additional advantages in using this method lie in its pragmatic value in terms of ease of data collection, and the built-in provision of control group data: since stress scores are on a continuous scale, comparisons between high and low stress groups are possible without the need to locate specific high-risk and control samples.

Notwithstanding the improved empirical rigor and pragmatic value of the more recent scales, the life events method has been criticized on conceptual and theoretical grounds. A major problem has to do with the difficulty in making inferences regarding causality. Although life stress measures typically correlate significantly with adjustment, there is potentially a problem of confounded measurement, since many items on life events measures (e.g., failing a grade at school) may themselves be manifestations of maladjustment.

In attempts to address the issue of causality, several studies have examined correlations with adjustment of two types of life events: those over which the individual could not have had any control (and which could not be realistically viewed as consequences of maladjustment), and those over which respondents had some degree of control. Results of these investigations indicate significant relationships between stress and adjustment in children, even when only those events beyond the respondent's control were considered (Gersten, Langner, Eisenberg, & Simcha-Fagan, 1977; Sandler & Block, 1979). Such findings on uncontrollable events suggest that while correlations between life events scores and adjustment may sometimes be inflated due to the inclusion of events which might be manifestations of maladjustment, these correlations are not simply artifactual (Thoits, 1983).

Another approach to examining issues of cause-and-effect has been to use the cross-lagged correlation method, which involves examining the extent to which life events at Time 1 might predict adjustment at Time 2, as opposed to the converse. The use of this technique has indicated that while stress can play an important role in maladjustment, the presence of adjustment problems can also lead to experiences of negative life events (Cohen, Burt, & Bjorck, 1987; Compas & Wagner, 1985; Compas, Howell, Phares, Williams, & Giunta, 1989; Compas, Wagner, Slavin, & Vannatta, 1986; Swearingen & Cohen, 1985). Further, the apparent bidirectional relationship between life stress and adjustment may, in some cases, result from the common influence of a third variable (Johnson & Bradlyn, 1988).

A final concern with life stress measures is the fact that although significant correlations have generally been found between stress and adjustment, the magnitude of these correlations is typically between .30 and .40. The low values of the correlations have sometimes been seen as reflecting deficits in measures of life events (Johnson & Bradlyn, 1988). However, the correlational values obtained may reflect the actual magnitude of the stress-adjustment relationship. Simple linear models of development are now widely viewed as being less adequate in predicting development than are transactional models, which posit that there is a reciprocal influence between the organism and the environment, and that development proceeds out of these mutual influences (Bronfenbrenner, 1986; Horowitz, 1989; Sameroff & Chandler, 1975). In risk research, studies that have explored the impact on adjustment of child attributes and environmental factors, in addition to life stress, have yielded multiple correlation coefficients between .60 and .80 (Garmezy, Masten, & Tellegen,1984; Luthar, in press; Seifer & Sameroff, 1987; Wertlieb, Weigel, Springer, & Feldstein, 1989), accounting for a considerably greater proportion of the variance in adjustment as compared to that predicted by life stress alone.

In conclusion, research using the life events method has yielded some promising results. While existing life events measures retain several conceptual and methodological limitations, studies employing rigorous research procedures—which allow for cause-effect interpretations—have been judged as providing strong evidence that life stress does play an important role in adjustment (Monroe & Peterman, 1988). Findings such as these support the continued use of life events questionnaires to assess stress in empirical research.

Small events or hassles. A second approach to operationalizing stress in studying resilience has been to assess relatively minor stresses that characterize everyday life. According to this viewpoint, hassles—or the irritating, frustrating experiences that occur in everyday transactions with the environment—are a useful measure of life stress, and predictive of various adjustment outcomes. The use of hassles as an index of stress has grown largely from the efforts of Lazarus and his colleagues (Lazarus, 1980, 1984; Lazarus & Cohen, 1977).

Lazarus's group has strongly argued for the superiority of hassles over life events as indices of stress. This claim is based in part on commonly noted limitations of life events methodology, such as the failure to consider the individual significance of events, and the low power to predict adjustment and health (Lazarus, 1984). In addition, it has been argued that compared to major life events, small events are somewhat less heterogeneous in meaning, since they refer to smaller units of behavior. Small events or hassles are also better suited to prospective studies of causal relationships between stress and adjustment, given their relatively high frequency of occurrence over short time intervals. Similarly, such events can be experimentally manipulated far more easily than can major stressors (Zautra, Guarnaccia, Reich, & Dohrenwend, 1988). Finally, research on small events may provide information about the processes through time by which life events affect health and adjustment outcomes. Conceivably, major life events could operate by affecting the person's pattern of daily hassles, so that hassles might be critical mediators in the relationship between life events and health (Kanner, Coyne, Schaefer, & Lazarus, 1981; Zautra et al., 1988).

Empirical research suggests that, among adults, hassles scores may be more strongly related to various outcome variables than are major life event scores

(DeLongis, Coyne, Dakof, Folkman, & Lazarus, 1982; Kanner et al., 1981). In predicting outcomes, a substantial relationship has been found to remain for hassles, even after the shared effect due to life events is removed. Conversely, the relationship between life events and outcomes, after partialling out the effects of hassles, has been found to be either weaker or nonsignificant (DeLongis et al., 1982; Kanner et al., 1981).

Methodological concerns require that findings of these studies be interpreted with caution. A major source of error in the relationships found between hassles and outcomes is confounded measurement between the predictor (event items) and the criterion (psychological health) (Dohrenwend, Dohrenwend, Dodson, & Shrout, 1984; Dohrenwend & Shrout, 1985). For example, even items such as "thoughts about death" or "fear of rejection" are similar to items commonly found on measures of psychological distress.

In response to comments about potential confounds between hassles and outcomes, Lazarus and colleagues have contended that stress lies not in the environmental input, but in the person's appraisal of the relationship between that input and the person's resources to cope with the demands posed (Lazarus, DeLongis, Folkman, & Gruen, 1985). While supporting this statement from a theoretical viewpoint, other researchers have argued that what is needed is separate measurement of event occurrence and the individual's evaluation of that event (Cohen, 1988; Green, 1986).

Technology for assessing hassles among children is still in its earliest stages (Kanner, Harrison, & Wertlieb, 1985; Wertlieb et al., 1989). A recent study (Wertlieb et al., 1989) used maternal reports of daily hassles, in addition to a life events scale for children, as indices of stress. Results indicated that daily hassles and negative life events both made independent, statistically significant contributions to variation in children's behavior symptoms, indicating the usefulness of both major and minor events as measures of stress.

Specific life stresses. A third approach to operationalizing stress of high-risk conditions in research on resilience has been to use specific stressful life experiences. A variety of life events and family circumstances have been utilized within this approach, ranging from severe disasters such as war and floods (Garmezy & Rutter, 1985), to sociodemographic and familial stressors such as economic deprivation (Sameroff, Seifer, Barocas, Zax, & Greenspan, 1987; Werner & Smith, 1982), institutionalization (Rutter & Quinton, 1984), parental divorce (Wallerstein, 1983), and parental psychopathology (Garmezy, 1974).

A common limitation in earlier studies using specific life stressors is the absence of control groups (Fisher, Kokes, Cole, Perkins, & Wynne, 1987). While studies focusing exclusively on high-risk samples do offer some insights into predictors of adjustment, they leave unanswered the important question of whether levels of competence in children labeled resilient are comparable to competence levels among well-functioning children in the general population. There is evidence indicating that may not, in fact, be the case. For instance, a longitudinal study on the effects of compensatory education found clear-cut differences between economically disadvantaged children who received such intervention, and a comparison group who did not. At the same time, however, the educational intervention did not result in the disadvantaged children attaining the level of intellectual achievement displayed by children in nondisadvantaged groups (Abelson, Zigler, & DeBlasi, 1974).

A second difficulty in cross-sectional studies employing specific life stressors has to do with issues of causality. Most of these investigations do not provide data on children's levels of adjustment prior to the occurrence of a major stressor. Even with the presence of control groups, it is necessary to rule out the possibility that cohorts which differ in their exposure to major stresses (e.g., parental divorce or institutionalization) do not also differ in psychological functioning prior to this exposure. The need for such clarifications is clear from research on child abuse. Several investigators (Gelles, 1973; Parker & Collmer, 1976) have suggested that abused children can be particularly difficult to care for. Thus, it is not clear whether abuse is necessarily a stressor that results in maladjustment or, at least in some instances, whether having difficult temperaments causes children to be abused (Farber & Egeland, 1987).

On the surface, the use of single life circumstances as stressors may seem to circumvent a significant problem inherent in measures of major and minor life events, i.e., the combination of a heterogeneous mix of stressors. However, this is not necessarily the case. In their research on invulnerability, Seifer and Sameroff (1987) used what is often considered a straightforward risk factor: maternal mental illness. Two complications in the use of this variable were outlined by the authors. First, there was the need to identify which aspects of the global variable represented risk factors. Severity and chronicity of maternal mental illness were better predictors of clinical symptoms in children than was diagnosis. Second, a variable tapping subclinical aspects of mental health, i.e., maternal anxiety, was also strongly related to child competence. Based on these data, the authors concluded that even factors generally treated as simple indices of risk have their own complex internal structures which must be considered. Similar precautions have been noted with regard to another widely studied life circumstance, parental divorce. It has been noted that divorce consists of a complex series of events and stressors, and the multiplicity of events, as well as the context in which they occur, are important correlates of outcome (Masten, 1989).

Socioeconomic status as an index of stress. Socioeconomic status (SES) is among the most commonly investigated indices of stress. Studies have pinpointed specific factors that characterize low-SES families and that operate as high risk factors. Apart from low status parental occupation, these include low maternal education, large family size, membership in a minority group, and absence of one parent (Rutter & Quinton, 1977; Sameroff et al., 1987; West & Farrington, 1977).

The widespread use of SES as an index of environmental influences appears to be based on two factors: the conceptual and operational simplicity of models using this variable, and the quickness and ease with which it can be assessed (Bronfenbrenner, 1986). However, several factors limit the scientific value of using socioeconomic status as a measure of life stress.

Knowledge of an individual's socioeconomic status in itself yields no information on the process through which this aspect of the environment might affect development. As Zigler, Lamb, and Child (1982) have noted, for psychologists, the discovery of a relationship between social class membership and a particular expression of behavior is a meaningless one, until the sociological variable is reduced to psychological terms. Similarly, Bronfenbrenner (1986) has noted the restricted scope of studies that focus simply on a "social address," with no explicit consideration of intervening processes or structures through which environmental influences may operate. Consonant with these theoretical perspectives, there is evidence that children's competence levels are influenced more by what parents *do* in their interactions with them, than they are by the parents' status in terms of occupation, income, and other sociodemographic variables (Braithwaite & Gordon, in press; Wolf, 1966).

Another limitation of using low SES as a stressor is evident in findings that many economically deprived children are well able to adjust to this life circumstance and appear to be no different from their more advantaged peers (Garmezy, 1981; Garmezy & Nuechterlein, 1972). Further, variations in competence associated with SES are likely to be observed only within a certain range of socioeconomic levels. In other words, while high-SES children generally show adjustment superior to that of their low-SES peers, weak correlations between competence and SES are likely to be found both above and below certain "threshold" levels (Luthar, in press); within samples of either affluent or underprivileged children, therefore, SES is unlikely to be a very useful index of life stresses.

Multiple measures of stress or risk. In discussing difficulties in defining risk, Seifer and Sameroff (1987) noted that there is no definite criterion by which a particular variable is investigated as a risk factor, a protective factor, or merely a measure related to the outcome in question. For example, while in their own research they used low SES as a potential risk factor, other investigators (Masten, 1989; Werner & Smith, 1982) have included high SES among variables investigated as potential protective factors. Seifer and Sameroff pointed out that this issue represents a logical dilemma. One might assume that any factor associated with poor child outcomes was a risk factor; however, this would leave no room to identify variables that protect against stress, since such variables—being predictors of adjustment—would also constitute risk factors. At the other extreme, one might opt for a rigidly circumscribed, small set of measures as representing risk, e.g., parental mental illness (Seifer & Sameroff). An acceptable rationale for the selection of a few measures over several others, however, would be difficult to construct.

Given this dilemma, Seifer and Sameroff argued for the inclusion of variables at different levels of individual, family, or societal organization as potential risk factors, incorporating the different systems that affect developmental processes. Thus, in their own research, they examined maternal mental health, parental perspectives on child development, family stress (including negative life events and family size), and socioeconomic status as potential risk factors. Although in their study the amount of variance explained varied, there was no single risk factor that accounted for all the significant variance in the outcome variable (IQ). Put differently, when the effect of any one risk factor was partialled out, the variance explained by the remaining risk variables was significant in all cases, attesting to the value of exploring multiple indices of risk from different areas.

The inclusion of multiple risk indices is being seen increasingly in research on resilience. Studies have used measures of life events as well as hassles (Dohrenwend, Zautra, Lennon, & Marbach, 1985; Gersten et al., 1977; Wertlieb, Weigel, & Feldstein, 1987; Wertlieb et al., 1989), and life event scales along with more specific stress indices such as low SES (Garmezy, Masten, & Tellegen,1984; Luthar, in press). The simultaneous consideration of multiple indices of risk is invaluable in helping define more completely the concept of risk which, in turn, is a prerequisite to achieving a sound understanding of the concept of resilience.

Outcome Measures: Maladjustment vs. Competence

Frequently, researchers have used the absence of psychopathology, or of maladaptive behavior, as an indicator of resilience against high-risk conditions (Mednick & Schulsinger, 1968; Rutter, 1982; Rutter & Quinton, 1984). Over the last two decades, developmental psychopathologists have increasingly explored the concept of "invulnerability," rather than focusing predominantly on vulnerability and maladjustment. Recent investigations on risk and vulnerability have tended more frequently to use aspects of health and competence as outcome measures, correcting empirical psychologists' traditional neglect of successful adaptation under adverse conditions (Garmezy & Tellegen, 1984).

Several researchers have argued for the use of social competence as the measure of choice in assessing levels of overall adjustment (Garmezy et al., 1984; Masterpasqua, 1989; Zigler & Trickett, 1978). With regard to definitions of social competence, two major criteria have been delineated, at least one of which should be reflected in measures of the construct: the success of the person in meeting societal expectations, and aspects of the individual's personal development or self-actualization (Zigler & Trickett, 1978).

Earlier studies on stress-resistance have frequently operationalized social competence levels on the basis of observable, behavioral criteria that represent success in meeting expectations of society. Investigations with children, for example, have often used ratings by teachers, parents, or peers, as well as academic achievement scores, in assessing competence (Garmezy et al., 1984; Luthar, in press; Masten, Morison, Pellegrini, & Tellegen, in press; O'Grady & Metz, 1987; Parker, Cowen, Work, & Wyman, 1990). The assumption in using such indices is that manifest competence on such behavioral dimensions reflects good underlying coping skills (Garmezy & Masten, 1986). Further, "broad-band" assessments via the use of multiple measurement modalities (e.g., ratings by peers and teachers, and academic scores) have served to buttress the validity of the competence construct (Waters & Sroufe, 1983).

In research on stress resistance, the shift toward focusing on competence rather than on maladjustment is laudable, representing as it does a somewhat more positive outlook on development and adjustment. There is, however, a major caveat in endorsing this approach. It does not allow for the fact that, despite competence on behavioral indices, individuals may have a variety of other psychological difficulties, such as depression or anxiety. Various theoretical arguments indicate this possibility, and there is some empirical evidence in its support.

A distinction commonly made by developmental psychopathologists (Achenbach & Edelbrock, 1978) is between action-oriented, "externalizing" symptoms (e.g., acting out and aggressive behavior) and thought-oriented, "internalizing" ones (e.g., depression and anxiety). It is possible that so-called "resilient" children's reactions to their stressful experiences are primarily of an internalizing nature, expressed in more covert symptoms such as depression or anxiety. This argument rests on two empirically based findings. First, the literature in developmental psychopathology indicates that, at higher levels of development, pathology tends to be expressed more often in internalizing symptoms, rather than in externalizing, "undercontrolled" behavioral disturbances (Achenbach & Edelbrock, 1983; Cohen, Gotlieb, Kershner, & Wehrspann, 1985; Cohen, Kershner, & Wehrspann, 1985; Zigler & Glick, 1986). Secondly, children identified as stress-resistant are generally at high developmental levels, as reflected, for instance, in their greater intellectual maturity (Masten, 1989; Masten et al., in press).

Given the above reasoning, the question at issue is whether profiles of resilient children on measures of depression would parallel their profiles on behavioral measures, showing them, again, to have superior adjustment levels. Addressing this issue, Luthar (in press) compared levels of internalizing symptoms among resilient adolescents (high stress, high competence) and two other groups: low stress/high competence and high stress/low competence. Results indicated that children identified as resilient had significantly higher scores on depression and anxiety as compared to those who were also high in competence but were from low stress backgrounds. Further, statistically comparable depression and anxiety levels were found among the so-called resilient children and those at the *lower extreme* in social competence (i.e., those in the high stress/low competence group). In spite of their impressive social competence, therefore, the "stress-resistant" adolescents were clearly not emotionally untroubled.

Similar findings on internalizing symptoms were obtained in a study of urban elementary school children (Parker et al., 1990). Within this investigation, levels of depression and anxiety were compared among stress-resilient (SR) and stress-affected (SA) children. Despite the superior behavioral competence of SR as compared to SA children, the resilient group did not show similar advantages in self-rated levels of depression or anxiety.

Clinical studies of resilient individuals provide further support for the presence of underlying symptoms. In describing an "invulnerable" adult, Peck (1987) noted that this individual's strong drive toward mastery, while invaluable in personal survival against odds, also periodically brought him into contact with high risk which he was unable to master, resulting in overwhelming anxiety or depression. Similar suggestions have been made in other clinical reports (Miller, 1979). Data such as these underscore the need for researchers to be cognizant of distinctions between adaptive behavior and emotional health in studying children who do well despite stress.

THEORETICAL MODELS OF VULNERABILITY AND RESILIENCE

Recent works have illustrated the importance of making conceptual distinctions between factors that are ameliorative against stress, based on the processes through which they influence adaptation. Garmezy et al. (1984) outlined three models describing the impact of personal attributes and stress on adjustment. The *compensatory* model is a simple additive one, wherein stressors tend to lower levels of competence, whereas various personal attributes help to improve adjustment levels. The operative mechanism, therefore, is a simple counteractive one. The *protective versus vulnerability* model implies an interactive relationship between stress and personal attributes in predicting adjustment. A protective function is implied if, for example, individuals with high levels of a trait are relatively unaffected by increasing stress, whereas those low on the trait show declines in competence with increasing stress levels. Conversely, in a vulnerability process, individuals with high levels of a certain attribute are more susceptible to increasing stress than are those low on the attribute. Finally, the *challenge* model hypothesizes a curvilinear relationship between stress and adjustment, so that stressors could actually enhance competence, providing that levels of stress are not too high.

Similar distinctions between compensatory and protective factors have been noted by other authors. Rutter (1987), for instance, pointed out the differences between "risk mechanisms" (which lead directly to disorder) and "vulnerability" or "protective" processes. The latter have an impact on adjustment by virtue of their *interactions with risk variables*, instead of (or in addition to) having direct effects on their own.

The identification of a statistically significant interaction effect is generally considered evidence of a buffering or moderating effect in the relationship between stress and adjustment (Kessler, 1983; Rutter, 1987). However, several difficulties arise in the search for interaction effects in resilience research, including the need for relatively large sample sizes, and the complexities of interpreting significant effects (Masten, 1989). Further, the predictive power of models involving interaction effects does not seem to be very impressive. Data provided by various studies (Garmezy et al., 1984; Luthar, in press; Masten, Garmezy, Tellegen, Pellegrini, Larkin, & Larsen, 1988; Wertlieb et al., 1989) suggest that if models using only main effects were compared to those including significant interaction terms as well, the increase in variance accounted for would typically be small, yielding, for example, increments from 62% to 66% (Garmezy et al., 1984) or from 45% to 50% (Luthar, in press). The relatively small increase in variance explained with the inclusion of interaction effects has led some authors to suggest that, although these effects do provide evidence for moderators against the effects of stress, their failure to enhance the predictive power of the model significantly may indicate that the more parsimonious model of simple main effects (the compensatory model) is also useful to consider (Wertlieb et al., 1989).

While the literature contains a great deal of information on factors that directly promote positive or negative health, so far there is comparatively little understanding of protective or buffering processes. The mechanisms involved in interaction effects are still incompletely understood; empirical studies have only recently begun to investigate effects that involve not evasion of a risk, but successful engagement and coping with it (Rutter, 1987). Findings of some of these studies are presented below.

PROTECTIVE MECHANISMS

On the basis of previous research in the area, Garmezy (1985) has identified three categories of factors that protect against stress: 1) dispositional attributes of the child, 2) family cohesion and warmth, and 3) the availability and use of external support systems by parents and children.

In the context of *dispositional attributes of the child*, genetic and constitutional factors have frequently been found to serve protective functions. Antecedents of resilience are likely to be found in ways in which the infant responds to environmental change, can be comforted, equilibrates physiological responses, and modifies sleep-wakefulness states (Block & Block, 1980). Temperamental features have also been found to operate in protective and vulnerability processes. Wertlieb et al. (1989) found three aspects of temperament to moderate the effects of stress: distractibility, threshold (level of stimulation required to elicit a discernible response), and approach (nature of responses to novel stimuli). Children with adverse temperaments are more likely than are other children to be the target of parental irritability, criticism, and hostility (Rutter, 1978). Protective aspects of gender have been identified by research indicating that, in comparison to girls, boys are more vulnerable to out-of-home day care (Gamble & Zigler, 1986), and that they react to stressful family circumstances with greater emotional and behavioral disturbances (Rutter, 1982).

Intellectual ability is one of the most widely investigated moderator variables in resilience research. However, the ways in which intelligence interacts with stress in predicting adjustment are still incompletely understood. Some investigations have indicated that intellectual ability shows protective effects (Kandel et al., 1988; Masten et al., 1988; Werner & Smith, 1982). For instance, Garmezy et al. (1984) found that, when faced with increasing levels of stress, bright children did not show the declines in social competence that were demonstrated by less intelligent children. Other studies, however, have failed to find significant interactions between intelligence and risk in predicting adjustment (White, Moffitt, & Silva, 1989). Still other investigations have yielded the somewhat counterintuitive finding that intelligence can sometimes operate as a vulnerability factor (Luthar, in press; Masten, 1982). In the Luthar study, intelligence was positively related to competence indices at low levels of stress. When stress levels were high, however, the intelligent children appeared to lose their advantage, and demonstrated competence levels more similar to those of less intelligent youngsters. Findings such as these have been interpreted via the argument that more intelligent children tend to have higher levels of sensitivity to their environments, which may heighten their susceptibility to stressors (Zigler & Farber, 1985). Given the widely differing findings across existing studies, however, it is clear that a great deal more research is required to understand the conditions under which intelligence operates as a protective factor, a vulnerability factor, or is simply uninvolved in interactions with stress.

The role of humor in resilience is suggested by exploratory analyses (Masten, 1982) showing that highly stressed, competent children had higher scores on humor generation than did children who were highly stressed but less competent. Protective aspects of social skills have been indicated by various investigations. Interaction effects obtained between interpersonal awareness and stress indicated that increasing stress was associated with decreasing competence, but only among children with low interpersonal awareness (Pellegrini, 1980). As compared to stress-affected elementary school children, those who are stress-resilient have been found to have higher levels of empathy, as well as more effective social problem solving skills and coping strategies (Parker et al., 1990). Finally, in a study involving adolescents, social expressiveness was found to be a protective factor (Luthar, in press).

An internal locus of control has been found to serve protective functions among children (Murphy & Moriarty, 1986; Parker et al., 1990), adolescents (Luthar, in press), and young adults (Werner, 1989). In their longitudinal study of stress-resistance, Werner and Smith (1982) found that resilient youngsters had high faith in their control over their environment (reflecting an internal locus of control), as opposed to believing that the external environment was random and immutable. In a somewhat similar vein, planning for marriage, a variable representing tendencies to exercise foresight and to take active steps to deal with environmental challenges, was protective for women who had been raised in institutions. Formerly institutionalized women who exercised planning were less likely to marry deviant men (criminals or men with a psychiatric disorder) than were those low in planning; among a group of controls, planning was not related to the choice of deviant versus nondeviant spouses (Rutter & Quinton, 1984).

The importance of *familial factors* in resilience has been indicated by several studies. Data on the development of ego-resilience through childhood indicate that while ego-brittle children come from homes marked by discord and conflict, ego-resilient children have parents who are competent, integrated, loving, patient, and compatible, and who have shared values (Block, 1971). A good relationship with at least one parental figure can protect against the risks associated with family discord (Rutter, 1979) and child abuse (Hunter & Kilstrom, 1979). Another investigation revealed that maternal competence in parenting served protective functions for girls in middle childhood (Masten et al., 1988). The significance of parental values and beliefs in resilience is indicated by the fact that among underprivileged families, parents' beliefs in opportunities through education can help children to attain considerable success and competence in their adult lives (Comer, 1988). The longitudinal study by Werner and Smith (1982) indicated various protective aspects of family functioning, which are considered in some detail in the following section.

The family has been found to serve important protective functions for individuals during adulthood as well. Among adult women who had been institutionalized as children, the presence of a supportive spouse exercised a protective function in influencing the quality of the women's parenting (Quinton, Rutter, & Liddle, 1984; Rutter & Quinton, 1984). Similar protective processes associated with the presence of intimate relationships or marital support have been found by other investigators (Brown & Harris, 1978; Parker & Hazdi-Pavlovic, 1984).

With regard to the *use of support systems*, the third category of protective factors outlined by Garmezy (1985), the literature indicates that positive outcomes tend to be associated with high use by high-risk children and their families. Resilient youngsters appear to be skillful at choosing and identifying with resilient models and sources of support (Murphy & Moriarty, 1976; Pines, 1979). Rather than seeking professional help, however, these youngsters more often tend to have a network of informal relationships that include friends of the same age, older friends, ministers, members of church youth organizations, and in some cases, teachers (Werner & Smith, 1982; Braithwaite & Gordon, in press).

A study of high-risk adolescents (Cauce, Felner, & Primavera, 1982) explored the protective functions of three dimensions of social support: family (parents, other relatives), formal (counselors, teachers, clergy), and informal (other adults, peers). The perceived helpfulness of these three support dimensions varied by sex, grade, and ethnic background. Interestingly, informal social support was related to better peer self-concept but was also associated with *lower* academic adjustment, indicating the potential protective as well as negative adaptive impact of different social support dimensions.

Studies have indicated that positive school experiences (academic or nonacademic) can serve protective functions. In an investigation by Rutter and colleagues, positive school experiences were found to be related to levels of planning for work and marriage among women who had been institutionalized as children, but were unrelated to planning among the control group (Rutter & Quinton, 1984).

The availability of supports for parents can strongly affect coping skills among high-risk families. For instance, the relationship between life stresses and illness has been found to be moderated by the presence of social supports from intrafamilial and extrafamilial sources (Wertlieb et al., 1987). A study of child neglect among low-income families revealed that treatment of the child was influenced by conditions such as the quality of housing and the presence or absence of a telephone, as well as factors such as the existence of a network of family and friends and church attendance (Giovannoni & Billingsley, 1970). Another study (Hunter & Kilstrom, 1979) revealed that the presence of social supports was among the significant factors differentiating parents who repeated an intergenerational cycle of child abuse from parents who did not. Finally, there is an abundance of literature that intervention programs that offer support services to high-risk children and their families can be of great benefit in terms of providing protective functions and promoting positive outcomes (see reviews by Berrueta-Clement, Schweinhart, Barnett, Epstein, & Weikart, 1984; Consortium for Longitudinal Studies, 1983; Copple, Cline, & Smith, 1987; Price, Cowen, Lorion, & Ramos-McKay, 1988; Seitz, in press).

LONGITUDINAL STUDIES OF RESILIENCE

Much of the extant research on resilience has utilized concurrent or retrospective designs. Although such studies can provide useful insights into factors that moderate the effects of stress, they preclude definitive conclusions regarding the causal relationships between stressors and developmental outcomes. The importance of longitudinal data is apparent in results of prospective studies indicating that phenomena associated with resilience show considerable variability over different points on the developmental continuum.

The 30-year study of resilient individuals conducted by Werner and colleagues (Werner, 1989; Werner & Smith, 1982) illustrates that the relative impact of different protective and risk factors changes at various life phases. For instance, males in their sample showed greater vulnerability than females during the first decade of life and less during the second, with another shift appearing at the beginning of the third decade. Similarly, different aspects of family functioning assumed varying levels of importance as protective factors over the course of childhood and adolescence. During childhood, for example, significant predictors of resilience included the presence of alternative caregivers in the household—the presence of the father (for boys) and the mother's long-term employment (for girls). During late adolescence, significant discriminators included the individual's perception of the quality of his or her relationship with the family, especially with the father, and the absence of maternal mental health problems in the case of girls (Werner & Smith, 1982).

Longitudinal studies also help to address the question of whether resilience shows continuity over time. In a study by Farber and Egeland (1987), levels of competence were assessed among abused and neglected children on five occasions between 12 and 42 months. Results indicated that, within the abused group, there was a subset of children who appeared competent at each stage of assessment. However, there was a decrease in the percentage of these children between 12 months and preschool. While 22 of 41 abused children were competent at 12 months, only 4 of 18 who were tested remained competent at preschool. In commenting on these findings, the authors predicted that if the home situation of these few survivors remained abusive, maladaptive behavior would be manifest during the early school years. In fact, a later study employing similar methods revealed that children who had been resilient during their first five years, and at the first grade level at elementary school, showed a substantial decline in functioning by the time they reached the third grade (Egeland & Kreutzer, in press).

Based on their longitudinal data on abused children, Farber and Egeland (1987) also made the important distinction between competent behavior and emotional health. They cited observational data on individual "invulnerable" children, illustrating that, in spite of their apparently good coping strategies and adaptive behavior, these children may not be emotionally healthy. These data are consonant with findings of cross-sectional studies cited earlier (Luthar, in press; Parker et al., 1990) indicating that high behavioral competence is not necessarily paralleled by superior adjustment on measures of internalizing symptoms of psychopathology.

Similar questions are raised by data from Werner's sample. At the age of 30, 62 of the original sample of 72 resilient individuals were located for follow-up assessments. The 30-year interview data revealed that most of these individuals were coping successfully with their adult responsibilities, as they had coped well with demands during childhood and adolescence. However, not all of these individuals were happy or satisfied with their lives. At the same time, the proportion of self-reported health problems was significantly higher among the high-risk resilient individuals than among the low-risk comparison group. These health problems often appeared related to stress (e.g., back problems, dizziness, ulcers), particularly among men. In addition, some of the resilient males showed difficulties in establishing intimate, committed relationships in their adult years (Werner, 1989).

IMPLICATIONS FOR RESEARCH

Based on the review of extant research on childhood resilience, various directions for future research are apparent. Several important questions remain unanswered in the context of operational definitions of the central constructs, stress and competence. In addition, greater clarity is needed with regard to the processes via which the effects of stressors are moderated, and with regard to the continuity with which the effects of moderators are seen over time.

In operationalizing the pivotal construct of stress, research on childhood resilience has tended to rely heavily on life events measures. While the life events approach has several advantages, some methodological issues clearly require further exploration. For instance, additional research is needed on the issue of controllability of events. Some researchers have advocated the inclusion of only uncontrollable events in studies on resilience (Gersten et al., 1977; Masten et al., 1988), since these are relatively unlikely to be confounded with indices of maladjustment. However, the use of an approach of this kind can lead to its own set of problems. Existing life event measures contain a mix of both controllable and uncontrollable events. Scores based on a subset of uncontrollable events would not only be restricted in range (Luthar, in press), but would also have uncertain psychometric properties, since marked reduction of items on any scale can affect its reliability and validity (Carmines & Zeller, 1979).

The development of psychometrically sound measures of uncontrollable life events would constitute a considerable contribution to the field. In addition, it would be useful to have prospective data that compare, across the two types of life event scores, a) the magnitude of relations with indices of childhood adjustment, b) the stability of these correlations over time, and c) questions of cause and effect, i.e., the extent to which life event scores predict adjustment, as opposed to the other way around.

Another issue that warrants further empirical attention concerns the clarification of how small events may be linked to major life stresses. Significant correlations between the two types of stressors have been found in various studies (Dohrenwend et al., 1985; Sensenig, 1985). Even when spuriousness has been controlled for (through eliminating item redundancy), substantial correlations remain (Zautra et al., 1988). Such findings suggest the utility of exploring whether small events might, in fact, mediate in the relationships found between life events and various adjustment indices.

A final recommendation in the context of operationalizing stress has to do with the use of multifaceted definitions of the variable. The need to include different stress indices in resilience research is implied within current theoretical paradigms on development (Bronfenbrenner, 1986; Horowitz, 1989; Sameroff & Chandler, 1975), as well as in empirical findings indicating that a variety of stressors can correlate significantly and independently with a single aspect of adjustment (Seifer & Sameroff, 1987).

The operationalizing of competence, the second major construct involved in resilience research, gives rise to similar questions. There is a need to examine the merits, and the possible pitfalls, of the current tendency to define resilience based solely on behavioral indices of competence. Additional evidence is required to replicate (or refute) findings which suggest that, despite their manifest competence, apparently resilient children may be emotionally troubled.

As pointed out by Farber and Egeland (1987), there are ethical issues to consider when disseminating the view that certain children are invulnerable to severe life stresses. The reliance on one-time assessments which indicate behavioral competence despite stress is not just insufficient to label a child as being resilient. More seriously, it could affect intervention and prevention programming. Children most likely to receive mental health services are those whose symptoms present management problems for authority figures. High-achieving youngsters who suffer from emotional problems are unlikely to receive such services without conclusive empirical evidence demonstrating that they, too, might struggle with distress despite their adaptive behavior. Prospective studies are, therefore, vital in order to establish whether children who appear resilient continue to do well not only in terms of adaptive behavior, but also on indices of emotional health.

In the context of factors that moderate the effects of life stress, some variables, such as internal locus of control, have been consistently found to be involved in protective processes against life stress. One useful direction for future research would be to focus on designing intervention strategies aimed at fostering the development of such protective attributes among high-risk populations.

Results on some moderator variables explored have shown considerable variations across studies on resilience. In some instances, inconsistencies in results may reflect the effects of differing developmental or sociodemographic influences across investigations. For instance, although intelligence may serve protective functions among preadolescents facing high stress (e.g., Masten et al., 1988), inner-city adolescents— facing greater freedom from the home and school—may tend to use their talents in arenas other than educational achievement (Luthar, in press). Additional research utilizing samples belonging to different age and SES groups can help to pinpoint developmental and environmental forces that may be associated with differential effects of moderator variables.

In conclusion, research on resilience in childhood has yielded several important insights over the last few decades. Building upon the existing knowledge base, future empirical endeavors can help to develop theoretical models that are increasingly complex, and that incorporate the effects of multiple forces operating at the levels of stress, competence, and the moderating processes involved in resilience. In future studies on resilience, the use of multifaceted approaches to assess stress and competence, the inclusion of developmental and sociodemographic factors in research paradigms, and the exploration of resilience in prospective designs can, together, be invaluable in terms of informing theory, as well as in yielding specific directions for future intervention programs and social policy initiatives.

REFERENCES

Abelson, W. D., Zigler, E., & DeBlasi, C. L. (1974). Effects of a four-year follow through program on economically disadvantaged children. *Journal of Educational Psychology, 66,* 756–771.

Achenbach, T., & Edelbrock, C. (1978). The classification of child psychopathology: A review and analysis of empirical efforts. *Psychological Bulletin, 85,* 1275–1301.

Achenbach, T., & Edelbrock, C. (1983). *Manual for the Child Behavior Checklist.* Burlington, VT: Department of Psychiatry, University of Vermont.

Anthony, E. J. (1987). Risk, vulnerability, and resilience: An overview. In E. J. Anthony & B. J. Cohler (Eds.), *The invulnerable child* (pp. 3–48). New York: Guilford Press.

Berrueta-Clement, J. R., Schweinhart, L. J., Barnett, W. S., Epstein, A. S., & Weikart, D. P. (1984). Changed lives: The effects of the Perry Preschool Program on youths through age 19. *Monographs of the High/Scope Educational Research Foundation,* No. 8.

Block, J. (1971). *Lives through time.* Berkeley, CA: Bancroft Books.

Block, J. H., & Block, J. (1980). The role of ego-control and ego-resiliency in the organization of behavior. In W. A. Collins (Ed.), *Development of cognition, affect, and social relations: The Minnesota Symposia on Child Psychology,* Vol. 13 (pp. 39–101). Hillsdale, NJ: Lawrence Erlbaum.

Braithwaite, R. L., & Gordon, E. W. (in press). *Success against the odds.* Howard University Press.

Bronfenbrenner, U. (1986). Ecology of the family as a context for human development: Research perspectives. *Developmental Psychology, 22,* 723–742.

Brown, G. W., & Harris, T. O. (1978). *Social origins of depression: A study of psychiatric disorders in women.* London: Tavistock Publications.

Carmines, E. G., & Zeller, R. A. (1979). *Reliability and validity assessment.* Newbury Park, CA: Sage Publications.

Cauce, A. M., Felner, R. D., & Primavera, J. (1982). Social support in high-risk adolescents: Structural components and adaptive impact. *American Journal of Community Psychology, 10,* 417–428.

Coddington, R. D. (1972). The significance of life events as etiologic factors in the diseases of children: A study of a normal population. *Journal of Psychosomatic Research, 16,* 205–213.

Cohen, L. H. (1988). Measurement of life events. In L. H. Cohen (Ed.), *Life events and psychological functioning: Theoretical and methodological issues* (pp. 11–30). Newbury Park, CA: Sage Publications.

Cohen, L., Burt, C., & Bjorck, J. (1987). Life stress and adjustment: Effects of life events experiences by young adolescents and their parents. *Developmental Psychology, 23,* 583–592.

Cohen, N. J., Gotlieb, H., Kershner, J., & Wehrspann, W. (1985). Concurrent validity of the internalizing and externalizing patterns of the Achenbach Child Behavior Checklist. *Journal of Consulting and Clinical Psychology, 53,* 724–728.

Cohen, N. J., Kershner, J., & Wehrspann, W. (1985). Characteristics of social cognition in children with different symptom patterns. *Journal of Applied Developmental Psychology, 6,* 277–290.

Comer, J. (1988). *Maggie's American dream.* New York: New American Library.

Compas, B. E., Davis, G. E., Forsythe, C. J., & Wagner, B. (1987). Assessment of major and daily stressful events during adolescence: The Adolescent Perceived Events Scale. *Journal of Consulting and Clinical Psychology, 55,* 534–541.

Compas, B. E., Howell, D. C., Phares, V., Williams, R. A., & Giunta, C. T. (1989). Risk factors for emotional/behavioral problems in young adolescents: A prospective analysis of adolescent and parental stress and symptoms. *Journal of Consulting and Clinical Psychology, 57,* 732–740.

Compas, B. E., & Wagner, B. M. (1985). *Reciprocal relationships of life events and daily hassles with psychological symptoms: A prospective study.* Paper presented at the Annual Convention of the American Psychological Association, Los Angeles.

Compas, B. E., Wagner, B. M., Slavin, L. A., & Vannatta, K. (1986). A prospective study of life events, social support, and psychological symptomatology during the transition from high school to college. *American Journal of Community Psychology, 14,* 241–257.

Consortium for Longitudinal Studies. (1983). *As the twig is bent . . . .* Hillsdale, NJ: Lawrence Erlbaum.

Copple, C. E., Cline, M. G., & Smith, A. N. (1987). *Path to the future: Long-term effects of Head Start in the Philadelphia school district.* Washington, D C: U. S. Dept. of Health and Human Services.

DeLongis, A., Coyne, J. C., Dakof, G., Folkman, S., & Lazarus, R. S. (1982). Relationship of daily hassles, uplifts, and major life events to health status. *Health Psychology, 1,* 119–136.

Dohrenwend, B. S., & Dohrenwend, B. P. (1978). Some issues in research on stressful life events. *Journal of Nervous and Mental Diseases, 166,* 7–15.

Dohrenwend, B. S., Dohrenwend, B. P., Dodson, M., & Shrout, P. (1984). Symptoms, hassles, social supports, and life events: Problems of confounded measures. *Journal of Abnormal Psychology, 93,* 222–230.

Dohrenwend, B. P., & Shrout, P. (1985). "Hassles" in the conceptualization and measurement of life stress variables. *American Psychologist, 40*, 780–785.

Dohrenwend, B. P., Zautra, A. J., Lennon, M. C., & Marbach, J. J. (1985). *Small events in life stress processes.* Symposium presentation, American Psychological Association meeting, Los Angeles.

Egeland, B., & Kreutzer, T. (in press). A longitudinal study of the effects of maternal stress and protective factors on the development of high risk children. In E. M. Cummings, A. L. Greene, & K. H. Karraker (Eds.), *Life-span perspectives on stress and coping.* New York: John Wiley.

Farber, E. A., & Egeland, B. (1987). Invulnerability among abused and neglected children. In E. J. Anthony & B. J. Cohler (Eds.), *The invulnerable child* (pp. 253–288). New York: Guilford Press.

Fisher, L., Kokes, R. F., Cole, R. E., Perkins, P. M., & Wynne, L. C. (1987). Competent children at risk: A study of well-functioning offspring of disturbed parents. In E. J. Anthony & B. J. Cohler (Eds.), *The invulnerable child* (pp. 211–228). New York: Guilford Press.

Gamble, T. J., & Zigler, E. (1986). Effects of infant day care: Another look at the evidence. *American Journal of Orthopsychiatry, 56*, 26–42.

Garmezy, N. (1974). Children at risk: The search for the antecedents of schizophrenia. Part I. Conceptual models and research methods. *Schizophrenia Bulletin, 8*, 14–90.

Garmezy, N. (1981). Children under stress: Perspectives on antecedents and correlates of vulnerability and resistance to psychopathology. In A. I. Rabin, J. Aronoff, A. M. Barclay, & R. Zucker (Eds.), *Further exploration in personality.* New York: Wiley-Interscience.

Garmezy, N. (1985). Stress-resistant children: The search for protective factors. In J. E. Stevenson (Ed.), *Recent research in developmental psychopathology* (pp. 213–233). Oxford: Pergamon Press.

Garmezy, N., & Masten, A. S. (1986). Stress, competence, and resilience: Common frontiers for therapist and psychopathologist. *Behavior Therapy, 17*, 500–521.

Garmezy, N., Masten, A. S., & Tellegen, A. (1984). The study of stress and competence in children: A building block for developmental psychopathology. *Child Development, 55*, 97–111.

Garmezy, N., & Nuechterlein, K. H. (1972). Invulnerable children: The fact and fiction of competence and disadvantage. *American Journal of Orthopsychiatry, 42*, 328–329. (Abstract)

Garmezy, N., & Rutter, M. (1985). Acute reactions to stress. In M. Rutter & L. Hersov (Eds.), *Child and adolescent psychiatry: Modern approaches.* London: Blackwell Scientific Publications.

Garmezy, N., & Tellegen, A. (1984). Studies of stress-resistant children: Methods, variables and preliminary findings. In F. J. Morrison, C. Lord, & D. P. Keating (Eds.), *Applied Developmental Psychology* (Vol. 1). New York: Academic Press.

Gelles, R. (1973). Child abuse as psychopathology: A sociological critique and reformulation. *American Journal of Orthopsychiatry, 43*, 611–621.

Gersten, J. C., Langner, T. S., Eisenberg, J. S., & Simcha-Fagan, O. (1977). An evaluation of the etiological role of stressful life-change events in psychological disorders. *Journal of Health and Social Behavior, 18,* 228–244.

Giovannoni, J., & Billingsley, A. (1970). Child neglect among the poor: A study of parental adequacy in families of three ethnic groups. *Child Welfare,* 196–204.

Green, B. L. (1986). On the confounding of "hassles," stress and outcome. *American Psychologist, 41,* 714–715.

Holmes, T., & Rahe, R. (1967). The Social Readjustment Rating Scale. *Journal of Psychosomatic Research, 11,* 213–218.

Horowitz, F. D. (1989). *The concept of risk: A reevaluation.* Invited address to the Society for Research in Child Development, Kansas City, MO.

Hunter, R., & Kilstrom, N. (1979). Breaking the cycle in abusive families. *American Journal of Psychiatry, 136,* 1320–1322.

Johnson, J. H. (1986). *Life events as stressors in childhood and adolescence.* Newbury Park, CA: Sage Publications.

Johnson, J. H., & Bradlyn, A. S. (1988). Life events and adjustment in childhood and adolescence: Methodological and conceptual issues. In L. H. Cohen (Ed.), *Life events and psychological functioning: Theoretical and methodological issues* (pp. 64–95). Newbury Park, CA: Sage Publications.

Johnson, J. H., & McCutcheon, S. M. (1980). Assessing life stress in older children and adolescents: Preliminary findings with the Life Events Checklist. In I. G. Sarason & C. D. Spielberger (Eds.), *Stress and anxiety* (Vol. 7). Washington, DC: Hemisphere.

Kandel, E., Mednick, S. A., Kirkegaard-Sorensen, L., Hutchings, B., Knop, J., Rosenberg, R., & Schulsinger, F. (1988). IQ as a protective factor for subjects at high risk for antisocial behavior. *Journal of Consulting and Clinical Psychology, 56,* 224–226.

Kanner, A. D., Coyne, J. C., Schaefer, C., & Lazarus, R. S. (1981). Comparison of two modes of stress measurement: Daily hassles and uplifts versus major life events. *Journal of Behavioral Medicine, 4,* 1–39.

Kanner, A. D., Harrison, A., & Wertlieb, D. (1985). *The development of the children's hassles and uplifts scale: A preliminary report.* Paper presented at a meeting of the American Psychological Association, Los Angeles.

Kessler, R. C. (1983). Methodological issues in the study of psychosocial stress. In H. B. Kaplan (Ed.), *Psychosocial stress: Trends in theory and research.* New York: Academic Press.

Lazarus, R. S. (1980). The stress and coping paradigm. In C. Eisdorfer, D. Cohen, & A. Kleinman (Eds.), *Conceptual models for psychopathology* (pp. 173–209). New York: Spectrum.

Lazarus, R. S. (1984). Puzzles in the study of daily hassles. *Journal of Behavioral Medicine, 7,* 375–389.

Lazarus, R. S., & Cohen, J. B. (1977). Environmental stress. In I. Altman & J. F. Wohlwill (Eds.), *Human behavior and the environment: Current theory and research* (pp. 89–127). New York: Plenum Press.

Lazarus, R. S., DeLongis, A., Folkman, S., & Gruen, R. (1985). Stress and adaptational outcomes: The problem of confounded measures. *American Psychologist, 40*, 770–779.

Luthar, S. (in press). Vulnerability and resilience: A study of high-risk adolescents. *Child Development*.

Masten, A. S. (1982). *Humor and creative thinking in stress-resistant children*. Unpublished doctoral dissertation, University of Minnesota.

Masten, A. S. (1989). Resilience in development: Implications of the study of successful adaptation for developmental psychopathology. In D. Cicchetti (Ed.), *The emergence of a discipline: Rochester Symposium on Developmental Psychopathology* (Vol. 1, pp. 261–294). Hillsdale, NJ: Lawrence Erlbaum.

Masten, A. S., Garmezy, N., Tellegen, A., Pellegrini, D. S., Larkin, K., & Larsen, A. (1988). Competence and stress in school children: The moderating effects of individual and family qualities. *Journal of Child Psychology and Psychiatry, 29*, 745–764.

Masten, A. S., Morison, P., Pellegrini, D., & Tellegen, A. (in press). Competence under stress: Risk and protective factors. In J. Rolf, A. S. Masten, D. Cicchetti, K. Neuchterlein, & S. Weintraub (Eds.), *Risk and protective factors in the development of psychopathology*. New York: Cambridge University Press.

Masterpasqua, F. (1989). A competence paradigm for psychological practice. *American Psychologist, 44*, 1366–1371.

Mednick, S. A., & Schulsinger, F. (1968). Some premorbid characteristics related to breakdown in children with schizophrenic mothers. In D. Rosenthal & S. S. Kety (Eds.), *The transmission of schizophrenia*. Elmsford, NY: Pergamon Press.

Miller, A. (1979). *The drama of the gifted child*. New York: Basic Books.

Monroe, S. (1982). Life events assessment: Current practices, emerging trends. *Clinical Psychology Review, 2*, 435–453.

Monroe, S. M., & Peterman, A. M. (1988). Life stress and psychopathology. In L. H. Cohen (Ed.), *Life events and psychological functioning: Theoretical and methodological issues* (pp. 31–63). Newbury Park, CA: Sage Publications.

Murphy, L. B., & Moriarty, A. E. (1976). *Vulnerability, coping, and growth*. New Haven, Yale University Press.

O'Grady, D., & Metz, J. R. (1987). Resilience in children at high risk for psychological disorder. *Journal of Pediatric Psychology, 12*, 3–23.

Parker, R., & Collmer, C. (1976). Child abuse: An interdisciplinary analysis. In E. M. Hetherington (Ed.), *Review of Child Development Research* (Vol. 5). Chicago: University of Chicago Press.

Parker, G. R., Cowen, E. L., Work, W. C., & Wyman, P. A. (1990). *Test correlates of stress-resilience among urban school children*. Manuscript submitted for publication.

Parker, G., Hazdi-Pavlovic, D. (1984). Modification of levels of depression in mother-bereaved women by parental and marriage relationships. *Psychological Medicine, 14*, 125–135.

Peck, E. C. (1987). The traits of true invulnerability and posttraumatic stress in psychoanalyzed men of action. In E. J. Anthony & B. J. Cohler (Eds.), *The invulnerable child* (pp. 315–360). New York: Guilford Press.

Pellegrini, D. (1980). *The social-cognitive qualities of stress-resistant children.* Unpublished doctoral dissertation, University of Minnesota.

Pines, M. (1979, January). Superkids. *Psychology Today,* pp. 53–63.

Price, R. H., Cowen, E. L., Lorion, R. P., & Ramos-McKay, J. (Eds.). (1984). *14 ounces of prevention: A case book for practitioners.* Washington, D C: American Psychological Association.

Quinton, D., Rutter, M., & Liddle, C.(1984). Institutional rearing, parenting difficulties, and marital support. *Psychological Medicine, 14,* 107–124.

Rutter, M. (1978). Early sources of security and competence. In J. S. Bruner & A. Garten (Eds.), *Human growth and development.* London: Oxford University Press.

Rutter, M. (1979). Protective factors in children's responses to stress and disadvantage. In M. W. Kent & J. E. Rolf (Eds.), *Primary prevention of psychopathology:* Vol. 3. *Social competence in children* (pp. 49–74). Hanover, NH: University Press of New England.

Rutter, M. (1982). Epidemiological-longitudinal approaches to the study of development. In W. A. Collins (Ed.), *The concept of development, Minnesota symposia on child psychology* (Vol. 15). Hillsdale, NJ: Lawrence Erlbaum.

Rutter, M. (1987). Psychosocial resilience and protective mechanisms. *American Journal of Orthopsychiatry, 57,* 316–331.

Rutter, M., & Quinton, D. (1977). Psychiatric disorder: Ecological factors and concepts of causation. In H. McGurk (Ed.), *Ecological factors in human development.* Amsterdam: North-Holland.

Rutter, M., & Quinton, D. (1984). Long-term follow-up of women institutionalized in childhood: Factors promoting good functioning adult life. *British Journal of Developmental Psychology, 18,* 225–234.

Sameroff, A. J., & Chandler, M. J. (1975). Reproductive risk and the continuum of caretaking casualty. In F. D. Horowitz (Ed.), *Review of child development research* (Vol. 4, pp. 187–244). Chicago: University of Chicago Press.

Sameroff, A. J., Seifer, R., Barocas, R., Zax, M., & Greenspan, S. (1987). Intelligence Quotient scores of 4-year-old children: Social-environmental risk factors. *Pediatrics, 79,* 343–350.

Sandler, I. N., & Block, M. (1979). Life stress and maladaptation of children. *American Journal of Community Psychology, 7,* 425–439.

Seifer, R., & Sameroff, A. J. (1987). Multiple determinants of risk and invulnerability. In E. J. Anthony & B. J. Cohler (Eds.), *The invulnerable child* (pp. 51–69). New York: Guilford Press.

Seitz, V. (in press). Intervention programs for impoverished children: A comparison of educational and family support models. *Annals of Child Development.*

Sensenig, P. E. (1985). *Restraint and overeating in response to stress.* Unpublished doctoral dissertation, Arizona State University, Tempe.

Swearingen, E. M., & Cohen, L. H. (1985). Measurement of adolescents' life events: A Junior High Life Experiences Survey. *American Journal of Community Psychology, 13,* 69–85.

Tausig, M. (1982). Measuring life events. *Journal of Health and Social Behavior, 23,* 52–64.

Thoits, P. (1983). Dimensions of life events that influence psychological distress: An evaluation and synthesis of the literature. In H. Kaplan (Ed.), *Psychosocial stress: Trends in theory and research* (pp. 33–103). New York: Academic Press.

Wallerstein, J. S. (1983). Children of divorce: Stress and developmental tasks. In N. Garmezy & M. Rutter (Eds.), *Stress, coping and development in children*. New York: McGraw-Hill.

Waters, E., & Sroufe, L. A. (1983). Social competence as a developmental construct. *Developmental Review, 3*, 79–97.

Werner, E. E. (1989). High-risk children in young adulthood: A longitudinal study from birth to 32 years. *American Journal of Orthopsychiatry, 59*, 72–81.

Werner, E. E., & Smith, R. S. (1982). *Vulnerable but invincible: A study of resilient children*. New York: McGraw-Hill.

Wertlieb, D., Weigel, C., & Feldstein, M. (1987). Stress, social support, and behavior symptoms in middle childhood. *Journal of Clinical Child Psychology, 16*, 204–211.

Wertlieb, D., Weigel, C., Springer, T., & Feldstein, M. (1989). Temperament as a moderator of children's stressful experiences. In S. Chess, A. Thomas, & M. E. Hertzig (Eds.), *Annual progress in child psychiatry and child development: 1988*. New York: Brunner/Mazel.

West, D. J., & Farrington, D. P. (1977). *The delinquent way of life*. London: Heinemann Educational Books.

White, J. L., Moffitt, T. E., & Silva, P. A. (1989). A prospective replication of the protective effects of IQ in subjects at high risk for juvenile delinquency. *Journal of Consulting and Clinical Psychology, 57*, 719–724.

Wolf, R. (1966). The measurement of environments. In A. Anastasi (Ed.), *Testing problems in perspective* (pp. 491–503). Washington, DC: American Council on Education.

Zautra, A. J., Guarnaccia, C. A., Reich, J. W., & Dohrenwend, B. P. (1988). The contribution of small events to stress and distress. In L. H. Cohen (Ed.), *Life events and psychological functioning: Theoretical and methodological issues* (pp. 123–148). Newbury Park, CA: Sage Publications.

Zigler, E., & Farber, E. A. (1985). Commonalities between the intellectual extremes: Giftedness and mental retardation. In F. Horowitz & M. O'Brien (Eds.), *The gifted and talented: Developmental perspectives*. Washington, DC: American Psychological Association.

Zigler, E., & Glick, M. (1986). *A developmental approach to adult psychopathology*. New York: John Wiley.

Zigler, E. F., Lamb, M. E., & Child, I. L. (1982). *Socialization and personality development* (2nd ed.). New York: Oxford University Press.

Zigler, E., & Trickett, P. K. (1978). IQ, social competence, and evaluation of early childhood intervention programs. *American Psychologist, 33*, 789–798.

Zimmerman, M. (1983). Methodological issues in the assessment of life events: A review of issues and research. *Clinical Psychology Review, 3*, 339–370.

12

Promoting Competent Young People in Competence-Enhancing Environments: A Systems-Based Perspective on Primary Prevention

Roger P. Weissberg

Yale University, New Haven, Connecticut

Marlene Caplan

University of London, England

Robin L. Harwood

National Institute of Child Health and Human Development, Washington, D.C.

Recent studies indicate that 15–22% of American children and adolescents suffer from diagnosable mental disorders. Researchers estimate that 25–50% engage in risk behaviors for negative health and behavior outcomes, such as drug abuse, unwanted pregnancy, AIDS, delinquency, and school dropout. The prevalence of problem behaviors, as well as current social trends, demands that effective primary prevention programs be developed and disseminated. This article reviews successful family-, school-, and community-based prevention efforts aimed at reducing the incidence and severity of children's psychosocial problems. High-quality, comprehensive, competence-promotion programs that focus on both children and their socializing environments represent the

Reprinted with permission from the *Journal of Consulting and Clinical Psychology*, 1991, Vol. 59, No. 6, 830–841. Copyright © 1991 by the American Psychological Association, Inc.

We gratefully acknowledge the support provided by the William T. Grant Foundation and the New Haven Public School System. We also appreciate the enormous intellectual contributions to this article made by Alice S. Jackson and the members of the William T. Grant Foundation Consortium on School-Based Social-Competence Promotion: Kenneth A. Dodge, Maurice J. Elias, J. David Hawkins, Leonard A. Jason, Philip C. Kendall, Cheryl A. Perry, Mary Jane Rotheram-Borus, and Joseph E. Zins.

> *state of the art in prevention. Establishing enduring, preventive interventions requires increased attention to program design, implementation, and institutionalization.*

During the late 1940s, the field of clinical psychology had the opportunity to decide how it could best contribute to what was defined as a staggering mental health service delivery crisis (Raimy, 1950). Large numbers of World War II veterans returned home with mental health problems, and there were not enough services available for those who needed them. Sarason's (1981) sociohistorical analysis describes how clinical adult psychology responded to this challenge by allying itself with what was then the prevailing ethos in American medicine and psychiatry. He questions the justification of psychology's chosen emphasis on individual treatment at the expense of a preventive orientation and wonders whether today's psychology could be more responsive to societal needs if it had made a primary commitment instead to collaborating with families, schools, and communities in establishing mental health promotions strategies for young people.

For better or worse, clinical child psychology has generally replicated the structure and function of clinical adult psychology (Walker & Roberts, 1983). Professionals direct their efforts primarily to the assessment, diagnosis, and treatment of disturbed children, rather than to the implementation and evaluation of systems-based approaches for promoting competence and preventing psychological dysfunction. This article shares significant recent advances in research and practice geared toward improving the quality of life for many troubled children and their families. Despite these important gains, however, it remains clear that traditional mental health resources are insufficient to address the needs of all children who experience emotional and behavioral problems.

This article discusses the value of working proactively with families, the educational system, and communities to enhance the psychological, social, and physical health of children. We argue that a dual focus on promoting competent young people and creating competence-enhancing environments is essential both to prevent behavior problems in children and to improve the functioning of those who already suffer from such difficulties. We address the following key issues: (a) What are the nature and extent of behavior problems presently experienced by young people? (b) What implications do research findings regarding the prevalence and common predictors of behavior problems have for conducting preventive interventions in the context of families, schools, and communities? (c) Is there empirical evidence to indicate that such programs can be beneficial? (d) What key elements enable successful prevention programs to produce long-term positive effects? (e) What are important next steps in prevention research and practice, and what role should mental health professionals play in these developments?

EXTENT OF CHILDHOOD PROBLEM BEHAVIORS AND THE NEED FOR PRIMARY PREVENTION

Recent epidemiological data suggest that 15–22% of the nation's 63 million children and adolescents have mental health problems severe enough to warrant treatment (Costello, 1990; National Advisory Mental Health Council, 1990; Tuma, 1989; Zill & Schoenborn, 1990). Given the links between maladjustment in childhood and a variety of negative psychosocial outcomes in adulthood, one feels concern both for the current suffering of this afflicted group and for the future generation of adults that our society is producing. Unfortunately, it has been estimated that fewer than 20% of the young people with mental health problems currently receive appropriate services (Tuma, 1989).

In addition to concerns about the high prevalence of mental health disorders, educators, health professionals, and the business community have expressed alarm about the growing number of young people who engage in behaviors that put them at high risk for negative psychosocial health and behavior outcomes such as drug abuse, teen pregnancy, AIDS, delinquency, and school dropout (e.g., Committee for Economic Development, 1987; Gans, Blyth, Elster, & Gaveras, 1990). Recent estimates indicate that 25% of the 28 million 10- to 17-year-olds in America are extremely vulnerable, and an additional 25% are moderately vulnerable, to the negative consequences of engaging in multiple high-risk social and health behaviors (Dryfoos, 1990; Report of the Task Force on Education of Young Adolescents, 1989). Although the remaining 50% are at low risk for engaging in such behaviors, they may nonetheless need strong and consistent support to avoid such involvement.

Recently, the National Association of State Boards of Education and the American Medical Association jointly issued *Code Blue: Uniting for Healthier Youth* (National Commission on the Role of the School and the Community in Improving Adolescent Health, 1990), which expressed grave concern about the current unprecedented adolescent health crisis in our nation. *Code Blue*, a phrase used in hospitals to signal a life-threatening emergency, calls on diverse personnel to rush to a patient's bedside and collaborate to save the patient's life. By analogy, the Commission indicated that the country's state of adolescent health constitutes a national emergency that poses serious economic and social ramifications. For the first time, young people are less healthy and less prepared to assume responsible places in our society than were their parents. This is especially worrisome inasmuch as society is more complex and competitive than ever before.

The widespread health and behavior problems of America's young people are due, in large part, to significant changes that have occurred during the past few decades in families, schools, neighborhoods, and the media. Major social, environmental, and economic changes include increased poverty rates among children, dramatic alterations in family composition and stability, the breakdown of traditional neighborhoods and extended families, reduced amounts of meaningful and supportive personal contact between young people and positive adult role models, changing demographics resulting in large numbers of economically and educationally disadvantaged young people entering school, the proliferation of health-damaging media messages, inadequate housing, unsafe neighborhood environments, and societal attitudes and behaviors that hurt ethnic minorities (Cherlin, 1988).

Given such difficult societal conditions, we are faced with critical questions concerning the most realistic, cost-effective ways to meet the psychological, social, and health needs of our young people. In particular, it appears that traditional treatment approaches can address the needs of only a small proportion of children in need. First, there is an enormous discrepancy between the number of available service providers and children who require help (Tuma, 1989). Second, although many mental health professionals make use of effective screening and early identification methods coupled with timely intervention, the mental health system continues to be dominated by a passive-receptive stance toward treatment (Cowen, Gesten, & Weissberg, 1980). That is, treatment typically begins after an individual seeks or is encouraged to get help for serious dysfunctional behavior that has developed over several years. At that point, appropriate services are very expensive, usually requiring a great deal of expertise and sustained involvement. Ironically, because the prognosis for successful outcomes in such instances is unfavorable, one could argue that a major portion of our scarce mental health resources is being devoted too late and in a cost-ineffective manner toward a small segment of people who may show few benefits. Finally, mental health interventions are often overly child-centered and thus pay inadequate attention to the settings (e.g., family, school, and community) that create and perpetuate a child's difficulties.

Recognition of these concerns has prompted calls for wide-spread primary prevention programming to promote childhood competence and thus reduce the incidence of young people who develop mental health problems (e.g., Report of the Task Panel on Prevention, 1978). Primary prevention strategies differ from traditional treatment approaches with respect to the targeting and timing of their intervention practices. In particular, they are (a) systems- and group-oriented rather than targeted to individuals; (b) directed primarily toward essentially healthy people who are not currently suffering any disability due to the condition being prevented, although targets may appropriately include those who are epidemiologically at risk for negative behavioral outcomes; and (c) concerned with promoting health, building competencies, and establishing supportive systems and settings as a protection against dysfunction (Cowen, 1986; Elias & Branden, 1988).

DEBATE REGARDING THE ROLE OF PRIMARY PREVENTION

There is considerable debate regarding the specific achievements of primary prevention in the field of mental health, as well as the role that mental health professionals should play in these efforts (Marlowe & Weinberg, 1985). Some scholars focus on the growing number of studies demonstrating the positive effects that prevention programs can have on children's social and health behavior (e.g., Dryfoos, 1990; Price, Cowen, Lorion, & Ramos-McKay, 1988; Schorr, 1988). However, in spite of these findings, others emphasize that evaluations of these programs fail to demonstrate that major functional mental illnesses, or even less severe diagnosable mental disorders, have been prevented (Lamb & Zusman, 1982; Shaffer, 1989).

Disagreements between advocates and critics of primary prevention are due, in large part, to differences at the level of basic assumptions about what constitutes mental disorder and the appropriate scope of activity for mental health professionals (Ford, 1985). For instance, critics of primary prevention often distinguish sharply between normative problems of living and diagnosable mental illness, in terms of both causation and implications for treatment. They give priority to reducing the prevalence of serious mental disorders and suggest that this can be achieved by identifying and treating underlying biological causes (Lamb & Zusman, 1982; Shaffer, 1989). Furthermore, they point out that there are already more children than we can serve who are in need of direct treatment and that limited resources cannot be diverted from treatment to prevention programs. Thus, they contend that children with mental disorders would be best served if mental health professionals functioned within their traditional boundaries of training and expertise (e.g., the assessment, diagnosis, and treatment of patients suffering from mental disorders).

In contrast, primary prevention advocates tend to emphasize greater continuity between the causes of and the appropriate responses to psychosocial health and behavior problems. On the basis of the belief that psychological and environmental factors interact powerfully with biological predispositions to affect behavioral competence or disorders, they contend that the prevention of dysfunction requires attention to multiple contributors to the child's growth and that intervening early in multiple child contexts is of equal or greater importance than treating the child (Rutter, 1982; Sameroff, 1991). Thus, nontraditional approaches to mental health enhancement—such as family support, school-based competence promotion, and social policy reform—are deemed an important part of mental health practice (Albee, 1983). Recognizing that diverse intervention strategies (educational, legal, media, etc.) can be used in varied contexts to enhance the adaptive growth and development of children, primary prevention advocates also highlight the importance of multidisciplinary collaboration to promote positive mental health (Jason, Hess, Felner, & Moritsugu, 1987).

REASONS FOR TARGETING MULTIPLE PROBLEM BEHAVIORS AND FOCUSING ON KEY SOCIALIZING CONTEXTS

Recent research in behavioral epidemiology indicates that mental health problems often co-occur with social problems like school failure or delinquency, as well as with health problems such as substance abuse (Donovan, Jessor, & Costa, 1988; Elliott, Huizinga, & Menard, 1989). In addition, there are common personality, behavioral, and environmental factors that are associated with an increased probability of these negative outcomes. Examples of such psychosocial risk factors are residence in a neighborhood that is deprived and disorganized, poor and inconsistent family management practices and communication, school failure and low expectations for achievement, poor peer relations, and early age of initiation of problem behaviors (Dryfoos, 1990). In contrast, protective mechanisms include a neighborhood with informal resources and supports, a cohesive family, ongoing contact with a caring adult, peer models for conventional behavior, self-esteem and a positive social orientation, good school performance, and adaptive coping skills (Cowen & Work, 1988; Garmezy, 1985; Rutter, 1987).

These findings challenge mental health professionals to broaden the outcomes they are trying to affect, as well as the intervention approaches used to achieve them. Dryfoos (1990) argued that the emergence of common predictors of multiple problem behaviors lends force to the perspective that interventions should focus more on the predictors of the behaviors, which are amenable to intervention, than on the behaviors themselves. She suggested, for example, that enhancement of early schooling and the prevention of school failure should be given high priority not only by those who want to lower the dropout rate, but also by those interested in preventing substance abuse, unwanted pregnancy, and conduct problems.

According to Perry and Jessor (1985), effective family-, school-, and community-based preventive interventions have potential to affect four different but interrelated domains of health: psychological health (subjective sense of well-being); social health (role fulfillment and social effectiveness); personal health (realization of individual potential); and physical health (physical-physiological functioning). Similarly, Zigler and Berman (1983) cautioned that it is a mistake to evaluate the effectiveness of early interventions with one construct such as IQ or a single diagnosable mental disorder. They argued instead for multidimensional assessments of children's social competence because such programs have potential to improve physical health, cognitive ability, academic achievement, social interaction skills, and various indicators of motivation and emotional functioning. In addition, they highlighted the value of evaluating molar educational outcomes (e.g., being in mainstream rather than in special-education classrooms; completing high school) and behavioral outcomes (e.g., incidence of delinquency or unwanted teen pregnancy, being self-supporting rather than on welfare). Although researchers must clarify relations among these variables and various mental disorders, these variables clearly constitute important criteria by which to assess the effects of mental-health treatment or prevention efforts with young people.

With regard to intervention, Ford (1985) noted that adopting a *competence perspective* might serve to maximize areas of common ground between critics and advocates of primary prevention. Competence refers to the behavioral effectiveness of one's transactions with the environment, as well as to one's sense of personal well-being in diverse aspects of life. Competence deficits, on the other hand, are reflected not only in diagnosable mental disorders, but also in difficulties with certain aspects of functioning such as social relationship problems, failure to achieve in school, involvement in health-damaging risk behaviors, and low self-esteem. The competence perspective asserts that mental health interventions—whether restorative or preventive—should be, and in fact are, primarily concerned with building behavioral competence and feelings of efficacy in diverse aspects of life.

In closing, the identification of common predictors of multiple problem behaviors and findings about the multifactorial causation of psychological, social, and health problems support the view that effective prevention or treatment approaches require attention to the key socializing contexts in which children grow—specifically, the family and the school (Dryfoos, 1990; Rutter, 1982). Children are most likely to function effectively and feel competent when (a) they have opportunities to be actively involved with and to contribute meaningfully to their family and school; (b) they have the skills, motivation, and information to succeed in these settings; and (c) their social systems and socializing agents (e.g., parents, teachers, peers) consistently reinforce their positive, adaptive behavioral performance (Hawkins & Weis, 1985). Following this framework, we propose that family-, school-, and community-based prevention programs will be most effective when they attempt both (a) to enhance children's capacities to coordinate skills, prosocial values, and information in order to cope adaptively with society's social tasks, challenges, and stresses and (b) to create environmental settings and resources that support the development of young people's positive personal, social, and health behavior (Weissberg, Caplan, & Sivo, 1989). It is also important to recognize that both the family and the school are situated within broader community, national, and cultural contexts (Bronfenbrenner, 1979). Because of this, interventions aimed at the family and the school must be both culturally sensitive and coordinated with larger community and national reform efforts. Only by coordinating with these broader contexts can prevention efforts produce positive, lasting changes in young people and their socializing contexts.

RESEARCH EVIDENCE REGARDING THE EFFICACY OF PRIMARY PREVENTION

During the last decade, literature focusing on the evaluation of prevention programs for children and adolescents has expanded dramatically (e.g., Bond & Compas, 1989; Dryfoos, 1990; Kazdin, 1991; Lorion, 1989; Mueller & Higgins, 1988; Price et al., 1988; Schorr, 1988; Zins & Forman, 1988). Although there are many promising demonstrations of beneficial prevention efforts, it is also true that many attempts at primary prevention fail to produce lasting behavior changes (e.g., Bangert-Drowns, 1988). This outcome may be due to the fact that many of these so-called prevention programs are unrealistically short, are poorly implemented, or fail to intervene simultaneously with the child and his or her socializing contexts. Establishing effective prevention programs involves a complex set of tasks, and it is counterproductive to overpromise what prevention can achieve or to oversimplify the difficulties involved in developing and implementing such efforts (Price & Lorion, 1989; Weissberg et al., 1989). At this time, the field will advance from research that clarifies why certain programs accomplish or fail to accomplish their goals.

This section selectively reviews illustrative prevention programs that have had positive behavioral effects for young people and then describes elements that appear critical for their success. We have selected carefully evaluated models that have realistic length, substance, and scope. Most focus explicitly on enhancing the competence of both children and their socializing environments. In addition, these models are well-designed, and there is considerable advocacy for their broader dissemination. For children under the age of 5 years, high-quality family support and early childhood education programs have produced long-term benefits (Price et al., 1988). For older children, the most promising strategies involve multiyear, school-based, social-competence and health-education programs with peer, parent, school-support, and community components (Perry, Klepp, & Sillers, 1989; Weissberg, 1991).

Family Support Programs

In family support programs, specially trained community members or professionals provide ongoing support to families during pregnancy, infancy, and early childhood. The major goals of family support are to promote nurturing and attentive parenting, parents' personal development and psychological well-being, and ultimately, healthy child development. In contrast to social service delivery systems that are oriented toward ameliorating crises, family support programs attempt to empower parents to help themselves and their children (Zigler & Black, 1989). We describe two exemplars of family support programs, the Yale Child Welfare

Research Project (Provence & Naylor, 1983) and the Houston Parent Child Development Center (Johnson, 1988), to illustrate this program model and its potential effects.

The Yale Child Welfare Research Project provided four interrelated services to 17 impoverished pregnant women expecting a firstborn child through 30 months postpartum. These included (a) 28 supportive home visits by a psychologist, social worker, or nurse that focused on solving practical problems such as obtaining more adequate food and housing or making decisions about future educational, career, and family goals; (b) 13–17 well-baby exams by a pediatrician; (c) an average of 13 months of center-based day care; and (d) 7–9 regularly scheduled developmental examinations. A 10-year follow-up study revealed that intervention mothers, relative to control mothers, obtained more education, were more likely to be employed, chose to bear fewer children, and were more active in seeking information about their child from classroom teachers. Although the two groups of children were comparable on IQ and achievement test performance, control boys were absent more often, rated by teachers as having more serious acting-out problems, and required an average of $1,120 more per year in special school services than did program children (Seitz, Rosenbaum, & Apfel, 1985). Although these findings suggest that family support combined with quality day care has considerable potential as a general model for preventive intervention, results from this study should be replicated with a larger sample, and greater attention must be paid to identifying the intervention components or mechanisms that contribute to improved maternal and child functioning.

The Houston Parent-Child Development Center offered a two-stage, 2-year program for Mexican Americans that required 550 hr of family involvement beginning when a child was 1 and ending at age 3 (Johnson, 1988). During the first year, mothers were visited in the home by a paraprofessional for twenty-five 90-min sessions focusing on information about child development, parenting skills, and using the home as a learning environment. During Year 2, mothers came to the Center four mornings per week for classes on child management and family communication skills while their children attended nursery school. In a 5- to 8-year follow-up study involving 139 second- through fifth-graders, program children performed better on a standardized achievement test and were rated by teachers as less aggressive and hostile and more considerate (Johnson & Walker, 1987). The Houston project has the methodological strengths of using a very large sample size and random assignment to groups. A high subject attrition rate, both during the intervention and at follow-up (primarily as a result of families moving out of the area), limits the generalizability of these positive findings to less mobile families.

Several other longitudinal studies demonstrate the long-term positive effects of family support on impoverished children and families (e.g., Infant Health and Development Program, 1990; Olds, 1988). In addition, Pierson (1988) reported that family support and early childhood programming positively affected the school performance and behavior of children of varying socioeconomic levels. The present research challenge is to identify more clearly the mechanisms by which such benefits are produced. This is a complicated task inasmuch as it appears that successful support services must be comprehensive, multifaceted, and flexible in order to be effective (Schorr, 1988). Seitz (1991) cautioned that family contacts per se do not guarantee parent involvement or improved child development. The timing of family contacts, the characteristics of the service provider, and the content of intervention activities are key variables to assess in future studies.

Early Childhood Education

Early childhood education may be broadly defined as any group program for children under age 5 that provides them with knowledge and social competence required for normal development or success in school (Haskins, 1989). This broad description includes a range of programs in terms of location (e.g., home day care, community center, or school) and educational approach (e.g., child-initiated learning, teacher-directed instruction). Research findings from the High/Scope Perry Preschool Study (Schweinhart & Weikart, 1988) and the Consortium for Longitudinal Studies (Lazar, Darlington, Murray, Royce, & Snipper, 1982) demonstrate that *high-quality* preschool programs can produce positive, enduring changes in children's social and behavioral functioning. On the basis of these positive research findings, there is growing national support for the widespread dissemination of early childhood education programs (e.g., Committee for Economic Development, 1987). In particular, the U.S. Department of Health and Human Services, Public Health Service (1990) recommended by the year 2000 that the country "achieve for all disadvantaged children and children with disabilities access to high quality and developmentally appropriate preschool programs that help prepare children for school, thereby improving their prospects with regard to school performance, problem behaviors, and physical health" (p. 254). Furthermore, Public Law 99-457, focusing on provision of early interventions for young handicapped and high-risk children, is providing a major impetus for early childhood services.

However, it should be emphasized that lasting benefits of early childhood education have been achieved only by high-quality programs characterized by a developmentally appropriate curriculum, based on child-initiated activities; teaching teams that are knowledgeable in early childhood development and receive ongoing training and supervision; class size limited to fewer than twenty 3- to 5-year-olds with at least two teachers; administrative leadership that includes support of the program; systematic efforts to involve parents as partners in their child's education, as well as sensitivity to the noneducational needs of the child and family; and evaluation procedures that are developmentally appropriate (Schweinhart &

Weikart, 1988). These characteristics of program design and implementation appear to be central ingredients of most successful prevention efforts (Weissberg et al., 1989). In contrast, there is ample evidence to suggest that early childhood education programs of lesser quality do not result in such positive effects (Haskins, 1989).

Between 1962 and 1967, the High/Scope Perry Preschool Project served low-income Black 3- and 4-year-old children with IQ scores between 70 and 90 (Schweinhart & Weikart, 1988, 1989). Program evaluators randomly assigned 58 children to a preschool group and 65 children to a control group. The classroom program involved five 90-min classes a week for 7 months per year over a 2-year period. Classroom groups had 25 children and four well-trained teachers who implemented the High/Scope Early Childhood Curriculum, an educational approach that promotes intellectual, social, and physical development through child-initiated learning activities. In addition, teachers made weekly 90-min home visits to involve parents as partners in their child's education. Longitudinal follow-up data on children up to age 28 indicate that program children, relative to control subjects, showed stronger commitment to schooling, higher academic achievement, lower rates of grade retention, fewer placements in special education (16% vs. 28%), lower rates of classification of mental impairment (15% vs. 35%), better high school graduation rates (67% vs. 49%), fewer arrests (31% vs. 51%), higher employment (50% vs. 32%), and lower use of welfare assistance (19% vs. 41%).

Other high-quality programs have also promoted multiple competencies and prevented problem behaviors in children. Most notably, the Consortium for Longitudinal Studies evaluated the long-term effects of 11 preschool programs (including the Perry Preschool Project) on 2,008 experimental and control children between ages 9 and 19. Program children were less likely to be retained or to require special education. In addition, they were more achievement-oriented, and their parents had higher educational and occupational aspirations than did the parents of control children. Although for some programs the results were stronger than for others, findings also suggested that these programs have potential to affect rates of delinquency and crime, teen pregnancy, welfare use, and employment (Royce, Darlington, & Murray, 1983). One limitation of early childhood education research to date involves the paucity of longitudinal studies that compare the differential long-term effects of various educational approaches. The importance of this research question has been highlighted by Schweinhart and Weikart (1988), who reported suggestive findings that programs that emphasize child-initiated learning activities may have more positive long-term behavioral affects than those that emphasize teacher-directed instruction.

In summary, although early intervention projects were initially conceptualized as programs to help children at risk for school failure, these results clearly have implications for primary prevention in mental health. Many school-related variables (e.g., poor achievement motivation, low aspirations and expectations for educational accomplishment, poor school performance, and school dropout) are risk factors for a variety of later problem behaviors, including substance abuse, unwanted teen pregnancy, conduct problems, depression, and suicide (Elliott et al., 1989). Early school failure and placement in special education are two critical markers that constitute major turning points in the lives of many children, with long-term implications for future adjustment (Dryfoos, 1990; Hawkins, Doueck, & Lishner, 1988; Maughan, 1988). Thus, early childhood education could be viewed as an innovative mental health strategy that affects many risk and protective factors for diverse problem behaviors. The strongest effects are in the domain of behavioral conduct, although it will be instructive for investigators to broaden their future assessments to include measures of depression and anxiety.

There is considerable debate about why these early interventions produced long-term effects. One causal model suggests that preschool education promotes cognitive and social skills that result in greater school readiness and a smoother transition to kindergarten. Subsequently, this preparation leads to positive responses by kindergarten teachers, which foster more improved student attitudes about schooling and better school performance in later grades; and school success, in turn, serves as a protective factor to prevent behavioral maladjustment and delinquency (Schweinhart & Weikart, 1988). An alternative set of explanations emphasizes the importance of changing parents' behaviors or restructuring their social expectations as primary mechanisms to positively affect the adjustment of children (Sameroff, 1991). For example, it is possible that extensive home visitations in high-quality preschool programs enhance parental competence and involvement, leading parents to become more adept socializers and to have more realistic expectations regarding their children's performance as well as the teachers and schools that serve them. These changes, in turn, provide firmer foundations for improved family functioning and child behavior. Overall, programs that focus on both children and their socializing environments appear to produce the most long-lasting gains (Seitz, 1991). However, future research must clarify the differential benefits that are achieved when parents participate actively or are less meaningfully involved in their child's early education.

Although high-quality, comprehensive early interventions appear to promote long-term competencies, researchers have noted that relying too heavily on any one time period or any one context for preventive interventions is a mistake (Zigler & Berman, 1983). Furthermore, although these early interventions produced significant gains in program relative to control students, the number of children experiencing school and social difficulties is still considerably higher than acceptable. For these reasons, as children and adolescents face the complex challenges inherent in growing up, it is necessary to create ongoing educational experiences and supports that promote their continued positive social and behavioral development.

Comprehensive School-Based Social-Competence and Health Education

The educational system offers the most efficient and systematic means available to promote the psychological, social, and physical health of school-age children and adolescents. Schools are compulsory institutions that have significant and sustained contact with most children during formative years of personality development (Rutter, Maughan, Mortimore, & Ouston, 1979). They have the potential to be especially well-suited sites to teach life skills and to prevent social maladaptation and health-damaging behavior. Under the right circumstances, learning activities may be introduced and environments can be created to support the development of health-protective skills, attitudes, values, and behaviors. Many psychological disorders and problem behaviors either have their roots in or may be exacerbated by a child's school experiences (Maughan, 1988; Rutter, 1982). School-based interventions are needed both to prevent the development of dysfunction and to improve the functioning of all children (i.e., those with and without health and behavior problems).

Currently, school administrators and teachers are both receptive to and ambivalent about providing prevention programming. On the one hand, public pressure to raise achievement test scores and to increase academic competitiveness raises concern whenever limited curriculum time is devoted to activities that are not directly related to traditional academic content areas. On the other hand, educators recognize that enhancing children's mental and physical health will improve their ability to learn and achieve academically as well as their capacity to become responsible citizens and productive workers. Recently, there has been considerable advocacy for school-based programming to promote children's psychological and physical health, especially as a result of public health concerns about substance abuse, AIDS, and antisocial behavior (DeFriese, Crossland, Pearson, & Sullivan, 1990; Zins & Forman, 1988). Given this advocacy, there is a splendid opportunity for prevention program developers and researchers to introduce programming of sufficient scope and length to produce long-term positive behavioral outcomes. This section briefly reviews research that supports establishing ecologically valid, kindergarten to high school social-competence and health education programs that include peer, parent, school support, and community components.

A case for multiyear, multicomponent prevention programs that address multiple problem behaviors. Classroom-based social-competence promotion programs to enhance students' psychological and physical health represent the most commonly implemented and evaluated school-based prevention approach (Bond & Compas, 1989; Dryfoos, 1990; Zins & Forman, 1988).[1] Programs that produce short-term

---

[1] Due to space limitations, we are not able to review other promising prevention programs that have been developed, such as individually oriented counseling services, mentoring programs, and health clinics (Dryfoos, 1990; Zabin, 1990); coping-skills and support programs for high-risk populations,

benefits have been established for children in preschool and kindergarten (Shure & Spivack, 1988), elementary school (Elias et al., 1986; Rotheram-Borus, 1988; Weissberg et al., 1981), middle school (Botvin & Tortu, 1988; Weissberg & Caplan, 1991), and high school (Eisen, Zellman, & McAlister, 1990). Most of these efforts have been brief (i.e., less than 1 year), single-method, single-level intervention strategies. Unfortunately, there is little evidence to suggest that such programs promote behavioral improvements that will last for several years postintervention (Dryfoos, 1990). Currently, there is growing recognition that more sustained comprehensive interventions may be required to produce lasting behavioral gains in school-age children and adolescents (Mueller & Higgins, 1988; Schorr, 1988; Zigler & Berman, 1983). Creating multiyear, classroom-based skills training approaches at the core of larger multilevel-systems efforts to promote social competence and health is a particularly promising direction for prevention research.

A variety of classroom-based health promotion strategies have been evaluated, including programs that provide information about the consequences of engaging in certain high-risk behaviors, as well as programs that emphasize generic personal and social skills training. Research suggests that knowledge-only programs have minimal effects on children's behaviors (Botvin & Tortu, 1988; Tobler, 1986). In contrast, programs that teach generic, broadly applicable personal and social competencies—such as self-control, stress management, problem solving, decision making, communication, peer resistance, and assertiveness—have yielded significant benefits at least 1-year postintervention in broad areas of personal competence, such as social adjustment, assertive behavior, aggressive behavior, peer sociability, and coping with stressors (Elias et al., 1986; Gesten et al., 1982; Rotheram-Borus, 1988; Shure & Spivack, 1988).

In spite of these positive effects, generic skills training programs do not consistently produce positive outcomes in more problem-specific domains, such as substance use or high-risk sexual behavior (Caplan & Weissberg, 1989; Durlak, 1983). Combining general personal and social skills training—for example, in prob-

---

such as children of alcoholic parents or divorcing parents (Emshoff, 1989; Pedro-Caroll & Cowen, 1985); training teachers to use proactive classroom management, interactive teaching, and cooperative learning methods to promote academic achievement, positive classroom behavior, and bonding to school (Hawkins et al., 1988; Slavin, 1983); and reorganizing school settings into smaller units (e.g., homerooms, grade clusters, and schools within schools) to provide increased student support, especially during times of transition from one school to another (Felner & Adan, 1988). Recently, investigators have combined the most effective of these programming elements to establish multicomponent individual and environmental school-based interventions that (a) promote students' academic and social competence (Gottfredson, 1986; Slavin, Madden, Karweit, Livermon, & Dolan, 1990) and (b) involve parents, teachers, mental health staff, and administrators in collaborative decision making about setting academic and social goals for students (Comer, 1988). Ultimately, a multifaceted array of school-based prevention strategies will be needed to address the diverse needs of today's young people. Educators, policymakers, and researchers will have to work together to determine the most effective ways to coordinate these varied efforts.

lem solving and decision making—with attempts to affect student knowledge, attitudes, and behavioral competence in specific domains appears to be a very promising approach for preventing specific problem behaviors (Botvin & Tortu, 1988; Caplan et al., in press). However, because research findings suggest children have limited capacities to transfer and generalize skills, attitudes, and information for handling stressors in one domain to address problems in another (Dodge, Pettit, McClaskey, & Brown, 1986), a major task for future research involves developing skills-attitude-information training models that target multiple problem areas in the context of the same intervention.

Recent research suggests that multiple years of classroom-based social-competence-promotion training may be required to produce long-term improvements in students' behavior (e.g., Botvin, Baker, Dusenbury, Tortu, & Botvin, 1990; Connell & Turner, 1985; Perry et al., 1989; Weissberg, 1989). For example, Weissberg and Caplan (1991) trained middle-school teachers to implement a curriculum focusing on impulse control, stress management, a six-step social information processing model for resolving problems, and behavioral social skills training. Evaluation results with 421 early adolescents indicated that program students, relative to control subjects, improved in problem-solving skills, prosocial attitudes toward conflict resolution, teacher-rated impulse control and peer sociability, and self-reported delinquent behavior. During the following year, teachers conducted booster training with a sample of seventh-grade students who participated in the initial intervention. Weissberg (1989) assessed the long-term impact of 2 years (i.e., in sixth and seventh grade) versus 1 year (i.e., in sixth or seventh grade) versus no training on students' problem-solving skills and adjustment during the fall of eighth grade. Students with 2 years of training, but not those with 1, showed significant gains relative to the no-treatment control group.

Although brief classroom-based programs may produce short-term behavioral gains, it appears unrealistic to expect such efforts to have lasting effects. Furthermore, it is unclear precisely how many hours of instruction are needed to promote robust improvements in children's health-related knowledge, attitudes, and behavior. Although relatively few hours of instruction can produce large effects for knowledge acquisition, 40–50 hr may be necessary to establish stable effects for all three domains (Connell, Turner, & Mason, 1985). These findings suggest that researchers need to design and evaluate more substantial (e.g., 40–50 hr) multiyear interventions in order to test adequately the extent to which classroom-based social-competence-promotion programs can produce long-term preventive effects.

School-based programs that focus independently on the child or environment are not as effective as those that simultaneously educate the child and instill positive changes in the environment. Consequently, a word must be said regarding *person-centered* versus *ecologically oriented* skills training programs. Training programs may appropriately be considered person-centered when skills are taught in the absence of creating environmental supports for continued skill application in daily interactions. In contrast, ecologically oriented programs emphasize not only the teaching of skills, but also the creation of meaningful real-life opportunities to use skills and the establishment of structures to provide reinforcement for effective skill application. From this perspective, the success of skills training programs may depend largely on their attention to changing socialization patterns and supports in the intervention setting (Elias & Weissberg, 1989). For example, ecologically oriented problem-solving programs try to introduce a common social information processing framework that children and teachers can use to communicate more effectively about problem situations (Shure & Spivack, 1988; Weissberg & Caplan, 1991). In other words, they try to change not only the child's behavior, but also the teacher's behavior, the relationship between the teacher and child, and classroom and school-level resources and procedures to support adaptive problem-solving efforts (Weissberg et al., 1989).

In line with the ecological perspective, Pentz et al. (1989) contended that many school-based prevention programs may not produce significant and sustained behavioral changes because of a lack of integration between school-based training with community-based interventions, the mass media, and other environmental influences outside of school that conflict with the concepts taught in school. They proposed that multilevel, multicomponent prevention efforts that coordinate the efforts of multiple socializing influences—including parents, peers, community leaders, local school and government administrators, and mass media programmers—may be needed to produce long-term social, psychological, and health benefits. Specifically, Pentz et al. (1989) developed a substance abuse prevention program that combined 10 sessions of classroom-based peer-resistance skills training, 10 homework sessions interviewing parents and family members about issues related to drug abuse prevention, mass media programming, and community organization. Outcome analyses with 22,500 sixth- and seventh-grade students indicated significantly lower prevalence rates for alcohol, cigarette, and marijuana use for the program participants compared with control subjects. Positive effects were sustained 3 years following the classroom intervention with low-risk and high-risk subjects showing significant reductions in tobacco and marijuana use (Johnson et al., 1990).

Perry et al. (1989) evaluated effects from a 5-year school-based behavioral education program, for students moving from 6th through 10th grade, conducted in the context of a communitywide intervention to promote cardiovascular health. The primary program goals involved social skills training to enhance students' ability to resist pressures to engage in health-compromising behaviors as well as to generate health-enhancing alternatives, changing peer group norms, and providing alternative healthy role models. All programs used peer leaders, who were elected by their classmates and trained by community staff, as key trainers of new skills and information within the classroom setting. Reported findings, which focused on the intervention's impact on smoking, indicated that 13.1% of program students compared with 22.7% of control children were current smokers.

Perry et al. (1989) and Pentz et al. (1989) have demonstrated the potential efficacy of multiyear, multicomponent school-based interventions—that involve parents, peers, and the surrounding community—to prevent substance abuse. A crucial next step in research is to determine whether these models can be used to prevent multiple social and psychological problem behaviors in the context of the same intervention. There is growing support for planned, sequential, comprehensive health education in kindergarten through Grade 12 that (a) emphasizes personal and social skills training; (b) promotes positive social values and health attitudes; and (c) provides honest, relevant information about health issues such as substance abuse, sex, AIDS, violence, family life, and mental health (DeFriese et al., 1990; National Commission on the Role of the School and the Community in Improving Adolescent Health, 1990; Report of the National Mental Health Association's Commission on the Prevention of Mental-Emotional Disabilities, 1986). Most notably, the U.S. Department of Health and Human Services, Public Health Service (1990) proposed by the Year 2000 that at least 75% of the nation's schools provide high-quality comprehensive health education.

Weissberg (1991) suggested that effectively implementing carefully evaluated comprehensive social-competence and health education (C-SCAHE) that targets the prevention of multiple problem areas is an urgently needed educational reform for the 1990s. Although this approach has potential to benefit many young people, there are potential barriers that could undercut the efficacy of such programming. Most notably, health education historically has emphasized conveying science information and facts at the expense of focusing on skills training to effect changes in health practices. Secondly, such programs have traditionally focused on issues related to physical health more than social or psychological health. C-SCAHE, in highlighting the dual importance of both *social competence* and *health*, calls for a better instructional balance between these areas.

Researchers and practitioners must attend more to issues of program design, implementation, and institutionalization. Attention to multiple aspects of program development—design, implementation, and institutionalization—is also of critical importance in establishing beneficial, enduring, school-based primary prevention programs (Weissberg et al., 1989). In terms of design, effective programming must focus simultaneously on (a) enhancing children's personal and social skills, attitudes and values, and domain-specific knowledge and (b) creating socializing systems at multiple levels to promote positive youth development. Programs must promote a sense of shared values, culture, and support among students, school staff, parents, and the larger community. This integration underscores the importance of coordinating classroom-, school-, and community-level programming efforts.

Regardless of a program's quality, its potential for positive effects is diminished when program implementers are poorly trained, have inadequate organizational support for program delivery, or lack the necessary skills to provide effective training. Well-designed programs that are implemented with low integrity may appear ineffective, when in fact they are quite beneficial (see Botvin et al., 1990; Connell et al., 1985). School systems must provide time and resources for proficient staff training, ongoing supervision, on-site coaching, and program monitoring in order to ensure implementation integrity (Hall & Hord, 1987).

It must also be noted that many initially successful interventions fail to sustain their impact in future years (Berman & McLaughlin, 1978). Thus, researchers must identify organizational practices and system-level policies or structures that enable successful programs to endure with continued positive effects (McLaughlin, 1990). Institutionalizing successful school-based programs requires that they be adapted to the ecology of the school and community in which they occur (Price & Lorion, 1989). For C-SCAHE programming to endure, it is critical to design a clearly articulated kindergarten through 12th-grade curriculum scope and sequence; determine where such training fits in the overall instructional program at the building level; ensure that the training approaches and content comply with state and federal guidelines and policies; and develop a solid infrastructure of school system supports for effective program implementation, monitoring, and improvement. Ultimately, a comprehensive program that targets multiple problem behaviors has greater potential to endure in school settings than have discrete, ad hoc, short-term categorical interventions that target the prevention of single problem behaviors (DeFriese et al., 1990).

The need to continue C-SCAHE with clinical treatment services. Multiyear, multicomponent, competence-promotion programs—involving the child, classroom, school organization, and larger community setting—are most promising as primary prevention strategies because they have excellent potential to influence children's skills, attitudes, and social and health behaviors. At the same time, it is important to recognize that these programs are not panaceas. Although some high-risk children may benefit from program participation, there are many who will still require additional treatment to reduce psychological maladjustment and enhance their behavioral functioning. An important part of C-SCAHE will involve training program implementers to recognize when high-risk children have additional needs for treatment and to refer those individuals for the appropriate services they need. Following the perspective that school-based intervention strategies should be reinforced by parents, the peer group, and the community, we deem it equally important to coordinate intervention strategies used in prevention programs and clinical treatment to produce more powerful intervention packages for high-risk children. Illustratively, cognitive-behavioral and social-skills treatment approaches that promote children's self-control and problem solving appear to be very compatible with the competencies taught in classroom-based programs (e.g., Kendall & Braswell, 1985). It seems important to compare the effects of classroom training versus clinical treatment versus a combined package to determine their differential effects on children already experiencing behavior problems.

CONCLUSION

This article describes several prevention efforts that attempt to promote competent young children and competence-enhancing environments. There is substantial evidence to indicate that these programs, when implemented effectively, can produce lasting behavioral benefits for young people; however, it may take considerable time before research convincingly resolves whether such improvements will actually reduce the incidence of mental disorders. If these prevention programs improve the social functioning, academic performance, and health behavior of large numbers of children, then the investment of resources seems well spent—especially inasmuch as young people with diagnosable disorders can participate and benefit from them.

Mental health professionals must decide what roles they will play in the prevention field. Examples of constructive participation may involve taking the lead or collaborating to establish innovative, multidisciplinary, multicomponent prevention programs or coordinating one's treatment efforts more closely with family-, school-, and community-based prevention efforts. In contrast, refraining from any participation until prevention research definitively demonstrates that these programs lower the incidence of diagnosable mental disorders could seriously limit the meaningful contributions that a professional might offer in addressing the needs of many children and adolescents at risk for psychosocial health and behavior problems.

In 1930, the White House Conference on Children and Youth expressed concern about the potential unintended negative consequences of professional specialization:

> To the doctor, the child is a typhoid patient; to the playground supervisor, a first baseman; to the teacher, a learner of arithmetic. At different times, he may be different things to each of these specialists, but rarely is he a whole child to any of them. (cited in U.S. Department of Health, Education, and Welfare, 1967, p. 9)

Each mental health professional will have to decide whether to characterize and treat children only within the context of mental-emotional disorders or to expand their perceptions to incorporate the multiple aspects of children's functioning and environmental circumstances. This article supports Sarason's (1981) notion that mental health professionals should forge a stronger collaboration with families, schools, and communities in order to provide high-quality, comprehensive prevention programming to more children and youth. The critical question to address is not whether prevention programs work, but how they can be conducted most effectively.

REFERENCES

Albee, G. W. (1983). Psychopathology, prevention, and the just society. *Journal of Primary Prevention, 4*, 5–40.

Bangert-Drowns, R. L. (1988). The effects of school-based substance abuse education: A meta-analysis. *Journal of Drug Education, 18*, 243–264.

Berman, P., & McLaughlin, M. W. (1978). *Federal programs supporting educational change: Vol. 8. Implementing and sustaining innovations.* Santa Monica, CA: Rand Corporation.

Bond, L. A., & Compas, B. E. (Eds.). (1989). *Primary prevention and promotion in the schools.* Newbury Park, CA: Sage.

Botvin, G. J., Baker, E., Dusenbury, L., Tortu, S., & Botvin, E. M. (1990). Preventing adolescent drug abuse through a multimodal cognitive-behavioral approach: Results of a 3-year study. *Journal of Consulting and Clinical Psychology, 58*, 437–446.

Botvin, G. J., & Tortu, S. (1988). Preventing adolescent substance abuse through life skills training. In R. H. Price, E. L. Cowen, R. P. Lorion, & J. Ramos-McKay (Eds.), *14 ounces of prevention: A casebook for practitioners* (pp. 98–110). Washington, DC: American Psychological Association.

Bronfenbrenner, U. (1979). *The ecology of human development: Experiments by nature and design.* Cambridge, MA: Harvard University Press.

Caplan, M., & Weissberg, R. P. (1989). Promoting social competence in early adolescence: Developmental considerations. In B. H. Schneider, G. Attili, J. Nadel, & R. P. Weissberg (Eds.), *Social competence in developmental perspective* (pp. 371–385). Boston: Kluwer.

Caplan, M., Weissberg, R. P., Grober, J. H., Sivo, P. J., Grady, K., & Jacoby, C. (in press). Social-competence promotion with inner-city and suburban young adolescents: Effects on social adjustment and alcohol use. *Journal of Consulting and Clinical Psychology.*

Cherlin, A. J. (1988). *The changing American family and public policy* . Washington, DC: Urban Institute Press.

Comer, J. P. (1988). Educating poor minority children. *Scientific American, 259*, 42–48.

Committee for Economic Development. (1987). *Children in need: Investment strategies for the educationally disadvantaged.* New York: Author.

Connell, D. B., & Turner, R. R. (1985). The impact of instructional experience and the effects of cumulative instruction. *Journal of School Health, 55*, 324–331.

Connell, D. B., Turner, R. R., & Mason, E. F. (1985). Summary of the findings of the School Health Education Evaluation: Health promotion effectiveness, implementation, and costs. *Journal of School Health, 55*, 316–323.

Costello, E. J. (1990). Child psychiatric epidemiology: Implications for clinical research and practice. In B. B. Lahey & A. E. Kazdin (Eds.), *Advances in clinical child psychology* (Vol. 13, pp. 53–90). New York: Plenum Press.

Cowen, E. L. (1986). Primary prevention in mental health: Ten years of retrospect and ten years of prospect. In M. Kessler & S. E. Goldston (Eds.), *A decade of progress in primary prevention* (pp. 3–45). Hanover, NH: University Press of New England.

Cowen, E. L., Gesten, E. L., & Weissberg, R. P. (1980). An interrelated network of preventively oriented school-based mental health approaches. In R. H. Price & P. Politzer (Eds.), *Evaluation and action in the community context* (pp. 173–210). New York: Academic Press.

Cowen, E. L., & Work, W. C. (1988). Resilient children, psychological wellness, and primary prevention. *American Journal of Community Psychology, 16*, 591–607.

DeFriese, G. H., Crossland, C. L., Pearson, C. E., & Sullivan, C. J. (1990). Comprehensive school health programs: Current status and future prospects. *Journal of School Health, 60*(4).

Didge, K. A., Pettit, G. S., McClaskey, C. L., & Brown, M. M. (1986). Social competence in children. *Monographs of the Society for Research in Child Development, 51*(2, Serial No. 213).

Donovan, J. E., Jessor, R., & Costa, F. (1988). The syndrome of problem behavior in adolescence: A replication. *Journal of Consulting and Clinical Psychology, 56*, 762–765.

Dryfoos, J. G. (1990). *Adolescents at risk: Prevalence and prevention.* New York: Oxford University Press.

Durlak, J. A. (1983). Social problem-solving as a primary prevention strategy. In R. D. Felner, L. A. Jason, J. N. Moritsugu, & S. S. Farber (Eds.), *Preventive psychology: Theory, research, and practice* (pp. 31–48). New York: Pergamon Press.

Eisen, M., Zellman, G. L., & McAlister, A. L. (1990). Evaluating the impact of a theory-based sexuality and contraceptive education program. *Family Planning Perspectives, 22*, 261–271.

Elias, M. J., & Branden, L. R. (1988). Primary prevention of behavioral and emotional problems in school-aged populations. *School Psychology Review, 17*, 581–592.

Elias, M. J., Gara, M., Ubriaco, M., Rothbaum, P. A., Clabby, J. F., & Schuyler, T. (1986). Impact of a preventive social problem-solving intervention on children's coping with middle-school stressors. *American Journal of Community Psychology, 14*, 259–275.

Elias, M. J., & Weissberg, R. P. (1989). School-based social-competence promotion as a primary prevention strategy: A tale of two projects. *Prevention in Human Services, 7*, 177–200.

Elliott, D. S., Huizinga, D., & Menard, S. (1989). *Multiple problem youth: Delinquency, substance use, and mental health problems.* New York: Springer-Verlag.

Emshoff, J. G. (1989). A preventive intervention with children of alcoholics. *Prevention in Human Services, 7*, 225–254.

Felner, R. D., & Adan, A. M. (1988). The School Transition Environment Project: An ecological intervention and evaluation. In R. H. Price, E. L. Cowen, R. P. Lorion, & J. Ramos-McKay (Eds.), *14 ounces of prevention: A casebook for practitioners* (pp. 111–122). Washington DC: American Psychological Association.

Ford, M. E. (1985). Primary prevention: Key issues and a competence perspective. *Journal of Primary Preventions, 5*, 264–266.

Gans, J. E., Blyth, D. A., Elster, A. B., & Gaveras, L. L. (1990). *America's adolescents: How healthy are they?* Chicago: American Medical Association.

Garmezy, N. (1985). Stress-resistant children: The search for protective factors. In J. E. Stevenson (Ed.), *Recent research in developmental psychopathology* (pp. 213–233). Oxford, England: Pergamon Press.

Gesten, E. L., Rains, M., Rapkin, B. D., Weissberg, R. P., Flores de Apodaca, R., Cowen, E. L., & Bowen, R. (1982). Training children in social problem-solving skills: A competence building approach, first and second look. *American Journal of Community Psychology, 10*, 95–115.

Gottfredson, D. C. (19886). An empirical test of school-based environmental and individual interventions to reduce the risk of delinquent behavior. *Criminology, 24*, 705–731.

Hall, G. E., & Hord, S. M. (1987). *Change in schools: Facilitating the process.* Albany, NY: State University of New York Press.

Haskins, R. (1989). Beyond metaphor: The efficacy of early childhood education. *American Psychologist, 44*, 274–283.

Hawkins, J. D., Doueck, H. J., & Lishner, D. M. (1988). Changing teaching practices in mainstream classrooms to improve bonding and behavior of low achievers. *American Educational Research Journal, 25*, 31–50.

Hawkins, J. D., & Weis, J. G. (1985). The social development model: An integrated approach to delinquency prevention. *Journal of Primary Prevention, 6*, 73–97.

Infant Health and Development Program. (1990). Enhancing the outcomes of low-birthweight, premature infants: A multisite randomized trial. *Journal of the American Medical Association, 263*, 3035–3042.

Jason, L. A., Hess, R. E., Felner, R. D., & Moritsugu, J. (Eds.). (1987). Prevention: Toward a multidisciplinary approach. *Prevention in Human Services, 5*(2), 1–309.

Johnson, C. A., Pentz, M. A., Weber, M. D., Dwyer, J. H., Baer, N., MacKinnon, D. P., Hansen, W. B., & Flay, B. R. (1990). Relative effectiveness of comprehensive community programming for drug abuse prevention with high-risk and low-risk adolescents. *Journal of Consulting and Clinical Psychology, 58*, 447–456.

Johnson, D. L. (1988). Primary prevention of behavior problems in young children: The Houston Parent-Child Development Center. In R. H. Price, E. L. Cowen, R. P. Lorion, & J. Ramos-McKay (Eds.), *14 ounces of prevention: A casebook for practitioners* (pp. 44–52). Washington, DC: American Psychological Association.

Johnson, D. L., & Walker, T. (1987). Primary prevention of behavior problems in Mexican-American children. *American Journal of Community Psychology, 15*, 375–385.

Kazdin, A. E. (1991). *Prevention of conduct disorder* (Preliminary report of the National Conference on Prevention Research). Bethesda, MD: National Institute of Mental Health.

Kendall, P. C., & Braswell, L. (1985). *Cognitive-behavioral therapy for impulsive children.* New York: Guilford Press.

Lamb, H. R., & Zusman, J. (1982). The seductiveness of primary prevention. In F. D. Perlmutter (Ed.), *New directions for mental health services: Mental health promotion and primary prevention* (Vol. 13, pp. 19–30). San Francisco: Jossey-Bass.

Lazar, I., Darlington, R., Murray, H., Royce, J., & Snipper, A. (1982). *The lasting effects of early education: A report from the Consortium for Longitudinal Studies, 47*(2-3; Serial No. 195).

Lorion, R. P. (Ed.). (1989). Protecting the children: Strategies for optimizing emotional and behavioral development. *Prevention in Human Services, 7*, 1–275.

Marlowe, H. A., & Weinberg, R. B. (Eds.). (1985). Is mental illness preventable? Pros and cons. *Journal of Primary Prevention, 5*, 200–313.

Maughan, B. (1988). School experiences as risk/protective factors. In M. Rutter (Ed.), *Studies of psychosocial risk: The power of longitudinal data* (pp. 200–220). New York: Cambridge University Press.

McLaughlin, M. W. (1990). The Rand Change Agent Study revisited: Macro perspectives and micro realities. *Educational Researcher, 19*, 11–16.

Mueller, D. P., & Higgins, P. S. (1988). *Funders' guide manual: A guide to prevention programs in human services—Focus on children and adolescents.* St. Paul, MN: Amherst H. Wilder Foundation.

National Advisory Mental Health Council. (1990). *National plan for research on child and adolescent mental disorders.* Washington, DC: National Institute of Mental Health.

National Commission on the Role of the School and the Community in Improving Adolescent Health. (1990). *Code Blue: Uniting for healthier youth.* Alexandria, VA: National Association of State Boards of Education.

Olds, D. L. (1988). The Prenatal/Early Infancy Project. In R. H. Price, E. L. Cowen, R. P. Lorion, & J. Ramos-McKay (Eds.), *14 ounces of prevention: A casebook for practitioners* (pp. 9–23). Washington, DC: American Psychological Association.

Pedro-Carroll, J. P., & Cowen, E. L. (1985). The Children of Divorce Intervention Program: An investigation of the efficacy of a school-based prevention program. *Journal of Consulting and Clinical Psychology, 53*, 603–611.

Pentz, M. A., Dwyer, J. H., MacKinnon, D. P., Flay, B. R., Hansen, W. B., Wang, E. Y. I., & Johnson, C. A. (1989). A multi-community trial for primary prevention of adolescent drug abuse: Effects on drug use prevalence. *Journal of the American Medical Association, 261*, 3259–3266.

Perry, C. L., & Jessor, R. (1985). The concept of health promotion and the prevention of adolescent drug abuse. *Health Education Quarterly, 12*, 169–184.

Perry, C. L., Klepp, K., & Sillers, C. (1989). Community-wide strategies for cardiovascular health: The Minnesota Heart Health Program youth program. *Health Education Research, 4*, 87–101.

Pierson, D. E. (1988). The Brookline Early Education Project. In R. H. Price, E. L. Cowen, R. P. Lorion, & J. Ramos-McKay (Eds.), *14 ounces of prevention: A casebook for practitioners* (pp. 24–31). Washington, DC: American Psychological Association.

Price, R. H., Cowen, E. L., Lorion, R. P., & Ramos-McKay, J. (Eds.). (1988). *14 ounces of prevention: A casebook for practitioners.* Washington, DC: American Psychological Association.

Price, R. H., & Lorion, R. P. (1989). Prevention programming as organizational reinvention: From research to implementation. In D. Shaffer, I. Philips, & N. B. Enzer (Eds.),

Prevention of mental disorders, alcohol and other drug use in children and adolescents (pp. 97–124). Washington, DC: Office for Substance Abuse Prevention.

Provence, S., & Naylor, A. (1983). *Working with disadvantaged parents and children: Scientific issues and practice.* New Haven, CT: Yale University Press.

Raimy, C. V. (Ed.). (1950). *Training in clinical psychology.* Englewood Cliffs, NJ: Prentice-Hall.

Report of the National Mental Health Association Commission on the Prevention of Mental-Emotional Disabilities. (1986). *The prevention of mental-emotional disabilities.* Alexandria, VA: National Mental Health Association.

Report of the Task Force on Education of Young Adolescents. (1989). *Turning points: Preparing American youth for the 21st century.* Washington, DC: Carnegie Council on Adolescent Development.

Report of the Task Panel on Prevention. (1978). *Task panel reports submitted to the President's Commission on Mental Health* (Vol. 4, pp. 1822–1863). Washington, DC: U.S. Government Printing Office.

Rotheram-Borus, M. J. (1988). Assertiveness training with children. In R. H. Price, E. L. Cowen, R. P. Lorion, & J. Ramos-McKay (Eds.), *14 ounces of prevention: A casebook for practitioners* (pp. 83–97). Washington, DC: American Psychological Association.

Royce, J. M., Darlington, R. B., & Murray, H. W. (1983). Pooled analyses: Findings across studies. In Consortium for Longitudinal Studies (Ed.), *As the twig is bent: Lasting effects of preschool programs* (pp. 411–459). Hillsdale, NJ: Erlbaum.

Rutter, M. (1982). Prevention of children's psychosocial disorders: Myth and substance. *Pediatrics, 70,* 883–894.

Rutter, M. (1987). Psychosocial resilience and protective mechanisms. *American Journal of Orthopsychiatry, 57,* 316–331.

Rutter, M., Maughan, B., Mortimore, P., & Ouston, J. (1979). *Fifteen thousand hours: Secondary schools and their effects on children.* Cambridge, MA: Harvard University Press.

Sameroff, A. J. (1991). *Prevention of developmental psychopathology using the transactional model: Perspectives on host, risk agent, and environmental interactions* (Preliminary report of the National Conference on Prevention Research). Bethesda, MD: National Institute of Mental Health.

Sarason, S. B. (1981). An asocial psychology and a misdirected clinical psychology. *American Psychologist, 36,* 827–836.

Schorr, L. B. (1988). *Within our reach: Breaking the cycle of disadvantage.* New York: Anchor Press.

Schweinhart, L. J., & Weikart, D. P. (1988). The High/Scope Perry Preschool Program. In R. H. Price, E. L. Cowen, R. P. Lorion, & J. Ramos-McKay (Eds.), *14 ounces of prevention: A casebook for practitioners* (pp. 53–65). Washington, DC: American Psychological Association.

Schweinhart, L. J., & Weikart, D. P. (1989). The High/Scope Perry Preschool Study: Implications for early childhood care and education. *Prevention in Human Services, 7,* 109–132.

Seitz, V. (1991). Intervention programs for impoverished children: A comparison of educational and family support models. *Annals of Child Development, 7,* 73–103.

Seitz, V., Rosenbaum, L. K., & Apfel, N. H. (1985). Effects of family support intervention: A 10-year follow-up. *Child Development, 56,* 376–391.

Shaffer, D. (1989). Prevention of psychiatric disorders in children and adolescents: A summary of findings and recommendations from Project Prevention. In D. Shaffer, I. Philips, & N. B. Enzer (Eds.), *Prevention of mental disorders, alcohol and other drug use in children and adolescents* (pp. 443–456). Washington, DC: Office for Substance Abuse Prevention.

Shure, M. B., & Spivack, G. (1988). Interpersonal cognitive problem solving. In R. H. Price, E. L. Cowen, R. P. Lorion, & J. Ramos-McKay (Eds.), *14 ounces of prevention: A casebook for practitioners* (pp. 69–82). Washington, DC: American Psychological Association.

Slavin, R. E. (1983). *Cooperative learning.* New York: Longman.

Slavin, R. E., Madden, N. A., Karweit, N. L., Livermon, B. J., & Dolan, L. (1990). Success for all: First-year outcomes of a comprehensive plan for reforming urban education. *American Educational Research Journal, 27,* 255–278.

Tobler, N. S. (1986). Meta-analysis of 143 adolescent drug prevention programs: Quantitative outcome results of program participants compared to a control of comparison group. *Journal of Drug Issues, 16,* 537–567.

Tuma, J. M. (1989). Mental health services for children: The state of the art. *American Psychologist, 44,* 188–199.

U. S. Department of Health and Human Services, Public Health Service. (1990). *Healthy people 2000: National health promotion and disease prevention objectives.* Washington, DC: U.S. Government Printing Office.

U. S. Department of Health, Education, and Welfare. (1967). *The story of the White House Conference on Children and Youth.* Washington, DC: Author.

Walker, C. E., & Roberts, M. C. (Eds.). (1983). *Handbook of clinical child psychology.* New York: Wiley.

Weissberg, R. P. (1989, April). *A follow-up study of school-based social-competence promotion for young adolescents.* Symposium presentation at the Biennial Meeting for the Society for Research in Child Development, Kansas City, MO.

Weissberg, R. P. (1991). Comprehensive social-competence and health education (C-SCAHE): An urgently needed educational reform for the 1990s. *Child, Youth, and Family Services Quarterly, 14,* 10–12.

Weissberg, R. P., & Caplan, M. (1991). *Promoting social competence and preventing antisocial behavior in young urban adolescents.* Manuscript submitted for publication.

Weissberg, R. P., Caplan, M. Z., & Sivo, P. J. (1989). A new conceptual framework for establishing school-based social-competence promotion programs. In L. A. Bond & B. E. Compas (Eds.), *Primary prevention and promotion in the schools* (pp. 255–296). Newbury Park, CA: Sage.

Weissberg, R. P., Gesten, E. L., Carnrike, C. L., Toro, P. A., Rapkin, B. D., Davidson, E., & Cowen, E. L. (1981). Social problem-solving skills training: A competence building intervention with second- to fourth-grade children. *American Journal of Community Psychology, 9*, 411–423.

Zabin, L. S. (1990). Adolescent pregnancy and early sexual onset. In B. B. Lahey & A. E. Kazdin (Eds.), *Advances in clinical child psychology* (Vol. 13, pp. 247–281). New York: Plenum Press.

Zigler, E., & Berman, W. (1983). Discerning the future of early childhood intervention. *American Psychologist, 38*, 894–906.

Zigler, E., & Black, K. B. (1989). America's family support movement: Strengths and limitation. *American Journal of Orthopsychiatry, 59*, 6–19.

Zill, N., & Schoenborn, C. A. (1990). Developmental, learning, and emotional problems: Health of our nation's children, United States, 1988. *Advance data from vital and health statistics* (No. 190). Hyattsville, MD: National Center for Health Statistics.

Zins, J., & Forman, S. G. (1988). Mini-series on primary prevention: From theory to practice. *School Psychology Review, 17*(4), 539–634.

Part III

DEVELOPMENTAL DISORDERS

In the first paper in this section, Bregman and Hodapp provide an elegant summary of the impact of advances in medical technology on our understanding of the etiology, phenomenology, and psychopathology of mental retardation. The past decade has seen an increased appreciation of the importance of biomedical factors in the etiology of retardation, particularly mild retardation. Improvements in diagnostic precision rest not only on increasingly sophisticated genetic and neuroimaging techniques, but also on increased attention to the influence of perinatal risk factors.

Advances in human genetics have implications for more than the diagnosis and treatment of mental retardation and co-occurring psychiatric conditions. Initial studies of patterns of psychological functions and their developmental course in etiology homogeneous groups of retarded individuals have been encouraging in revealing specific profiles of strengths and weaknesses in a variety of areas and conditions. Nevertheless, in some single-gene disorders, including beta-thalasemia and Lesch-Nyhan syndrome, a variety of different genetic abnormalities among affected individuals including single-base substitutions, microdeletions, insertions, and duplications—have been found to result in clinical phenotypes that are essentially invariant. Conversely, an identical genetic abnormality, as among the hyperperphenylalanimemia syndromes, can result in essentially no clinical symptoms or in classic phenylketonuria. Clarification of the causes of genetic and phenotypic heterogeneity will be of importance to the further understanding of factors underlying normal and pathological cognitive, social, and adaptive development.

The next two papers in this section are concerned with the communicative and socioemotional functioning of autistic children. It is widely recognized that speaking autistic children have particular difficulty with the pragmatics of language—that is, the functional uses of language in a social context. Tager-Flusberg and Anderson's study examines the ways in which young autistic children are able to respond in a contingent or topically related way while engaged in conversation with their mothers. Four spontaneous language samples generated during play with mothers were obtained at four-month intervals for one year from six autistic and six Down's syndrome children, initially matched for chronological age and mean length of utterance. The language samples were analyzed in accordance with whether the child's verbalization directly followed the adult's communication—an adjacent response; whether the response was topically related—a contingent response; and whether the response did or did not add new information. The analyses of developmental trends are of particular interest. The conversational skills of autistic and Down's syndrome children whose mean length of utterance is between one and two words are very similar. However, significant differences between the groups emerge at later stages of language development. As mean length of utterance increases, children with Down's syndrome become better able to maintain an established topic of conversation and to contribute more novel and substantive material to the ongoing discussion. Autistic children show no such developmental changes. Increases in mean length of utterance are not accompanied by advances in discourse ability. The frequency of contingent responses does not increase, and autistic children do not begin to add new information to the topic of discourse. The failure of young autistic children to share information even though they have acquired the linguistic ability to do so may reflect early deficits in the development of a "theory of mind" as the authors suggest. In addition, the findings are illustrative of the complex relationship between delay and deviance in the development of autistic children.

The weight of recent research evidence supports that view that autistic persons have particular deficits in the processing of socioemotional information. Hobson's critical review of studies of autistic individuals' perception and understanding of emotion provides an excellent summary of this rapidly growing area of investigation. Sources of difficulty in the design and interpretation of experiments directed toward the exploration of emotionality in autism are thoroughly discussed. Particular attention is focused on the problems of devising control tasks and the selection of appropriate control groups. Awareness of differences regarding these issues assists in the reconciliation of discrepant findings. Hobson suggests that experimental studies are of greatest value in dissecting the patterns of association and dissociation among a cluster of autistic individuals' abilities and disabilities. However, the generalization of the results of experiments to naturalistic situations is limited and does not resolve whether demonstrated emotional deficits are a cause or a consequence of autistic children's impaired interpersonal relations.

The final paper in this section on developmental disorders summarizes currently available information on clinical manifestations, etiology, prevalence, pathogenesis, and treatment of the Rett syndrome. First described in 1966, Rett syndrome is reported to affect only females. The syndrome, characterized by a progressive loss of cognitive and motor skills and the development of stereotypic hand movements, is thought to afflict as many as 10,000 girls in the United States. However, fewer than 1200 have been identified thus far, which is most likely a consequence of a failure to differentiate the syndrome from other developmental disorders, specifically autism. The syndrome can be distinguished from other developmental disorders clinically, but its etiology thus far has excluded explanation, although a genetic basis is probable. Future investigation into the etiology and pathogenesis of Rett syndrome will also contribute to the further understanding of genotype/phenotype relations.

13

Current Developments in the Understanding of Mental Retardation Part I: Biological and Phenomenological Perspectives

Joel D. Bregman, M.D.

Emory University, Atlanta, Georgia

Robert M. Hodapp, Ph.D.

Yale University, New Haven, Connecticut

During the past decade, noteworthy advances have taken place within the field of mental retardation. The application of advanced biological techniques in such areas as molecular genetics and neuroimaging has substantially improved our ability to identify the biological factors that underlie the origin and pathogenesis of an increasing number of mental retardation syndromes. Refined genetic and psychosocial assessments have highlighted the impressive degree of heterogeneity that is present within and across many mental retardation syndromes, stimulating increasing interest and study. This, the first of a two-part review, will focus on recent developments in biological and phenomenological aspects of mental retardation.

During the past several decades, clinical and research endeavors in the field of mental retardation have spanned a broad range of topics. Areas of active interest have included biological and psychosocial aspects of origin and pathogenesis, the patterns and longitudinal course of social and cognitive development, educational and vocational training and remediation, and the assessment and treatment of emo-

Reprinted with permission from the *Journal of the American Academy of Child and Adolescent Psychiatry*, 1991, Vol. 30, No. 5, 707–719. Copyright ©1991 by the American Academy of Child and Adolescent Psychiatry. This research was supported in part by Yale Mental Health Clinical Research Center and National Institute of Mental Health grant 30929, and the John Merck Fund.

tional and behavioral disturbances, to name just a few. This paper will highlight the application of some current biological techniques and psychological approaches to the study of mentally retarded children and adults. In addition, several controversial viewpoints will be presented that challenge some time-honored notions and beliefs.

The first section of the paper will focus on selected biological issues, including etiological factors underlying mild cognitive impairment, neurodevelopmental outcome of very low birthweight preterm infants, noteworthy advances in human genetics, and the application of neuroimaging techniques. The second section of the paper will present two particularly important areas in psychological research: the differential functioning of specific etiological groups and the developmental approach to mental retardation. Several common themes that cut across these diverse areas of investigation and clinical care will be noted, including an appreciation for the significant degree of variability present within this population and the likelihood that developmental disorders of specific cause may be associated with specific phenotypic profiles. Several mental retardation syndromes, including Down syndrome (DS), fragile X syndrome, and Prader-Willi syndrome (PWS), have been the subject of particular study and will serve to illustrate the latter theme.

BIOLOGICAL TOPICS

Overview of Medical Risk Factors and Mild Cognitive Impairment

As medical technology becomes more and more sophisticated, an increasing proportion of mentally retarded children and adults are discovered to have a medical basis for their cognitive and adaptive impairments. Among individuals with mild cognitive impairments (representing three-fourths of the mentally retarded population), socioeconomic disadvantage traditionally has been regarded as the salient etiological factor. However, detailed assessments of many such children often reveal the influence of subtle, but nonetheless significant, biological factors, such as small chromosomal abnormalities, rare genetic syndromes, subclinical lead intoxication, nutritional deficiencies, and exposure to a host of adverse perinatal risks (including prematurity and low birth weight, maternal smoking, alcohol and drug ingestion, etc.). A surprisingly high frequency of biological abnormality has been reported among children with relatively mild intellectual impairments. Two recent studies examined epidemiologically representative samples of Swedish and British children with borderline intellectual functioning and mild mental retardation (Hagberg et al., 1981; Lamont and Dennis, 1988). A medical risk factor was judged to be responsible for the presence of intellectual impairment among 30% to 42% of the 295 children. The majority of the children in the British study experienced perinatal trauma, whereas approximately 20% demonstrated a genetic cause for their cognitive deficits (polygenic factors excluded). In an additional 37% of the cases, biological factors may have been contributory. Interestingly, for 39% of the children who had convincing evidence of a medical cause, both parents had received special education. If the search for a specific biological cause had been curtailed after obtaining the family history, the true contribution of medical factors would have been underestimated.

Prematurity and Low Birth Weight

In future years, the contribution of perinatal risk factors may become more important as the increasing sophistication of medical technology improves the survival of very premature, low birth-weight infants without entirely eliminating neurological sequelae. Ongoing longitudinal studies assessing the neurodevelopmental functioning of such children have been focusing on the identifying medical and psychosocial factors that are predictive of future disability. Findings should improve the accuracy of prognostic judgments and help to identify the most appropriate types of early developmental intervention.

In conducting studies of this nature, it is important to establish the predictive validity of developmental assessments administered during the first months of life. Several investigators have reported strong associations between early neurodevelopmental functioning and later neurological integrity and intellectual ability among both developmentally impaired and nonimpaired infants and children. Scores on neurodevelopmental assessments performed on more than 300 premature infants between 9 and 12 months of age accurately predicted general neurological and intellectual outcome at 4 to 7 years of age in more than 85% of cases (Largo et al., 1990; Ross et al., 1986; Stewart et al., 1989; Williams et al., 1987). Predictions were particularly accurate for children who developed major neurodevelopmental impairment and those who maintained a normal level of functioning. It remains unclear whether subtle deficits in later childhood can be predicted with this degree of accuracy. The strength of the association between testing periods was unaffected by the type of population (term and preterm infants, those later identified as mentally retarded) or by the choice of assessment instrument used either initially or at follow-up (e.g., Griffiths, Bayley, and McCarthy developmental scales, Stanford-Binet, WISC-R, etc.).

Several investigators have studied the differential outcome of infants manifesting varying degrees of neurological risk. Gestational age and birth weight have been significantly correlated with neurological and intellectual outcome during the school-age years (Largo et al., 1989; Mazer et al., 1988). In addition, the effects of neurological insults (e.g., intracranial hemorrhage, integrity of cerebral blood flow) sustained by preterm infants on later neurodevelopmental functioning have been studied by a number of investigators. A particularly reliable prognostic sign is the ultrasound documentation of intracranial hemorrhage during the early neonatal period. Preterm infants who sustain intracranial hemorrhage manifest inferior neuromotor and cognitive functioning at 2 to 5 years of age when compared with preterm infants who escape this neurological complication (Bozynski et al., 1984; Williams et al., 1987). This appears to be particularly true for infants who manifest signs of abnormality (e.g., ventriculomegaly, periventricular abnormalities) that persist beyond term gestational age. An association between the severity of the hemorrhage and the degree of later neurodevelopmental impairment has been reported. For example, of 221 preterm, low birth-weight infants evaluated by Szymonowicz et al. (1986) and De La Costello et al. (1988), less than 5% of those with normal neonatal ultrasounds exhibited serious neurodevelopmental disability at 2- and 4-year follow-up. This contrasts with more than 70% of those with signs of significant abnormality on neonatal ultrasound (e.g., intracerebral hemorrhage, periventricular leukomalacia, hydrocephalus). Between one-fourth and one-third of neonates with intermediate degrees of abnormality on ultrasound went on to develop developmental difficulties. The integrity of cerebral blood flow (CBF) has also been identified as a potential early prognostic sign of developmental outcome. Preterm infants who manifest increased CBF (perhaps reflecting increased vascular compliance secondary to ischemia) are more likely to exhibit later neurodevelopmental abnormality than are those who manifest normal CBF (Van Bel et al., 1989).

The influence of socioeconomic status on the development of preterm infants has also received preliminary study. Positive correlations between variables reflecting socioeconomic disadvantage and measures of cognitive, language, and perceptual functioning during childhood have been reported, primarily among preterm infants with fewer and less severe medical and neurological risk factors (Cohen et al., 1986; Largo et al., 1989, 1990). These findings indicate that a wide range of factors influence the outcome of at-risk premature infants and lend strong support for the involvement of preterm infants and their families in intensive early intervention programs.

Human Genetics

Genetic abnormalities may be responsible for the developmental delays manifested by more than one-fourth of children and adolescents referred for evaluation (Fryns, 1987). In most surveys, DS and fragile X syndrome account for as many as one-third of the identified genetic cases. The mechanism(s) by which genetic abnormalities cause mental retardation remains unclear. Absent genetic material (e.g., chromosomal deletions) may fail to supply a gene product necessary for normal morphogenesis, whereas additional genetic material (e.g., chromosomal trisomies) may result in the overproduction of a gene product that interferes with development. In general, the greater the amount of missing or additional genetic material, the more serious the outcome. However, there also are circumstances (e.g., deletions of chromosome 4) in which a small deletion may produce a greater degree of mental retardation than a larger one (Baraitser, 1986). The proportion of cells containing a chromosomal abnormality (mosaicism) is also correlated with the degree of intellectual impairment, but here again, the association is not absolute. Current investigations have been focusing on the necessity of having inherited a complete set of genetic material from each parent (genomic imprinting). Our understanding of the genetic mechanisms that underlie mental retardation are decidedly rudimentary and will undoubtedly expand as research continues.

During the past 15 years, major strides have been made in the field of human genetics. For well over 75 heredity disorders, the responsible (mutant) genes have been located and cloned, and for at least one-half of this number, closely-linked deoxyribonucleic acid (DNA) markers have been identified (Antonarakis, 1989). Advances in genetic diagnosis, carrier detection, and prenatal counseling have stemmed largely from the development of three particular procedures, high-resolution banding techniques, specialized culture media procedures, and recombinant DNA.

Cytogenetic banding techniques. During recent years, karyotyping techniques have become increasingly sophisticated. Procedures using cells arrested at the prometaphase stage of cell division now allow for the identification of approximately 1,000 separate chromosomal bands. This level of resolution, which involves several dozen to several hundred genes, has made it possible to link more than 120 clinically recognizable mental retardation syndromes with specific genetic lesions (typically, very small partial deletions, duplications, and translocations) (Fryns, 1987). As molecular genetic techniques become applicable to increasingly larger portions of the genome, microdeletion syndromes are likely to be identified with greater frequency.

Culture media techniques. Another cytogenetic advance involves the use of specialized culture media for a detection of certain types of chromosomal lesions, particularly fragile sites. Fragile sites are short segments of a chromosome that have a tendency to break when exposed to culture media deficient in specific nutrients. The breaks occur at specific and predictable locations within a given individual and family and usually follow Mendelian patterns of transmission. One group of fragile sites, the so-called folate sensitive fragile sites are of particular importance. These sites become visible when the cells are grown in folate-deficient culture media. The site affecting the long arm of the X chromosome, fragile Xq27.3, is the only fragile site that has been associated with a clinical syndrome (fragile X syndrome). The molecular genetic lesion that underlies the syndrome remains unknown. One hypothesis holds that specific regions of DNA may be particularly sensitive to normal fluctuations in the available pool of thymidine or deoxycytidine, resulting in abnormal chromosomal condensation.

Molecular genetic techniques. During the past 10 years, molecular genetic procedures have developed at a rapid pace. This has allowed for the expansion of numerous genetic disorders, including the single gene defects that underlie inborn errors of amino acid metabolism, endocrine disorders, and lysosomal storage diseases (many of which are associated with mental retardation) (Antonarakis, 1989). The accuracy of carrier detection and prenatal diagnosis has been improved substantially by the use of molecular genetic procedures.

Two major types of molecular lesions or mutations can be detected by recombinant DNA techniques: gross abnormalities (deletions, insertions, rearrangements) and abnormalities of one to several contiguous nucleotides (point mutations). For situations in which the precise mutation or gene is unknown but the locus and mode of inheritance are, indirect detection through the use of linkage analysis can be fruitful. This involves the use of either known markers or restriction fragment length polymorphisms (RFLPs). The development of RFLP procedures has been particularly significant, because they exploit the natural variability present in the DNA base sequence. There are about 10^7 clinically silent variations in each individual's DNA. These nonpathological DNA polymorphisms are present in more than 1% of the population and are transmitted in Mendelian fashion to succeeding generations. RFLPs can be exploited diagnostically when they are closely linked to the disease locus of interest and can be tracked differentially through maternal and paternal sides of the family. It then may be possible to determine the likelihood that a particular family member has inherited the disease locus. This procedure may be followed for carrier detection and prenatal diagnosis.

The three methodologies described above are often used together to increase the sensitivity of genetic diagnosis. They have been of particular importance in the identification of microdeletions and fragile sites that underlie a number of well-recognized clinical syndromes (Table 1).

Genotypic and phenotypic heterogeneity. As knowledge about genetic disorders increases, the degree of genetic and phenotypic heterogeneity associated with these syndromes becomes more apparent. This holds true for chromosomal abnormalities and single gene defects, alike. The clinical breadth and severity of a circumscribed, well-defined genetic abnormality may vary widely across affected individuals. Furthermore, clinically distinct syndromes can result from apparently identical genetic lesions (e.g., PWS and Angelman syndromes [AS]).

Insights regarding genetic heterogeneity at the molecular level have resulted from extensive study of several well-characterized single gene disorders, including beta-thalassemia and Lesch-Nyhan syndrome. Both of these disorders have been associated with a variety of different genetic abnormalities among affected individuals, including single-base substitutions, microdeletions, insertions, and duplications identified through the use of recombinant DNA techniques. Despite this impressive degree of genetic heterogeneity, the clinical phenotypes remain essentially invariant (Avery and First, 1989; Yang et al., 1984). The converse of this also occurs; a sin-

TABLE 1.
Clinical Syndromes Associated with Chromosomal Deletions and Fragile Sites

Syndrome	Chromosome	Abnormality	Reference
Prader-Willi	15q11-q13	Deletion	Butler, 1990
			Magenis et al., 1990
Angelman	15q11-q13	Deletion	Magenis et al., 1990
			Williams et al., 1990
DiGeorge	22q11	Deletion	Schinzel, 1988
			Fryns, 1987
Wilm's tumor, aniridia, gonadoblastoma	11p13	Deletion	Schinzel, 1988
			Fryns, 1987
Fragile X	Xq27	Fragile site	Webb et al., 1986

gular genetic abnormality can result in phenotypic heterogeneity. For example, among the hyperphenylalaninemia syndromes, an apparently identical genetic abnormality can result in essentially no clinical symptoms or in classic phenylketonuria.

Several other disorders have received particular attention during recent years because they have contributed substantially to our understanding of the factors that mediate genetic expression. One such condition, PWS, was first described in 1956 and includes a variable phenotypic profile involving hypotonia and feeding difficulties in infancy, short stature, genital abnormalities in males, delayed onset of puberty, varying degrees of intellectual impairment, and compulsive food-seeking behavior and obesity. High-resolution banding and molecular genetic techniques have revealed a microdeletion of the chromosome 15q11/12 site among up to 80% of the 450 PWS patients studied thus far (Butler, 1990; Fryns, 1987; Schinzel, 1988). AS, a phenotypically distinct disorder first described in 1965, includes severe mental retardation, aphasia, a stiff and jerky gait, seizures, and paroxysms of laughter. Interestingly, approximately 60% of the AS cases studied to date have demonstrated a microdeletion at the same site of chromosome 15 as that found in PWS (Imaizumi et al., 1990; Magenis et al., 1990). For both PWS and AS, the great majority of cases have been sporadic; reoccurrence among siblings has been noted in less than 4% of cases. Microdeletions have been found among sporadic but not among familial cases. Recent studies have indicated that in virtually all sporadic cases studied to date, the deleted chromosome in PWS patients has been of paternal origin, whereas that in AS patients has been of maternal origin. Furthermore, Nicholls et al. (1989) have described six sporadic cases (two confirmed) of deletion negative PWS in which the probands inherited two different cytogenetically normal chromosome 15s from their mother (maternal heterodisomy). It was hypothesized that the absence of a paternal contribution of genes from this chromosomal region led to the PWS phenotype rather than a mutation of specific genes. This unifying explanation of the genetic basis of both deletion positive and deletion negative cases of PWS and AS has been described as the phenomenon of genomic imprinting and will be discussed below.

Fragile X syndrome, an X-linked disorder with a prevalence of approximately 1 per 1,000 male subjects (Webb et al., 1986) ranks second to DS as the most common genetic cause of mental retardation. Clinical features include subtle facial dysmorphism, macroorchidism, cognitive and language impairment, and a high rate of psychopathology—principally attention deficit hyperactivity disorders and pervasive developmental disorders. The significant degree of genetic and phenotypic variability associated with fragile X syndrome serves as a model for many other genetic disorders. Even with the use of techniques that enhance cytogenetic expression (e.g., the addition of methotrexate or 5-fluorodeoxyuridine to the tissue culture media), the fragile X site is visible in only a small proportion of the X chromosomes (often less than 10%). This is particularly true for phenotypically normal male and female carriers, in the majority of whom cytogenetic evidence of the fragile X site is absent entirely. Even among those with the highest rates of expression (usually severely affected male individuals), fewer than one-half of the cells reveal the fragile site. Molecular genetic techniques using RFLPs are now being used successfully in some pedigrees, thereby enhancing carrier detection and prenatal diagnosis (Murphy et al., 1986).

Fragile X syndrome is also associated with a significant degree of phenotypic variability involving a range of physical, cognitive, linguistic, and behavioral features. Approximately 20% of male subjects and 75% of heterozygous female subjects exhibit no discernible clinical features of the syndrome yet remain capable of transmitting the genetic abnormality to their children (Webb et al., 1981). In addition, it has been observed that the siblings, daughters, and grandsons of nonpenetrant transmitting male subjects are less likely to be affected than are corresponding family members of affected male subjects.

Investigators have sought explanations for the genetic and phenotypic variability associated with the disorders described above. There has been an active search for the factors that determine the phenotypic expression of a chromosome 15q11-q13 microdeletion (PWS vs. AS) and those that influence the penetrance and expressivity of fragile X syndrome. A number of possible explanations have been offered, including the differences in the combinations of abnormal recessive alleles at separate but closely linked loci (Imaizumi et al., 1990) or in the expression of unmasked genes on nondeleted chromosomes as a result of differences in gene order along the chromosome (Williams et al., 1990). The most likely explanation, however, involves genomic imprinting, the differential modification of parental chromosomes during gametogenesis such that gene function is altered (Magenis et al., 1990; Nicholls et al., 1989; Williams et al., 1990). In several animal models (for example, the mouse), the inheritance of haploid gametes from both parents is essential for normal development. Some alleles, in fact, are lethal if both copies are inherited from only one parent. It has been hypothesized that imprinting reflects the degree to which segments of DNA are methylated during gametogenesis (a gender specific process). Methylation serves to regulate the transcriptional process, and when critical regulatory genes are affected, significant modifications in phenotypic expression might result. In the case of PWS and AS, the lack of paternally or maternally derived alleles of chromosome 15 may result in a missing gene product or a failure to offset a deleterious gene product normally produced by the missing chromosome. In the case of fragile X syndrome, it has been suggested that a permutation may be inherited by nonpenetrant male subjects (Pembrey et al., 1986). The permutation, itself, is of no clinical significance. However, once the affected X chromosome is transmitted to a daughter and undergoes X inactivation and subsequent reactivation (Lyon hypothesis), the permutation may permanently inhibit reactivation of the segment of DNA that surrounds it. This *imprinted*, nonfunctional DNA segment may then be responsible for producing the fragile X phenotype. Several other genetic disorders are thought to be affected by genomic imprinting, because their onset and severity are known to be influenced by the gender of the transmitting parent (Table 2). In fact, imprinting may be responsible for the patterns of penetrance and expressivity observed in a large number of disorders, including neuropsychiatric disorders, such as bipolar disorder.

Down syndrome and dementia. Fresh insights regarding how genetic mechanisms may underlie cognitive impairment have been generated by research exploring the relationship between DS and dementia of the Alzheimer's type (AD). Since the late 17th century, it has been observed that the cognitive and adaptive functioning of many DS individuals deteriorates during middle age, suggestive of an early onset form of dementia. Although most available research has documented definitive signs of dementia in only about one-half of middle-aged individuals with DS (Cutler et al., 1985; Karlinsky, 1986; Schellenberg et al., 1989), careful longitudinal studies suggest that the development of dementia may be universal within the DS population (Evenhuis, 1990). During the past 60 years, numerous studies have documented the presence of Alzheimer's-like neuropathological abnormalities at autopsy (e.g., senile plaques (SP) and neurofibrillary tangles (NT)) in essentially all DS individuals older than 40 years of age who, thus far, have been examined (Karlinsky, 1986; Mann, 1988; Wisniewski et al., 1985). There are many clinical and neuropathological similarities between middle-aged DS individuals and those with AD, including an increased prevalence of dementia with advancing age, a relatively selective accumulation of SPs and NTs in the cerebral cortex and limbic system, a significant correlation between the degree of clinical and neuropathological changes, a reduction in central cholinergic and noradrenergic activity, and the extracellular deposition of beta-amyloid protein (BAP) within SPs. These findings have caused some investigators to propose that similar genetic mechanisms may underlie the dementing process that affects both DS and AD. There is some evidence in support of this proposal. Some studies have found an increased incidence of DS within the families of AD probands, especially those with an early age of onset (< 60 years). The early onset form of AD tends to be familial (FAD), the latter representing as many as one-third of AD cases (Cutler et al., 1985; Karlinsky, 1986). Preliminary studies have reported linkage between dementia and the q11.2-21 region of chromosome 21 in some families with FAD (Schellenberg et al., 1989; Van Camp et al., 1989). This locus is relatively close to, but not identical with, the region critical for the development of the DS phenotype (21q22) (Klunk and Abraham, 1988) and to the regions coding for BAP and for superoxide dismutase (SOD-1, an enzyme that scavenges superoxide radicals and hydrogen peroxide). These hypothetical linkages are intriguing, nonetheless. Early reports suggest that individuals with DS have 1.5 times the level of precursor BAP in serum and 2 times

TABLE 2.
Genetic Disorders Thought to Be Affected by Genomic Imprinting

Syndrome	Chromosome	Clinical Finding	Parental Origin
Huntington's Chorea[a, c]	4	Earlier, more severe	Paternal onset
Wilm's tumor[a, c]	11	Greater prevalence	Maternal
Prader-Willi[a, c]	15	Presence of syndrome	Paternal
Angelman[a, c]	15	Presence of syndrome	Maternal
Myotonic dystrophy[c]	19	More severe	Maternal
Neurofibromatosis type I[b]	17	Greater severity	Maternal
Fragile X[c]	X	Increased penetrance and expressivity	Maternal

[a] Nicholls et al. (1989).
[b] Rodenhiser et al. (1989).
[c] Williams et al. (1990).

TABLE 3.
Neurological Disorders Identifiable by Neuroimaging Techniques

Congenital malformations (e.g., agenesis of the corpus callosum)
Congenital infections (e.g., toxoplasmosis, cytomegalovirus)
Inherited metabolic disorders (e.g., leukodystrophies—Krabbe's syndrome)
Hydrocephalus
Brain stem lesions (e.g., Arnold Chiari malformation)
Intracranial vascular abnormalities (e.g., hemorrhage, thrombosis)
Intracranial tumors

[a] Based on information from Roach et al. (1987).

that in brain tissue as compared with AD patients and normal controls, perhaps reflecting the extra complement of chromosome 21 (Rumble et al., 1989). In addition, there also appears to be an elevation in red blood cell SOD-1, which may lead to an imbalance in antioxidant defense mechanisms and an increase in potentially toxic oxygen radicals (Percy et al., 1990).

These findings have generated a number of hypotheses regarding the relationship among DS, AD, and cognitive impairment. For example, the clinical and neuropathological changes of DS and AD might result from genetically mediated defects in the microtubular structures of the cell, thereby predisposing to chromosomal instability and non-disjunction. If this were to affect the regulatory genes involving SOD-1, the accumulation of potentially toxic metabolites might result (Cutler et al., 1985; Karlinsky, 1986; Klunk and Abraham, 1988).

Neuroimaging. During the past 15 years, major advances have been made in the identification of abnormalities in central nervous system (CNS) structure and function through the development of neuroimaging modalities, such as computed tomography (CT), magnetic resonance imaging (MRI), and positron emission tomography (PET). These techniques offer the potential of enhancing our understanding of the pathogenic mechanisms that underlie the cognitive and adaptive impairments manifested by individuals with developmental disorders.

Neuroimaging has been instrumental in delineating the CNS manifestations of a variety of neurological disorders (Table 3), many of which are associated with mental retardation. With its high degree of resolution and superior visualization of white matter, MRI has been of particular benefit in the diagnosis of congenital malformations and infections. CT and MRI have also been most important in the diagnosis and follow-up of children and adults with neurocutaneous syndromes, such as neurofibromatosis, tuberous sclerosis, and Sturge-Weber syndrome (Braffman et al., 1988). Severe learning disorders (including mental retardation) are often associated with these syndromes. The neurocutaneous disorders are accompanied by a variety of NS abnormalities, including neoplasms (e.g., neurofibromas, malignancies), abnormal proliferations of indigenous tissue (e.g., hamartomas), hydrocephalus, and vascular lesions (e.g., hemangioblastomas). Diagnosis and prognosis are often dependent on the careful identification of these CNS abnormalities through neuroimaging. In addition, periodic reimaging can be lifesaving in many cases, because successful treatment of critically located lesions often depends on early detection.

CT and MR imaging techniques have also been applied to the study of mildly retarded and nonretarded autistic individuals. Although some studies have reported normal findings (Creasey et al.,1986; Garber et al., 1989; Rumsey et al., 1988), others have uncovered noteworthy abnormalities, including enlarged ventricles, small caudate nuclei, altered cerebral and ventricular asymmetries, and hypoplasia of the cerebellar vermis (e.g., Campbell et al., 1982; Courchesne et al., 1988; Gaffney et al., 1989; Jacobson et al., 1988). It has been hypothesized that abnormalities in these and associated regions may result from a neuropathological process operative during the first months of gestation (e.g., aberrant neuronal migration) (Courchesne et al., 1988). Confirmation of this hypothesis awaits further research.

Functional assessments, such as PET, are becoming increasingly employed in research investigations. For example, PET has been used to identify seizure foci among developmentally impaired infants and children, to determine cerebral metabolic rates and blood flow in preterm infants with intraventricular and intracerebral hemorrhages, and to localize neurological deficits in language and motor functions (e.g., aphasia, apraxia) (Chugani et al., 1989; Cutler, 1986).

Another area of increasing interest has been the study of individuals with developmental disorders. PET scanning has been performed on samples of children with mental retardation. As a group, these children exhibit *reduced* cerebral metabolic rates for glucose (CMRglc), the magnitude of which correlates with the degree of mental retardation (Chugani et al., 1987). Individuals with particular developmental syndromes also have been studied, including those with DS. Compared with control subjects, young adults with DS exhibit hypermetabolism, whereas older DS individuals exhibit hypometabolism, particularly within the parietal and temporal lobes, similar to that observed in AD (Cutler, 1986; Schapiro et al., 1988). Preliminary evidence suggests that reductions in CMRglc precede the development of clinically significant deteriorations in neuropsychological functioning. Normal subjects maintain an invariant pattern of CMRglc across a wide age range, spanning 21 to 83 years (Cutler, 1986; Schapiro et al., 1988).

Hypermetabolism has also been observed in association with other developmental conditions. In children with Sturge-Weber syndrome, hypermetabolism occurs within the affected hemisphere very early in life, followed by hypometabolism as the disease progresses (Chugani et al., 1989). It has been hypothesized that hypermetabolism early in the course of these developmental syndromes may result from abnormal, redundant circuitry or alterations in cellular metabolic processes.

Preliminary evidence suggests that autistic adults also may manifest a general increase in CMRglc as well as a reduction in the functional association typically observed between different brain regions, including the frontal and parietal lobes (Horwitz et al., 1988; De Volder et al., 1987; Rumsey et al., 1985). These reduced associations may reflect abnormalities in directed attention and sensorimotor functioning often observed in autism.

Thus, imaging techniques offer the potential of revealing differential patterns of structural and functional abnormality present among developmental disorders of varying cause.

PHENOMENOLOGY

In recent years, psychological research in mental retardation has explored two new directions. The first extends knowledge about the psychological functioning of different etiological groups, and the second elaborates and expands the so-called developmental approach to mental retardation.

Individual Etiological Groups

Traditional research approaches involving mentally retarded individuals separate groups on the basis of the degree rather than the cause of the impairment. For example, typical contrasts might involve mildly versus severely retarded children or retarded versus nonretarded children of either the same mental or chronological age. However, the body of literature that compares the functioning of individuals with mental retardation of different causes has been expanding. DS and fragile X syndrome have attracted particular interest. For these and several other causes of mental retardation, we are rapidly approaching specific profiles of strengths and weaknesses in a variety of areas.

Down Syndrome. DS, the most extensively studied mental retardation syndrome, has been associated with specific patterns of language, cognitive, and social development (Cicchetti and Beeghly, 1990).

Language. There is general agreement that language functioning represents a relative developmental weakness for children with DS. Recent work indicates, however, that only certain aspects of language development are deficient. Grammar has been identified as an area of particular weakness, and pragmatics (social usage) as an area of particular strength. Indeed, when matched on overall grammatical ability, DS children out perform nonretarded children on pragmatic tasks involving topic maintenance and turn taking during conversation (Leifer and Lewis, 1984).

Social skills. The social skills of DS children appear to be highly developed (consistent with findings for language pragmatism). The social quotients of these children surpass their intelligence quotients between the age range of 4 and 17 years

(Cornwell and Birch, 1969). However, there may be a limit to this relative strength in social skills, because *most* higher-level social and adaptive behaviors require linguistic sophistication. Recent findings based on the Vineland Adaptive Behavior Scales indicate particular strengths in socialization (e.g., interpersonal cooperation, respect for social rules and convention) relative to functioning in the area of daily living skills (e.g., personal care, domestic tasks, and community responsibilities) (Sparrow, 1989, pers. commun.).

Affect. Most studies have found that DS children exhibit a muted affect in comparison with nonretarded children of the same mental age. For example, DS infants smile in response to stimuli that evoke laughter in nonretarded infants, and whimper in response to stimuli that evoke crying in their counterparts (Cicchetti and Sroufe, 1976). This muted affect may be related to the hypotonicity frequently manifested by these children. Interestingly, the degree of hypotonicity has been correlated with the degree of impairment in cognitive and adaptive functioning (Cicchetti and Sroufe, 1976; Cullen et al., 1981).

Attention. DS children seem to have particular difficulty in regulating their gaze to gather information. During play, they are more likely to focus on a single stimulus than to visually scan the environment (Krakow and Kopp, 1982). In addition, although they often look toward their mothers, they rarely make eye contact for the purpose of communicating interest in a shared event (so-called "referential eye contact") (Jones, 1980). Deficiencies in scanning and referential eye contact lessen the richness of both social and nonsocial environmental contacts and reduce the ability of these children to extract information from the environment (Kopp, 1983).

Rates of development. The rate of intellectual development manifested by children with DS appears to decrease over time. Although some researchers question this finding, most studies reveal a progressive decline in IQ scores during various developmental epochs (e.g., infancy, the period of language acquisition, and the preschool and school-age years) (Dunst, 1988; Fowler, 1984; Morgan, 1979; Reed et al., 1980). Hypotheses for this developmental phenomenon are discussed below.

Fragile X Syndrome

Psychological research involving children (especially male) with fragile-X syndrome has been growing at a rapid pace (Dykens and Leckman, 1990).

Cognitive functioning. Studies have found that fragile X children experience relative strengths in simultaneous (gestalt) processing and relative weaknesses in sequential (bit-by-bit) processing (Dykens et al., 1987a; Kemper et al., 1988). In addition, with the exception of mathematics, performance on achievement tests (particularly vocabulary) has been strong. Interestingly, children with DS do not appear to manifest this pattern of higher simultaneous and lower sequential processing (Pueschel et al., 1987).

Language. Deficits in language functioning have been described among male subjects with fragile X syndrome, including rapid, perserverative speech patterns. Recent work suggests that many of these linguistic problems may be secondary to deficits in sequential processing. For example, deficiencies have been found in grammar but not in vocabulary (Marans et al., 1989). Sequential deficits also appear in the speech patterns of fragile X subjects. Abnormalities occur in the articulation of word strings, phrases, sentences, and repetitive syllables (Marans et al., 1987) but not in the articulation of single words (Klasner and Hagerman, 1987).

Adaptive behavior. In contrast with DS individuals, those with fragile X syndrome exhibit strengths in daily living skills relative to functioning in communication and socialization domains (Dykens et al., 1987b, 1989a; Wolf et al., 1987). Within the daily living sphere, personal skills (e.g., toileting, grooming) and domestic skills (e.g., cooking, cleaning) are more highly developed than community skills (e.g., money management, telephone use).

Rates of development. The rate of intellectual development of fragile X syndrome male subjects declines over time (Hagerman et al., in press; Lachiewicz et al., 1987). However, the pattern of this decline differs from that exhibited by children with DS. Among the majority of fragile X male subjects, decrements in IQ are most noticeable during the pubertal years, particularly between the ages of 10 and 15 (Dykens et al., 1989b). The specific mechanism responsible for this finding has not yet been identified, however. Small decrements in IQ also appear to occur during the school-age years, especially among boys with higher initial IQs (Hodapp et al., 1990).

These findings suggest that mental retardation syndromes of differing origin may be associated with distinct profiles of cognitive, linguistic, and adaptive functioning as well as with unique patterns of intellectual development. The few studies that have directly compared different etiological groups support this concept of syndrome-specific functioning. The language characteristics of children with fragile X syndrome, DS, and autism have been differentiated. Wolf-Schein et al. (1987) found that fragile X subjects exhibit more jargon, perseveration, echolalia, and inappropriate and tangential language than DS subjects. Ferrier (1987) reported that eliciting utterances and partial self-repetitions was most characteristic of fragile X subjects, dysfluent speech was most characteristic of DS subjects, and multiple inappropriate utterances most characteristic of autistic subjects. Marans et al. (1989) described strengths in vocabulary and weaknesses in grammar among both fragile X and DS subjects, although the differences were more striking for the former group. Similar differences between DS and fragile X syndrome children may also be present in tests of intellectual abilities (Leckman et al., 1989).

Based on this etiologically specific approach, individuals with nonspecific forms of mental retardation (those who form the lower tail of the normal distribution of intelligence) should exhibit a relatively even pattern of cognitive performance (similar to that of nonretarded children of the same mental age). At present, the functioning of children with nonspecific mental retardation on Piagetian tasks supports the hypothesis; performance is similar to that of mental age-matched nonretarded children (Weisz et al., 1982). However, the functioning of this group on tasks of information processing tends to negate the hypothesis. Approximately half of the studies reveal that children with nonspecific mental retardation perform more poorly than mental age-matched peers on tasks of selective attention, concept usage, discrimination, and incidental learning (Weiss et al., 1986). The mentally retarded children manifest either a specific cognitive deficit in information processing above and beyond their slower rate of development (Mundy and Kasari, 1990) or a task-specific decrement in motivation (Weisz, 1990).

Several methodological difficulties affect comparative research involving different etiological populations. One involves the ability to identify subjects with truly nonspecific forms of mental retardation. At present, this is primarily a process of exclusion and is limited by the sensitivity of current diagnostic techniques to identify specific etiological groups. Another obstacle is the reality that the prevalence of many mental retardation syndromes is low, making it difficult to attain sufficiently large subject groups. In fact, some etiologies have different subgroups that may differ among themselves (e.g., trisomy 21, mosaicism, and translocation types of DS). Finally, there often are vast differences in levels of functioning among individuals with identical disorders. Despite these difficulties, there do appear to be profiles of ability that are specific to different etiological groups (Burack et al., 1988, 1990).

Developmental Approach to Mental Retardation

The developmental approach to mental retardation was originally proposed in the late 1960s (Zigler, 1969). It posits that although retarded children manifest a slower rate and lower final level of development, their overall pattern of cognitive growth remains similar to that of nonretarded children. In particular, mentally retarded children are hypothesized to follow universal sequences of development (the similar sequence hypothesis) and to perform identically with nonretarded children of the same mental age on cognitive-linguistic tasks (the similar structure hypothesis). Although these hypotheses were originally restricted to nonorganic causes of retardation, they have recently been expanded to include a variety of different etiological groups (Hodapp et al., 1990a).

The field of developmental psychology has expanded to include the study of the unfolding interaction between the child and the social environment. Such study has found expression in the transactional model of development, mother-child interaction, and family systems theory. Application to work with retarded children and their families has also begun and will be discussed later.

Sequences and rates of development. With a renewed interest in the contexts of development, many developmental psychologists have begun questioning the notion of universal, invariant sequences of development (Bronfenbrenner et al., 1986). In general, the sequential nature of development seems to be related to the type of development studied and to the period in childhood during which it occurs. Processes considered to be more biologically mediated (e.g., motor functioning, cognition) tend to begin early in life and to follow a sequential pattern of development (McCall, 1981; Scarr-Salapatek, 1975). Social, cultural, and moral behaviors, on the other hand, appear to be influenced by environmental determinants to a greater extent than are processes such as cognition (Miller, 1986). The development of mentally retarded children is consistent with these findings. During infancy, for example, children with retardation of diverse origin follow universal stages of sequential cognitive development (Cicchetti and Mans-Wagener, 1987; Dunst, in press). Patterns of social development, however, may depend more heavily on the characteristics of specific etiologically related groups. For example, whereas normally developing children begin to express object-related needs and social functions (e.g., greetings) at the same point in development, autistic children express object-related needs first and social functions at a much later point, if at all (Wetherby, 1986).

Similarly, rates of developmental growth appear to vary among mentally retarded children from different etiological groups. For instance, children with DS exhibit a progressive decrease in their rate of development beginning in infancy. McCall et al. (1977) have identified 2, 8, 13, and 21 months as the ages during infancy at which the nature of intelligence changes qualitatively. At each of these points, DS children encounter difficulty in comprehending new cognitive tasks and appear to lose developmental ground (Dunst, 1988; in press; Kopp and McCall, 1982). In contrast, most boys with fragile X syndrome exhibit little change in their developmental rate until the time of puberty. Between the ages of 10 and 15, they too, begin to experience a slowing in their rate of intellectual growth (Dykens et al., 1989b; Hodapp et al., 1990b).

Cross-domain relationships. Influenced by Piagetian theory, researchers in the 1960s and early 1970s believed that children perform equally on all domains within a given level of cognitive development. Recent work, however, has revealed performance discrepancies across domains among some children, thereby casting doubt on the concept of cross-domain homogeneity. Despite this, there do appear to be several cross-domain relationships that hold for nonretarded and several retarded populations. These relationships involve areas of functioning that share a similar underlying structure and have been termed "local homologies of shared origin" (Bates et al., 1979; Mundy et al., 1982). For example, McCune-Nicholich and Bruskin (1982) have found that symbolic play and early language develop in tandem for nonretarded children. Prelinguistic children mouth or handle objects, children in the one-word stage engage in single-schemed play (e.g., using a toy cup to "drink"), and children beginning two-word sentences (early stage I language) combine simple schemes, such as feeding a doll, then grooming it. Identical relationships between levels of symbolic play and early language have also been found in children with DS (Hill and McCune-Nicholich, 1981) and with autism (Mundy et al., 1987), suggesting that such relationships occur among all children.

Mother-child interactions. During recent years there has been much study of mutuality and reciprocity in social interactions between children and their parents. These studies have shown that mothers simplify their speech and modulate their behavior to match the child's level of functioning. At the same time, mothers help their children to perform by structuring the environment, attracting the child's attention, breaking difficult tasks into component parts, and in other ways providing what has been called a "social scaffold" for the child. Subsequent studies involving retarded children and their mothers have revealed both similarities and differences. For example, mothers of DS children are similar to those of nonretarded children in their level of grammatical complexity, use of key words, and use of a high-pitched voice (Rondal, 1977). However, these and other mothers of handicapped children tend to be more controlling and didactic in their interactions (Cardoso-Martins and Mervis, 1985; Jones, 1980). These differences in the style of interactions (but not the structure) may be related to different perceptions of the child and to emotional reactions (the so-called "mourning reactions") experienced by mothers of retarded children (Blacher, 1985; Hodapp, 1988).

Family systems. Related to this interest in mother-child relations is the burgeoning interest in families and the process of change that occurs as children develop. The presence of a retarded child is currently thought to constitute a stressor within the family system; one, however, that is buffered by the financial and emotional resources available to the family (Crnic et al., 1983; Gallagher et al., 1983). Factors associated with more adaptive family functioning include economic advantage, the presence of both parents within the household, marital success, and the availability of social support (Beckman, 1983; Farber, 1959; Friedrich, 1979; Suelzle and Keenan, 1981). Recent studies have focused on the functioning of siblings of handicapped children. As a group, siblings do not appear to be at particular risk for the development of psychiatric disturbance (Lobato, 1983). However, several factors do predispose to maladjustment, including the status of eldest female or same-gender sibling (Cleveland and Miller, 1977), difficulties on the part of parents in accepting the handicapped child's condition, the lack of a clear cause for the mental retardation, and the need for intensive parental care and attention directed toward the handicapped child (McHale et al., 1984). It appears that some siblings experience resentment and anger as a result of growing up with a retarded child (Grossman, 1972), whereas others become more empathic, altruistic, idealistic, and tolerant (Cleveland and Miller, 1977; Grossman, 1972).

DISCUSSION

The work of the past decade has highlighted the complexity of biological and psychological aspects of mental retardation. Advances in biological medicine have made it possible to identify the putative cause of mental retardation among an increasing number of affected children. Greater attention to the influence of perinatal risk factors and increased sophistication of medical technology (e.g., metabolic assay procedures, neuroimaging techniques, genetic assessments) have contributed to improved diagnosis. An important task for the future will be the development of more sophisticated procedures for judging the relative importance of biological and psychosocial vulnerabilities that underlie cognitive impairment. In addition, it will be important to identify the psychosocial variables that serve a protective function among biologically predisposed individuals.

Given the pace of technological progress, it is likely that an increasing number of infants with serious perinatal risks will survive the neonatal period. Accordingly, it will become increasingly important to identify infants at risk for the development of future disability so that appropriate early intervention can be instituted. Although infants at risk for severe intellectual impairment can be identified by existing evaluation procedures, those destined to develop mild to moderate degrees of disability cannot. Therefore, improvements must be made in the sensitivity and predictive accuracy of neurodevelopmental assessment techniques.

Recent advances in human genetics have been impressive. However, as our knowledge base has expanded, so has our appreciation for the complexity of the processes involved in genetic expression. For instance, although an increasing number of mental retardation syndromes have been linked to relatively subtle and specific genetic abnormalities, very little is known about the factors and mechanisms directly responsible for the development of cognitive impairment. Straightforward explanations, such as the apparent size of a chromosomal lesion, or at a molecular level, the degree of under- or overproduction of a gene product do not fully explain the presence and degree of cognitive impairment. We are just beginning to uncover other potential factors, such as genomic imprinting and complex interactions among regulatory gene systems. Recent investigations have suggested that a common genetic abnormality may underlie the cognitive impairment of DS and AD. Relatively close linkage has been established among the loci responsible for DS, AD, and the gene products, BAP and SOD-1. However, the linkage is not close enough to fully explain the clinical associations. In addition, only a portion of AD appears to be familial, and only a portion of familial cases are associated with DS. Clearly, more complex mechanisms must be operative. Clarification of the causes of such genetic and phenotypic heterogeneity may lead to greater understanding of the factors that underlie normal as well as abnormal cognitive, social, and adaptive development.

A similar set of issues surrounds the development of advanced neuroimaging techniques. Recent findings have stimulated the development of new ideas regarding the structural basis and pathophysiology of several retardation syndromes. However, questions regarding the validity and the specificity of such findings must still be answered (e.g., associations between cerebellar abnormalities and autism on MRI and between temperoparietal hypometabolism and DS and AD on PET, etc.). Future research directions might include the adoption of more highly standardized neuroimaging procedures and the study of more homogeneous clinical populations. Such endeavors might help determine the specificity of findings for developmental groups of different origin and pathogenesis.

Research in developmental psychology has revealed the significant variability in cognitive, linguistic, and adaptive functioning that occurs across etiologically distinct retardation syndromes. Such work has also indicated that the behavioral profiles associated with these distinct syndromes may be specific and discriminating. An area that has received increasing interest is the cross-fertilization of knowledge about human development gleaned from the study of mentally retarded and nonretarded populations. Such cross fertilization may increase our appreciation for the degree of rigidity versus plasticity of developmental sequences, the nature of cross-domain relations, and the effects that different sequences or relations might have on further development. An example of this approach is the recent application of family systems theory to the study of families with mentally retarded children.

Although much has been learned during the past 10 to 15 years, we are just beginning to understand basic issues in mental retardation. Thoughtful, systematic research offers the hope of increasing our understanding not only of mental retardation, but also of those processes that underlie the physiological, cognitive, and psychological aspects of normal development.

REFERENCES:

Antonarakis, S. E. (1989), Diagnosis of genetic disorders at the DNA level. *N. Engl. J. Med.*, 320:153–163.

Avery, M. E. & First, L. R. (1989), Molecular genetics. In: *Pediatric Medicine*, eds. M. E. Avery & L. R. First. Baltimore: Williams & Wilkins, 1989.

Baraitser, M. (1986), Chromosomes and mental retardation. *Psychol. Med.*, 16:495–497.

Bates, E., Benigni, L., Bretherton, I., Camaioni, L. & Volterra, V., (1979), *The Emergence of Symbols*. New York: Academic Press.

Beckman, P. (1983), Influence of selected child characteristics on stress in families of handicapped infants. *Am. J. Ment. Defic.*, 19:150–156.

Blacher, J. (1985), Sequential stages of parental adjustment to the birth of a child with handicaps: fact or artifact? *Ment. Retard.*, 22:55–68.

Bozynski, M. E., et al. (1984), Two year longitudinal followup of premature infants weighing less than 1,200 grams at birth: sequelae of intracranial hemorrhage. *J. Dev. Behav. Pediat.*, 5:346–352.

Braffman, B. H., Bilaniuk, L. T., & Zimmerman, R. A. (1988), The central nervous system manifestations of the phakomatoses on MR. *Radiol. Clin. North Am.*, 26:773–799.

Bronfenbrenner, U., Kessel, F., Kessen, W. & White, S. (1986), Toward a critical social history of developmental psychology: a propadeutic discussion. *Am. Psychol.*, 41:1218–1230.

Burack, J. A., Hodapp, R. M. & Zigler, E. (1988), Issues in the classification of mental retardation: differentiating among organic etiologies. *J. Child Psychol. Psychiatry*, 29:765–779.

————————————(1990), Technical note: toward a more precise understanding of mental retardation. *J. Child Psychol. Psychiatry*, 31:471–475.

Butler, M. G. (1990), Prader-Willi syndrome: current understanding of cause and diagnosis. *Am. J. Med. Genet.*, 35:319–332.

Campbell, M., Rosenbloom, S., Perry, R. et al. (1982), Computerized axial tomography in autistic children. *Am. J. Psychiatry*, 139:510–512.

Cardoso-Martins, C. & Mervis, C. (1985), Maternal speech to prelinguistic children with Down Syndrome. *Am. J. Ment. Defic.*, 89:451–458.

Chugani, H. T., Phelps, M. E., Light, R. K. & Mazziotta, J. C. (1987), Metabolic correlates of mental retardation in children determined with FDG positron emission tomography (PET). *J. Cereb. Blood Flow Metab.*, 7:S533.

————Mazziotta, J. C. & Phelps, M. E. (1989), Sturge-Weber syndrome: a study of cerebral glucose utilization with positron emission tomography. *J. Pediatr.*, 114:244–253.

————Mans-Wagener, L. (1987), Sequences, stages, and structures in the organization of cognitive development in infants with Down syndrome. In: *Infant Performance and Experience: New Findings with the Ordinal Scales*, eds. I. Uzgiris & J. McV. Hunt. Urbana: University of Illinois Press.

————Sroufe, L. A. (1976), The relationship between affective and cognitive development in Down's Syndrome children. *Child Dev.*, 47:920–929.

Cleveland, D. & Miller, N. (1977), Attitudes and life commitments of older siblings of mentally retarded adults: an exploratory study. *Ment. Retard.*, 3:38–41.

Cohen, S. E., Parmelee, A. H., Beckwith, L. & Sigman, M. D. (1986), Cognitive development in preterm infants: birth to 8 years. *J. Dev. Behav. Pediat.*, 7:102–110.

Cornwell, A. & Birch, H. (1969), Psychological and social development in home-reared children with Down's Syndrome (mongolism). *Am. J. Ment. Defic.*, 74:341–350.

Courchesne, E., Yeung-Courchesne, R., Press, G. A., Hesselink, J. R. & Jernigan, T. L. (1988), Hypoplasia of cerebellar vermal lobules VI and VII in autism. *N. Engl. J. Med.*, 318:1349–1354.

Creasey, H., Rumsey, J. M., Schwartz, M., Duara, R., Rapoport, J. L. & Rapoport, S. I. (1986), Brain morphometry in autistic men as measured by volumetric computed tomography. *Arch. Neurol.*, 43:669–672.

Crnic, K., Friedrich, W. & Greenberg, M. (1983), Adaptation of families with mentally retarded children: a model of stress, coping, and family ecology. *Am. J. Ment. Defic.*, 88:125–138.

Cullen, S., Cronk, C., Pueschel, S., Schnell, R., & Reed, R. (1981), Social development and feeding milestones of young Down Syndrome children. *Am. J. Ment. Defic.*, 85:410–415.

Cutler, N. R. (1986), Cerebral metabolism as measured with positron emission tomography (PET) and [^{18}F] 2-deoxy-D-glucose: healthy aging, Alzheimer's disease and Down syndrome. *Prog. Neuropsychopharmacol. Biol. Psychiatry*, 10:309–321.

————Heston, L. L., Davies, P., Haxby, J. V. & Schapiro, M. B. (1985), Alzheimer's disease and Down's syndrome: new insights. *Ann. Intern. Med.*, 103:566–578.

De La Costello, A. M., Hamilton, P. A., Baudin, J. et al. (1988), Prediction of neurodevelopmental impairment at four years from brain ultrasound appearance of very preterm infants. *Dev. Med. Child Neurol.*, 30:711–722.

De Volder, A., Bol, A., Michel, C., Congneau, M. & Goffinet, A. M. (1987), Brain glucose metabolism in children with the autistic syndrome: positron tomography analysis. *Brain Dev.*, 9:581–587.

Dunst, C. J. (1990), Sensorimotor development of infants with Down Syndrome. In: *Children with Down Syndrome: A Developmental Perspective*, eds. D. Chiccetti & M. Beeghly. New York: Cambridge University Press.

————(1988), Stage transitioning in the sensorimotor development of Down's syndrome infants. *J. Ment. Defic. Res.*, 32:405–410.

Dykens, E. M. & Leckman, J. F. (1990), Developmental issues in fragile X syndrome. In: *Issues in the Developmental Approach to Mental Retardation*, eds. R. M. Hodapp, J. A. Burack & E. Zigler. New York: Cambridge University Press.

————Hodapp, R. M. & Leckman, J. F. (1989a), Adaptive and maladaptive functioning in institutionalized and noninstitutionalized fragile X males. *J. Am. Acad. Child Adolesc. Psychiatry*, 28:427–430.

————————Ort, S., Finucane, B., Shapiro, L. & Leckman, J. F. (1989b), The trajectory of cognitive development in males with fragile X syndrome. *J. Am. Acad. Child Adolesc. Psychiatry*, 28:422–426.

————————Leckman, J. F. (1987a), Strengths and weaknesses in the intellectual functioning of males with fragile X syndrome. *Am. J. Ment. Defic.*, 92:234–236.

————Leckman, J. F., Paul, R. & Watson, M. (1987b), The cognitive, behavioral, and adaptive functioning of fragile X and non-fragile X retarded men. *J. Autism Dev. Discord.*, 18:41–52.

Evenhuis, H. M. (1990), The natural history of dementia in Down's syndrome. *Arch. Neurol.*, 47:263–267.

Farber, B. (1959), The effects of a severely retarded child in family systems. *Monogr. Soc. Res. Child Dev.*, 24:2.

Ferrier, L. (1987), *A comparative study of the conversational skills of fragile X, autistic, and Down Syndrome individuals.* Unpublished doctoral dissertation, Boston University (Abstracts International DA8715419).

Fowler, A. (1984), *Language acquisition of Down's Syndrome children: Production and comprehension.* Unpublished doctoral dissertation, University of Pennsylvania (Abstracts International DA8505068).

Friedrich, W. (1979), Predictors of coping behavior of mothers of handicapped children. *J. Consult. Clin. Psychol.*, 47:1140–1141.

Fryns, J. P. (1987), Chromosomal anomalies and autosomal syndromes. *Birth Defects*, 23:7–32.

———Jacobs, J., Kleczkowska, A. & Van den Berghe, H. (1984), The psychological profile of the fragile X syndrome. *Clin. Genet.*, 25:131–134.

Gaffney, G. R., Kuperman, S., Tsai, L. Y. & Minchin, S. (1989), Forebrain structure in infantile autism. *J. Am. Acad. Child Adolesc. Psychiatry*, 28:534–537.

Gallagher, J. J., Beckman, P. J. & Cross, A. H. (1983), Families of handicapped children: sources of stress and its amelioration. *Except. Child.*, 50:10–19.

Garber, H. J., Ritvo, E. R., Chiu, L. C., Griswold, V. J., Kashanian, A., Freeman, B. J. & Oldendorf, W. H. (1989), Magnetic resonance imaging study of autism: normal fourth ventricle size and absence of pathology. *Am. J. Psychiatry*, 146:532–534.

Grossman, F. (1972), *Brothers and Sisters of Retarded Children*. Syracuse, NY: Syracuse University Press.

Hagberg, B., Hagberg, G., Lewerth, A. & Lindberg, U. (1981), Mild mental retardation in Swedish school children. *Acta Paediatr. Scand.*, 70:445–452.

Hagerman, R., Schreiner, R., Kemper, M., Wittenberger, M., Zahn, B. & Habicht, K. (in press), Longitudinal IQ changes in fragile X males. *Am. J. Med. Genet.*

Hill, P. & McCune-Nicholich, L. (1981), Pretend play and patterns of cognition in Down's syndrome infants. *Child Dev.*, 23:43–60.

Hodapp, R. M. (1988), The role of maternal emotions and perceptions in interactions with young handicapped children. In: *Parent-Child Interaction and Developmental Disabilities*, ed. K. Marfo. New York: Praeger.

———Burack, J. A. & Zigler, E. (Eds.) (1990a), *Issues in the Developmental Approach to Mental Retardation*. New York: Cambridge University Press.

———Dykens, E. M., Hagerman, R., Schreiner, R., Lachiewisc, A., Gullion, C. & Leckman, J. F. (1990b). Developmental implications of changing trajectories of IQ in males with fragile X syndrome. *J. Am. Acad. Child Adolesc. Psychiatry*, 29:214–219.

Hopper, P. (1989). *Sibling relations in families with an autistic child*. Paper submitted for publication.

Horwitz, B., Rumsey, J. M., Grady, C. L. & Rapoport, S. I. (1988), The cerebral metabolic landscape in autism. *Arch. Neurol.*, 45:749–755.

Imaizumi, K., Fumio, T., Kuroki, Y., Naritomi, K., Hamabe, J. & Niikawa, N. (1990), Cytogenetic and molecular study of the Angelman syndrome. *Am. J. Med. Genet.*, 35:314–318.

Jacobson, R., Le Couteur, A., Howlin, P. & Rutter M. (1988), Selective subcortical abnormalities in autism. *Psychol. Med.*, 18:39–48.

Jones, O. (1980), Prelinguistic communication skills in Down's syndrome and normal infants. In: *High-Risk Infants and Children: Adult and Peer Interactions.* eds. T. Field, S. Soldberg, D. Stern & A. Sostek. New York: Academic Press.

Karlinsky, H. (1986). Alzheimer's disease in Down's syndrome. *J. Am. Geriatr. Soc.*, 34:728–734.

Kemper, M. B., Hagerman, R. & Altshul-Stark, D. (1988), Cognitive profiles of boys with fragile X syndrome. *Am. J. Med. Genet.*, 30:191–200.

Klasner, E. & Hagerman, R. (1987), *Speech and language characteristics and intervention strategies with fragile X patients.* Paper presented at the First National Fragile X Conference, Denver, CO.

Klunk, W. E. & Abraham, D. J. (1988), Filamentous proteins in Alzheimer's disease: new insights through molecular biology. *Psychiatr. Dev.*, 2:121–152.

Kopp, C. (1983), Risk factors in development. In: *Handbook of Child Psychology, Vol. 2, Infancy and Developmental Psychobiology*, ed. P. Mussen. New York: Wiley.

————McCall, R. (1982), Predicting later mental performance for normal, at risk, and handicapped infants. In: *Lifespan Development and Behavior*, Vol. 4, eds. P. Baltes & O. Brim. New York: Academic Press.

Krakow, J. & Kopp, C. (1982), Sustained attention in young Down syndrome children. *Topics in Early Childhood Special Education*, 2:32–42.

Lachiewicz, A., Gullion, C., Spiridigliozzi, G. & Aylsworth, A. (1987), Declining IQs of young males with fragile X syndrome. *Am. J. Ment. Defic.*, 92:272–278.

Lamont, M. A. & Dennis, N. R. (1988), Aetology of mild mental retardation. *Arch. Dis. Child.*, 63:1032–1038.

Largo, R. H., Pfister, D., Molinari, L. et al. (1989), Significance of prenatal, perinatal and postnatal factors in the development of AGA preterm infants at five to seven years. *Dev. Med. Child Neurol.*, 31:440–456.

————Graf, S., Kundu, S., Hunziker, U. & Molinari, L. (1990), Predicting developmental outcome at school age from infant tests of normal, at-risk and retarded infants. *Dev. Med. Child Neurol.*, 32:30–45.

Leckman, J., Hodapp, R., Dykens, E., Sparrow, S., Zelinsky, D. & Ort, S. (1989), *Evidence for specific profiles of cognitive processing among fragile X males.* Paper presented at the Fourth International Workshop on the Fragile X Syndrome and X-Linked Mental Retardation, New York.

Leifer, J. & Lewis, M. (1984), Acquisition of conversational response skills by young Down Syndrome and nonretarded young children. *Am. J. Ment. Defic.*, 88:610–618.

Lobato, D. (1983), Siblings of handicapped children: a review. *J. Autism Dev. Disord.*, 13:347–364.

Magenis, R. E., Toth-Fejel, S., Allen, L. J. et al. (1990), Comparison of the 15q deletions in Prader-Willi and Angelman syndromes: specific regions, extent of deletions, parental origin, and clinical consequences. *Am. J. Med. Genet.*, 35:333–349.

Mann, D. M. A. (1988), The pathological association between Down syndrome and Alzheimer disease. *Mech. Aging Dev.*, 43:99–136.

————Paul, R. & Leckman, J. (1987), *Speech and language profiles in males with fragile X syndrome.* Paper presented at the American Speech and Hearing Association Conference, New Orleans, LA.

Marans, W., Hodapp, R. & Leckman, J. (1989, April). *Syndrome specific language profiles: a comparison of fragile X and Down Syndrome males.* Paper presented to the 1989 International Fragile X Conference, Denver, CO.

Mazer, B., Piper, M. C. & Ramsay, M. (1988), Developmental outcome in very low birthweight infants 6 to 36 months old. *J. Dev. Behav. Pediatr.*, 9:239–297.

McCall, R. B. (1981), Nature-nurture and the two realms of development: a proposed integration with respect to mental development. *Child Dev.*, 52:1–12.

———Eichorn, D. & Hogarty, P. (1977), Transitions in early mental development. *Monogr. Soc. Res. Child Dev.*, 38.

McCune-Nicholich, L. & Bruskin, C. (1982), Combinatorial competency in symbolic play and language. In: *The Play of Children*, eds. D. Pepler & K. Rubin. New York: Karger.

McHale, S., Simeonnson, R. & Sloan, J. (1984), Children with handicapped brothers and sisters. In: *The Effects of Autism on the Family*, eds. E. Shopler and G. Mesibov. New York: Plenum.

Miller, J. (1986), Early cross-cultural commonalities in social explanation. *Developmental Psychology*, 22:514–520.

Morgan, S. (1979), Development and distribution of intellectual and adaptive skills in Down syndrome children: implications for early intervention. *Ment. Retard.*, 17:247–249.

Mundy, P. & Kasari, C. (1990), The similar structure hypothesis and differential rate hypothesis in mental retardation. In: *Issues in the Developmental Approach to Mental Retardation*, eds. R. M. Hodapp, J. A. Burack & E. Zigler. New York: Cambridge University Press.

———Seibert, J. & Hogan, A. (1982), Relationships between sensorimotor and early communication abilities in developmentally delayed children. *Merrill-Palmer Quarterly*, 30:33–48.

———Sigman, M., Ungerer, J. & Sherman, T. (1987), Nonverbal communication and play correlates of language development in autistic children. *J. Autism Dev. Disord.*, 17:349–364.

Murphy, P. D., Watson, M. S., Kidd, K. K. & Breg, W. R. (1986), Molecular approaches to carrier detection and prenatal diagnosis of the fragile X syndrome. *Pediatr. Res.*, 20:269A.

Nicholls, R. D., Knoll, J. H. M., Butler, M. G., Karam, S. & Lalande, M. (1989), Genetic imprinting suggested by maternal heterodisomy in non-deletion Prader-Willi syndrome. *Nature*, 342:281–285.

Pembry, M. E., Winter, R. M. & Davies, K. E. (1986), Fragile X mental retardation: current controversies. *Trends in Neurosciences,* Feb:68–62.

Percy, M. E., Dalton, A. J., Markovic, V. D., McLachlan, D. R. C., Hummel, J. T., Rusk, A. C. M. & Andrews, D. F. (1990), Red cell superoxide dismutase, glutathione peroxidase and catalase in Down syndrome patients with and without manifestations of Alzheimer disease. *Am. J. Med. Genet.*, 35:459–467.

Pueschel, S. M., Gallagher, P., Zartler, A. & Pezzullo, J. (1987), Cognitive and learning profiles in children with Down Syndrome. *Res. Dev. Disabil.*, 8:21–37.

Reed, R., Pueschel, S., Schnell, R. & Cronk, C. (1980), Interrelationships of biological, environmental, and competency variables in young children with Down syndrome. *Applied Research in Mental Retardation*, 1:161–174.

Roach, E. S., Smith, T., Terry, C. V., Riela, A. R. & Laster, D. W. (1987), Magnetic resonance imaging in pediatric neurologic disorders. *Journal of Clinical Neurology*, 2:111–116.

Rodenhiser, D. I., Coulter-Mackie, M. B., Singh, S. M. & Jung, H. H. (1989), Genomic imprinting as a possible contribution to variable expression in neurofibromatosis type I NFI. *Am. J. Hum. Genet.*, 45(4 suppl):A215.

Rondal, J. (1977), Maternal speech in normal and Down's syndrome children. In: *Research to Practice in Mental Retardation*, Vol. 2, ed. P. Mittler. Baltimore: University Park Press.

Ross, G., Lipper, E. G. & Auld, P. A. (1986), Early predictors of neurodevelopmental outcome of very low birthweight infants at three years. *Dev. Med. Child Neurol.*, 28:171–179.

Rumble, B., Retallack, R., Hilbich, C. et al. (1989). Amyloid A4 protein and its precursor in Down's syndrome and Alzheimer's disease. *N. Engl. J. Med.*, 320:1446–1452.

Rumsey, J. M., Duara, R., Grady, C., Rapoport, J. L., Margolin, R. A., Rapoport, S. I. & Cutler, N. R. (1985), Brain metabolism in autism. *Arch. Gen. Psychiatry*, 42:448–455.

———Creasey, H., Stepanek, J. S., Dorwart, R., Patronas, N., Hamburger, S. D. & Duara, R. (1988), Hemispheric asymmetries, fourth ventricular size, and cerebellar morphology in autism. *J. Autism Dev. Discord.*, 18:127–137.

Scarr-Salapatek, S. (1975), An evolutionary perspective on infant intelligence: species patterns and individual variations. In: *Origins of Intelligence*, ed. M. Lewis. New York: Plenum.

Schapiro, M. B., Ball, M. J., Grady, C. L., Haxby, J. V., Kaye, J. A. & Rapoport, S. I. (1988), Dementia in Down's syndrome: cerebral glucose utilization, neuropsychological assessment, and neuropathology. *Neurology*, 38:938–942.

Schellenberg, G. D., Bird, T. D., Wijsman, E. M., Moore, D. K. & Martin, G. M. (1989), The genetics of Alzheimer's disease. *Biomed. Pharmacother.*, 43:463–468.

Schinzel, A. (1988), Microdeletion syndromes, balanced translocations, and gene mapping. *J. Med. Genet.*, 25:454–462.

Stewart, A. L., Costello, A. M., Hamilton, P. A. et al. (1989), Relationship between neurodevelopmental status of very preterm infants at one and four years. *Dev. Med. Child Neurol.*, 31:756–765.

Suelzle, M. & Keenan, V. (1981), Changes in family support networks over the life cycle of mentally retarded persons. *Am. J. Ment. Defic.*, 86:267–274.

Szymonowicz, W., Yu, V. Y., Bajuk, B. & Astbury, J. (1986), Neurodevelopmental outcome of periventricular haemorrhage and leukomalacia in infants 1250 g or less at birth. *Early Hum. Dev.*, 14:1–7.

Van Bel, F., den Duden, L., van de Bor, M., Stijnen, T., Baan, J. & Ruys, J. H. (1989), Cerebral blood-flow velocity during the first week of life of preterm infants and neurodevelopment at two years. *Dev. Med. Child Neurol.*, 31:320–328.

Van Camp, G., Stinissen, P., Van Hul, W., Backhovens, H., Wehnert, A., Bandenberge, A. & Van Broeckhoven, C. (1989), Selection of human chromosome 21-specific DNA probes for genetic analysis in Alzheimer's dementia and Down syndrome. *Hum. Genet.*, 83:58–60.

Webb, G. C., Rogers, J. G., Pitt, D. B., Halliday, J. & Theoald, T. (1981), Transmission of fragile (X) (q27) site from a male. *Lancet*, 2:1231–1232.

Webb, T. P., Bundey, S. E., Thake, A. I. & Todd, J. (1986), Population incidence and segregation ratios in the Martin-Bell Syndrome. *Am. J. Med. Genet.*, 23:573–580.

Weiss, B., Weisz, J. & Bromfield, R. (1986), Performance of retarded and nonretarded persons on information-processing tasks: further tests of the similar structure hypothesis. *Psychol. Bull.*, 100:157–175.

Weisz, J. R. (1990), Cultural-familial Mental Retardation: a developmental perspective on cognitive performance and "helpless" behavior. In: *Issues in the Developmental Approach to Mental Retardation*, eds. R. M. Hodapp, J. A. Burack & E. Zigler. New York: Cambridge University Press.

———Yeates, K. & Zigler, E. (1982), Piagetian evidence and the developmental-difference controversy. In: *Mental Retardation: The Developmental-Difference Controversy*, eds. E. Zigler & D. Balla. Hillsdale, NJ: Erlbaum.

Wetherby, A. (1986), Ontogeny of communicative functions in autism. *J. Autism Dev. Disord.*, 16:295–316.

Williams, C. A., Zori, R. T., Stone, J. W., Gray, B. A., Cantu, E. S. & Ostrer, H. (1990), Maternal origin of 15q11-13 deletions in Angelman syndrome suggests a role for genomic imprinting. *Am. J. Med. Genet.*, 35:350–353.

Williams, M. L., Lewandowski, L. J., Coplan, J. & Deugenio, D. B. (1987), Neurodevelopmental outcome of preschool children born preterm with and without intracranial hemorrhage. *Dev. Med. Child Neurol.*, 29:243–249.

Wisniewski, K. E., Wisniewski, H. M. & Wen, G. Y. (1985), Occurrence of neuropathological changes and dementia of Alzheimer's disease in Down's syndrome. *Ann. Neurol.*, 17:278–282.

Wolf, P., Gardner, J., Lappen, J., Paccia, J. & Schnell, R. (1987, December), *Social adaptation and behavior in males with Fragile X syndrome.* Paper presented at the First National Fragile X Conference, Denver, CO.

Wolf-Schein, E., Sudhalter, V., Cohen, I. (1987), Speech-language and fragile X syndrome: initial findings. *Journal of the American Speech-Language Hearing Association*, 35–38.

Yang, T. P., Patel, P. I., Chinault, A. C. et. al. (1984), Molecular evidence for a new mutation at the HPRT locus in Lesch-Nyhan patients. *Nature*, 310:412–414.

Zigler, E. (1969), Developmental versus differences theories of mental retardation and the problem of motivation. *Am. J. Ment. Defic.*, 73:536–566.

14

The Development of Contingent Discourse Ability in Autistic Children

Helen Tager-Flusberg and Marcia Anderson

University of Massachusetts, Boston

This study investigated communicative competence in autistic children. Six autistic boys were matched to six children with Down syndrome on age and language level. For each child four samples of spontaneous speech over the course of 1 year were analysed. Child utterances were coded for adjacency, contingency and various categories of continent discourse that either did or did not add new information. Autistic children were found to be more non-contingent, and to show no development change in their contingent discourse, especially in categories of contingent discourse that added new information.

INTRODUCTION

Over the past decade it has become widely recognized that autistic children's primary area of language dysfunction lies in that domain of pragmatics—or the functional uses of language in a social context (e.g. Baltaxe, 1977; Fay & Mermelstein, 1982; Paul, 1987; Schopler & Mesibov, 1985; Tager-Flusberg, 1981, 1989). This perspective on the language deficit in autism takes on special significance when it is viewed in relation to the other cognitive and social impairments that are the hallmark of this pervasive developmental disorder (Caparulo & Cohen,

Reprinted with permission from the *Journal of Child Psychology and Psychiatry,* 1991, Vol. 32, No. 7, 1123–1134. Copyright © 1991 by The Association for Child Psychology and Psychiatry.

This research was generously supported by a grant from the National Institute of Child Health and Human Development (RO1 HD 18833). Portions of these data were presented in 1988 at the Symposium for Research on Child Language Disorders, Madison, Wisconsin. Some of the analyses were carried out as part of an undergraduate honors thesis submitted by the second author to the Department of Psychology at the University of Massachusetts at Boston. We appreciate the help provided by Therese Baumberger, Susan Calkins, Ann Chadwick-Dias, Tina Nolin and Gail Andrick in preparing the transcripts and we extend our sincere gratitude to the children and their families who participated in the study.

1977; Baron-Cohen 1988) For this reason it is important to identify more precisely the particular aspects of pragmatic functioning that are specifically impaired in autism in order to advance our theoretical understanding of the nature of the psychological deficit in autism.

Kanner's original papers on autism included descriptions of the children's language, especially some of the aberrant features such as echolalia, pronominal reversals and repetitive questioning, as non-communicative (Kanner, 1943, 1946); and subsequent work supported this view (e.g. Creak, 1972; Ricks & Wing, 1975). More recently, as research on pragmatic aspects of language and communication has grown (cf. Bates, 1976; Bruner, 1975; Keenan, 1974), a different perspective has been placed on autistic children's language. Within this newer framework, even the peculiar features of autistic children's language have been interpreted in a more positive way, as an effort toward communicating with others. Primant's research on both immediate and delayed echolalia has enriched our understanding of the variety of messages that are communicated through this form of language (Prizant & Duchan, 1981; Prizant & Rydell, 1984; see also, McEvoy, Loveland & Landry, 1988). Other forms of repetitive speech, including excessive questioning or other idiosyncratic phrases, have also been shown to serve a primarily communicative role (Coggins & Frederickson, 1988; Hurtis, Ensrud & Tomblin, 1982). Thus we no longer view autistic children's communicative abilities in an all-or-none fashion (Wetherby, 1986); rather these abilities lie on a continuum both within and across children at different levels of functioning.

A number of studies have investigated factors that influence autistic children's communicative competence. Wetherby and Prutting (1984), who studied four autistic children at the early stages of language development, found that they used a limited range of communicative functions: those that served *environmental* ends, to gain a desired object or action. Their subjects rarely used language to serve a *social* function, such as gaining attention or showing off, in contrast to matched normal controls. Both the situational context (Mermelstein, 1983) and conversational partner (Bernard-Opitz, 1982; McHale, Simeonsson, Marcus & Olley, 1980) have been shown to influence the communicative level of autistic children. The more structured the situation, the more communicative the autistic child will be. Similarly, autistic children will be more communicative with people that they know well, such as their mother (Bernard-Opitz, 1982) or a familiar teacher (McHale *et al.*, 1980).

One important aspect of communicative competence is the ability to maintain and develop a topic of discourse. Autistic children have been found to be quite deficient in this area because they either do not respond to adult initiations or they do so in a non-topically related way (Ball, 1978; Paccia-Cooper, Curcio & Sacharko, 1981; Tager-Flusberg, 1982). Nevertheless, at least some of the time the autistic subjects in these studies were able to respond appropriately to their conversational partner. Curcio and Paccia (1987) found that one factor influencing this discourse ability was the linguistic environment: if adults asked conceptually simple yes/no questions that were related to the child's previous utterance, autistic children were more likely to be able to maintain the ongoing topic of conversation.

The primary goal of this study was to extend this line of research on communicative competence in autism by investigating the ways in which autistic children are able to respond in a continent, or topically related, way while engaged in conversation with their mothers. Research by Bloom and her colleagues has shown that as young normally developing children become more proficient linguistically, they are more likely to respond contingently to their mothers' utterances, and to do so in more advanced ways by adding new information to the topic of discourse (Bloom, Rocissano & Hood, 1976). We were particularly interested in studying the development of this aspect of discourse ability in a group of autistic children to see whether they would show the same changes in their communicative competence as do normal children.

In order to distinguish deficits in this area of language functioning that are specific to autism from those that may be related to delays in language acquisition, we included a control group of children with Down syndrome, who were the same ages and at the same levels of linguistic competence as the autistic children at the start of the study. Children with Down syndrome provide a particularly interesting contrast to autistic children in that it is a genetic condition that is almost never associated with autism (cf. Wakabayashi, 1979). Unlike autistic children, they are generally described as being highly sociable and responsive in communicative situations (Leifer & Lewis, 1984; Loveland, Tunali, McEvoy & Kelley, 1989), and do not share similar impairments in social-cognitive development (Baron-Cohen, Leslie & Frith, 1985, 1986).

METHOD

Subjects

The subjects for this study included six children with autism and six children with Down syndrome who were part of a larger study on language acquisition (Tager-Flusberg *et al.*, 1990). The autistic subjects, all boys, were diagnosed using DSM-III criteria and current proposals for defining the syndrome (Cohen, Paul & Bolkmar, 1987; Denckla, 1986), including onset prior to 30 months; gross and sustained impairments in socialization and social relationships; delay and deficits in language development; and repetitive or obsessive behaviors.

The autistic children lived with their families and attended special programs in school or at home. Their socio-economic status ranged from lower to upper middle class. The children all had some spontaneous language at the start of the study.

Their non-verbal IQs were assessed using the Leiter International Performance Scale (Leiter, 1974) and five of the six boys fell in the normal or low-normal range of intellectual functioning.

The Down syndrome children, four boys and two girls, were selected to match the autistic children on chronological age and language level, using mean length of utterance (MLU) at the time of the first sample for this study. They too lived at home, attended special programs and came from families with similar educational and socio-economic backgrounds as the autistic subjects. The Down syndrome children's scores on the Leiter indicated that they were not matched on non-verbal IQ or mental age levels.

Details about the two groups of subjects are shown in Table 1. t-Tests confirmed that the two groups were well matched on age [$t(10) = 0.34$] and MLU [$t(10) = 0.07$] at the time of the first sample. The autistic subjects, however, had significantly higher non-verbal IQ scores than the Down syndrome subjects [$t(10) = 4.32$, $p<.001$].

Collection and Preparation of Language Samples

Spontaneous speech samples were collected in the children's homes while they interacted with their mothers, in play or other loosely structured activities selected by the mothers. The sessions, lasting about 1 hour, were recorded using video- and audio-cassette equipment by two researchers. Written transcripts were later prepared from the audiotapes. The transcripts were then checked using the videotapes, and detailed context notes about the ongoing non-verbal activity were added. The transcripts of the language samples were typed into computer files, using the SALT

TABLE 1.
Subject characteristics

	Autistic					Down Syndrome			
Child	Age (years; months)	IQ*	MLU Sample 1	MLU Sample 4	Child	Age (years; months)	IQ	MLU Sample 1	MLU Sample 4
Stuart	3;4	61	1.17	1.90	Charlie	3;3	46	1.21	1.43
Roger	4;1	105	2.86	3.28	Kate	4;1	65	2.98	4.03
Brett	5;8	108	3.74	3.91	Penny	5;3	63	3.36	4.14
Mark	7;7	75	1.46	2.12	Martin	5;4	47	1.63	2.21
Rick	4;7	94	1.73	2.79	Billy	5;9	49	1.93	2.51
Jack	6;9	91	3.03	2.84	Jerry	6;9	54	2.86	3.32
M	5;4	89	2.37	2.81		5;1	54	2.33	2.94
S.D.	1;8	18	0.99	0.73		1;3	8	0.86	1.07

*Non-verbal IQ score.

format (Miller & Chapman, 1985) to facilitate coding and analysis. More details about the procedures used to collect and prepare the language samples can be found in Tager-Flusberg *et al.* (1990).

Coding

For each child four language samples were taken at 4-monthly intervals providing data across the span of 1 year. MLU was computed for each sample based on 100 consecutive intelligible spontaneous utterances, using the SALT program. Each sample was then assigned to one of Brown's language stages on the basis of MLU: Stage 1, 1.0–1.9; Stage 2, 2.0–2.4; Stage 3, 2.5–2.9; Stage 4, 3.0–3.4; Stage 5, over 3.5

The samples were coded for the use of contingent speech using a hierarchical coding scheme that was adapted from one developed by Bloom *et al.* (1976). At the first level, each child's utterance was coded for adjacency, that is, its relation to a prior adult utterance. All child utterances were coded into one of the following three categories.

Adjacent: Child utterance follows immediately after an adult utterance addressed to child.

Non-adjacent: Child utterance does not follow immediately after adult utterance; may follow child utterance, after an adult utterance with intervening pause, vocalizations, or an adult utterance not addressed to child.

Unintelligible: Child utterance is either fully or partially unintelligible.

Only adjacent utterances were then coded at the next level for their relation to the topic of the previous adult utterance. The following categories were used to code adjacent utterances.

Imitation: Child utterance is exact or partial repetition of prior adult utterance. It maintains the topic but is not different from the adult utterance.

Contingent: Child utterance maintains topic of prior adult utterance without being a simple imitation.

Non-contingent: Child utterance does not relate to topic of prior adult utterance.

The following is an example from an autistic subject who was playing with toy animals:

Mother: See the horse running?
Child: Look at the Susan.
(Child shifts away from the animals and mentions the visitor present.)

At the third level, all contingent utterances were coded further to distinguish the different ways in which the child maintained the ongoing topic of discourse, in addition to simple imitation. The following categories were used.

Yes/No: One word yes/no (or equivalent) responses.

Routines: Includes standard social routines (e.g. thank you, good night), verbal games, songs, TV talk, etc.

Recode: Repetition of prior adult utterance with some alteration in form; however, no additions or changes in meaning.

The following is an example from a Down syndrome child who was also playing with toy animals:

Mother: I think that's his tail.

Child: Yeah, a tail.

Self-recode: Repetition of child's own prior utterance after intervening adult acknowledgement, with alterations in form but not in meaning.

An example from an autistic child is:

Child: Have a paintbrush please.

Mother: No.

Child: I want the paintbrush.

Wh-response: Simple noun phrase response to adult test wh-questions.

For example, from an autistic child:

Mother: What color is the milkball?

Child: It's white.

Expansion: Adds information to topic and content of prior adult utterance.

An example from a Down syndrome subject is:

Mother: You're invited to a concert, yeah.

Child: And need a ticket for get in concert.

Self-expansion: Adds information to topic of child's own prior utterance after intervening *adult acknowledgement.*

Alteration: Adds information by opposing some aspect of content of adult prior utterance.

For example, from a Down syndrome subject who is trying on a paper mask she made:

Mother: This is a man?
Child: No, it's a lady.
Expatriation: Adds information to topic of prior adult utterance and introduces new
  related topic.

Another example from a Down syndrome child who is discussing a TV program:

Mother: Oh I'm glad a black dog came along and saved the bunny.
Child: No, hunter shoot him.

RESULTS

The data from each level of the coding scheme were analysed for developmental
trends as well as for comparisons between the groups. The first level of the coding
scheme distinguished between adjacent and non-adjacent utterances. In their study
of normal children Bloom *et al.* (1976) found that at all MLU stages there was more
adjacent speech than non-adjacent speech. Figure 1 presents the data on adjacency
as a percentage of the total number of intelligible utterances from our autistic and
Down syndrome subjects. Bloom *et al.*'s (1976) findings for their four normal subjects at stages 1, 2 and 5 are also included on the graph. Overall, the groups look
very similar to one another, although, at all stages, normal children are less adjacent
and more non-adjacent than the autistic and Down syndrome children.

The autistic and Down syndrome children were compared in their adjacency
using a multivariate analysis of variance (MANOVA) on data transformed with an
arcsin transformation for proportional data (Snedecor & Cochran, 1967). Neither

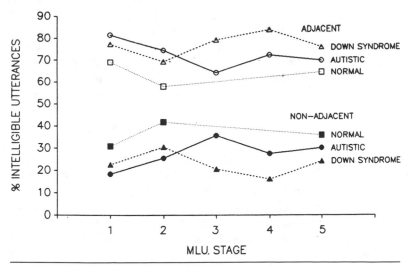

Figure 1. Distribution of adjacent and non-adjacent utterances.

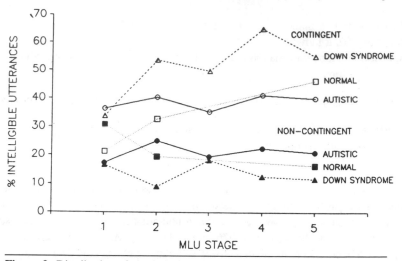

Figure 2. Distribution of contingent and non-contingent utterances.

the main effect of group [$F(1, 46) = 1.40$] nor the interaction between group and adjacency variables [$F(2, 45) = 1.13$] were significant.

We then analysed the children's adjacent utterances for contingent responding, as a percentage of total intelligible utterances. The data for contingent and non-contingent utterances are presented in Fig. 2, again including Bloom *et al.*'s (1976) data on normal children. At all stages the Down syndrome and autistic children are more contingent than non-contingent. In contrast, the normal children at stage 1 used more non-contingent speech. From stage 2 on, the Down syndrome children were highest in their use of contingent speech, and lowest in their use of non-contingent speech. the autistic children appear more similar to Bloom *et al.*'s normal children in their overall use of contingent speech; however, unlike either the normal or the Down syndrome children, they do not show an increase in the use of contingent speech with growth in MLU.

Table 2 shows the overall means and standard deviations for the different types of adjacent utterances for the Down syndrome and autistic children. A MANOVA on arcsin-transformed data yielded a significant interaction effect between group and contingency variables [$F(2,45) = 6.48$, $p<.005$], and there were significant univariate effects on contingent responses [$F(1, 46) = 5.71$, $p<.03$] and non-contingent responses [$F(1, 46) = 7.4$, $p<.01$], confirming that the Down syndrome children were more contingent in their speech than the autistic children. There were no significant univariate effects on imitation [$F(1, 46) = 0.01$].

The final level of analysis focused on the ways in which the children maintained

TABLE 2.

Means (and standard deviations) for categories of adjacent speech for
autistic and Down syndrome subjects

	Autistic		Down Syndrome	
	M	(S.D.)	*M*	(S.D.)
Non-contingent	20.1*	(5.6)	14.6	(7.1)
Contingent	38.1	(13.3)	48.5	(15.5)
Imitation	16.1	(12.8)	14.9	(10.6)

*Percentage of total intelligible utterances.

the ongoing topic of discourse. Children could reply in a topic-related way to their mother's prior utterance in a variety of ways, including imitation and nine different categories of contingent responses. Of these, five categories were identified as not adding significant new information; yes/no, routine, recode, self-recode, and wh-response. According to Bloom *et al.* (1976) imitation should also be included as a category of topic-related responding that adds no new information. The other four categories did provide new information to the ongoing topic of discourse, including expansion, self-expansion, alternative and expatiation. Bloom *et al.* (1976) found that the latter group, particularly expansions, were the most important developmentally. In general, as children's MLU grew, they were more likely to respond contingently by adding new information.

Table 3 presents the data from the autistic and Down syndrome children for the categories of topic-related responses that do, and do not, add new information.

TABLE 3.

Means (and standard deviations) for categories of topic-related responses
for autistic and Down syndrome children

	Autistic		Down Syndrome	
	M	(S.D.)	*M*	(S.D.)
No new information				
Yes/No	12.2*	(10.4)	27.9	(15.5)
Routine	7.9	(6.6)	2.9	(2.7)
Recode	5.3	(2.6)	4.5	(2.4)
Self-recode	4.1	(3.2)	2.9	(2.0)
Wh-response	29.3	(9.9)	14.3	(8.3)
Imitation	28.9	(17.8)	24.8	(19.1)
New information				
Expansion	7.8	(4.5)	16.6	(10.2)
Self-expansion	2.2	(2.1)	2.3*	(1.8)
Alternative	1.9	(2.7)	3.2	(2.1)
Expatiation	0.3	(0.8)	0.7	(0.9)

*Percentage of topic-related adjacent utterances.

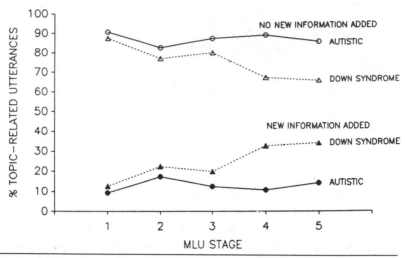

Figure 3. Distribution of topic-related utterances that do and do *not* add new information.

Figure 3 presents a developmental summary of these two sets of responses. Across these sets of response categories, autistic children did not appear to change with growth in MLU. This contrasts sharply with the Down syndrome children who, like normal children, showed a general increase in topic-related responses that add new information, as they became more advanced linguistically. Among specific categories of responses that do not add information, autistic children only showed declines over time in imitation, while the Down syndrome children declined in imitation and wh-responses. None of the categories of responses that add new information increased over time for autistic children, whereas the Down syndrome children showed significant increases in the use of expansions.

A MANOVA on arcsin-transformed data, comparing the two groups of children on the categories of topic-related responses that did not add new information, showed a significant main effect of group: $F(1, 46) = 5.34, p<.03$; and an interaction effect: $F(4, 43) = 7.3, p<.0001$. Significant univariate effects were found for yes/no responses [$F(1, 46) = 11.96, p<.002$], which were more prevalent among the Down syndrome children, and for Wh-responses [$F(1,46) = 9.68, p<.004$] and routines [$F(1,46) = 10.97, p<.002$], which were more prevalent among the autistic children.

The MANOVA comparing the groups on responses that did new information was not significant [$F(3,44) = 2.0$]. Significant univariate effects on expansions [$F(1,46) = 6.33, p<.02$] and expatiations [$F(1,46) = 5.31, p<.03$] were found, indicating that these categories were more prevalent among the Down syndrome children. No significant differences were found in the children's uses of alternatives and self-expansions, which were very infrequent among all the subjects.

DISCUSSION

The findings from this study are quite revealing about the ways in which autistic children compare to other populations of children in the acquisition of discourse skills. We found evidence that when autistic children interact with their mothers, they look quite similar to both Down syndrome and normally developing children who are at the same levels of language development, for certain aspects of conversational skill, especially at the early stages. On the other hand, those autistic children whose language advanced more begin to look different from the control groups in quite significant ways. While the numbers of subjects within each of the groups represented in this study are small, we found fairly consistent developmental patterns. Nevertheless, we need to be cautious about the conclusions to be drawn, given the limitations in sample sizes.

In certain respects, for example, turn-taking ability, autistic children are no different from Down syndrome children: there are no differences in their use of adjacent utterances (cf. Paccia-Cooper *et al.*, 1981; Tager-Flusberg, 1982). Moreover, at the early stages of language development, when MLU is less than 2.0, autistic children are also similar in contingent topic-related discourse, and even in their use of particular categories of contingent discourse. Here, then, we have evidence that high-functioning autistic children who are beginning to learn how to speak may not be particularly impaired in these aspects of their discourse abilities, at least when they are interacting with their mothers in a highly familiar environment.

Significant differences between the groups of children emerge at later stages of linguistic development. The patterns of development for normal and Down syndrome children show that, while there are no changes in the proportion of speech that is adjacent to their conversational partner's, as structural aspects of their language advance these children become more contingent in their speech, indicating that they are more able to maintain an established topic of conversation. The Down syndrome children appear to be even more adjacent and contingent than language-matched, normally developing children, which supports the impression these children give for being very sociable and interactive. Furthermore, as their language advances, both normal and Down syndrome children increase in their use of expansions and other categories of topic-related discourse that add new information; thus they contribute more novel and substantive material to the ongoing discussion. Thus, developmentally we see that normal and Down syndrome children change the content of their communications, telling more interesting and novel information to their mothers.

In sharp contrast, we see from Figs 2 and 3 that the autistic children show no such developmental changes. Their developmental patterns are essentially flat: advances in structural aspects of language are not paralleled by advances in discourse abilities. This lack of developmental change means that, as their language advances, autistic children look increasingly more different from both normal and Down syndrome children in both the content and style of their communications.

These significant differences between autistic children and other populations, that emerge at later linguistic stages, are particularly striking when we look at the ways in which the children maintain the conversational topic. Autistic children do not begin adding new information to the topic of discourse by expanding, challenging, or introducing new related topics. Instead, the data on differences in the use of various categories of contingent discourse suggest that autistic children continue relying on developmentally primitive ways of maintaining a topic, such as routines, recodings, and simple responses to test questions, even though they may have acquired the linguistic ability to contribute to the conversation in more interesting and advanced ways. In other words, structurally their language becomes more sophisticated while its content does not change. The relative paucity of expansions and other categories of discourse that add new information to the ongoing topic suggests that autistic children do not develop the understanding that they can be a source of new knowledge for their mothers.

How might such a problem in learning to converse in more advanced ways by relating novel information connect to other deficits of autistic children? One current hypothesis is that autistic children are significantly impaired in the acquisition of a so-called "theory of mind" (Baron-Cohen *et al.*, 1985; Frith, 1989); that is, they have particular deficits in understanding mental states, both their own and others'. A number of experiments provide considerable support for this view (e.g. Baron-Cohen, 1989a,b; Baron-Cohen *et al.*, 1985, 1986; Leslie & Frith, 1988; Perner, Frith, Leslie & Leekam, 1989), which is of special importance in that this proposal has the potential to directly link the social, cognitive and language deficits that are specific to autism (cf. Baron-Cohen,1988; Leslie, 1987). These studies have found that autistic children are deficient in a number of different domains which reflect a developing theory of mind, for example, conceiving false beliefs (Baron-Cohen *et al.*, 1985, 1986), distinguishing mental and physical entities, or appearance and reality (Baron-Cohen, 1989b), and understanding sources of knowledge (Leslie & Frith, 1988; Perner *et al.*, 1989).

A child who does not understand that people have mental states would not appreciate that various people can have access to different information or knowledge. On this view, then, autistic children may fail to realize that they know something that their mother does not and that they could inform her of something new. Such an impairment would lead to serious disturbances in communication, as has been hypothesized by Frith (1989). This particular interpretation about the source of autistic children's communicative problems is consistent with the specific pattern of results that we found in this study. Thus, the clearest difference to emerge between our autistic and Down syndrome children was that the autistic children failed to develop those categories of discourse that add new information to the topic of discourse, supporting the view that their conversational impairment stems from a lack of knowledge that people communicate by exchanging information, or indeed, that people have access to different information.

There is, we believe, a direct relationship between the particular deficits in discourse ability that we identified in this study, and the proposed deficit in autism in developing a theory of mind. Even before the age when normal children acquire a rich understanding of false belief, appearance-reality, and sources of knowledge, their language demonstrates the acquisition, at the least, of an 'implicit' theory of mind (Bretherton & Beeghly, 1982; Feldman, 1988; Shatz, Wellman & Silber, 1983). Our data suggest that autistic children show specific impairments even at these early stages in acquiring the conceptual understanding of mental states in themselves and other people, which show up in the paucity of the content of their communications. Future research will need to focus on the roots of these problems and other ways in which the language deficits in autistic children might be linked to deficits in acquiring a theory of mind.

REFERENCES

Ball, J. (1978). A pragmatic analysis of autistic children's language with respect to aphasic and normal language development. Unpublished doctoral dissertation, Melbourne University.

Baltaxe, C. A. M. (1977). Pragmatic deficits in the language of autistic adolescents. *Journal of Pediatric Psychology, 2*, 176–180.

Baron-Cohen, S. (1988). Social and pragmatic deficits in autism: cognitive or affective? *Journal of Autism and Developmental Disorders, 18*, 379–402.

Baron-Cohen, S. (1989b). Are autistic child's theory of mind, a case of specific developmental delay. *Journal of Child Psychology and Psychiatry, 30*, 285–298.

Baron-Cohen, S. (1989b). Are autistic children "behaviorists"? An examination of their mental-physical and appearance-reality distinctions. *Journal of Autism and Developmental Disorders, 19*, 579–600.

Baron-Cohen, S., Leslie, A. M. & Frith, U. (1985). Does the autistic child have a 'theory of mind'? *Cognition, 21*, 37–46.

Baron-Cohen, S., Leslie, A. M. & Frith, U. (1986). Mechanical, behavioral, and intentional understanding, of picture stories in autistic children. *British Journal of Developmental Psychology, 4*, 113–125.

Bates, E. (1976). *Language and contest: the acquisition of pragmatics.* New York: Academic Press.

Bernard-Opitz, V. (1982). Pragmatic analysis of the communicative behavior of an autistic child. *Journal of Speech and Hearing Disorders, 47*, 99–109.

Bloom, L., Rocissano, L. & Hood, L. (1976). Adult-child discourse: developmental interaction between information processing and linguistic knowledge. *Cognitive Psychology, 8*, 521–552.

Bretherton, I. & Beeghly, M. (1982). Talking about internal states: the acquisition of an explicit theory of mind. *Developmental Psychology, 18*, 906–921.

Bruner, J. S. (1975). The ontogenesis of speech acts. *Journal of Child Language, 2*, 1–19.

Caparulo, B. & Cohen, D. J. (1977). Cognitive structures, language, and emerging social competence in autistic and aphasic children. *Journal of the American Academy of Child Psychiatry, 15*, 620–644.

Coggins, T. E. & Frederickson, R. (1988). The communicative role of a highly frequent repeated utterance in the conversations of an autistic boy. *Journal of Autism and Developmental Disorders, 18*, 687–694.

Cohen, D. J., Paul, R. & Volkmar, F. R. (1987). Issues in the classification of pervasive developmental disorders and associated conditions. In D. J. Cohen & A. M. Donnellan (Eds), *Handbook of autism and pervasive developmental disorders* (pp. 20–40). New York: Wiley.

Creak, M. (1972). Reflections on communication and autistic children. *Journal of Autism and Childhood Schizophrenia, 2*, 1–8.

Curcio, F. & Paccia, J. (1987). Conversations with autistic children: contingent relationships between features of adult input and children's response adequacy. *Journal of Autism and Developmental Disorders, 17*, 81–93.

Denckla, M. B. (1986). New diagnostic criteria for autism and related behavioral disorders—guidelines for research protocols. *Journal of the American Academy of Child Psychiatry, 25*, 221–224.

Fay, D. & Mermelstein, R. (1982). Language in infantile autism. In S. Rosenberg (Ed.), *Handbook of applied psycholinguistics* (pp. 393–428). Hillsdale NJ: Erlbaum.

Feldman, C. F. (1988). Early forms of thought about thoughts: some simple linguistic expressions of mental state. In J. W. Astington, P. L. Harris & Dr. R. Olson (Eds), *Developing a theory of mind* (pp. 126–137). New York: Cambridge University Press.

Frith, U. (1989). *Autism: explaining the enigma.* Oxford: Basil Blackwell.

Hurtig, R., Ensrud, S. & Tomblin, J. B. (1982). The communicative function of question production in autistic children. *Journal of Autism and Developmental Disorders, 12*, 57–69.

Kanner, L. (1943). Autistic disturbances of affective contact. *Nervous Child, 2*, 217–250.

Kanner, L. (1946). Irrelevant and metaphorical language in early childhood autism. *American Journal of Psychiatry, 103*, 242–246.

Kennan, E. O. (1974). Conversational competence in children. *Journal of Child Language, 1*, 163–183.

Leifer, J. S. & Lewis, M. (1984). Acquisition of conversational response skills by young Down syndrome and nonretarded young children. *American Journal of Mental Deficiency, 88*, 610–618.

Leiter, (1974). International Performance scale. In O. Buros (Ed.), *Tests in print II: index to tests, test reviews and the literature of specific tests.* Highland Park, NJ: Gryphone.

Leslie, A. M. (1987). Pretence and representation. The origins of 'theory of mind'. *Psychological Review,* **94,** 412–426.

Loveland, K. A., Tunali, B., McEvoy, R. E. & Kelley, M. L. (1989). Referential communication and response adequacy in autism and Down's syndrome. *Applied Psycholinguistics,* **10,** 301–313.

McEvoy, R. E., Loveland, K. A. & Landry, S. H. (1988). The functions of immediate echolalia in autistic children: a developmental perspective. *Journal of Autism and Developmental Disorders,* **18,** 657–668.

McHale, S. M., Simeonsson, R. J., Marcus, L. M. & Olley, J. G. (1980). The social and symbolic quality of autistic children's communication. *Journal of Autism and Developmental Disorders,* **10,** 299–310.

Mermelstein, R. (1983). The relationship between syntactical and pragmatic development in autistic, retarded, and normal children. Paper presented at the Eighth Annual Boston University Conference on Language Development, Boston, MA, October 1983.

Miller, J. & Chapman, R. (1985). *Systematic analysis of language transcripts: user's guide.* Madison WI: University of Wisconsin Language Analysis Laboratory.

Paccia-Cooper, J., Curcio, F. & Sacharko, G. (1981). A comparison of discourse features in normal and autistic language. Paper presented at the Sixth Annual Boston University Conference on Language Development, Boston, MA, October 1981.

Paul, R. (1987). Communication. In D. J. Cohen & A. M. Donnellan (Eds), *Handbook of autism and pervasive developmental disorders* (pp. 61–84). New York: Wiley.

Perner, J., Frith, U., Leslie, A. M. & Leekam, S. (1989). Exploration of the autistic child's theory of mind: knowledge, belief, and communication. *Child Development,* **60,** 689–700.

Prizant, B. M. & Duchan, J. F. (1981). The functions of immediate echolalia in autistic children. *Journal of Speech and Hearing Disorders,* **46,** 241–249.

Prizant, B. & Rydell, P. J. (1984). Analysis if functions of delayed echolalia in autistic children. *Journal of Speech and Hearing Research,* **27,** 183–192.

Ricks, D. & Wing, L. (1975). Language, communication, and the use of symbols in normal and autistic children. *Journal of Autism and Childhood Schizophrenia,* **5,** 191–221.

Schopler, E. & Mesibov, G. (Eds.) (1985). *Communication problems in autism.* New York: Plenum.

Shatz, M., Wellman, H. & Silber, S. (1983). The acquisition of mental verbs: a systematic investigation of first references to mental state. *Cognition,* **14,** 301–321.

Snedecor, G. W. & Cochran, W. G. (1967). *Statistical methods.* Ames, IA: Iowa State University Press.

Tager-Flusberg, H. (1981). On the nature of linguistic functioning in early infantile autism. *Journal of Autism and Developmental Disorders,* **11,** 45–56.

Tager-Flusberg, H. (1982). Pragmatic development and its implications for social interaction in autistic children. In D. Park (Ed.), *The proceedings of the 1981 international conference on autism* (pp. 103–107). Washington, DC: NSAC.

Tager-Flusberg, H. (1989). A psycholinguistic perspective on language development in the autistic child. In G. Dawson (Ed.), *Autism: Nature, Diagnosis and Treatment* (pp. 92–115). New York: Guilford.

Tager-Flusberg, H., Calkins, S., Nolin, T., Baumberger, T., Anderson, M. & Chadwick-Dias, A. (1990). A longitudinal study of language acquisition in autistic and Down syndrome children. *Journal of Autism and Developmental Disorders,* **20,** 1–21.

Wakabayashi, S. (1979). A case of infantile autism associated with Down's syndrome. *Journal of Autism and Developmental Disorders,* **9,** 31–36.

Wetherby, A. M. (1986). Ontogeny of communicative functions in autism. *Journal of Autism and Developmental Disorders,* **16,** 295–316.

Wetherby, A. M. & Prutting, C. (1984). Profiles of communicative and cognitive-social abilities in autistic children. *Journal of Speech and Hearing Research,* 27, 364–377.

15

Methodological Issues for Experiments on Autistic Individuals' Perception and Understanding of Emotion

R. Peter Hobson

University College, London England

The purpose of this paper is to consider problems that arise in design-ing and interpreting experimental investigations of autistic children's capacities for perceiving and understanding emotion, and to offer a review of published studies. Attention is drawn to some strengths and limitations of the experimental approach in this domain.

> Sweet is the lore which nature brings;
> Our meddling intellect
> Misshapes the beauteous forms of things
> —We murder to dissect.

Wordsworth: *The Tables Turned*

INTRODUCTION

In 1943, Kanner suggested that autistic children "have come into the world with innate ability to form the usual, biologically provided affective contact with people" (p. 250). During the two decades from 1960 to 1980, this potentially illuminating proposal was largely eclipsed by accounts in which cognitive or language dysfunc-tion featured as *the* essential feature of autism. One reason for this change in ori-entation was that a scientific technology for assessing children's cognitive and

Reprinted with permission from the *Journal of Child Psychology and Psychiatry,* 1991, Vol. 32, No. 7, 1135–1158. Copyright © 1991 by the Association for Child Psychology and Psychiatry.

I thank Beate Hermelin, Anthony Lee, Janet Ouston and Catherine Buckley for wrestling with me wrestling with these problems over recent years.

language abilities was at hand, and studies comparing autistic and non-autistic subjects on standardized IQ tests came to establish that important group differences emerge on measures of these kinds (e.g. DeMyer, Barton & Norton, 1972; Gillies, 1965; Lockyer & Rutter, 1970; Tubb, 1966). In the vanguard of the 'cognitive' movement, however, were two investigators of unusual originality and perspicacity, Beate Hermelin and Neil O'Connor, who undertook studies that were more ambitious in style; they selected autistic and specially targeted control subjects (normal, retarded, and perceptually handicapped), and employed specifically designed matching and control procedures with a view to teasing out the cognitive and linguistic processes that differentiate autistic and non-autistic children (see Hermelin & O'Connor, 1970; O'Connor & Hermelin, 1978, for summaries of this early work). What emerged was hard evidence that autistic children do have special, and probably unique, intellectual handicaps.

Yet the findings from such studies in no way justified confidence that those cognitive impairments which are characteristic of autism are 'basic' in the sense of being primary and underived from other psychological factors in development, nor 'basic' in the sense of underlying the children's remaining, and especially social-affective, disabilities. Very recently, the thrust of a fresh theoretical and methodological initiative has helped to propel Kanner's original thesis into the limelight once more (Fein, Pennington, Markowitz, Braverman & Waterhouse, 1986; Hermelin & O'Connor, 1985; Hobson, 1982, 1989a; Mundy & Sigman, 1989; Rutter, 1983). The purpose of this paper is to consider some methodological considerations that have special importance for this research programme, and to review the experimental studies reported to date.

It is fitting to begin by reflecting on the place of experimental approaches to the study of interpersonal transactions and relationships (e.g. Hinde, 1979). If science is the 'art of the soluble' (Medawar, 1967), then experimental psychologists working on autism are faced with a dilemma: do we confine ourselves to what is easily measurable and thereby shun such manifestly important issues as the qualities of human relatedness between one individual and another, or do we try to dissect out the components of organically constituted interpersonal relations and permit our 'meddling intellect' to misshape the very form of our subject matter? The experimental method requires that subjects be studied under rigorously controlled conditions, yet human relatedness usually involves exchanges between people which have highly intricate, dynamic forms, both for the experience and behaviour of each individual participant and for the interpersonal 'system' considered as such. How then might we apply the experimental method to such facets of human psychology?

I shall simplify this discussion by confining myself to the issue of autistic children's understanding of other people's bodily affective expressions. The place to begin is with a conceptual analysis of what 'understanding' means in this context. Just as knowledge admits of degrees (Hamlyn, 1978), so there are many levels of understanding. For instance, an individual might grasp *something* of the difference between, say, a person's smile and a frown, without that 'something' amounting to more than a recognition that what will follow is likely to be more agreeable in the former than in the latter case. An adequate understanding would entail a good deal more, not only about the causes and patterning of emotional expressions and behaviour, but also about the ways in which expressions are indeed 'expressive' of personal, subjective experience. It follows that an investigator of autism might target any one of a number of facets of 'emotional meaning' as a focus for research. I shall dwell on four possible options for experimental study, in order to illustrate problems that arise in choosing stimulus materials and response measures, and in devising control tasks. En route, I shall make reference to some psychometric difficulties which studies in this area are likely to encounter.

ON EMOTIONAL RESPONSIVENESS TO OTHERS' EMOTIONS

I shall begin with the plausible suggestion that a child can only come to understand other people's feelings and related subjective states of mind through his or her own capacity to react with coordinated feelings to expressions of feeling in others, that is, by sensing the impact of others' emotional states. Suppose one wanted to test whether a person frowning or smiling, or uttering a soothing voice or a scream, or making a threatening or comforting gesture has the same kind of emotional impact on autistic as on non-autistic children. An investigator would have to consider whether it makes sense to isolate the 'stimulus' facial, vocal or gestural expressions, divorced from their natural contexts in human exchanges, and whether it is feasible to present each expression or combination of expressions in a manner sufficiently standardized to make group comparisons feasible. Suppose one overcomes such problems and resolved the ethical issues. What should one take as a response measure?

A major difficulty arises because we are trying to evaluate autistic children's emotional responses to other people's expressions of feeling, but the manifestations of such responsiveness in autistic children's own expressions and behaviour are likely to be muted or idiosyncratic (Hertzig, Snow & Sherman, 1989; Langdell, 1981; Macdonald *et al.*, 1989; Ricks & Wing, 1975; Snow, Hertzig & Shapiro, 1987; Yirmiya, Kasari, Sigman & Mundy, 1989). How can an observer judge the significance of autistic children's expressions, if the normal coordinated patterns of expression and behaviour might be absent or aberrant in these children? One approach might be to study whether seemingly "normal" expressions occur in their customary behavioural and situational contexts—and studies by Dawson, Hill, Spencer, Galpert and Watson (1990) and Kasari, Sigman, Mundy and Yirmiya (1990) indicate that autistic children's smiles rarely occur along with eye contact in situations of joint attention or in response to their mothers' smiles. Even in other circumstances, to presume that an autistic child's 'smile-like' (but often not infectiously 'smile-like') facial expression means quite the same as a non-autistic child's smile would be to presume too much. Rather, one would require independent evidence of what exactly the children's bodily expressions signified, and perhaps in some cases whether they signified 'affective' responses at all.

Consider the experiment conducted by Ricks (1979). Ricks tape-recorded the spontaneous vocalizations of young autistic, non-autistic retarded and normal children in situations that the researcher designed to be those of requesting, frustration, greeting and pleased surprise. He then asked mothers to listen to the tape-recordings, and to identify which of the children's sounds came from which situations. Whereas all parents were able to recognize the contexts from which normal infants' signals were derived, but found it difficult to identify particular infants, the parents of autistic children could identify their own children *vis-á-vis* non-autistic retarded children, *and* could recognize the contexts with which their own children's cries were associated—but they were confused by the vocalizations of autistic children other than their own. Each autistic child's vocalizations were quite idiosyncratic. How are we to interpret these results? Consider the relation between a given autistic child's vocalization and a particular context, for instance, the lighting of a sparkler firework to cause surprise. If we focus upon this relation alone, it might be either that the vocalization was the child's idiosyncratic expression of surprise, or that for this child the sparkler evoked not surprise but instead some other kind of idiosyncratic emotional reaction. It is impossible to decide between these alternatives without recourse to judgements of other expressions or actions of the child, expressions and actions that are likely to present ambiguities of their own.

The point is that, when we judge the meaning of normal children's reactions, any one of a set of naturally coordinated 'cues' may serve as an adequate basis for judgement. To the extent that such 'cues' are abnormal or in coordinated in autistic children, our judgements may require the careful appraisal of multiple sources of evidence for what expressions mean, and such judgements may ultimately prove tentative and provisional. I would even suggest that one important test of the quality and meaning of autistic children's expressions is to evaluate the subjective experiences of normal people who engage with the children, in that the 'feel' of such experiences may reveal much about the abnormal patterning and communicative value of what transpires. There is clearly a need for circumspection when we interpret the expressive behaviour of autistic individuals.

ON THE UNDERSTANDING OF COORDINATED
EXPRESSIONS OF EMOTION

In the above discussion of actual and imagined experiments in relatively 'real-life' contexts, I have focused upon the problem of arriving at response measures that can be interpreted with confidence. It is a problem that occurs in a different form in the next kind of study I shall consider. In this case, the hypothesis to be adopted is that autistic children are impaired in perceiving the ways in which other people's different emotional expressions are associated with one another and with appropriate kinds of emotion-inducing event. For example, do they grasp how an angry face tends to accompany an angry voice and threatening posture, and usually occurs in response to anger-inducing situations? The issues are related to those already considered, in so far as normal children might well link the different expressions together by perceiving or 'affectively sensing' how each of the expressions is indeed expressive of a higher order feature of mental life, namely, the other person's feeling itself.

(a) The Design of Index Tasks

In order to examine whether children recognize how expressions 'hold together,' one obvious approach is to begin by dismantling whole-body expressions into component parts, such that facial expressions are divorced from vocalizations and gestures. Children can then be given the task of putting a face to a bodily gesture or vocalization or emotion-inducing situation. Such cross-modal (face-to-voice), cross-expression (face-to-gesture) and cross-situation (face-to-context) tasks are especially valuable because they require subjects to have some understanding of the meaning of the different expressions. Whereas in single-modality tasks such as faces-to-faces matching, perceptual features common to different faces may allow for successful 'non-emotional' performance strategies, such meaning-independent approaches are not likely to avail when highly diverse task materials are to be coordinated. There are, however, problems with the method. In particular, it does not follow from the fact that an individual, perhaps an infant, sees various expressions as expressive of some single state, that the individual will necessarily have the ability to abstract the 'meaning' of separated expressions and perform the highly contrived task of putting Humpty Dumpty together again (but see Walker, 1982; Walker-Andrews, 1988, for evidence that, under special conditions, normal 6-month-olds can show abilities of this kind). Nor does it follow that if another individual, say an autistic child, fails to 'sense' the emotional content common to a given facial expression and gesture, then that child will be unable to fit together static images of faces and gestures, jig-saw fashion. The reason is that there might be more than one reason for failing or more than one strategy for succeeding in this form of task. Indeed, the very artificiality of the tasks and the peculiarities of the task materials create conditions that are almost 'depersonalized' and sapped of emotional impact, to the extent that an *unnatural* strategy of matching body configurations might prove most successful for the tasks in hand. In other words, there is a danger of creating a setting in which one subject's intuitive emotional sensitivity might confer little advantage over another subject's emotionally insensitive but cognitively effective classification abilities.

At this point it is worth reviewing the rationale behind our presenting emotional-related task materials to autistic individuals. Such materials are being employed not to provide a quantitative estimate of real-life emotion recognition *per se,* but rather to test for group differences between autistic and non-autistic subjects. The underlying assumption is that, notwithstanding the artificiality of the experimental procedures, real-life emotion recognition abilities do contribute to the ease with which non-autistic children accomplish the tasks. If there were a dearth of such abilities in autistic children, therefore, then they would for this reason find the tasks more difficult than non-autistic control subjects. Given that truly interpersonal perceptiveness and sensitivity to feelings might make but a modest contribution to subjects' judgements of the highly abstracted task materials, one might anticipate that the group differences would be quantitatively small, but if they were consistent and in the predicted direction (i.e. with autistic subjects performing less well), then this would support the underlying hypothesis concerning autistic children's impairments in emotional recognition, it follows from this rationale that the aim should be to present materials that are as life-like and feeling-full as possible, so that there is maximal gain for subjects who can pick up the affective quality of the expressions being judged.

It is for these reasons that there is much to be said for employing videotape and audiotape presentations of emotional expressions (Frijda, 1953). A child can be affectively moved by 10-second sequences of a face on the television monitor or by brief audiotaped vocalizations, in a way that is very rare when the child looks at a photograph. Videotape and audiotape presentations introduce other difficulties, however. If one wishes to present 'pure' gestures, then the videotaped person will need to have a masked face. If one wishes to present 'pure' contexts for emotion, for instance depicting on videotape a person being surprised by something falling on top of him, then the person must apprehend the event only at the climax of the sequence, which must then be cut immediately if gestural reactions are not to confuse the picture—and it takes only a split-second of the person *not* reacting to convey that something odd is happening, and to influence one's judgement about his feelings. Then there is the familiar problem of selecting appropriate response measures. If subjects are asked to name the feelings expressed by the person on videotape, there is a possibility that poor performance will reflect specifically language-related disabilities rather than those pertaining to emotion recognition *per se.* If they are asked to choose photographs of facial expressions, then they may perform poorly for the reason that they are failing to attend to or discriminate amongst the relatively subtle perceptual features of the static photographs, rather than failing to grasp the meanings of the more 'alive' and obviously contrasting videotaped images that are supposed to be the focus of study. In addition, there is the problem of overcoming the potentially confounding influence of memory task demands, given that the children need to have time to consider their interpretation of transient videotaped events that have run their course.

The resolution of such difficulties may not be possible except through a piecemeal approach in which one and then another response measure is adopted. For example, one might conduct a preliminary training procedure in which subjects have to learn to match schematic drawings of expressive faces with a series of 'live' emotionally expressive faces on videotape. This would encourage all subjects to attend to the 'meaning' rather than the specific perceptual configurations of both videotaped and drawn faces, and would establish that they can discriminate among the schematic faces for the succeeding parts of the task. Given the obvious problems that might attend the use of drawings, however, photographed faces would also have to be used to corroborate any findings. Then there would be a need to 'freeze' the videotaped gestures and contexts in drawings or photographs, so that subjects could reflect on their choice of a face for each sequence of dynamic events. In case the results reflected subjects' abilities with facial drawings and photographs *per se,* one would need to test subjects for their abilities to coordinate non-facial expressions, for example, gestures with vocalizations. It would also be well to ascertain that the children could grasp non-emotional meanings in the videotaped scenes. It will be evident that such methodological maneouvres go only some way to screen out possible non-emotion-specific sources of task difficulty, and that the role of control tasks remains critically important.

Considerations like these should determine the form of the 'index tasks' to test for the coordination of emotional expressions. I shall now consider two critical aspects of experimental design that apply to this as they do to most other forms of experiment on emotion recognition in autism: the design of control tasks and the selection of control subjects.

(b) The Design of Control Tasks

I shall not dwell on the problems of devising control tasks that are adequate in terms of level of difficulty, reliability, and so on, since these routine psychometric matters have been thoroughly reviewed elsewhere (Chapman & Chapman, 1973). Even when subjects' understanding of the coordination of only two modes of expression is studied—for instance, facial and vocal expressions—the design of a sufficient range and quality of control tasks is a (perhaps *the*) major challenge. The principal reason has to do with the nature of emotional expressions. For instance, a given person's face may alter to only a minor degree in perceptible form, yet undergo a major alteration in its emotional meaning. Although there are other human attributes with comparable characteristics—the changes that accompany ageing, for example (e.g. Shaw & Pittenger, 1977)—there are very few non-human attributes in which modest changes in visual appearance correspond with changes in acoustic properties and with major changes in meaning. Strictly, the items or events featured in a control task should also undergo changes in visual appearance which include a significant dynamic component, and the changes in meaning should be reversible and signify changes in state. Otherwise, the uncontrolled non-emotion-specific variables might be responsible for differences in group performance.

The possible influence of non-emotion-specific factors in causing group differences is what makes control tasks necessary, of course. The purpose of the experimental approach is to test for group differences that reflect emotion-specific recognition abilities and disabilities. It would be mistaken to interpret autistic children's difficulties on emotion recognition tasks as difficulties with 'emotion recognition' *per se,* if they were failing to comply with such general task demands as those of memory, cross-modal matching, the recognition of 'meaning,' the understanding of abstract task materials, and so on. Or would it? I suggest that, in fact, much depends on the degree of task specificity **and** emotion-independence of the 'general' disabilities in question, and, more importantly, on the details of the hypothesis being tested and of the inferences being drawn. Suppose, for example, autistic children were poor at coordinating the visual and acoustic characteristics of a range of 'abstract' qualities and events, including expressions of emotion. If such results reflected an impairment in real-life psychological capacities, rather than simply reflecting task-specific difficulties, then we might infer that autistic children *do* have emotion recognition deficits, but that these seem to be one expression of a more general underlying 'cognitive' dysfunction. (Such a view has been propounded by Scheerer, Rothmann & Goldstein, 1945, for example.) On the other hand, the impact of such a cognitive disability in the particular domain of emotion recognition might have its own, specifically emotion-related repercussions for development, for instance in autistic children's capacity to derive a concept of persons with their own mental life (Hobson, 1990a, b). The point is that the degree of specificity that one needs to establish through experiment is closely related to the hypothesis that one is testing. It is *not* the case that emotion recognition deficits have to be independent of, or more severe than, all the other deficits of autistic children. It *is* the case that experiments in this domain need to establish that performance on a given form of task is not emotion-independent, i.e., it is not the case that one could replace the strictly emotional-related parts of the task with just about anything else, and achieve the same results.

It may be worthwhile to anchor the above rather abstract considerations with specific examples of control tasks. To illustrate the best efforts of colleagues and myself with regard to tests in which children chose photographed facial expressions for emotionally expressive voices (Hobson, Ouston & Lee, 1988a), one of our batch of control tasks required subjects to select photographs for the recorded sounds of six reversible states of a single substance, water—a stream, a waterfall, a lake, a shower, a fountain and the sea—and another involved the sounds and photographs of a person engaged in different kinds of 'walking'—running downstairs, walking on shingle, walking on a pavement, walking on rubble, running on a pavement, and walking on snow. If these tasks were approximately equal in difficulty to the emotion recognition tasks, we argued, and if autistic subjects were as proficient as control subjects in matching such non-emotional sounds and photographs but performed less well in coordinating the voices and faces of emotional expressions, then there would be evidence of at least some specificity to their difficulties in the social-affective domain. Even here, as I have noted, the degree of specificity would remain open to question—for example, the 'abstractness' of emotions, rather than their emotionality *per se*, might account for any group differences that were observed (how abstract are types of walking?). Ultimately, the resolution of such doubts would await further studies which included appropriate control conditions.

(c) The Selection of Control Subjects

There are two choices to be made in the selection of control subjects. The first is to decide whether control subjects are to be normal children, non-autistic mentally retarded subjects, individuals with receptive developmental language disorder, or children from some alternative diagnostic group. The second, closely related issue concerns the choice of matching procedures. In both cases, the most important point is that one cannot control for everything at the same time. In the long run, therefore, there is no substitute for repeating experiments with control subjects from different diagnostic groups, so that one can sift out the relative contribution of chronological age (CA), mental age (MA), specific aspects of language disability, possible perceptual abnormalities, and so on. Having said this, there are serious disadvantages in choosing MA-matched normal children as the sole or principal control group, unless the autistic subjects happen to have a normal level (if not profile) of intelligence. If the autistic subjects have some degree of general mental retardation, then normal control subjects will be lower in CA as well as higher in IQ, and it becomes impossible to disentangle whether the source of group differences on the index *and*/or control tasks has to do with either of these characteristics, rather than with the 'non-autistic' versus 'autistic' diagnostic contrast. This is especially problematic when control subjects are very young, for very young children may make errors for a wide variety of task-related as well as developmental reasons. Largely on these grounds, Prior (1979) has argued that many claims for specific impairments in autistic individuals are questionable because the control groups tested have been inadequate to exclude the possibility that the findings reflected autistic subjects' developmental delays. For many purposes, therefore, it is most appropriate to begin by testing non-autistic mentally retarded control subjects who are matched with autistic subjects for CA and MA (and therefore IQ), since this increases the likelihood that group differences are indeed autism-specific. It is of further interest if a study includes a group of matched normal children, but that is because the contrast between the normal and the *non*-autistic retarded subjects is revealing for the effects of generalized cognitive impairment on task performance. Such effects will also play a role in autistic children's difficulties, but it is only in this indirect way that normal children's performance illuminates the deficits associated with autism.

The situation needs to be analysed in far more detail than this, however. For the sake of argument, I shall consider the simplest case, in which autistic and non-autistic retarded subjects are matched for CA and 'MA' on an individual basis. The most obvious complication is that a given level of performance on a task purporting to measure 'MA' need not indicate that the matched groups are at all comparable on those 'general' intellectual abilities that may be important for constraining task performance. For example, it is widely recognized that autistic individuals not only have a radically abnormal profile of performance on the WISC (e.g. Bartak, Rutter & Cox, 1975), but they also achieve higher scores on the full-scale WISC than on the Peabody Picture Vocabulary Test (Dunn, 1965; Lockyer & Rutter, 1970). This means that if autistic subjects are systematically matched according to the full-scale WISC, then in most cases they will be systematically *un*matched on various sub-scales of the WISC, and particularly in certain of their verbal abilities. Or again, autistic subjects matched on the British Picture Vocabulary Test (Dunn, Dunn & Whetton, 1982) are likely to perform better than non-autistic control subjects on a 'non-verbal' test such as Raven's matrices (Raven, 1960, 1965; see, for example, Hobson, Ouston & Lee, 1988a). Even within the very loosely defined domains of 'verbal' and 'performance' (non-verbal) ability, a given score may reflect very different processes underlying performance in autistic and non-autistic subjects, and such processes may be highly pertinent for the interpretation of results from emotion recognition tasks (a matter to be discussed and illustrated later).

Even if for certain purposes it is justifiable to treat 'verbal ability' and 'performance ability' as coherent sets of abilities that are roughly comparable across autistic and non-autistic individuals, there still exists the thorny problem of which measure to employ for matching subjects in experiments on emotion recognition. There are two separate considerations here. The first has to do with the abilities required for real-life 'emotion recognition,' or for the perception and/or understanding of the way that people's expressions of emotion are coordinated with each other. The second has to do with the abilities required to comply with specifically task-related, and perhaps 'emotion-unrelated,' demands of the experimental procedure. In the kinds of expression-coordinating tasks under consideration, for example, subjects have to sustain attention, register and remember what they see and hear, comprehend what it means to choose a schematic or photographed face, and so on. If one now questions whether 'verbal' or 'performance' ability is either necessary or sufficient, or of marked or negligible importance, for success in such tasks, the answer is by no means self-evident. In at least certain groups of individuals engaged in certain forms of emotion recognition task, performance appears to be relatively independent of language and more closely related to holistic, right cerebral hemisphere processing (Buck, 1982; Tucker, 1981). On the other hand, it takes little imagination to think of ways that language-related conceptualization might assist with either 'real-life' understanding of emotions and/or with the mastery of non-specific task demands. If one matches autistic subjects according to non-verbal ability, therefore, it is difficult to exclude the possibility that they might achieve low scores because of their low language ability, so that either (a) it is true that they have real-life emotion recognition deficits, but these are a function of more generalized language impairments, and/or (b) they do not have such deficits, but perform poorly on the tasks because they are at a disadvantage in meeting non-specific, emotion-independent task demands.

The most obvious way to circumvent this difficulty is to match subjects according to verbal ability. There are serious problems with this strategy, however. Suppose it is *not* the case that language-related, non-specific task demands are constraining performance and therefore determining the patterns of scores (a matter that might be decided by employing specifically language-impaired non-autistic control subjects). Generally speaking, autistic children's language abilities are amongst the most impaired of their cognitive capacities (e.g. Bartak *et al.*, 1975; Gillies, 1965). If one is going to ascribe deficits in emotion recognition to autistic children only if they are *more* impaired in this regard than on language-related tests, then one is setting a very stringent criterion for what are to count as deficits. Indeed, one may be setting an inappropriate criterion. Suppose it proved to be the case that verbal MA-matched autistic and non-autistic subjects achieved similar scores on emotion recognition tasks, as in fact has been the case in a number of published studies (to be discussed later). In this case, to focus on the absence of group differences would be to discount the discrepancy between autistic subjects' low scores on emotion recognition tasks and their relatively higher scores on measures of 'non-verbal' ability (e.g., Braverman, Fein, Lucci & Waterhouse, 1989; Hobson, 1986a,b: Ozonoff, Pennington & Rogers, 1990; Tantam, Monaghan, Nicholson & Stirlin, 1989)—a discrepancy which might be the critical pointer to abnormalities in the social-affective realm. The crucial question would be whether subjects' levels of verbal ability were determining task performance—and this could not simply be presumed on the strength of a correlation between verbal MA and emotion recognition scores. Indeed, if the importance of language ability were such as to justify matching according to verbal MA, then to the extent that language-related ability determined task performance, it might also put constraints on the emotion recognition scores of lower ability control subjects and obscure group differences that would otherwise be evident.

The second difficulty with matching according to verbal ability is more subtle, but if anything more important. Suppose, once again, that autistic and non-autistic subjects matched for CA and verbal MA performed with roughly equal success on tests of emotion recognition. It should not be assumed that it is verbal ability that determines emotion recognition ability, whether in tasks or in real-life, when it might equally be the case that autistic children's language disabilities arise wholly or in part from problems that can be traced back to early deficits in recognizing and reacting to emotions in others. Although this claim might appear to be implausible, it is easy to overlook how greatly the learning and use of language is dependent upon the existence of meanings and frames of reference shared between a child and other people, and these in turn rely heavily on the child's awareness of people with minds of their own (e.g. Baron-Cohen, 1988; Hobson, 1989a). If emotional responsivity and awareness makes an important contribution to a child's capacity to share with others (Hobson, 1989b; Mundy & Sigman, 1989), then even serious language impairments in autistic children might reflect developmental sequelae to primary social-affective deficits. A study by Mundy, Sigman and Kasari (1990) lends weight to this suggestion, in that language development in their sample of young autistic children was predicted by a measure of gestural non-verbal joint attention 1 year previously, but *not* by measures of initial language score or IQ (in contrast with the situation for non-autistic retarded control subjects). It is even conceivable that linguistic sequelae might be more severe or more prominent than the original deficits which caused them. Therefore, to match according to verbal ability might be to 'control out' at least a portion of the variance attributable to group differences in emotion recognition ability. Comparisons between children with autism and those with specific language impairments which are not due to emotion-related deficits might be especially revealing here, for the reason that in this control group 'verbal' and 'emotion-related' abilities might *not* be correlated. The essential point is that a correlation between two abilities in autistic and/or control subjects does not establish the nature of the connectedness between the abilities in either group of children, nor indeed whether a connection exists at all (see Hobson *et al.*, 1988a, for further discussion of this point).

The upshot of this argument is that far greater emphasis needs to be placed on subjects' relative abilities on emotion recognition tasks *vis-á-vis* specially designed control tasks, than on any observed group similarities adjudged with reference to often ambiguously determined performance on relatively non-specific matching tasks, such as the British Picture Vocabulary Scale (see Hobson & Lee, 1989, and later discussion). There are also additional strategies that may be helpful in examining whether or not the potential hazards of each kind of matching procedure do in fact apply in a given set of studies. For example, if one matches autistic and control subjects according to scores on Raven's matrices (Raven, 1960, 1965), a relatively 'non-verbal' measure, one should seek for evidence that language-related task demands might be rendering the task incomprehensible to autistic subjects. If very few subjects are found to be responding randomly on the emotion recognition tasks, and if they tackle control tasks of similar design with great ease, then it becomes less plausible that language-related task demands are rendering the task an 'emotion-independent' linguistic challenge. In other words, it should be possible to screen subjects for their ability to meet basic language-related and other non-specific task demands, such that matching according to non-verbal measures becomes a rational and for certain purposes an appropriate methodological approach. Ultimately, of course, it is desirable to measure the disparities and cor-relations among a range of cognitive abilities and indices of emotion recognition ability from a variety of differently designed tasks, or preferably to match subjects according to different abilities on different occasions.

(d) The Interpretation of Results

We are now in a position to appraise the results from experiments that have been conducted on autistic children's understanding of the ways that people's emotional expressions are coordinated with one another. My own early studies in this domain (Hobson, 1987a,b) incorporated many of the design features noted earlier—relatively 'live' videotaped and audiotaped materials were presented; these were truly representative of different emotions; subjects indicated their judgements by choosing both schematic and photographed faces and subsequently drawn gestures, and so on—but the major limitations were that (a) the control task was not equated with the index task for level of difficulty, and ceiling effects rendered this non-emotion condition a 'screening' task for subjects' ability to meet basic task demands, rather than a true control task; (b) the principal control group comprised normal subjects, although a smaller non-autistic retarded group also took part; and (c) the principal matching procedure involved the use of Raven's matrices, a non-verbal measure, so that the possible influence of autistic children's language disabilities was largely untested. The findings were that there *were* group differences in the expected direction, with autistic subjects performing less well than the matched normal children on all parts of the emotions task, and less well than the matched non-autistic retarded children on all but the 'contexts' condition; nearly all the autis-tic children were not responding randomly on the emotions tasks; and the autistic as well as non-autistic children could easily master the general task demands, as indicated by their near-ceiling performance on the non-emotion screening tasks and their ability to predict the 'non-emotional' implications of videotaped scenes. The principal conclusion was that autistic children had difficulties in coordinating expressions of emotion (for whatever underlying reason, and with whatever degree of specificity), to a degree that was out of keeping with their non-verbal (Raven's) abilities.

We followed up this result with a more elaborate study on face-to-voice expression matching (Hobson *et al.*, 1988a). In this case, autistic and non-autistic retarded subjects were individually matched according to verbal ability and CA, and a range of carefully constructed control tasks with appropriate levels of difficulty were included (examples were given earlier in this paper). Once again, the results were that, relative to nonautistic retarded control subjects, the autistic subjects performed less well on the emotion tasks than on the non-emotion tasks. On the other hand, when the two verbal MA-matched groups were compared on the emotion tasks considered in isolation, the group difference was not significant. Similarly Prior, Dahlstrom and Squires (1990) found no significant group differences in cross-modal emotion matching tasks designed on the model of my own earliest videotape tasks, which thus included only screening tasks rather than appropriately difficult control tasks, which thus included only screening tasks rather than appropriately difficult control tasks for non-emotion matching. The most important point here, one that these authors curiously failed to emphasize as being in contrast with my own earlier experiments, is that autistic and non-autistic retarded subjects' emotion recognition performance was evaluated in relation to performance on a 'verbal' matching task, the Peabody Picture Vocabulary Test. In this respect, therefore, the Prior *et al.* (1990) results conform with those reported in Hobson *et al.* (1988a), except that only in the latter study were there control tasks adequate to reveal the significant group-by-task interaction.

An investigation by Ozonoff *et al.* (1990) also included a sound-to-photograph cross-modal matching task alongside a non-emotional control task. This study failed to provide evidence for specificity in autistic children's impairments in cross-modal affect matching. Although these results need to be weighed carefully, the experiment of Hobson *et al.* (1988a) had the following methodological advantages over that by Ozonoff *et al.* (1990): non-autistic retarded rather than normal control subjects were employed, and very close individual subject-to-subject matching according to CA as well as (BPVS) verbal ability was achieved, removing the potential confounding effects on task performance of control subjects' much younger ages and higher IQs; the subject groups were much larger (21 subjects per group in Hobson *et al.*, 1988a, rather than 13 or 14 subjects per group in Ozonoff *et al.*, 1990); Hobson *et al.* (1988a) tested a broader range of emotions, and control tasks were selected to represent items in relatively homogeneous sets of non-emotion objects and events; the range of scores on both the emotion and non-emotion tasks was wider and less near 'ceiling' than in the study by Ozonoff *et al.* (1990) and overall performance was more similar across diagnostic groups—whereas in Ozonoff *et al.*'s (1990) study the autistic subjects tended to perform less well than control subjects on both emotion and non-emotion tasks, there was a cross-over in profiles of performance in the study by Hobson *et al.*, with autistic subjects scoring (non-significantly) higher than control subjects on the non-emotion tasks and (non-significantly) lower on the emotion tasks, to yield a significant group-by-task interaction. Having stated this, it is important to acknowledge that in these experiments, the differences between autistic and non-autistic subjects' performance on emotion-related *vis-á-vis* emotion-unrelated tasks were quantitatively small, even when qualitatively significant. The principal issues to be addressed are whether one would require group contrasts that were quantitatively more impressive before ascribing a perceptual-affective deficit to autistic children, and whether such an ascription can be discounted by the finding that verbal MA-matched autistic and non-autistic subjects are not significantly different when one reviews their performance on tests of coordinating emotional expressions in isolation from that on psychometrically adequate control tasks. The latter of these issues has already been discussed at some length; the former may be approached by evaluating the present results alongside those from different kinds of emotion recognition study, and it is to these that I now turn.

ON ATTENTIVENESS TO AND DISCRIMINATION OF EMOTIONAL EXPRESSIONS

It is often helpful to design studies in which tasks are presented that do not have a correct or incorrect solution, but which afford subjects the opportunity to tackle problems in different ways that might reveal important group differences. Not all of the following experiments fall into this category, but a number of them involve attempts to get beneath the surface of 'raw scores' in order to appraise the processes or 'strategies' that underlie subjects' performance. This may be particularly helpful in sorting out whether group differences arise because of developmental 'deviance' or delay. I have already referred to the importance of such methodology when investigators are presenting single-modality tasks such as those of face-matching, for the reason that similar levels of task performance may be achieved in every different ways by autistic and non-autistic children. What we really need to know is whether or not there are group differences in sensitivity to the 'emotional' content of the task materials.

For this section of the paper, the underlying hypothesis is that either through innate neuropsychological faculties or through abilities sharpened by attentiveness to bodily characteristics, non-autistic children are especially adept at discriminating the facial, vocal or other bodily expressions of others, but that autistic children are abnormal in their relative inability to discriminate and/or attend to such expressions. Here I shall illustrate the methodological points by proceeding directly to a review of specific experiments. Weeks and Hobson (1987) conducted a study with 15 autistic and 15 non-autistic retarded subjects, individually matched for chronological age, sex, and performance on three subtests of the verbal scale of the WISC-R. Subjects were given a task of sorting photographs to 'go with' one or the other of a pair of target photographs showing the head and shoulders of individuals who differed in three, two or one of the following respects: sex, age, facial expression of emotion, and the type of hat they were wearing. The principal statistically significant finding was that the majority of non-autistic children sorted according to people's facial expressions ("happy" versus 'non-happy') before they sorted according to type of hat (floppy versus woollen), but most autistic children gave priority to sorting by type of hat. Moreover, when in the course of the experiment the number of contrasting features in the target photographs was progressively reduced, all 15 non-autistic children sooner or later sorted by emotional expression without being told to do so, but only six of the 15 autistic children did this ($p = 0.0003$, Fisher's exact test). Finally, five the 15 autistic children but none of the 15 non-autistic children failed to sort consistently by facial expression when given explicit instructions to do so.

Only after we had completed this experiment did we discover that Jennings (1973) had conducted a similar (not identical) unpublished study which yielded results that were comparable to our own. Jennings (1973) tested 11 autistic and 11 non-autistic retarded children aged between 5 and 14 years, group-matched for age and verbal ability on the Peabody Picture Vocabulary Test, together with normal children aged 3–7 years, on a task designed by Savitsky and Izard (1970) in which subjects had to point to which two out of three photographs were the same or almost the same. There were 96 such groups of three photographs, and each 'triad' showed one particular individual with either (a) the same expression (either happiness, sadness, fear or anger) in all photographs, but wearing a hat in only two out of the three photographs (24 triads), (b) wearing the same hat in all photographs, but with two faces showing the same emotional expression and the third with a neutral expression (24 triads), or (c) one face with an emotional expression but with no hat, one face with the same emotional expression and a hat, and the third with a neutral expression and a hat (48 triads). The first result was that autistic but not control subjects performed significantly better than pairing by hats (condition a) than in pairing by emotional expressions (condition b). This was due to autistic children's superior performance in the former task rather than lower scores in the latter task; the three groups' similar scores in sorting by 'emotions' when these were the only cue provided indicates that the autistic children could *discriminate* the expressive faces from neutral faces (by whatever perceptual strategy), a fact that is relevant for interpreting the subsequent finding. The second result was that in the 'strategy choice trials' (condition c), the autistic children paired significantly more often on the basis of hats and less often on the basis of emotional expressions than did either of the control groups (in fact, the autistic children paired on the basis of emotion about one-quarter as often as either control group, and we have seen how this could not be attributed to a failure in discriminating the expressions). Jennings also conducted a simple emotion recognition study in which each emotionally expressive face was paired (twice) with a neutral face, and subjects were asked to "point to the one who is . . . happy/afraid of something/mad at somebody/*or* sad or unhappy," and in this very simple task autistic subjects performed less well than control subjects but to a non-significant degree.

It is worth emphasizing that the group differences in these tasks occurred with small groups of subjects matched both for CA and *verbal* ability. The tasks illustrate how one may need to 'fine-tune' the content of emotion-related materials presented to autistic subjects. One has to ensure that both emotion-related and emotion-unrelated features are sufficiently prominent to serve as bases for sorting photographs, and that neither kind of feature is so prominent as to completely overshadow the presence or relevance of the other. More important and more problematic than this is the need to reduce the likelihood that emotion-related features are being registered in a 'non-emotion-related' manner. The point is that one cannot determine whether what *we* call an emotion-related feature is 'emotional-related' for subjects, especially for autistic subjects, even when it happens that the subjects do attend to the feature in question.

This principle may be relevant for interpreting the results from a second class of studies, namely those comprising photographic facial affect matching tasks, in some of which there have appeared to be modest or non-significant emotion-specific group differences. For example, Braverman *et al.* (1989) tested autistic and normal control subjects on three well-piloted choice-from-sample photograph matching tasks. A non-social control task involved matching objects photographed in different views, a non-affective social task involved matching differently photographed faces by identity, and the affect task involved matching photographed faces (some with different identities) according to emotional expression. The principal results were that the children with pervasive developmental disorder performed significantly less well than non-verbal MA-matched normal children on affect matching tasks, but less well only to a non-significant degree when compared with verbal MA-matched (and therefore younger) normal children. Given that the normal control children were as young as 3 years 3 months old (mean age 5 years 4 months), it is quite possible that this factor may have introduced additional task-related constraints on their performance. An additional finding was that unlike non-verbal MA-matched normal children, those with pervasive developmental disorder were impaired on affect matching relative to their own performance on object matching (the differences on identity matching were suggestive but non-significant), a result that seemed to indicate at least a moderate degree of specificity to these subjects' emotion recognition deficits.

The investigation by Ozonoff *et al.* (1990), also limited by the use of young normal rather than non-autistic retarded control subjects, employed relatively simple (e.g. happy versus sad) photographic affect and identity matching tasks that were not equated for difficulty and that yielded some near-ceiling scores, and

photographic match-from-sample tasks similar to those of Braverman *et al.*
(1989). There were no significant group-by-task interactions when subjects were
matched for their spontaneous mean length of utterance. As the authors noted,
however, this matching procedure may not be appropriate, given that it assesses
spontaneous social interaction as well as language development. When subjects
were matched according to non-verbal MA, the group differences on emotion
sorting were highly significant and those on identity sorting were noon-
significant (although for these relatively small groups of subjects, the interaction
here was also non-significant); and on the photographic match-to-sample tasks,
autistic subjects were similar to control subjects on object matching, but impaired
on identity as well as affect matching tasks. Given the reservations expressed by
Ozonoff *et al.* (1990) about the evidence for specific emotion perception deficits
in autism, it is particularly notable that in a recent study employing a new, well-
designed facial matching task for emotions across photographs of different individuals with different intensities of emotion, these same investigators have
reported significant group differences between groups of autistic and Asperger
subjects and a heterogeneous group of CA- and verbal MA-matched non-autistic
control subjects (Ozonoff, Pennington & Rogers, 1991; Ozonoff, Rogers &
Pennington, 1991). Finally, Hertzig *et al.* (1989) included photograph matching
and 'selection' tasks (e.g. 'show me her happy face') amongst the tests they
administered to group-matched (Peabody) autistic, non-autistic retarded, and normal children. When compared with scores on 'activity'-related tasks (concerning
eating, drinking and sleeping), autistic subjects' scores on these particular affect-
related tasks revealed no specific impairment. The major drawback here was that
each affect-related task involved a restricted range of items, there being but a single item each involving angry, happy and sad facial expressions.

   Thus, although there has been a trend for autistic subjects to perform less well
than control subjects on emotion-related *vis-à-vis* emotional-unrelated tasks in
straightforward 'single-modality' facial matching tasks, statistically significant
group-by-task interactions have been an inconsistent finding. Given that the results
from Jennings (1973) and Weeks and Hobson (1987) were so striking, and given
the emotional face matching deficits in autistic subjects recently reported by
Ozonoff *et al.* (1991) we need to enquire how it could be that the results on photograph matching tasks are sometimes equivocal. The findings from a further face
matching task conducted by Hobson, Ouston and Lee (1988b) might help to resolve
this paradox. It will be recalled that Braverman *et al.* (1989) and Ozonoff *et al.*
(1990) employed a control task in which faces were matched by identity. So, too,
did our own independently designed study (Hobson *et al.*, 1988b). We found that
verbal MA-matched autistic and non-autistic retarded subjects were equally proficient in sorting full faces of different people according to the same emotions, and
equally proficient in sorting full faces of people with different emotions according

to their individual identities. Once again this might seem to be strong evidence against highly specific emotion recognition deficits in autism, at least with respect to facial expressions. However, we also gave the same tasks with the photographed faces having blanked-out mouths, and again with the faces having blank mouths and foreheads. The materials were designed so that even the latter photographs retained some 'feel' of the emotions in the faces. The results included a significant second-order interaction of diagnosis by condition (emotion, identity) and form of face (full-face, blank-mouth, blank-mouth-and-forehead): whereas on the identities task, the performance of the two groups showed a similar steady decline as the photographs became increasingly blanked-out, on the emotions task the performance of autistic subjects worsened more abruptly than that of control subjects as cues to emotion were progressively reduced. The autistic subjects seemed relatively unable to use the 'feel' in the faces to guide performance. Not only this, but correlations between individual subjects' scores on the identity and emotion tasks were higher for autistic than for non-autistic subjects, suggesting that the autistic subjects might have been sorting the expressive faces by 'non-emotional' perceptual strategies—a suggestion that is also in keeping with the pattern of autistic subjects' errors in the face matching study of Ozonoff *et al.* (1991). Finally, the whole task was repeated with upside-down faces—and here, the autistic subjects achieved significantly higher scores than control subjects in matching both 'identities' and 'emotions'!

The most important conclusion to be drawn from all this is that group similarities in scores on face matching or other simple emotion recognition tasks may not indicate similarities in the processes underlying task performance. If autistic and control subjects are tackling the tasks in fundamentally different ways, it may be mistaken to construe non-significant group contrasts as evidence for relatively normal emotion recognition abilities among autistic children. This point is more than hypothetical—there is evidence that it matters. The above findings are supported by those from the study by Tantam *et al.* (1989), who reported that autistic children performed unusually well in choosing labels for emotions in upside-down faces, relative to their performance on other emotion recognition tasks. Or again, Macdonald *et al.* (1989) reported that high-ability autistic subjects' ability to name emotions in expressive speech was relatively little affected when the speech was electronically filtered. The possibility arises that apparently conflicting evidence about emotion recognition deficits in autism may turn out not to be conflicting after all, once the contributions of non-emotion-related and truly emotion-related task strategies are differentiated. It may also prove that, in so far as autistic individuals accomplish 'emotional recognition' tasks, they may often be doing so in a manner that reflects a radically abnormal mode of 'recognition' rather than by processes suggestive of more straightforward developmental delay.

A third methodological approach to testing subjects'; ability to discriminate emotional expressions has been to ask the children to provide names for facial and vocal expressions of emotion. The most elaborate controlled study is that by Hobson *et a.* (1989), who asked subjects to give free-response labels for photographs of emotionally expressive faces and audiotape recordings of expressive voices, and also labels for photographs and sounds of non-emotional objects and events. Autistic subjects differed from verbal MA-matched non-autistic retarded and normal subjects in being relatively poor at naming feelings in both faces and voices *vis-á-vis* naming the images and sounds of non-personal objects. Similarly Tantam *et al.* (1989) reported that autistic and non-autistic retarded subjects matched for age and non-verbal (Raven's) ability were not significantly different in choosing names for photographed objects, but differed in their ability to select labels for emotions portrayed in upright photographed faces. Results from an uncontrolled pilot study by Scott (1985) suggested that subjects with Asperger's syndrome might have similar deficits. Or again, Hertzig *et al.* (1989) reported that in a task eliciting 'descriptions' of affect- and activity-related photographs ('how does she feel/what is she doing?'), autistic children were relatively poor at naming feelings. Thus it is in the context of experiments featuring non-emotional control tasks that most of the evidence for emotion-specific naming deficits in autism has been obtained.

On the other hand, Hobson *et al.* (1989) noted that when scores on their emotion naming tasks were considered in isolation, the group differences between BPVS-matched autistic and control subjects were no longer statistically significant. So, too, in the study by Braverman *et al.* (1989), children with autism who were matched with normal children according to non-verbal MA performed significantly less well than control subjects in tests of 'affect labelling' ('How does the person feel?') as well as 'affect comprehension' ('Show me the happy face'), but these group differences were more modest and no longer significant when subjects were matched according to verbal ability. Such results are also in keeping with the report by Szatmari, Bartolucci, Krames, Flett and Tuff (1989) that, when IQ was taken into account, autistic adolescents were not significantly different from normal-IQ control subjects in their ability to identify videotaped bodily expressions of emotion. Yet, as has been emphasized, there is a need to exercise caution in interpreting apparent group similarities when these are judged solely with reference to complexly determined performance on matching tasks. This suggestion receives empirical support from two further studies, one by Hobson and Lee (1989) to be discussed shortly, and the other by Macdonald *et al.* (1989). Macdonald *et al.* (1989) tested very high-ability autistic adults and control subjects for the ability to name emotions in expressive speech, and to name facial affect photographs, as well as to match them with contexts that might elicit each emotion. The autistic subjects were significantly poorer on each of these tasks than their non-verbal MA-matched control subjects, and in general these effects could *not* be attributed to discrepant verbal abilities across the subject groups. In this case, there was evidence for emotion-related naming difficulties which were out of keeping with autistic subjects' verbal disability.

Taken together, the findings from affect naming tasks offer substantial but not unequivocal support for the earlier evidence that there are specific emotion recognition deficits in autism.

ON UNDERSTANDING EMOTION-RELATED CONCEPTS

A potentially fruitful approach to the study of specifically emotion-related perceptual capacities is to adopt the perspective of genetic epistemology (Piaget, 1972). Genetic epistemology might be characterized as the study of the origins and development of knowledge or, strictly speaking, the study of the possibility of the growth of knowledge (Hamlyn, 1982). If we can identify concepts for which appropriately configured emotional sensitivity and experience are essential substrates or ingredients, then we would predict that in individuals who have profound dysfunction of affective organization and relatedness, such concepts will be specifically shallow or aberrant. The most obvious concept-dependent candidates for study are emotion words *per se,* but there is a complication here that relates to our earlier concerns with the specifically emotional-related content of task materials. The complication is that there are various kinds of meaning to emotion words, or to express this differently, a variety of criteria according to which emotion words may be learned (and taught). Even an individual with profound disorder in affect-perception and affective experience might come to appreciate certain uses and meanings of such words. As noted earlier, knowledge admits of degrees, and a child might learn that 'unhappy' is a word relevant to a tearful child, even if he or she had little comprehension of the subjective dimensions or perhaps the motivational implications of unhappiness. If this were the case, then only in certain circumstances or only to some degree would the child's conceptual limitations become apparent. It might even prove to be the case that concepts which seem to be emotion-unrelated, but from a developmental perspective are founded on earlier capacities for appropriate kinds of emotion-related experience, are more drastically impoverished than 'emotion' concepts themselves.

Consider the concept of 'persons', that is, the concept of human beings who have both bodily and mental attributes (Strawson, 1962). As previously argued elsewhere (Hobson, 1989a,b), autistic children's concepts of persons with their own subjective mental life may be deficient precisely by virtue of the children's failure to engage in reciprocal, affectively charged personal relations. If this is so, then one would predict that autistic children should fail to grasp concepts that capture particular aspects of people's subjective mental lives, such as notions of belief. There is recent evidence to suggest that such concepts are relatively lacking or deficient in autistic individuals (e.g. Baron-Cohen, 1989; Baron-Cohen, Leslie & Frith, 1985; Leslie & Frith, 1988; Perner, Frith, Leslie & Leekam, 1989). In so far as the concept of 'belief' might represent a developmentally advanced distillate of those aspects of subjective mental life that are first recognized through the perception of emotionally expressive behaviour, then a child's concept of people's beliefs may require a background of emotional-related understanding; and in so far as concepts of belief are unlike concepts of emotion in being more or less exclusively anchored to the child's understanding of the nature of subjectivity and consciousness, autistic children might be expected to manifest more striking conceptual imitations in relation to beliefs than in relation to emotions. In fact, Tager-Flusberg (1989) has reported that autistic children's spontaneous use of words referring to cognitive states such as belief is more markedly deficient than their use of emotion words. My purpose in citing these (controversial) points of theory is to emphasize how difficult it may be to evaluate evidence of the primacy of 'cognitive state' over 'emotion-related' conceptual deficits—much depends on the quality of the children's understanding of the emotion words.

The thrust of the argument is that group differences in the 'affective-personal' domain should be apparent in certain circumstances, but will not be apparent in others. The problem arises because it is not an easy matter to decide *a priori* under which natural or experimental conditions the extent of autistic children's abilities and disabilities will be revealed or concealed. Recent experiments have illustrated that emotion-related concepts *are* specifically impaired in autistic individuals. The evidence from tasks of naming or describing photographed facial and audiotaped vocal expressions of emotion has already been described. We have also noted evidence that autistic individuals have difficulty in matching expressions of emotion with contexts for the feelings expressed (Hobson, 1986a; MacDonald *et al.*, 1989; see also, Dawson & Fernald, 1987). In a recent study by Baron-Cohen (1991), autistic and non-autistic mentally retarded subjects who achieved similar scores on the British Picture Vocabulary Scale (BPVS: Dunn *et al.*, 1982) were asked questions about very simple emotions (happiness and sadness) prompted by stereotyped situations or desires: the performance on 'situations' was at ceiling for each group, and the retarded subjects performed as poorly as autistic subjects on the 'desires' condition. Considering the reported ceiling effects on the former task and the complex relation between performance on the BPVS and on tests of emotion comprehension (especially tests that take the form of questions), Baron-Cohen's (1991) conclusion that his findings documented 'new areas of relatively intact social understanding in autism' may be premature. A more searching test of emotion-related conceptual understanding has been reported by Hobson and Lee (1989). Whereas non-autistic retarded subjects achieved similar scores on emotion-related items at roughly the same point on the British Picture Vocabulary Scale (Dunn *et al.*, 1982), individually matched autistic subjects with almost identical *overall* BPVS scores were specifically impaired on the emotion-related items. These items had been rated as 'emotion-related' by independent judges, and they included word-picture combinations in which the words to be judged were delighted, disagreement, greeting and snarling, as well as more obviously 'emotional' words such as horror and surprise. Moreover, the results could not be attributed to the abstract nature of such concepts, since autistic and non-autistic subjects were equally able to judge non-emotion-related abstract words *vis-á-vis* equally difficult 'concrete' words. Once again, therefore, this time at a conceptual level, significant group differences between autistic and non-autistic subjects were demonstrable specifically in the realm of emotional understanding. And once again, this time on a test of language ability that is widely employed as a matching procedure in experiments on autism, similar levels of overall performance belied different profiles of performance in autistic and non-autistic subjects, thereby obscuring potentially important emotional-related group contrasts even on a supposedly 'cognitive' test. Such findings illustrate how tentative one should be about using such a test as the sole benchmark for evaluating autistic subjects' performance on emotional-related tasks. They also indicate that in an experiment which involved autistic and non-autistic retarded subjects almost exactly matched for CA and 'verbal ability' on an individual basis, and which included emotion-related and (relatively) emotion-unrelated items of almost identical level and range of difficulty, autistic subjects demonstrated specific impairments in the affective domain.

CONCLUSIONS

I have tried to pinpoint some sources of difficulty for designing and interpreting experiments on autistic individuals' perception and understanding of emotion. I have also tried to indicate how easily we may be led astray when reviewing evidence in this domain. In particular, I have highlighted problems in evaluating the meaning of autistic children's own 'expressive' behaviour, in selecting appropriate control groups and matching procedures, in devising control tasks and interpreting their relevance for different kinds of experimental hypothesis, and in determining whether emotional-unrelated aspects of apparently emotion-related task materials or response measures might confound the results.

The considerations that arose in these methodological respects have led me to advance two more controversial theses. The first arises from the fact that experiments of the kinds reviewed here include forms of task that are highly contrived. In particular most task materials involve seriously 'degraded' representations of dynamic emotional-related interpersonal events. I believe that such experimental approaches are nevertheless warranted because they are being employed to test for specific group differences between closely matched groups of subjects. As such, they are likely to prove invaluable for dissecting out the patterns of association and dissociation amongst a cluster of autistic individuals' abilities and disabilities. On the other hand we need to acknowledge that in the domain of emotion recognition, differential task performance is a very crude index of group differences in subjects' real-life abilities and propensities (a point also made by Braverman *et al.,* 1989). It follows that, when testing the hypothesis of autism-specific impairments in emotion recognition and understanding, it is far less important to discover marked group differences than to find evidence of significant group contrasts in the expected direction on a range of different emotion recognition tasks, each of which might illustrate a separable facet of autistic individuals' abnormalities in attending to, discriminating, understanding or finding words for people's feelings or emotional-related states of mind. If this reasoning is correct, then there is the obvious implication that experiments which do not test relatively large, closely matched groups of subjects on appropriate index and control tasks might fail to yield significant findings, even though the results might be expected to manifest trends in the expected direction. The results from the studies cited here more or less conform to this pattern.

The second argument, linked to the first, is that providing the experimental design is adequate in relation to choice of control groups and control tasks, then findings indicative of significant differences between autistic and non-autistic subjects may be more telling than results which seem to reveal modest or insignificant group differences. Amongst the most important factors to bear in mind here are the different forms of interrelationship that may exist amongst the abilities required for succeeding on the matching measures, the index tasks and the control tasks, and the different 'strategies' or processes that may yield similar levels of performance in each of these areas.

These arguments bear upon the way we evaluate the evidence for or against specific emotion recognition deficits in autism. What they do not resolve is whether any such deficits are a source of an effect of autistic children's impaired interpersonal relations. Even if emotion-perceptual deficits are primary rather than secondary, they may not be the only or the essential universal feature of the children's impairments in the capacity for appropriately patterned 'non-verbal' communicative interaction with other people. If autism is best viewed as a profound disorder of *inter*personal relations (Hobson, 1989a, 1991), then it might be the case that certain children who have relatively intact *potential* for affective contact with others are nevertheless rendered autistic (or 'autistic-like') by other kinds of severe impediment to interpersonal perception and/or coordination (e.g. congenital blindness: Frailberg, 1977; Hobson, 1990a; Keeler, 1958).

Finally, it is necessary to return to the point with which I began in the Introduction, and to set experimental studies in context. Autistic children's inabilities to communicate and to share, including their incapacities for 'non-verbal' bodily anchored affective contact with other people, must surely feature amongst their cardinal abnormalities. In the broadest sense, it is a matter of methodology that, in our attempts to define autistic children's social-affective impairments, experimental evidence should complement and be complemented by our intuitive judgements of what is lacking or awry in the children's capacities for personal relatedness. I suggest that results from experiments on emotion recognition and understanding in autism are beginning to dovetail with and perhaps enrich the clinical insights of Kanner (1943) in this regard.

REFERENCES

Baron-Cohen, S. (1988). Social and pragmatic deficits in autism: cognitive or affective? *Journal of Autism and Developmental Disorders, 18,* 379–402.

Baron-Cohen, S. (1989). The autistic child's theory of mind: a case of specific developmental delay. *Journal of Child Psychology and Psychiatry, 30,* 285–297.

Baron-Cohen, S. (1991). Do people with autism understand what causes emotion? *Child Development, 62,* 385–395.

Baron-Cohen, S., Leslie, A. M. & Frith, U. (1985). Does the autistic child have a "theory of mind"? *Cognition, 21,* 37–46.

Bartak, L., Rutter, M. & Cox, A. (1975). A comparative study of infantile autism and specific developmental receptive language disorder. I. The children. *British Journal of Psychiatry, 1267,* 127–145.

Braverman, M., Fein, D., Lucci, D. & Waterhouse, L. (1989). Affect comprehension in children with pervasive developmental disorders. *Journal of Autism and Developmental Disorders, 19,* 301–316.

Buck, R. (1982). Spontaneous and symbolic nonverbal behaviour and the ontogeny of communication. In R. S. Feldman (Ed.), *Development of nonverbal behavior in children* (pp. 29–62). New York: Springer.

Chapman, L. J. & Chapman, J. P. (1973). *Disordered thought in schizophrenia.* New York: Appleton-Century-Crofts.

Dawson, G. & Fernald, M. (1987). Perspective-taking ability and its relationship to the social behavior of autistic children. *Journal of Autism and Developmental Disorders, 17,* 487–498.

Dawson, G., Hill, D., Spencer, A., Galpert, L. & Watson, L. (1990). Affective exchanges between young autistic children and their mothers. *Journal of Abnormal Child Psychology, 18,* 335–345.

DeMyer, M. K., Barton, S. & Norton, J. A. (1972). A comparison of adaptive, verbal and motor profiles of psychotic and non-psychotic subnormal children. *Journal of Autism and Childhood Schizophrenia, 2,* 359–377.

Dunn, L. M. (1965). *Expanded manual for the Peabody Picture Vocabulary Test.* Circle Pines, MN: American Guidance Service.

Dunn, L. M., Dunn, L. M. & Whetton, C. (1982). *British Picture Vocabulary Scale.* Windsor: NFER-Nelson.

Fein, D., Pennington, B., Markowitz, P., Braverman, M. & Waterhouse, L. (1986). Toward a neuropsychological model of infantile autism are the social deficits primary? *Journal of the American Academy of Child Psychiatry,* **25,** 198–212.

Fraiberg, S. (1977). *Insights from the blind.* London: Souvenir.

Frijda, N. H. (1953). *The understanding of facial expression of emotion. Acta Psychologica,* **9,** 294–362.

Gillies, S. (1965). Some abilities of psychotic children and subnormal controls. *Journal of Mental Deficiency Research,* **9,** 89–101.

Hamlyn, D. W. (1978). *Experience and the growth of understanding.* London: Routledge & Kegan Paul.

Hamlyn, D. W. (1982). What exactly is social about the origins of understanding? In G. Butterworth & P. Light (Eds), *Social cognition* (pp. 17–31). Brighton: Harvester.

Hermelin, B. & O'Connor, N. (1970). *Psychological experiments with autistic children.* Oxford: Pergamon Press.

Hermelin, B. & O'Connor, N. (1970). Logico-affective states and nonverbal language. In E. Schopler & G. B. Mesibov (Eds), *Communication problems in autism* (pp. 283–310). New York: Plenum Press.

Hertzig, M. E., Snow, M. E. & Sherman, M. (1989). Affect and cognition in autism. *Journal of the American Academy of Child Psychiatry,* **28,** 195–199.

Hobson, R. P. (1982). The autistic child's concept of persons. In D. Park (Ed.), *Proceedings of the* 1981 *International Conference on Autism, Boston, U.S.A.* (pp. 97–102). Washington DC: National Society for Children and Adults with Autism.

Hobson, R. P. (1986a). The autistic child's appraisal of expressions of emotion. *Journal of Child Psychology and Psychiatry,* **27,** 321–342.

Hobson, R. P. (1986b). The autistic child's appraisal of expressions of emotion: a further study. *Journal of Child Psychology and Psychiatry,* **27,** 671–680.

Hobson, R. P. (1989a). Beyond cognition: a theory of autism. In G. Dawson (Ed.), *Autism: nature, diagnosis, and treatment* (pp. 22–48). New York: Guilford.

Hobson, R. P. (1989b). On sharing experiences. *Development and Psychopathology,* **1,** 197–203.

Hobson, R. P. (1990a). On acquiring knowledge about people, and the capacity to pretend: response to Leslie. *Psychological Review,* **97,** 114–121.

Hobson, R. P. (1990b). Concerning knowledge of mental states. *British Journal of Medical Psychology,* **63,** 199–203.

Hobson, R. P. (1991). Social perception in high-level autism. In E. Schopler and G. Mesibov (Eds), *High-functioning individuals with autism.* New York: Plenum Press (in press).

Hobson, R. P. & Lee, A. (1989). Emotion-related and abstract concepts in autistic people: evidence from the British Picture Vocabulary Scale. *Journal of Autism and Developmental Disorders,* **19,** 601–623.

Hobson, R. P., Ouston, J. & Lee, A. (1988a). Emotion recognition in autism: coordinating faces and voices. *Psychological Medicine,* **18,** 911–923.

Hobson, R. P., Ouston, J. & Lee, A. (1988b). What's in a face? The case of autism. *British Journal of Psychology,* **79,** 441–453.

Hobson, R. P., Ouston, J. & Lee, A. (1989). Naming emotion in faces and voices: abilities and disabilities in autism and mental retardation. *British Journal of Developmental Psychology, 7,* 273–250.

Jennings, W. B. (1973). A study of the preference for affective cues in autistic children. Unpublished Ph.D. thesis, Memphis State University.

Kanner, L. (1943). Autistic disturbances of affective contact. *Nervous Child, 2,* 217–250.

Kasari, C., Sigman, M., Mundy, P. & Yirmiya, N. (1990). Affective sharing in the context of joint attention interactions of normal, autistic, and mentally retarded children. *Journal of Autism and Developmental Disorders, 20,* 87–100.

Keeler, W. R. (1958). Autistic patterns and defective communication in blind children with retrolental fibroplasia. In P. H. Hoch & J. Zubin (Eds), *Psychopathology of Communication.* New York/London: Grune & Stratton.

Langdell, T. (1981). Face perception: an approach to the study of autism. Unpublished Ph.D. thesis, University of London.

Leslie, A. M. & Frith, U. (1988). Autistic children's understanding of seeing, knowing and believing. *British Journal of Developmental Psychology, 6,* 315–324.

Lockyer, L. & Rutter, M. (1970). A five- to fifteen-year follow-up study of infantile psychosis. IV. Patterns of cognitive ability. *British Journal of Social and Clinical Psychology, 9,* 152–163.

Macdonald, H., Rutter, M., Howlin, P., Rios, P., Le Couteur, A., Evered, C. & Folstein, S. (1989). Recognition and expression of emotional cues by autistic and normal adults. *Journal of Child Psychology and Psychiatry, 30,* 865–877.

Mcdawar, P. B. (1967). *The art of the soluble.* New York: Barnes & Noble.

Mundy, P. & Sigman, M. (1989). Specifying the nature of the social impairment in autism. In G. Dawson (Ed.), *Autism: nature, diagnosis, and treatment* (pp. 3–21). New York: Guilford.

Mundy, P., Sigman, M. & Kasari, C. (1990). A longitudinal study of joint attention and language development in autistic children. *Journal of Autism and Developmental Disorders, 20,* 115–128.

O'Connor, N. & Hermelin, B. (1978). *Seeing and hearing and space and time.* London: Academic Press.

Ozonoff, S., Pennington, B. F. & Rogers, S. J. (1990). Are there emotion perception deficits in young autistic children? *Journal of Child Psychology and Psychiatry, 31,* 343–361.

Ozonoff, S., Pennington, B. F. & Rogers, S. J. (1991a). Executive function deficits in high-functioning autistic individuals. *Journal of Child Psychology and Psychiatry* (in press).

Ozonoff, S., Rogers, S. J. & Pennington, B. F. (1991b). Asperger's syndrome: evidence of an empirical distinction from high-functioning autism. *Journal of Child Psychology and Psychiatry* (in press).

Perner, J., Frith, U., Leslie, A. M. & Leekam, S. R. (1989). Exploration of the autistic child's theory of mind: knowledge, belief and communication. *Child Development, 60,* 689–700.

Piaget, J. (1972). *The principles of genetic epistemology* (translated by W. Mays). London: Routledge & Kegan Paul.

Prior, M. R. (1979). Cognitive abilities and disabilities in infantile autism: a review. *Journal of Abnormal Child Psychology, 7*, 357–380.

Prior, M. R., Dahlstrom, B. & Squires, T. I., (1990) .Autistic children;'s knowledge of thinking and feeling states in other people. *Journal of Child Psychology and Psychiatry, 31*, 587–601.

Raven, J. C. (1960). *The standard progressive matrices: sets A, B, C, D and E.* London: H. K. Lewis.

Raven, J. C. (1965). *The coloured progressive matrices: sets A, Ab, B.* London: H. K. Lewis.

Ricks, D. M. (1979). Making sense of experience to make sensible sounds. In M. Bullowa (Ed), *Before speech* (pp. 245–268). Cambridge University Press.

Ricks, D. M. & Wing ,L. (1975). Language, communication and the user of symbols in normal and autistic children. *Journal of Autism and Childhood Schizophrenia, 5*, 191–221.

Rutter, M. (1983). Cognitive deficits in the pathogensis of autism. *Journal of Child Psychology and Psychiatry, 24*, 513–531.

Savitsky, J. C. & Izard, C. E. (1970). Developmental changed in the use of emotion cues in a concept-formation task. *Developmental Psychology, 3*, 350–357.

Scheerer, M., Rothmann, E, & Goldstein, K, (1945). A case of "idiot savant" an experimental study of personality organization. *Psychological Monographs, 58*, (No. 269), 1-63.

Scott, D. W. (1985). Asperger's syndrome and non-verbal communication: a pilot study. *Psychological Medicine, 15*, 683–687.

Shaw, R. & Pittenger, J. (1977). Perceiving the face of change in changing faces: implications for a theory of object perception. In R. Shaw & J. Branford (Eds), *Perceiving, acting and knowing: toward an ecological psychology* (pp. 103–132). Hillsdale, NJ: Lawrence Erlbaum.

Snow, M. E., Hertzig, M. E. & Shapiro, T. (1987). Expression of emotion in young autistic children. *Journal of American Academy of Child and Adolescent Psychiatry, 26*, 838–838.

Strawson, P. F. (1962). Persons. In V. C. Chappell (Ed), *The philosophy of mind* (pp. 127–146). Englewood Cliffs, NJ: Prentice-Hall.

Szatmari, P., Bartolucci, G., Krames, L., Flett, G. & Tuff, I.(1989). The perception of non-verbal social information among adolescents with pervasive developmental disorders. Unpublished manuscript.

Tager-Flusberg, H. (1989). An analysis of discourse ability and internal state lexicons in a longitudinal study of autistic children. Paper presented at the Biennial Meeting of the Society for Research in Child Development, Kansas City.

Tantam, D., Monaghan, L., Nicholson, H. & Stirlin, J. 1989). Autistic children's ability to interpret faces: a research note. *Journal of Child Psychology and Psychiatry, 30*, 623–630.

Tubbs, V. K. (1966). Types of linguistic disability in psychotic children. *Journal of Mental Deficiency Research, 10*, 230–240.

Tucker, D. M. (1981). Lateral brain function, emotion, and conceptualization. *Psychological Bulletin,* **89,** 19–46.

Walker, A. S. (1982). Intermodal perception of expressive behaviors by human infants. *Journal of Experimental Child Psychology,* **33,** 514–535.

Walker-Andrews, A. S. (1988). Infants' perception of the affordances, of expressive behaviors. In C. Rovee-Collier (Ed.), *Advances in infancy research* (Vol. 5, pp. 173–221). Norwood, NJ: Ablex.

Weeks, S. J. & Hobson, R. P. (1987). The salience of facial expression for autistic children. *Journal of Child Psychology and Psychiatry,* **28,** 137–151.

Yirmiya, N., Kasari, C., Sigman, M. & Mundy, P. (1989). Facial expressions of affect in autistic, mentally retarded and normal children. *Journal of Child Psychology and Psychiatry,* **30,** 725–735.

16

Rett Syndrome: A Review of
Current Knowledge

Rick Van Acker
University of Illinois at Chicago

Rett syndrome was first described in 1966 by Andreas Rett. To date, this syndrome has been reported only to afflict females. The disorder is characterized by a progressive loss of cognitive and motor skills as well as the development of stereotypic hand movements, occurring after an apparently normal 6 to 18 months of development. Although Rett syndrome is thought to afflict as many as 10,000 girls in the United States, fewer than 1,200 have been identified thus far. A lack of awareness of this disorder is thought to play a critical role in the failure to differentially diagnose this syndrome. The present article presents a review of our current knowledge concerning this disorder. Information is provided related to the clinical manifestations, etiology, prevalence, pathogenesis, and treatment of the Rett syndrome.

Rett syndrome, at least in its classical form, is a phenotypically distinct progressive neurological disorder with a characteristic pattern of cognitive and functional stagnation and subsequent deterioration. The disorder was first described by Rett (1966, 1969) following his serendipitous discovery of a number of girls displaying strikingly similar behavioral characteristics and developmental histories. Unfortunately, Rett reported substantially increased levels of blood ammonia (hyperammonemia), a finding that was subsequently found only rarely associated with this disorder. This false lead, coupled with very limited exposure (Rett, 1977) of this information in the English language medical literature, resulted in a general failure to recognize Rett syndrome as a nosologic entity. In fact, the syndrome had been virtually overlooked until Hagberg, Aicardi, Dias, and Ramos (1983) published their report of 35 girls from France, Portugal, and Sweden with Rett syn-

Reprinted with permission from the *Journal of Autism and Developmental Disorders*, 1991, Vol. 21, No. 4, 381–406. Copyright © 1991 by the Plenum Publishing Corporation.

drome in the *Annals of Neurology*. This landmark account awakened the recognition and interest of clinicians and researchers and provided credit to Rett for his pioneering efforts on the disorder that bears his name.

CLINICAL MANIFESTATIONS

Individuals with Rett syndrome exhibit a characteristic course of development (Naidu, Murphy, Moser, & Rett, 1986). Prenatal and perinatal histories of these persons are generally unremarkable. Parents report normal physical and mental development for the first 7 to 18 months of life as evidenced by physical growth and psychomotor and verbal behavior (Gillberg, 1987). This apparently normal period of development is followed by a slowing or cessation of the acquisition of developmental milestones (e.g., walking in many cases). Rapid deterioration of behavior is evidenced by loss of acquired speech, voluntary grasping, and the purposeful use of the hands. The girls begin to exhibit a lack of sustained interest in persons or objects and demonstrate limited interpersonal contact, however, eye contact is maintained (Holm, 1985; Trevathan & Naidu, 1988; Witt-Engerstrom, 1987). This deterioration is typically accomplished by age 3, occurs within 1 year or less, and results in apparent severe to profound mental retardation and stereotyped behaviors. The developmental deterioration is accompanied by the onset of deceleration of head growth, coarse, jerky movements of the trunk and limbs, a stiff-legged, broad-based gait with rather short steps and swaying movements of the shoulders when ambulating (Coleman & Gillberg, 1985; Hanefield, 1985; Kerr & Stephenson, 1986; Naidu et al., 1986; Percy, Zoghbi, & Riccardi, 1985). A leading symptom of the syndrome involves stereotypic hand clasping, "hand washing," and hand-to-mouth movements similar to those displayed in Figure. 1 (Ishikawa et al., 1978; Leiber, 1985). As individuals with Rett syndrome approach adolescence they are frequently subject to increased spasticity and vasomotor disturbances of the lower limbs, possible loss of existing ambulation, scoliosis, and a diminished rate of growth. Facial grimacing, bruxism (teeth grinding), hyperventilation, apnea (breath holding), aerophagia (air swallowing), constipation, and seizure activity also sometimes accompany the syndrome (Trevathan & Naidu, 1988). Hagberg and Witt-Engerstrom (1986) proposed a staging system to facilitate the characterization of the disorder patterns and profiles from infancy through adolescence. Their system suggests four clinical stages and was derived from a synthesis of clinical observations over the years in 50 Swedish cases of Rett syndrome. The purpose of the staging system is to provide average guidelines for stage patterns thought to be of use when confronted with the diagnostic problems resulting from the complex symptomatology and longitudinal profile of the condition. Some points of nosologic interest for each of the various stages are presented.

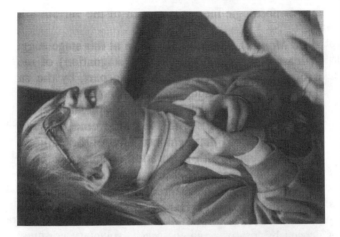

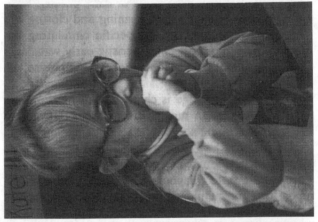

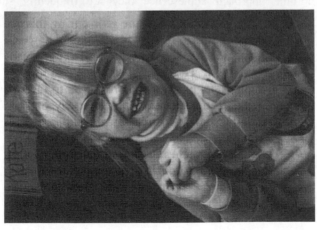

Figure 1. Stereotypic hand movements in Rett syndrome.

Stage 1 (Onset 6–18 Months).

The clinical profile at this stage sugggests a deterioration, or at least a general slowing down (stagnation) of motor development. This is often compensated or hidden, in part, by the rapid developmental speed of infancy. Thus, additional gross motor abilities often are learned during this stage but are delayed in their appearance. Some researchers have suggested that persons with Rett syndrome display significant abnormalities from birth and that demonstration of the pathogenesis simply becomes more noticeable with maturation (Nomura & Segawa, 1990). For example, Opitz and Lewin (1987) in a study of eight girls with Rett syndrome reported that to "variable degrees all patients showed evidence of congenital hypotonia" (p. 447). Hanefield (1985) also expressed the view that persons with Rett syndrome may have a "dyskinetic" disturbance of hand movement from birth. Excess levels of hand patting, waving, and involuntary movements including alternate opening and closing of the fingers, twisting of the wrists and arms, or nonspecific circulating hand-mouth movements appear to be the most characteristic early warning signals for the syndrome (Home, 1985; Kerry, Montague, & Stephenson, 1987; Witt-Engerstrom, 1987).

Stage 2 (Onset 1–3 Years).

This stage is characterized by the obvious loss of previously acquired abilities. In most individuals a relatively well-demarcated period of rapidly declining social interaction, stagnation or loss of acquired cognitive abilities, and loss of purposeful hand use and speech is evident. This deterioration frequently has been sufficiently dramatic to simulate a toxic or encephalitic state (Hagberg & Witt-Engerstrom, 1986). Parents frequently report that their children seem irritable and "spontaneous tantrums" are common. Stereotyped movements, often virtually continuous during waking hours, become a prominent symptom. Seizure activity is present in approximately one fourth of the girls during this stage.

Stage 3 (Onset 2–10 Years).

During this stage we find that persons with Rett syndrome display diminishing autistic symptomatology and improved social interaction is reported. The intellectual functioning of the girl with Rett syndrome during this stage is generally reported to fall within the severe to profound range of mental retardation. Spasticity or rigidity and scoliosis tend to progress and "jerky" truncal ataxia and apraxia becomes prominent.

Stage 4 (Onset 10 + Years).

Progressive muscle wasting, scoliosis, spasticity, and rigidity frequently are displayed during this final stage. Decreasing mobility and a number of late stage second neuron abnormalities (e.g., drop foot abnormalities, remarkably plantar-flexed feet) may require the use of a wheelchair. Seizure activity often becomes less problematic. Social interaction (eye contact) and attentiveness improve. Expressive and receptive language, however, are virtually nonexistent.

This four-stage clinical pattern and profile for Rett syndrome has been reported to be "a sometimes crude and a somewhat simplistic frame" for specifically characterizing and covering the whole profile in all cases (Hagberg & Witt-Engerstrom, 1986, p. 58). Transitions between stages are not uncommonly indistinct and there are often problems when one attempts to separate the stages accurately for research purposes (Philippart, 1986). Even so, the staging system has been found to be a useful instrument for a more systematic registration, thought, and approach to the complex clinical manifestations of individuals with the Rett syndrome and their changes. Although persons over the age of 25 have been identified, the oldest currently being 65 years of age (International Syndrome Association, 1990), little systematic research has been conducted with this group to provide information on the course of the disorder past adolescence.

DIAGNOSTIC CRITERIA AND DIFFERENTIAL DIAGNOSIS

Diagnostic criteria for inclusion and exclusion of Rett syndrome have been delineated (Hagberg, Goutieres, Hanefeld, Rett, & Wilson, 1985) and are presented in Table 1. Rett syndrome, to date, is exclusively described in female patients, nevertheless, the possibility of a male case cannot be ruled out. Some researchers (Coleman, 1990; Philippart, 1990), in fact, have presented case study reports of three males displaying behavioral symptoms and developmental histories similar to those reported for Rett syndrome. Thus, the male sex is not presently considered in the exclusionary criteria. The presentation of Rett syndrome differs considerably depending upon the stage and age of observation. For example, a child of 4 or 5 years of age with classical Rett syndrome can be correctly diagnosed with relative ease. The period during infancy, however, is frequently misinterpreted due to vague symptomology. Likewise, the late stage in adolescence displays a common, complex, multihandicapped picture of extreme severity with secondary contractures that resembles any number of disorders and, therefore, often misdiagnosed. The entire disease process must be recognized and considered to fully understand this condition (Trevathan & Naidu, 1988).

Only 11% of the estimated 8,000-10,000 girls in the united States afflicted with Rett syndrome have been identified thus far (Moser. 1986). Lack of awareness of

TABLE 1
Diagnostic Criteria for Rett Syndrome[a]

Necessary criteria
1. Apparently normal prenatal and perinatal period
2. Apparently normal psychomotor development through the first 6 months
3. Normal head circumference at birth
4. Deceleration of head growth between ages 5 months and 4 years
5. Loss of acquired purposeful hand skills between ages 6 and 30 months, temporally associated with communication dysfunction and social withdrawal
6. Development of severely impaired expressive and receptive language, and presence of apparent severe psychomotor retardation
7. Stereotypic hand movements such as hand wringing/squeezing, clapping/tapping, mouthing, and "washing"/rubbing automatisms appearing after purposeful hand skills are lost
8. Appearance of gait apraxia and truncal apraxia-ataxia between ages 1 and 4 years
9. Diagnosis tentative until 2 to 5 years of age

Supportive criteria
1. Breathing dysfunction
   a. Periodic apnea during wakefulness
   b. Intermittent hyperventilation
   c. Breath-holding spells
   d. Forced expulsion of air or saliva
2. EEG abnormalities
   a. Slow waking background and intermittent rhythmic slowing (3-5 Hz)
   b. Epileptiform discharges, with or without clinical seizures
3. Seizures
4. Spasticity often with associated development of muscle wasting and dystonia
5. Peripheral vasomotor disturbances
6. Scoliosis
7. Growth retardation
8. Hypotrophic small feet

Exclusion criteria
1. Evidence of intrauterine growth retardation
2. Organomegaly, or other signs of storage disease
3. Retinopathy or optic atrophy
4. Microcephaly at birth
5. Evidence of perinatally acquired brain damage
6. Existence of identifiable metabolic or other progressive neurologic disorder
7. Acquired neurologic disorders resulting from severe infections or head trauma

[a]Reproduced with permission from Trevathan and Naidu (1988).

this disorder on the part of physicians and clinicians is undoubtedly a major contributing factor to this state of affairs. Even when physicians are aware of the Rett syndrome, however, and accurate diagnosis is not always forthcoming. As mentioned above the vague symptomology associated with this disorder complicate the screen diagnosis, especially in the earliest stage. Table 2 presents some of the clinical characteristics and differential diagnosis often assigned to persons with Rett syndrome. The most common nonspecific diagnosis for children with Rett syndrome above age 1 is reported to be the infantile autistic syndrome (Olsson, 1987).

TABLE 2
Comparison of Rett Syndrome and Infantile Autism[a]

Rett syndrome
1. Normal development to 6 to 18 months
2. Progressive loss of speech and hand function
3. Profound mental retardation in all functional areas
4. Acquired microcephaly, growth retardation, decreased weight gain
5. Stereotypic hand movements always present
6. Progressive gait difficulties, with gait and truncal apraxia and ataxia; some may become nonambulatory
7. Language always absent
8. Eye contact present, and sometimes very intense
9. Little interest in manipulating objects
10. Seizures in at least 70% in early childhood (various seizure types)
11. Bruxism, hyperventilation with air-swallowing and breath-holding common
12. Choreoathetoid movements and dystonia may be present
Infantile autism
1. Onset from early infancy
2. Loss of previously acquired skills does not occur
3. More scatter of intellectual function. Visual-spatial and manipulative skills often better than apparent verbal skills
4. Physical development normal in the majority
5. Stereotypic behavior is more varied in manifestation and is always more complex; midline manifestations rare
6. Gait and other gross motor functions normal in first decade of life
7. Language sometimes absent; if present, peculiar speech patterns always present; markedly impaired nonverbal communication
8. Eye contact with others typically avoided or inappropriate
9. Stereotypic ritualistic behavior usually involves skillful but odd manipulation of objects or sensory self-stimulation
10. Seizures (usually temporal-limbic complex partial) in 25% in late adolescence and adulthood
11. Bruxism, hyperventilation, and breath-holding not typical
12. Dystonia and chorea not present[b]

[a]Reproduced with permission from Trevathan and Naidu (1988).
[b]Extrapyramidal signs may appear in some patients with autism after puberty.

In fact, many children with Rett syndrome seem to fulfill the necessary criteria sufficient to establish the diagnosis of infantile autism (Gillberg, 1987; Olsson, 1987; Olsson & Rett, 1985). Thus some researchers (Allen, 1988; Gillberg, 1989) argue that perhaps Rett syndrome might best be thought of as a subtype of autism or overlapping diagnostic entities. Recent research efforts (Naidu et al., 1990; Olsson, 1987; Olsson & Rett, 1985, 1990; Percy, Zoghbi, Lewis, & Jankovic, 1988), however, have identified some clinically important differences between the Rett syndrome (especially during the latter two stages) and other conditions with autism or autistic traits. A basic distinction between the two disorders can be made on the basis of motor behavioral analysis (Olsson & Rett, 1985, 1987; Percy et al., 1988). "Whereas autism represents a regression of verbal but not motor skills, Rett syndrome involves the apparently simultaneous regression of both skills" (Percy et al., 1988, p. S67). Children with Rett syndrome reportedly differ from children with infantile autism with respect to their respiratory pattern (displaying breath-holding, hyperventilation, and air-saliva expulsion), the presence of ataxia and apraxia, hypoactivity and a general slowness of movements, an absence of purposeful hand movement, and stereotyped hand movements including wetting hands with saliva, handwashing movements, continually bringing hands together, and flexing and stretching the middle finger joints (Giliberg, 1986; Olsson, 1987; Percy et al, 1988). Persons with Rett syndrome demonstrate a very restricted repertoire of movements that appear monotonous in both form and speech (Olsson & Rett, 1985). Van Acker (1987) reported that the stereotypic behaviors of persons with Rett syndrome were displayed in patterned sequences with significant conditional probabilities, whereas those of persons with infantile autism were displayed in a random fashion. Another critical feature that may help in the differential diagnosis of Rett syndrome and infantile autism has been presented by Budden (1986): Persons with Rett syndrome frequently develop appropriate speech before the onset of symptoms. On the other hand, children with autism differed from those with Rett syndrome in that they displayed overactivity, inappropriate vocalizations, and tended to replicate simple motor activities or complex movements within a rich repertoire of motor behavior (Percy et al., 1988).

Olsson (1987) reported that of the 14 criteria delineated by Rendle-Short (1969) as characteristic of autism, girls with Rett syndrome may display the following: (a) severe problems on contact with others; (b) acts as if deaf but responds actively and positively to music; (c) resists invitations to learn new things; (d) no fear of real dangers; (e) resistance to divergence from the familiar; (f) expression of wishes through gestures; (g) giggling and laughter without evident cause; (h) lack of eye contact; and (i) social isolation. Olsson (1987) suggested, however, that in the Rett syndrome there are more pronounced deviations (individual differences) with regard to these characteristics and "that some of the children with Rett syndrome fail to fulfill the criteria for infantile autistic syndrome by a long way" (p. 498). Furthermore, 5 of the Rendle-Short criteria were not seen in persons with Rett syndrome. These include: (a) predominant rejection of caressing and tenderness; (b) conspicuous physical hyperactivity in terms of continuous grabbing and concomitant locomobility; (c) excessive attachment to certain objects; (d) rotation of small objects; and (e) stereotypic playing habits. Olsson concluded that "although many children with the Rett syndrome fulfill the criteria for the infantile autistic syndrome, they do so in a qualitatively different way" (p. 498).

In a comparison of two boys with Heller's syndrome (disintegrative psychosis) and six girls with Rett syndrome, Burd, Fisher, and Kerbeshian (1989) reported persons afflicted with these disorders differed from children with classic autism.

Children with Heller dementia and Rett syndrome displayed normal prenatal and perinatal periods, followed by marked developmental regression after which they acquired few or no new skills. The authors suggested that these children should be distinguished from those with classic autism, and should be classified as "pervasive disintegrative disorder, Heller type" and "pervasive disintegrative disorder, Rett type."

In summary, one must acknowledge that considering the present concept of infantile autism as a behavioral syndrome, the initial differential diagnosis of Rett syndrome for some children may prove somewhat problematic. Infantile autism, however, is rare in females which means that the mere presence of severe autistic symptomology in a girl under the age of 2 would prompt the consideration or Rett syndrome in the differential diagnosis. One must also be aware, however, that "a large percentage of children with Rett syndrome age 0–6 months or older than 3–5 years are not autistic" (Olsson & Rett, 1987). Thus, physicians and clinicians alike must realize that the presence of an autistic behavioral syndrome is not an obligatory condition for a diagnosis of Rett syndrome (Olsson & Rett, 1987).

EPIDEMIOLOGY

There are, at this time, approximately 1,420 cases of the Rett syndrome worldwide registered with the International Rett Syndrome Association, with the following distribution: United States, 1,165; Canada, 65; Mexico, 3; and other foreign, 189 (International Rett Syndrome Association, 1990). The prevalence of the Rett syndrome has been studied, based upon the Swedish registry for mental retardation and surveys of neuropediatricians, in a part of southwestern Sweden comprising five counties and the city of Gothenburg (Hagberg, 1985). In a population of 315,469 children and adolescents, 6 to 17 years of age, 13 cases were detected, all girls. The corresponding prevalence was about 1 per 15,000 live female births. Recent information from Scotland, based upon records from the only child neurology referral service in a well-defined area, indicates that the prevalence rate might be somewhat higher; 1 per 12,000–13,000 (Kerr & Stephenson, 1986). Thus, Rett syndrome seems more common (almost twice as prevalent) among girls than phenylketonuria (PKU), a condition that is screened for in all neonates in the majority of developed countries (Hagberg, 1985). As progressive brain disorders and metabolic diseases together constitute only 5–6% (1.5–2.0 per 10,000 children) of the etiologies in severely mentally retarded persons, the Rett syndrome should be considered an important etiological factor in females. In fact, this syndrome might well be responsible for one fourth to one third of progressive developmental disabilities among girls (Hagberg, 1985).

Anecdotal case information reported from most parts of the world (e.g., Budden, 1986; Goutieres & Aicardi, 1985; Hanaoka, Ishikawa, & Kamoshita, 1985; Kerr

& Stephenson, 1986) supports the suggestion that the Rett syndrome does not seem to be a rare phenomenon and that it is more or less universal; additionally less than 2 per 100 cases of Rett syndrome display familial relationships (Zoghbi, 1988). Thus, the pattern of occurrence of Rett syndrome is quite dissimilar to that of traditional inborn errors of metabolism (e.g., glactosemia, Hartnup's disease, ketoaciduria, phenylketonuria) which often display strong geographical, ethnical, and familial accumulation.

ETIOLOGY

Although the Rett syndrome can be distinguished from other childhood developmental disabilities, and although systematically researched, the genesis of this disorder has eluded explanation. Rett syndrome, to date, has only been described in females. Additionally, a number of familiar cases (represented in Table 3) have been reported with a prominent pattern of commonality along maternal lines and complete concordance in monozygotic twins (Zoghbi, 1988). A genetic basis for this disorder, therefore, has been sought by several investigators (Gillberg,

TABLE 3
Familial cases in Rett Syndrome[a]

	No. of pairs
Monozygotic twins	
Both females afflicted	7
Only one female afflicted	0
Dizygotic twins (female/female)	
Both females afflicted	0
Only one female afflicted	3
Dizygotic twins (female/male)	
Female afflicted	7
Full sisters	6
Half-sisters	2
Full cousins	1
Second cousins	1
Second half-cousins	1
Aunt–niece	1
Great-grand aunt–niece	1
Sister and half-brother, both have children with Rett syndrome	1

[a]Modified from Zoghbi (1988) with information provided through the International Rett Syndrome Association (April 15, 1990).

Wahlstrom, & Hagberg, 1984, 1985; Hanefeld, Hanefeld, Wilischowski, & Schmidtke, 1986; Killian, 1986; Riccardi, 1986) but these efforts have been inconclusive. The hypothesis of X-linked new mutations which might cause early abortions of hemizygous male fetuses and a dominant phenotype in heterozygous females, however, seems the most likely genetic explanation of the Rett syndrome (Comings, 1986; Riccardi, 1986). Zoghbi (1988) suggested that the familial pattern showing the presence of more than one daughter with Rett syndrome in a family where the mother is apparently not affected could best be explained by the possibility of a nonrandom X chromosome inactivation in these mothers.

> It is possible that the X chromosome carrying the Rett gene is predominantly inactivated as a consequence of selection favoring cells in the X chromosome carrying the normal gene. During gametogenesis, however, this X chromosome is reactivated and the Rett gene is expressed in the female fetus, while the male fetus may be aborted. (p. 577)

Some support for this hypothesis was reported by Riccardi (1986).

Wahlstrom and his associates (Gilliberg, Wahlstrom, & Hagberg, 1985; Wahlstrom, 1985; Wahlstrom & Anvret, 1986) have suggested a convincing argument for an alternative two-step mutation explaining the epidemiological findings in the Rett syndrome. This hypothesis postulates that girls with the Rett syndrome would have an inherited mutated gene in one of the X chromosomes in addition to a somatic mutation at the same locus in the other X chromosome. An inherited mutated gene or a somatic cell mutation in a male zygote would result in an early abortion.

The evidence for a genetic etiology for the Rett syndrome is perhaps promising, but is obviously inconclusive at the present time. Future research is needed to enable us to identify if any of the present hypotheses are indeed valid. Ultimately the female-limited nature of the Rett syndrome may prove misleading in regards to the importance of the X chromosome. The research on the genetic basis of the Rett syndrome has been reviewed by Hillig (1985) and Zoghbi (1988).

PATHOPHYSIOLOGY

Although the pathogenesis of the Rett syndrome is unknown, one hypothesis is that symptoms results from an abnormality in the dopamine system, a neurotransmitter system that regulates the control of voluntary movements in the extrapyramidal system. This hypothesis, based on clinical findings suggestive of extrapyramidal dysfunction (Zoghbi, Percy, Glaze, Butler, & Riccardi, 1985), has led Nomura and her associates (Nomura, Segawa, & Higurashi, 1985) to speculate that as the disease progresses the dopamine system becomes hyperactive due to postsynaptic supersensitivity caused by hypoactive dopamine neurons. Abnormality in the dopamine system is supported by the finding of a decrease of biogenic amine metabolites in cerebrospinal fluid in six children with Rett syndrome, the most significant reductions being in homovanillic acid (HVA), the major dopamine metabolite (Zoghbi et al., 1985). An abnormality in this system is further supported by demonstration of decreasing binding of ^{3}H-spiperone, a ligand with high affinity for dopamine D2 receptors, in the putamen in an autopsy study (Riederer et al, 1985). Hand-mouth stereotypies, hypotonia, and ataxia similar to that seen in Rett syndrome are demonstrated in boys with the Lesch Nyhan syndrome, a disorder where all biochemical aspects of the function of dopamine neuron terminals in the corpus striatum have been found to be decreased up to 10–30% of control values in autopsy studies of three affected cases (Lloyd et al., 1981).

Recently, however, studies have failed to replicate the findings that the Rett syndrome is characterized by abnormal neurotransmitter levels. Unlike the six cases reported by Zoghbi et al. (1985) where norepinephrine and dopamine metabolites were reduced in comparison to control individuals, subjects in a more recent investigation (Harris et al., 1986) did not demonstrate a reduction in metabolites of either of these neurotransmitter substances. Reduction of dopamine D2 receptor binding in the putamen was not demonstrated in living subjects by *in vivo* positron emission tomography (PET) scanning as found by Riederer et al. (1985) with ^{3}H-spiperone in his autopsy study. Additionally, low normal receptor binding rather than dopamine receptor suspersensitivity was reported (in direct opposition to the results reported by Nomura et al., 1985). Similar findings are reported in a second study (Riederer et al, 1986). Preliminary biochemical analyses on plasma, urine cerebrospinal fluid, and postmortem brain areas indicated no disturbance of neurotransmitter function. These researchers suggest that undernutrition (a problem common to girls with the Rett syndrome) might influence the synthesis and turnover of these biogenic amines. An alternative hypothesis might suggest, however, that such a deficit might also be triggered as a primary consequence of the disease process.

Neuropathological studies in the Rett syndrome have been few. One brain autopsy from England (Harding, Tudmay, & Wilson, 1985), a forensic report from Vienna (Missliwetz & Depastas, 1985), the summary of eight autopsies done in Vienna by Jellinger and Seiteberger (1986), and a later single autopsy from Vienna (Brucke, Sofic, Killian, Rett, & Riederer, 1988) indicated that malnutrition was common before death, and that diffuse brain atrophy with a decrease in brain weight by 13.8–33.8% to that of age-matched controls is a common nonspecific finding. The degree of atrophy appears to be related to the duration of the disorder. No evidence of active degeneration disease, however, has been seen, and the whole brain seems to be affected by the atrophy. The most conspicuous specific finding was an underpigmentation of the substantia nigra which contained many fewer well-pigmented neurons for the age of the person (53–73%), and fewer pigmented granules per neuron, while the total number of nigral neurons and the triphasic substructure of neuromelanin were within the normal range. These findings were supported in a study of Lekman et al. (1989). Brucke et al. (1988) also reported low melanin content in the locus coeruleus. They suggest this lack of pigmentation serves as "evidence of a retardation in maturation of these neurons [in the substantia nigra and locus coeruleus] which possibly leads to a decreased synthesis rate of dopamine and a compensatory enhancement in its turnover rate" (p. 323). Increased levels of dopamine and serotonin metabolites in their subject support their hypothesis. The pathogenetic mechanisms of the morphologic brain lesions and their relations to clinical and neurochemical findings in Rett syndrome remain unknown and deserve further intensive investigations.

THERAPEUTIC INTERVENTION

To date there is no cure for the Rett syndrome, one can only treat the individuals' symptoms. Physical and occupational therapists play an important role in the care of girls with Rett syndrome (Hanks, 1986). Intensive therapy, while failing to alter the actual course of the disease, has been successful in addressing symptoms by maintaining or improving functional movement, mobility, preventing deformities, and keeping the girls in contingent contact with their environments. Although persons with Rett syndrome display numerous similarities, their specific therapeutic problems and responses to treatment vary dramatically (Hanks, 1986; Lieb-Lundell, 1988; Sponseller, 1989). The therapeutic intervention program, therefore, must be highly individualized for each person.

Apraxia and ataxia are frequently the earliest manifestations of motor problems in Rett syndrome. The girls display a marked fixing or locking of their joints into positions of stability to counter disruption in balance, inhibiting the ability to shift positions. Thus, the legs are often kept in wide abduction while sitting and standing (see Fig. 2), and weight shift is absent (Hanks, 1986). The girls often demonstrate expressions of agitation and fear in response to any movements not self-initiated. Similar voluntary movements, however, are not related to these stress reactions. Lieb-Lundell (1988) reported that "no amount of practice or exposure alters this response of fear to extrinsically initiated movement" (p. 533).

A number of therapeutic interventions have been successful in the treatment of apraxia-ataxia of: (a) use of the therapy ball, (b) balance-stimulating floor activities, (c) segmental rolling, and (d) rotation and weight shift activities (Hanks, 1986). Vestibular movement activities (e.g., merry-go-rounds, swings) have also been reported as helpful if the child tolerates this intervention (Hanks, 1986, p. 248). The resulting muscle imbalance may lead to severe contractures, especially distally (e.g., a downward pointing of the foot). This spasticity may also be responsible,

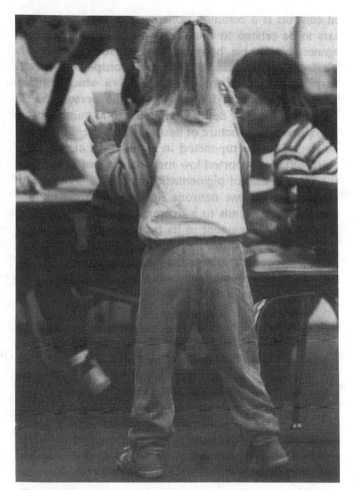

Figure 2. Legs in wide abduction to counter disruption in balance.

at least in part, for the high incidence of scoliosis in girls with Rett syndrome (Hanks, 1986; Sponseller, 1989).

Hydrotherapy emphasizing movement in the water, range of motion, and basic water skills has been helpful in the improvement of range of motion and the reduction of discomfort (Hanks, 1986; Lieb-Lundell, 1988; Schleichkorn, 1987). Tone reduction activities such as rotation, weight shift, and vibration have been reported to result in a temporary reduction of spasticity (Hanks, 1986).

Ambulation remains one of the critical skills to develop and maintain in persons with Rett syndrome. Many of the girls fail to develop this skill prior to Stage 2, while others lose this ability as part of the rapid motor degeneration. For these girls efforts to develop independent standing and ambulation must be stressed. Weight-bearing exercises, walking, and gait training have been successful (Hanks, 1986, 1989, 1990). Frequently, foot deformities (e.g., ankle pronation, plantar flexion inversion, and toe curling) must be corrected through the use of orthoplast shoe inserts, orthoses, inhibitive casts, and toe spreaders. Many of the commonly utilized assisting devices for ambulation (e.g., push-type walker) are of limited usefulness due to loss of purposeful hand function.

Girls that have the ability to ambulate must engage in activities that maintain this skill and promote stimulation of the joints and muscles (Kjoerholt & Salthammer, 1989). Walking and stair climbing should be a regular part of the daily routine to maximize these skills. Kjoerholt and Salthammer (1989) cautioned that therapists must be patient as the girls walk "very slowly and will often stop without any noticeable reason, probably due to apraxia" (p. 84).

Scoliosis (a side-to-side curvature of the spine) in the Rett syndrome is well documented (Hagberg et al., 1983; Hanks, 1986, 1989; Harrison & Webb, 1990; Loder, Lee, & Richards, 1989; Sponseller, 1989) and kyphosis (hunchback) is common (Rett, 1977; Sponseller, 1989). Unfortunately, there are no rigid guidelines to predict deformity or to recommend treatment. Standard criteria (e.g., sex or patient, curve pattern, onset of menarche) typically useful in the determination of an appropriate intervention strategy do not appear to be of use with this syndrome (Hennessy & Haas, 1988). Maintaining good spinal mobility through exercise, however, has been suggested (Hanks, 1986). For example, scoliosis results in a muscle imbalance in the area around the curve. The muscles on one side of the spinal column will be spastic and hypotonic musculature. The person often tends to lean towards the hypotonic side. Exercises designed to maximize her use of the muscles she avoids using are in order (e.g., feed and lead her by the hand on her hypotonic side). Good positioning is vital and strollers, wheelchairs, and high chairs should be fitted properly to produce a symmetrical sitting posture and an erect spine (Hanks, 1986; Kjhoerholt & Salthammer, 1989).

Seizure activity is not uncommon in persons with Rett syndrome. In fact, a study based upon the electroencephalogram (EEG) records of 44 persons with Rett syndrome found abnormal EEG tracings to be almost universal (Niedermeyer, Rett, Renner, Murphy, & Naidu, 1986). While no "typical" EEG pattern of the Rett syndrome was identified, "a monotonous type of rhythmical medium voltage slow activity, mostly in the 3–5 second range and of generalized character" (p. 196) was most commonly displayed (68.4%). Abnormal sleep patterns have also been noted. For example, Haas, Rice, Trauner, and Merritt (1986), reported the "presence of intermittent episodes of high amplitude bursts of spike wave or slow wave discharges followed by a brief period of relative suppression of background activity" (p. 238) during sleep. Robb, Harden, and Boyd (1989) reported that in their study of 52 girls with Rett syndrome, discharges, consisting of short waves or spikes, were a common feature. These discharges could be infrequent or almost continuous and characteristically were most prominent around the middle third of the head.

Pronounced EEG abnormalities were most often found between the ages of 3 to 10 years and tended to become less severe during the second decade of life (Niedermyer et al, 1986; Rett, 1986). Several clinicians (Adkins, 1986; Budden, 1986; Naidu et al, 1986; Philippart, 1986) agree that standard dosages of Tegretol (carbamazepine) constitute the best seizure management program. Hagberg (1985) warned, however, that many girls with Rett syndrome overreact and must therefore be taken off the medication.

Stereotyped hand movements represent one of the most distinguishing characteristics of the Rett syndrome. Hand wringing, hand washing, hand tapping, and hand-to-mouth movements are common stereotypies resulting in the loss of purposeful hand function. These movements appear to evolve with age, preceding from simple, rapid movements to a slower, more complex form and ultimately to slow, less complicated repetitive movements (Clare, 1986). The behavior is more remarkable under stressful situations and diminishes or disappears momentarily when changing posture or eating. In some of the girls, stereotypic movements exacerbated during periods of respiratory dysrhythmia (hyperventilation and apnea) (Kerr et al., 1990). Van Acker (1987) reported that while the proportion of time persons with Rett syndrome engaged in stereotyped hand movements appeared resistant to environmental manipulation, a 40% reduction in these movements was displayed by one girl when involved in computer-assisted instruction. Therefore, observations suggest that some variation in frequency and duration of stereotyped movements is related to age and environmental conditions. Attempts to modify the stereotyped behavior of persons with Rett syndrome by operant approaches and various medications such as L-dopa, haloperidol, 5-HTP, and various anticonvulsants, however, have been unrewarding thus far (Percy et al., 1985).

Splinting has been found to be successful in interrupting hand-to-mouth (Hanks, 1986) and hand wringing (Aron, 1990; Naganuma, 1988) movements, thus allowing the girls to direct their attention to tasks and persons in their environment and to reduce the risk of skin breakdown related to these high rate behaviors. Some persons with Rett syndrome have demonstrated improved functional hand use while splints were in use (Naganuma, 1988). Tuten and Miedaner (1989), however, were unable to replicate the effectiveness of hand splints. The two subjects involved in this study displayed no decrease in stereotyped hand wringing, nor any subsequent increase in functional hand use as a result of hand splint application. To date, no studies have demonstrated any maintenance effects of hand splints over time once the splints have been removed. Additionally, many persons with Rett syndrome are unable to tolerate the application of hand or arm splints for even short periods.

Berkson (1987) has suggested that the desire to control one's impact on his or her environment may play a critical role in the origin and maintenance of stereotyped behavior. One might suspect, therefore, that highly motivating activities that allow one to demonstrate a cause-and-effect relationship with their environment could possibly lead to a decrease in stereotyped behavior. Limited support for this hypothesis is available in the Rett syndrome literature. Hanks (1986) reported "toys that combine bright colors and sound and require input from the child are helpful in keeping the child involved with the environmental and making attempts to use her hands" (p. 250). Music therapy has also proved useful in the promotion of functional hand use. The music appears to increase the level of awareness and the instruments motivate efforts to reach out and interact (Wesecky, 1986). Battery-operated toys and computers modified to respond to an easily activated switch provide an almost limitless array of possibilities to not only decrease stereotyped behavior (Van Acker, 1987) but also increase functional hand use, communication, and cognitive development (Hanks, 1986; Sonseller, 1989; Zappella, 1986).

Feeding and nutrition is another area of concern in the treatment of girls with Rett syndrome. Their limited functional hand use frequently curtails attempts at self-feeding. Programs employing operant procedures, however, have sometimes proven effective in promoting finger-feeding and modified utensil use (Hanks, 1986; Sponseller, 1989). Many of the girls also display physiological problems related to excessive tongue thrusting, chewing, and swallowing. Proper positioning and tone reduction activities (if spasticity is the problem) are essential to reduce the risk of choking.

Perhaps more alarming, girls with Rett syndrome display a marked tendency to lose weight and some evidence suggests defects in carbohydrate (Clark et al., 1990; Haas & Rice, 1985; Haas et al, 1986), ascorbic acid, and glutathione (Sofic, Riederer, Killian, & Rett, 1987) metabolism. Malabsorption of critical nutrients and failure to benefit from adequate caloric intake must be considered when examining the malnutrition displayed in some persons with Rett syndrome (Missliwetz & Depastas, 1985). Haas and his associates (Haas & Rice, 1985; Haas et al, 1986) reported improved weight gain in conjunction with diminished stereotyped behavior and better seizure control when a high calorie, high fat ketogenic diet was implemented. A nutritionist should be available to consult with parents and program staff relative to diet if weight gain is a problem.

Constipation is a common problem experienced by persons with Rett syndrome. Many of the girls fail to consume adequate fluids and fiber which result in an impacted bowel (Hunter, 1987). Dietary measures (ingestion of high liquid content fruit, fiber, mineral oil, etc.) may prove adequate, although artificial laxatives, enemas, or suppositories are often required (Naidu et al, 1990).

Additional problematic behaviors and specific symptoms are frequently reported to accompany the Rett syndrome. For example, a significant portion of the girls engage in self-injurious behaviors. Self-biting, self-pinching, and self-hitting are the most common self-injurious behaviors reported in the literature. These behaviors are typically displayed (initially) during the second phase of the disorder and frequently cease during the second decade of life without intervention (Clare, 1986). Iwata, Pace, Willis, Gamache, and Hyman (1986) examined the self-injurious behavior of two girls with Rett syndrome. They reported that the hand biting of these girls appeared to "be related to organic predisposition rather than being shaped inadvertently by the environment" (p. 164). Interestingly, the hand biting of both girls was reduced through an operant procedure that involved a combination of differential reinforcement of alternative behavior (a food reinforcer provided for toy contact) and a 30-second hand restraint contingent upon hand biting. Thus, operant procedures may prove effective in the treatment of some of the behavioral characteristics of the Rett syndrome, however, maintenance of treatment effects has not been documented.

Irritability, aggressive behaviors (hitting others), and screaming/crying spells also frequently are reported during the period of rapid deterioration (Stage 2). These periods of tantrum most often occur without an apparent cause, may last for more than an hour, and may cease as abruptly as they began (Budden, 1987; Hunter, 1987; Naidu et al, 1986). Parents report that music, holding the child while rocking, short trips in the car, and warm baths most frequently calm their children (Sponseller, 199). Proper sleep and diet appear to minimize the level of irritability and severity of the tantrums in many children. For example, Budden (1987) reported that frequent high carbohydrate meals diminished irritability in two girls. Unfortunately, this irritability often extends well into the night, disrupting the sleep patterns of the child and increasing the probability of additional tantrums. Sleep may also be disturbed by periods of spontaneous laughing. Medications such as chloral hydrate, Tranzene (chlorazepate dipotassium) or Benadryl (dphenylhydramine hydrochloride) are found helpful to induce sleep (Budden, 1987). The use of water beds or electric blankets that provide added warmth also have been reported by parents to improve their child's ability to sleep (Sponseller, 1989).

EDUCATIONAL INTERVENTION

The cognitive profile typical of persons with Rett syndrome has not been clearly delineated. Much of the literature on Rett syndrome suggests that girls experience a true dementia involving cognitive and motor degeneration resulting in severe or profound mental retardation (Charnov, Stach, & Didonato, 1989; Naidu et al, 1986; Rolando, 1985). Charnov et al. (1989), for example, evaluated the developmental histories of 16 girls with Rett syndrome through parent interview (of preregression development) and current functioning assessment employing the Birth to Three Developmental Scale (Bangs & Dodson, 1979). In all developmental areas, they reported that the current functioning of each subject was substantially below that which the children were attributed to have achieved prior to the onset of the disorder. Interestingly, the current developmental skills profile mirrored that of the preregression skills. Additionally, the "preregression" pattern of development did not appear to represent normal development, suggesting that these children either displayed abnormal development from birth or that the age of onset for the disorder may be earlier than previously expected and affect areas of development, especially problem-solving skills, prior to the decline in motor skills.

There is some support, however, for a hypothesis of cognitive arrest or stagnation at the developmental level achieved at the age of onset of the condition in combination with a severe extrapyramidal movement and expressive language disorder as opposed to cognitive dementia (Hagberg & Witt-Engerstrom, 1986; Kerr & Stephenson, 1986; Stephenson & Kerr, 1987). Fontanesi and Haas (1988) evaluated the cognitive functioning of 18 girls with Rett syndrome. They administered the Vineland Adaptive Behavior Scales and the Bayley Scales of Adaptive Abilities in addition to examining medical and developmental histories and interviewing parents regarding the age their daughters attained developmental milestones. Their results indicated that "skills not dependent on either language or fine motor function are retained at a developmental level equivalent to the age of onset" (p. S23). Gross motor functioning, daily living skills, and object permanence were relatively preserved, while fine motor control and language functioning displayed substantial degeneration from preregression developmental levels. Further research is needed to gain a fuller understanding of the cognitive abilities of girls with Rett syndrome. If, for example, persons with Rett syndrome demonstrate a capability to learn that is greater than their capacity for fine motor or language functioning, then instructional techniques similar to those employed with children who have cerebral palsy and motor dysfunction might prove more effective than current educational approaches typically using operant shaping and prompting procedures designed for children with severe and profound handicaps (Fontanesi & Haas, 1988).

Communication programming with persons with Rett syndrome has received little empirical research. Formal testing suggests these girls to be at a presymbolic language level (International Rett Syndrome Association, 1990; Owen, 1990). Although, again, one cannot determine whether these results relate primarily to cognitive deficits or to an expressive language disorder. Numerous anecdotal reports exist, however, that suggest these girls may well understand more than they can express (Weisz, 1987).

Most successful communication programs take advantage of the communicative behaviors displayed by the girls (e.g., Donnellan, Mirenda, Mesaros, & Fassbender, 1984). Vocalizations, facial expression, gestures, walking towards a desired item or activity, and eye gaze are common communicative behaviors displayed by persons with Rett syndrome. Parents and educators must attune themselves to their child's communicative behavior and respond contingently to these signals. As with any child, the critical element in the development of a meaningful communication system depends upon the contingent interaction of the person and her environment (Lewis, Alessandri, & Sullivan, 1990). When others learn to detect the communicative behaviors and to respond to them in a systematic fashion, a formal and effective system of communication can be developed. Cause-and-effect relationships that allow the child to gain an understanding of their ability to impact their environment is essential for communication training. An awareness of cause-and-effect relationships may be enhanced through the use of simple switches to activate toys or computer monitors. Musical instruments have also been shown to promoted the child's desire to interact with their environment (Wesecky, 1986; Zapella, 1986).

Persons with Rett syndrome have been taught to employ communication systems that involve eye pointing, communication boards (pictures), facial expression, gestures, and the activation of switches. For example, one of the girls worked with tapped the page of a book to signal her desire to have the page turned. Building upon this communicative action, her teachers began to incorporate a series of large pictures that displayed the items she had available at any given meal time. The child was prompted to tap the picture of the desired food item prior to her obtaining a bite or sip of the particular items. This procedure proved effective and the student now has an expressive picture vocabulary of approximately 23 words (selected from a field of four pictures at any one time). Another parent has taken photographs of her daughter's facial and gestural communicative behaviors and developed a "dictionary" for those who interact frequently with the child (International Rett Syndrome Association, 1990).

Owen (1990) implemented a whole language (verbal and signed language) intervention program with four girls with Rett syndrome. Although her results failed to support the effectiveness of this intervention with this population, she reported that at least one of the girls was able to master a sign approximation that closely resembled the topography of one of her stereotyped movements. She suggested that perhaps these movements may lend themselves to an operant shaping procedure when systematically paired with contingent environmental stimuli. Given the importance of communication skills, further research is needed to identify the range of communication functioning in, and effective methods to teach improved communication skills to, persons with Rett syndrome.

Only a small percentage of the estimated 10,000 girls in the United States afflicted with the Rett syndrome has been identified thus far (Moser, 1986). Lack of awareness of this disorder on the part of physicians and clinicians is undoubtedly a major contributing factor to this state of affairs. Even when physicians are aware of the Rett syndrome, however, an accurate diagnosis is not always forthcoming. There is often a hesitation to accept, as a specific entity, a disorder for which there is no laboratory marker. In the absence of a specific chromosomal or biochemical marker, as was true of Down syndrome for the first 90 years after that disorder was recognized (Hutt & Gibby, 1976), the diagnosis of the Rett syndrome depends upon careful analysis of signs and symptoms. Further research into the cause, pathogenesis, defective treatment, and ultimately prevention of this disorder is sorely needed. As one of the slogans of the International Rett Syndrome Association states, "If we care today, we can cure tomorrow."

REFERENCES

Adkins, W. N. (1986). Rett syndrome at an institution for the developmentally disabled. *American Journal of Medical Genetics, 24*(Suppl. 1), 85–97.

Allen, D. A. (1988). Autistic spectrum disorders: Clinical presentation in preschool children. *Journal of Child Neurology, 3*(Suppl.), S48–S56.

Aron, M. (1990). The use and effectiveness of elbow splints in the Rett syndrome. *Brain and Development, 12*, 162–163.

Bangs, T., & Dodson, S. (1979). *Birth to Three Developmental Scale*. Hingham, MA: Teaching Resources Corp.

Berkson, G. (1987, August). *Three approaches to an understanding of abnormal stereotyped behaviors*. Paper presented at the American Psychological Association, New York.

Brucke, T., Sofic, E., Killian, W., Rett, A., & Riederer, P. (1988). Reduced concentrations and increased metabolism of biogenic amines in a single case of Rett syndrome: A postmortem brain study. *Journal of Neutral Transmission, 68*, 315–324.

Budden, S. S. (1986). Rett syndrome: Studies of 13 affected girls. *American Journal of Medical Genetics, 24*(Suppl. 1), 99–109.

Budden, S. S. (1987). The role of the physician in the care of the child with Rett syndrome. *Brain and Development, 9*, 532–534.

Burd, L., Fisher, W., & Kerbeshian, J. (1989). Pervasive disintegrative disorder: Are Rett syndrome and Heller dementia infantilis subtypes? *Developmental Medical Child Neurology, 31*, 609–616.

Charnov, E. K., Stach, B. A., & Didonato, R. M. (1989, November). *Pre and post onset developmental levels in Rett syndrome*. Paper presented at the American Speech-Language-Hearing Association Convention.

Clare, A. J. (1986). *Rett syndrome: Behind their eyes is more than they can show us*. Dissertation, Thames Polytechnic Incorporating Avery Hill College, Kent, U.K.

Clarke, A., Gardner, Medwin, D., Richardson, J., McGann, A., Bonham, J. R., Carpenter, K. H., Bhattacharya, S., Haggerty, D., Fleetwood, J. A., & Aynsley-Green, A. (1990). Abnormalities of carbohydrate metabolism and of OCT gene function in the Rett syndrome. *Brain and Development, 12*, 119–124.

Coleman, M. (1990). Is classical Rett syndrome ever present in males? *Brain and Development, 12*, 31–32.

Coleman, M., & Gillberg, C. (1985). *The biology of autistic syndromes* (pp. 45–50). New York: Praeger.

Comings, D. E. (1986). The genetics of Rett syndrome: The consequences of a disorder where every case is a new mutation. *American Journal of Medical Genetics, 24*(Suppl. 1), 383–388.

Donnellan, A. M., Mirenda, P. L., Mesaros, R. A., Fassbender, L. L. (1984). Analyzing the communicative functions of aberrant behavior. *Journal of the Association for Persons with Severe Handicaps, 9,* 210–212.

Fontanesi, J., & Haas, R. H. (1988). Cognitive profile of Rett syndrome. *Journal of Child Neurology, 3*(Suppl.), S20–S24.

Gillberg, C. (1986). Autism and Rett syndrome: Some notes on differential diagnosis. *American Journal of Medical Genetics, 24*(Suppl. 1), 127–131.

Gillberg, C. (1987). Autistic symptoms in Rett syndrome: The first two years according to mother reports. *Brain and Development, 9,* 499–501.

Gillberg, C. (1989). The borderland of autism and Rett syndrome: Five case histories to highlight diagnostic difficulties. *Journal of Autism and Developmental Disorders, 19,* 545–559.

Gillberg, C., Wahlstrom, J., & Hagberg, B. (1984). Infantile autism and Rett's syndrome: Common chromosomal denominator. *Lancet, 2,* 1094–1095.

Gillberg, C., Wahlstrom, J., & Hagberg, B. (1985). A "new" chromosome marker common to the Rett syndrome and infantile autism? The frequency of fragile sites at X P22 in 81 children with infantile autism, childhood psychosis and the Rett syndrome. *Brain and Development, 7,* 365–367.

Goutieres, F., & Aicardi, J. (1985). Rett syndrome: Clinical presentation and laboratory investigations in 12 further French patients. *Brain and Development, 7,* 305–306.

Haas, R., & Rice, M. L. A. (1985). Is Rett's syndrome a disorder of carbohydrate metabolism? Hyperpyruvic acidemia and treatment by ketogenic diet. *Annals of Neurology, 18,* 418.

Haas, R. H., Rice, M. A., Trauner, D. A., & Merritt, A. (1986). Therapeutic effects of a ketogenic diet in Rett syndrome. *American Journal of Medical Genetics, 24*(Suppl. 1), 225–246.

Hagberg, B. (1985). Rett syndrome: Swedish approach to analysis of prevalence and cause. *Brain and Development, 7,* 277–280.

Hagberg, B., Aicardi, J., Dias, K., & Ramos, O. (1983). A progressive syndrome of autism, dementia, ataxia, and loss of purposeful hand use in girls: Rett syndrome: Report of 35 cases. *Annals of Neurology, 14,* 471–479.

Hagberg, B., Goutieres, F., Hanefeld, F., Rett, A., & Wilson, J. (1985). Rett syndrome: Criteria for inclusion and exclusion. *Brain and Development, 7,* 372–373.

Hagberg, B., & Witt-Engerstrom, I. (1986). Rett syndrome: A suggested staging system for describing impairment profile with increasing age towards adolescence. *American Journal of Medical Genetics, 24*(Suppl. 1), 47–59.

Hanaoka, S., Ishikawa, N., & Kamoshita, S. (1985). Three cases of Rett syndrome. In S. Kamoshita (Ed.), *Abstracts for the workshop on Aicardi syndrome and Rett syndrome.* Tokyo: Dainippon Tosho.

Hanefeld, F. (1985). The clinical pattern of the Rett syndrome. *Brain and Development, 7,* 320–325.

Hanefeld, F., Hanefeld, U., Wilichowski, E., & Schmidtke, J. (1986). Rett syndrome—Search for genetic markers. *American Journal of Medical Genetics, 24*(Suppl. 1), 377–382.

Hanks, S. B. (1986). The role of therapy in Rett syndrome. *American Journal of Medical Genetics, 24*(Suppl. 1), 247–252.

Hanks, S. B. (1989, May). *Motor disabilities and physical therapy strategies in Rett syndrome.* Paper presented at the 5th Annual Conference of the International Rett Syndrome Association. Washington, D.C.

Hanks, S. (1990). Motor disabilities in the Rett syndrome and physical therapy strategies. *Brain and Development, 12,* 157–161.

Harding, B. N., Tudmay, A. J., & Wislon, J. (1985). Neuropathological studies in a child showing some features of the Rett syndrome. *Brain and Development, 78,* 342–344.

Harris, J. C., Wong, D. F., Wagner, H. N., Rett, A., Naidu, S., Dannals, R. F., Links, J. M., Batshaw, M. L., & Moser, H. W. (1986). Positron emission tomographic study of D2 dopamine receptor binding and CSF biogenic amine metabolites in Rett syndrome. *American Journal of Medical Genetics, 24*(Suppl. 1), 201–210.

Harrison, D. J., & Webb, P. J. (1990). Scoliosis in the Rett syndrome: Natural history and treatment. *Brain and Development, 12,* 154–156.

Havlak, C., & Covington, C. (1989). Motor function: Physical and occupational therapy strategies. In *Education and therapeutic intervention in Rett syndrome.* Ft. Washington, MD: International Rett Syndrome Association.

Hennessy, M. J., & Haas, R. H. (1988). The orthopedic management of Rett syndrome. *Journal of Child Neurology, 3*(Suppl.), S43–S47.

Hillig, U. (1985). On the genetics of the Rett syndrome. *Brain and Development, 7,* 368–371.

Holm, V. A. (1985). Rett syndrome: A case report from an audiovisual program. *Brain and Development, 7,* 297–299.

Hunter, K. (1987). Rett syndrome: Parents' views about specific symptoms. *Brain and Development, 9,* 535–538.

Hutt, M. L., & Gibby, P. G. (1976). *The mentally retarded child: Development, education, and treatment.* New York: Allyn and Bacon.

International Rett Syndrome Association. (1990). *Parent Idea Book: Managing Rett Syndrome.* Ft. Washington, MD: Author.

Ishikawa, A., Goto, T., Narasaki, M., Yokochi, K., Kitahara, H., & Fukuyama, Y. (1978). A new syndrome (?) of progressive psychomotor deterioration with peculiar stereotyped movement and autistic tendency: A report of three cases. *Brain and Development, 3,* 258.

Iwata, B. A., Pace, G. M., Willis, K. D., Gamache, T. B., & Hyman, S. L. (1986). Operant studies of self-injurious hand biting in the Rett syndrome. *American Journal of Medical Genetics, 24,* 157–166.

Jellinger, K., & Seiteberger, F. (1986). Neuropathology of Rett syndrome. *American Journal of Medical Genetics, 24*(Suppl. 1), 259–288.

Kerr, A. M., Montague, J., & Stephenson, J. B. P. (1987). The hands, and the mind, pre- and postregression, in Rett syndrome. *Brain and Development, 9,* 487–490.

Kerr, A., Southall, D., Amos, P., Copper, R., Samuels, M., Mitchell, J., & Stephenson, J.

(1990). Correlation of electroencephalogram, respiration, and movement in the Rett syndrome. *Brain and Development, 12,* 61–68.

Kerr, A., & Stephenson, J. B. P. (1986). A study of the natural history of Rett syndrome in 23 girls. *American Journal of Medical Genetics, 24,* 77–83.

Killian, W. (1986). On the genetics of Rett syndrome: Analysis of family and pedigree data. *American Journal of Medical Genetics, 24*(Suppl. 1), 369–376.

Kjoerholt, K., & Salthammer, E. (1989). Kjoerholt Salthammer Fysioterapi. In *Educational and therapeutic intervention in Rett syndrome.* Ft. Washington, MD: International Rett Syndrome Association.

Leiber, B. (1985). Rett syndrome: A nosological entity. *Brain and Development, 7,* 275–276.

Lekman, A., Witt-Engerstrom, I., Gottfries, J., Hagberg, B. A., Percy, A. K., & Svennerholm, L. (1989). Rett syndrome: Biogenic amines and metabolites in postmortem brain. *Pediatric Neurology, 5,* 357–362.

Lewis, M., Alessandri, S. M., & Sullivan, M. W. (1990). *Expectancy, loss of control and anger expression in young infants.* Report of the Institute for the Study of Child Development. Robert Wood Johnson Medical School Department of Pediatrics, New Brunswick, NJ.

Lieb-Lundell, C. (1988). The therapist's role in the management of girls with Rett syndrome. *Journal of Child Neurology, 3*(Suppl.), S31–S34.

Loder, R. T., Lee, C. L., & Richards, B. A. (1989). Orthopedic aspects of Rett syndrome: A multicenter review. *Journal of Pediatric Orthopedics, 9,* 557–562.

Lloyd, K. G., Hornykiewicz, O., Davidson, L., Shannak, K., Farley, I., Goldstein, M., Sibuya, M., Kelly, W. N., & Fox, I. H. (1981). Biochemical evidence of dysfunction of brain neurotransmitters in the Lesch-Nyhan syndrome. *New England Journal of Medicine, 305,* 1106–1111.

Missliewetz, J., & Depastas, G. (1985). Forensic problems in Rett syndrome. *Brain and Development, 7,* 326–328.

Moser, H. W. (1986). Preamble to the workshop on Rett syndrome. *American Journal of Medical Genetics, 24*(Suppl. 1), 1–20.

Naganuma, G. (1988). Motor function: Physical therapy strategies. In *Educational and therapeutic intervention in Rett syndrome.* Ft. Maryland, MD: International Rett Syndrome Association.

Naidu, S., Hyman, S., Piazza, K., Savedra, J., Perman, J., Wenk, G., Kitt, C., Troncoso, J., Price, D., Cassanova, M., Miller, D., Thomas, G., Niedermeyer, E., & Moser, H. (1990). The Rett syndrome: Progress report on studies at the Kennedy Institute. *Brain and Development, 12,* 5–7.

Naidu, S., Murphy, M., Moser, H. W., & Rett, A. (1986). Rett syndrome: Natural history in 70 cases. *American Journal of Medical Genetics, 24*(Suppl. 1), 61–72.

Niedermeyer, E., Rett., A., Renner, H., Murphy, M., & Naidu, S. (1986). Rett syndrome and the electroencephalogram. *American Journal of Medical Genetics, 249*(Suppl. 1), 195–200.

Nomura, Y., & Segawa, M. (1990). Clinical features of the early stage of the Rett syndrome. *Brain and Development, 12,* 16–19.

Nomura, Y., Segawa, M., & Hasegawa, M. (1984). Rett syndrome—Clinical studies and pathophysiological consideration. *Brain and Development, 6,* 475–486.

Nomura, Y., Segawa, M., & Higurashi, M. (1985). Rett syndrome—An early catecholamine and indolamine deficient disorder? *Brain and Development, 7,* 334–341.

Olsson, B. (1987). Autistic traits in the Rett syndrome. *Brain and Development, 9,* 491–498.

Olsson, B., & Rett, A. (1985). Behavioral observations concerning differential diagnosis between the Rett syndrome and autism. *Brain and Development, 7,* 281–289.

Olsson, B., & Rett, A. (1987). Autism and Rett syndrome: Behavioral investigations and differential diagnosis. *Developmental Medicine and Child Neurology, 29,* 429–441.

Olsson, B., & Rett, A. (1990). A review of the Rett syndrome with a theory of autism. *Brain and Development, 12,* 11–15.

Opitz, J. M., & Lewin, S. (1987). Rett syndrome—A review and discussion of syndrome delineation. *Brain and Development, 9,* 445–450.

Owen, V. E. (1990). *The use of a total communciation intervention to examine the communication skills in girls with Rett syndrome.* Unpublished doctoral dissertation, University of Illinois at Chicago.

Percy, A. K., Zoghbi, H. Y., Lewis, K. R., & Jankovic, J. (1988). Rett syndrome: Qualitative and quantitative differentiation from autism. *Journal of Child Neurology, 3*(Suppl.), S65–S67.

Percy, A. K., Zoghbi, H., & Riccardi, V. M. (1985). Rett syndrome: Initial experience with an emerging clinical entity. *Brain and Development, 7,* 300–304.

Philippart, M. (1986). Clinical recognition of Rett syndrome. *American Journal of Medical Genetics, 24*(Suppl. 1), 111–118.

Philippart, M. (1990). The Rett syndrome in males. *Brain and Development, 12,* 33–36.

Rendle-Short, J. (1969). Infantile autism in Australia. *Medical Journal of Australia, 2,* 245–249.

Rett, A. (1966). Ueber ein eigenartiges hirnatrophisches syndrom hyperammonamie im kindesalter. *Wiener Medizinische Wochenschrift, 116,* 723–738.

Rett, A. (1969). Ein zerebral-atrophisches Syndrom bei Hyperammonamie im Kindesalter. *Fortschritte der Mediziin, 87,* 507–509.

Rett, A. (1977). A cerebral atrophy associated with hyperammonaemie. In P.J. Vinken & G. W. Bruyn (Eds.) *Handbook of clinical neurology.* Amsterdam: North Holland.

Rett, A. (1986). History and general overview. *American Journal of Medical Genetics, 24*(Suppl. 1), 21–26.

Riccardi, V. M. (1986). The Rett syndrome: Genetics and the future. *American Journal of Medical Genetics, 24*(Suppl. 1), 389–402.

Riederer, P., Brucke, T., Sofic, E., Kienzl, E., Schnecker, K., Eng., D., Schay, V., Kryzik, P., Eng, D., Killian, W., & Rett, A. (1985). Neurochemical aspects of the Rett syndrome. *Brain and Development, 7,* 351–360.

Riederer, P., Wieser, M., Wichart, I., Schmidt, B., Killian, W., & Rett, A. (1986). Preliminary brain autopsy findings in progredient Rett syndrome. *American Journal of Medical Genetics, 24*(Suppl. 1), 305–315.

Robb, S. A., Harden, A., & Boyd, S. G. (1989). Rett syndrome: An EEG study in 52 girls. *Neuropediatrics, 20,* 192–195.

Rolando, S. (1985). Rett syndrome: Report of eight cases. *Brain and Development, 7,* 290–296.

Schleichkorn, J. (1987). Rett syndrome: A neurological disease largely undiagnosed here. *Physical Therapy Bulletin, 2,* 16–18.

Sofic, E., Riederer, P., Killian, W., & Rett, A. (1987). Reduced concentrations of ascorbic acid and glutathione in a single case of Rett syndrome: A postmortem brain study. *Brain and Development, 9,* 529–531.

Sponseller, P. D. (1989). *Orthopaedic problems in Rett syndrome.* Ft. Washington, MD: International Rett Syndrome Association.

Stephenson, J. B., & Kerr, A. M. (1987). Rett syndrome: Disintegration not dementia. *Lancet, 1,* 741.

Trevantahn, E., & Naidu, S. (1988). The clinical recognition and differential diagnosis of Rett syndrome. *Journal of Child Neurology, 3*(Suppl.), S6–S16.

Tuten, H., & Miedaner, J. (1989). Effect of hand splints on stereotypic hand behavior of girls with Rett syndrome: A replication study. *Physical Therapy, 69,* 1099–1103.

Van Acker, R. (1987). *Stereotypical responding associated with Rett syndrome: A comparison of girls with this disorder and matched subject controls without the Rett syndrome.* Doctoral Dissertation, Northern Illinois University, Dekalb.

Wahlstrom, J. (1985). Genetic implications of Rett's syndrome. *Brain and Development, 7,* 573–574.

Wahlstrom, J., & Anvret, M. (1986). Music therapy for children with Rett syndrome. *American Journal of Medical Genetics, 24*(Suppl. 1), 253–257.

Witt-Engerstrom, I. (1987). Rett syndrome: A retrospective pilot study on potential early predictive symptomatology. *Brain and Development, 9,* 481–486.

Zappella, M. (1986). Motivational conflicts in Rett syndrome. *American Journal of Medical Genetics, 24*(Suppl. 1), 143–151.

Zoghbi, H. (1988). Genetic aspects of Rett syndrome. *Journal of Child Neurology, 3*(Suppl.), S76–S78.

Zoghbi, H. Y., Percy, A. K., Glaze, D. G., Butler, I. J., & Riccardi, V. M. (1985). Reduction of biogenic amine levels in the Rett syndrome. *New England Journal of Medicine, 313,* 921–924.

PART IV
CLINICAL ISSUES

The four papers in this section address a group of issues of general interest to clinicians. Klinefelter's syndrome (KS), first described in 1942 in terms of endocrinologic findings, is now recognized as a sex chromosome anomaly characterized by a surplus of X chromosomes in phenotypic males. Early studies of XXY males produced results suggesting an increased risk for psychiatric disturbance, criminality, and mental retardation. Although these result were always suspect because they were derived form the investigation of clinical and/or institutionalized populations, the stereotype still persists to some degree. More recent studies of XXY boys identified in cytogenetic surveys conducted in eight centers throughout the world have produced reliable information regarding the growth and development of these boys during childhood and adolescence, much of which has been succinctly summarized by Mandoki and colleagues. It is clear that the diagnosis of KS does not denote an increased likelihood of criminality, psychopathology, or mental retardation. Conversely, the XXY male is most likely to be of normal intelligence, to be free of psychiatric disturbance, and to demonstrate no more criminality than observed in XY men when intelligence and socioeconomic status are controlled. Nevertheless, XXY boys commonly exhibit speech and language delays in early childhood and academic difficulties during the school years. Although no specific personality profile or behavioral pattern typifies the XXY male, common characteristics of temperament have been observed, including introversion, lack of assertiveness, withdrawal from group activities, and lower levels of activity. The mechanisms underlying the emergence of these cognitive and behavioral difficulties are not clearly understood, but it is recommended that the diagnosis be considered in boys with language difficulties, learning problems, and behavioral difficulties in association with lack of coordination, long limbs, increased height, and small penis and testes for age. Early intervention to address delays in neuromuscular, language, and cognitive development should be followed by testosterone treatment at about 12 years of age in order to facilitate normalization during the adolescent years.

Epidemiologically based investigation has clearly established that neurologic impairment is associated with an increased frequency of occurrence of psychiatric disorder. Epilepsy is the most prevalent neurologic disorder of childhood and adolescents. Kim, in reviewing the psychiatric aspects of epilepsy during the developmental period, notes that for the majority of affected children and adolescents who either recover spontaneously or are well managed medically, epilepsy is a

385

benign disease. Nevertheless, approximately one-third of manifest various difficulties, including lack of seizure control and academic, emotional, behavioral, and family problems. As a group, these children have a much higher rate of psychiatric disorder than do either healthy children or children with other chronic illnesses. Although the type of psychiatric disorder manifested in epileptic youths is not different from the range of psychiatric disorder found in the general population or among children with chronic medical illness, disruptive behavior disorders appear to be overrepresented. Moreover, when groups of children with the same psychiatric diagnosis, such as attention-deficit hyperactivity disorder (ADHD), are examined across different neurodevelopmental indices, problems with epileptic youths are seen to be more extensive and more severe than among those who are seizure-free. Kim's discussion of the treatment of children with comorbid epilepsy and psychiatric disorder includes a thoughtful consideration of the role of the psychiatrist as a member of an interdisciplinary treatment team.

In the next paper in this section, Mrazek and colleagues present empirical evidence of a statistical association between early parental behavior and a later increase in the incidence of asthma in a cohort of 150 children who were genetically at risk for the development of asthma. In this elegantly designed and conducted study, judgments of both parenting problems and maternal coping were made during a home visit when the infants were 3 weeks old using clinical interview techniques of demonstrated reliability. Respiratory status was monitored over the next two years with children classified as manifesting: (1) asthma (2) recurrent infectious wheezing (3) a single isolated wheezing episode or (4) no wheezing. Early problems in coping and parenting were associated with the later onset of asthmas at the $p<.001$ level of significance. Moreover, parents of children who developed asthma were also significantly more likely to have had difficulties when their infants were 3 weeks of age that those whose children developed infectious wheezing. Stressing that an association cannot be considered evidence of a causal link, this group of investigators thoughtfully consider a variety of explanatory hypotheses. The time-honored controversy between nature and nurture is appropriately redefined in terms of interactions between genetic predispositions and experience.

The final paper in this section is a systematic effort to consider adolescent suicidality from both a phenomonologic and a developmental perspective. Borst and colleagues investigate the relationship of ego development, age, gender, and diagnosis to suicidality among 219 adolescent inpatients. The Diagnostic Interview Schedule for Children provided the information base for the classification of subjects as suicide attempters or as nonsuicidal and for their categorization into three diagnostic groups: affective disorder, conduct disorder, or mixed conduct-affective-disorder. Lovenger's Washington University Sentence Completion Test was used to assess developmental maturity. This measure consists of 26 incomplete sentences, which, when reliably related for level of ego development, led to the characterization of subjects as preconformist (88%) and conformist (12%). The results indicate that gender (female), diagnosis (affective or mixed conduct-affective), and ego development (conformist) each contributed significantly to the prediction of suicide attempts. The model correctly predicted the suicidal status of 78.1% of the sample. The findings are interpreted as suggesting that although more mature ego states are generally more adaptive, in the presence of psychopathology they may be associated with very maladaptive and personally injurious behaviors. Paradoxically, a delay in the development of ego functions may function as a protective factor for suicide rather than as an additional suicide risk factor. At the very least, the examination of level of ego development represents an additional dimension for clinicians to consider when assessing suicidal risk.

17

A Review of Klinefelter's Syndrome in Children and Adolescents

Miguel W. Mandoki, Gavla S. Sumner, Robert P. Hoffman, and Daniel L. Riconda

University of Florida Health Science Center, Jacksonville

Klinefelter's syndrome (XXY syndrome) has been identified as the spectrum of phenotypic features resulting from a sex chromosome complement that includes two or more X chromosomes and one or more Y chromosomes. Cytogenetic surveys conducted across the world have identified a sizable population of XXY males, who have been studied extensively from the newborn period through adolescence. The longitudinal studies of these boys have produced an accurate and reliable account of the growth and development of the XXY male. There now exists a growing body of knowledge that suggests that XXY boys often experience language deficits, neuromaturational lag, academic difficulties, and psychological distress, which may be reduced or ameliorated by early identification, anticipatory guidance, and proper medical management.

Klinefelter's syndrome (47XXY) was first described by Klinefelter et al. (1942) in terms of endocrinological findings. With the advancement of cytogenetics, Klinefelter's syndrome (KS) is now recognized as a sex chromosome anomaly characterized by a surplus of X chromosomes in phenotypic males (Bradbury et al., 1956). The 47XXY complement is the most common chromosomal pattern in persons with KS; however, mosaic patterns (i.e., 46XY/47XXY) and on rare occasions KS variants (i.e., 48, XXXY) are observed. KS is estimated to affect between 1 in 500 and 1 in 1,000 live born males; two-thirds of whom are predominantly of the 47XXY karyotype (Polani, 1967; Hamerton et al., 1975).

Reprinted with permission from the *Journal of the American Academy of Child and Adolescent Psychiatry*, 1991, Vol. 30, No. 2, 167–172. Copyright ©1991 by the American Academy of Child and Adolescent Psychiatry.

Early studies of XXY males produced the disturbing findings of an increased risk for psychiatric disturbance, criminality, and mental retardation (MacLean et al., 1962; Forssman and Hambert, 1963; MacLean et al., 1968; Forssman, 1970; Nielsen, J., 1970; Hook, 1973; Witkin et al., 1976). However, the subjects of early investigations were often found in clinical or institutional settings and had exhibited a degree of pathology that had warranted admission to a mental hospital, prison, or mental/penal institution. The results of early investigations of institutionalized XXY males are considered highly questionable because of selection bias inherent in studies of institutionalized populations and associated problems in research methodology. The more recent studies of XXY boys identified in cytogenetic surveys conducted in eight centers throughout the world have produced reliable information regarding the growth and development of these boys during childhood and adolescence (Leonard et al., 1979, 1982; Nielsen et al., 1979, 1982, 1986; Ratcliffe et al., 1979, 1982b, 1986; Robinson et al., 1979b, 1982, 1986; Stewart et al., 1979, 1982b, 1986; Evans et al., 1982, 1986; Walzer et al., 1982, 1986; Leonard and Sparrow, 1986).

This report will review current knowledge of the genetic and endocrinological characteristics of KS as well as the psychological functioning of XXY males in childhood and adolescence.

GENETIC CHARACTERISTICS

KS is the result of a meiotic nondisjunction during gametogenesis of the egg or sperm. Sanger et al. (1977), in summarizing the data collected in studies of X-linked genes in individuals with sex chromosome abnormalities to determine the parent in which the nondisjunction occurred, reports that in 67% of the males with 47XXY karyotype, the abnormality was due to nondisjunction in the mother. There are no known predisposing factors that have been identified as causative or preventative. Studies have suggested that there is a significant increase in risk for 47XXY live births with advanced maternal age (Carothers and Fillippi, 1988).

Clinical impression can only raise the suspicion of the diagnosis of KS; the phenotype is so variable that the only symptom may be infertility in adulthood. Confirmation of this diagnosis can be achieved through karyotype analysis of peripheral blood or skin fibroblast. The buccal smear should not be used for confirmation but may be a useful screening tool.

Growth and Sexual Development

In summarizing the findings of prospective studies, Robinson et al. (1979a) report an increased incidence of congenital abnormalities among 47XXY infants. Eighteen percent of XXY males were found to have one or more congenital abnormalities as compared with one percent of their siblings. Minor congenital anomalies were observed in 26% of the XXY children as compared with 7% of their sibs.

The mean weight and height of XXY infants falls within the normal range at birth, although significantly lower birth weights have been observed by Ratcliffe et al. (1979) and Stewart et al. (1979) compared with controls and siblings. The head circumference of XXYs tends to be small (Stewart et al., 1982b) and remains so during childhood and adolescence (Ratcliffe et al., 1982a). As the XXY male increases in age, his height is found to be increasingly above normal; height velocity is significantly increased from the age of 5 compared with sibling controls, and there is a significant tendency to have proportionately long legs in childhood (Stewart et al., 1982a). The bone age of XXY boys has been found to be, on an average, two standard deviations below the mean until 8 years of age but approaches the mean at 12 years of age and may advance as much as 3 years within 1 chronological year with the onset of puberty (Stewart et al., 1986).

The sexual development of XXY boys is normal at birth and continues to be normal during prepubertal years; below average testicular volume and stretched penile length are often found in prepuberty but measure within the normal range for age (Stewart et al., 1982b). Ferguson-Smith (1959) reports that the prepubertal testes of XXY boys show a reduced number of germinal cells, and azoospermia is virtually the rule. The XXY adolescent demonstrates a normal progression of puberty at 13 to 15 years of age; however, testicular size increases slowly and remains well below the mean for age (Stewart et al., 1986). After the increase in testicular volume occurring in puberty, testicular growth ceases and later decreases in size (Robinson et al., 1986). The mean testicular volume of XXY adolescents is 3 ml, which is similar to the testicular size (usually less than 3.5 ml [Boisen, 1979]) of adult men with KS. Gynecomastia may be a significant problem for some adolescent and adult XXY males (Lancet, 1988).

NEUROENDOCRINE FUNCTIONING

The pituitary-gonadal functioning of XXY boys has been found to be normal during childhood; follicle-stimulating hormone (FSH) and luteinizing hormone (LH) values are within the normal range before the onset of puberty (at age 12) but are elevated at the age of 14 (Robinson et al., 1986). A rise in serum testosterone is observed in adolescence, but reaches a plateau after the age of 14 and does not rise above mid-normal range. The XXY boys are clearly hypergonadotropic by the age of 13 to 14 (Stewart et al., 1982b; Robinson et al., 1986). Beginning at puberty, a variety of abnormalities in the hypothalamic-pituitary-testicular axis are seen. Testosterone levels may be normal (Samaan et al., 1979) or low (Ratcliffe et al., 1982a). These levels are maintained by increased hypothalamic secretion of gonadotropin releasing hormone and pituitary secretion of LH and FSH because of decreased testosterone feedback on the hypothalamic pituitary axis (Ratcliffe et al., 1982a). The mean plasma LH response to Gn RH stimulation is increased, while the FSH response is diminished (De Behar et al., 1975). The hypersecretion of gonadotropin by the pituitary has been reported to lead to enlargement of the sella turcica (Samaan et al., 1979). There is also increased conversion of testosterone to estradiol (Garbrilove et al., 1980). The increased estradiol to testosterone ratio may account for the increased incidence of gynecomastia seen in patients with KS. Young adult XXY males have been found to have significantly higher LH and FSH and lower concentrations of testosterone compared with controls (Schiavi et al., 1978).

Testosterone Treatment

The success of testosterone treatment in producing improvement in the emotional and behavioral characteristics of XXY males has not been firmly established. Several authors have reported positive effects of testosterone treatment in XXY boys as related to learning and behavior (Annell et al., 1970; Johnson et al., 1970; Caldwell and Smith, 1972; Sorensen et al., 1981). Sorensen and his colleagues (1981) administered testosterone enanthate 100 mg intramuscularly every third week, and if no effect was found, increased the dosage to 200 mg. Ten of 11 boys treated reported increased vitality, zeal, and concentration ability. In contrast to the findings of Sorensen and his colleagues (1981), Stewart et al. (1986) found treatment of testosterone cypionate, 100 mg every 4 weeks, to have no effect on the behavior, personality, or school performance of XXY boys 13 to 15 years of age. The treatment was successful only in initiating puberty in those boys whose onset of puberty was delayed. Stewart and his colleagues (1986) did, however, suggest that testosterone treatment with more physiological doses of testosterone administered at more frequent intervals might produce beneficial effects on psychosocial adaptation, academic performance, and psychosexual adjustment. Significantly, Nielsen et al. (1988) report that testosterone cypionate and testosterone enanthate induce an increase in serum testosterone level for only 12 to 14 days. Therefore, the 4-week intervals between injections used by Stewart et al. (1986) were considered too long. Accordingly, Nielsen et al. suggest that the lack of significant effect of testosterone treatment found by Stewart et al. (1986) cannot be taken as evidence of lack of effect of testosterone treatment. Nielsen et al.'s (1988) follow-up study of 30 XXY adult males treated with testosterone indicated that 77% of the men were judged to have benefited from testosterone treatment. The men reported more endurance and strength, less fatigue, more activity, better working capacity, improved concentration, better learning ability, better mood, less irritability, less need for sleep, and better relations with others. Nielsen et al. (1988) recommend that testosterone treatment be offered to XXY boys, preferably at the age of 11 to 12 in an effort to promote normal pubertal development and to have a stabilizing effect on emotional development.

COGNITIVE DEVELOPMENT

Intelligence

The diagnosis of KS does not denote a specific level or category of intelligence. Studies of XXY males have identified individuals functioning within the above average to superior range of intelligence (Nielsen et al., 1982; Theilgaard, 1984; Robinson et al., 1986; Walzer et al., 1986). In summarizing prospective studies of XXY's identified at birth, Stewart et al. (1982a) report that only 18.7% of XXY boys studied had a full-scale IQ below 90; of those identified as having a depressed full-scale IQ, 47.5% had a decreased verbal IQ, which negatively impacted the full-scale score. The global intelligence of XXY boys has appeared below that observed in siblings and controls (Robinson et al., 1979a), but low IQs have mostly been found in the verbal areas; whereas, performance scores have not been found significantly reduced (Nielsen et al., 1979; Evans et al., 1982; Pennington et al., 1982; Stewart et al., 1982b, 1986; Walzer et al., 1982, 1986; Leonard and Sparrow, 1986; Ratcliffe et al., 1986; Netley, 1987; Graham et al., 1988). Decreased verbal IQs have also been observed in XXY adults (Theilgaard et al., 1971; Porter et al., 1988), which suggests that verbal deficits observed in childhood and adolescence continue into adulthood.

In summary, research findings indicate that XXY males are most often of normal intelligence, may demonstrate a slight deficit in global intelligence compared with controls that appears related to decreased verbal scores, and, overall, demonstrate a wide spectrum of IQ scores.

Language Development

XXY boys frequently demonstrate delayed speech and language development that may be detected as early as 2 to 2 1/2 years of age (Leonard et al., 1974, 1982; Bancroft et al., 1982). In summarizing the findings of sex chromatin surveys of newborns conducted between 1967 and 1974, Robinson et al. (1979a) report that half of the XXY boys studied demonstrated significantly delayed speech development compared with their siblings. The parents of young XXY boys report delayed speech and language development in their children, with deficits noted in sentence-building skills, speech and production, intonation and accent, or in finding specific words to express thoughts clearly (Walzer et al., 1982). Leonard et al. (1979, 1982) report a significantly decreased developmental rate of language among XXY boys aged 2 to 2 1/2 years that followed these boys into the school years. These children continued to demonstrate impaired language development at 8 to 9 years of age, exhibiting language deficits in the areas of articulation, comprehension, verbal abstraction, sequencing, and ability to clearly express a story idea.

Graham et al. (1988) find that XXY boys demonstrate impairment in expressive language, which appears related to a pattern of deficits including problems in rate and order processing of auditory stimuli, problems understanding complex grammatical constructions, and problems in oral language. Problems in oral language include deficits in morphology, word-retrieval abilities, and narrative construction. The results of Graham et al.'s study (1988) suggest that XXY boys are handicapped by auditory rate processing difficulties and auditory memory deficits with concomitant difficulties in expressive language. Their expressive language deficits appear to involve difficulties in word finding, syntax production, and narrative formulation.

The language deficits apparent in XXY children are also observed in adults. Theilgaard (1984), in a study of XXY males identified in a birth cohort of tall men in Copenhagen, found XXY adults to have difficulties in articulating and structuring verbal expression. Their weakness in verbalization was demonstrated by a lack of precision, incomplete sentences, vagueness, awkward word-construction, difficulty in word mobilization, and the use of words without a preestablished reference to what the words might designate. Additional evidence that the verbal deficits observed in XXY children may continue into adulthood is provided by Porter and her colleagues (1988); when XXY adults were compared with matched controls, the XXY males demonstrated significantly poor performance on three of four tests used to measure verbal ability. An analysis of WAIS-R Verbal Subtests indicated that none of the men with KS scored beyond the fiftieth percentile on any of the verbal subtests.

Motor Development

Motor development of XXY boys falls within the normal range; however, a tendency to poor gross motor coordination has been observed (Nielsen et al., 1979; Robinson et al., 1979a, 1982, 1986). Robinson et al. (1979b) find XXY boys to be motorially slow and awkward in infancy and early childhood, which is thought to be related to neuromaturational lag. The children studied by Robinson and his colleagues (1979b, 1982) demonstrated delayed neuromaturation. Poor gross and fine motor coordination was observed as well as visual-motor and sensory integration problems, which were manifested in difficulty with eye-hand coordination, distractibility, impulsivity, and short attention span. Balance and equilibrium difficulties were also evident. Interviews with parents of the XXY boys suggested that neuromuscular delays affected school performance in areas associated with writing skills, timed activities, and athletic activities with peers. The neuromaturational lag identified in early childhood is thought to persist well beyond these years by Robinson and his colleagues (1986), who found that their sample of XXY between the ages of 9 and 17 years achieved lower mean scores than controls on tasks involving gross and fine motor skills, coordination, speed and dexterity, and strength.

Educational Performance

The most consistent finding in the investigation of XXY males is that of poor school performance. Stewart et al. (1982a) report that all of the eight centers participating in chromosome surveys and studies of newborns have reported that educational problems are common in their samples (63.7% of the 58 XXY cases as compared with 26.3% of the controls). In summarizing the findings of longitudinal studies of boys with the sex chromosome aneuploidy XXY, Netley (1986) reports that 67.6% of the XXY boys were judged to have educational problems in comparison with 22.2% of matched controls.

Although of normal intelligence, XXY boys demonstrate poor reading and spelling skills (Stewart et al., 1979; Leonard et al., 1982; Ratcliffe et al., 1986; Netley, 1987; Graham et al., 1988). These children have been found to require exceptional education and to repeat a grade at a much greater rate than siblings or controls (Leonard et al., 1979, 1982; Robinson et al., 1982, 1986; and Stewart et al., 1982b, 1986). Reading difficulties are especially noted in XXY boys, with Ratcliffe et al. (1986) reporting that 66.7% of the boys that she and her colleagues studied required remedial teaching in reading. Robinson et al. (1986) reported that 50% of the XXY boys studied by his group appeared to have a specific dyslexia, and 11 of 14 boys had problems in reading.

In an investigation of the oral and written language abilities of XXY boys, Graham et al. (1988) found that these boys had difficulty mastering basic skills of word analysis, and that their problems in word analysis were associated with decreased accuracy and rate of oral reading and reduced comprehension of text-related material. The children's deficits in reading, word analysis, and spelling were found to be associated with the presence of oral language problems and decreased auditory processing abilities. Graham and his colleagues (1988) found that those XXY boys demonstrating language disorders in the preschool years also demonstrated disorders of reading and writing during the school years.

PERSONALITY AND BEHAVIOR

Although no specific personality profile or behavioral pattern typified the XXY male, common characteristics of temperament have been observed. The XXY boy is often described as introverted and quiet, less assertive, passive, demonstrating lower levels of activity compared with other children, and tending to withdraw from group activities (Nielsen et al., 1979, 1982; Stewart et al., 1982b, 1986). The XXY boy also exhibits immaturity to a significant degree and appears susceptible to anxiety (Nielsen et al., 1979; Stewart et al., 1979; Robinson et al., 1982, 1986).

The self-ratings of XXY adolescents, as studied by Ratcliffe et al. (1982a), find XXY boys rating themselves as more tender minded, apprehensive, and insecure compared with controls. They reported more problems with peer group relationships and less sexual interest in girls. Similar findings were reported in Theilgaard's (1984) study of young adult XXY males. These men rated themselves as more nervous, passive, dependent, and less assertive compared with controls. They also reported having difficulty making social contact with others and were less outgoing socially. They demonstrated less self-acceptance, lower levels of ambition and satisfaction, and decreased sexual libido. Ratcliffe et al. (1982a) and Theilgaard (1984) report lower masculinity scores among XXY males, as measured by the Bem's (1974) sex role inventory and the Thematic Apperception Test, respectively. Ratcliffe and her colleagues suggest that masculine attributes are generally socially desirable, and the significantly lower masculinity score of the XXY adolescent in the study could reflect reduced self-esteem. Theilgaard reports that the XXY males studied lacked a crystallized sense of masculinity and appeared to have difficulty living up to the masculine role. She suggests that the parents, siblings, and peers of XXY boys may fail to respond to these children in a manner which would sharpen their awareness of their male gender.

DISCUSSION

The data provided by longitudinal studies of XXY males identified in cytogenetic surveys of newborns and the controlled studies of noninstitutionalized XXY adults have clarified many of the misconceptions associated with an additional X chromosome. We now know that the diagnosis of KS does not denote an increased likelihood of criminality, psychopathology, or mental retardation. To the contrary, the XXY male is most likely to be of normal intelligence (Stewart et al., 1982a; Theilgaard, 1984) free of psychiatric disturbance (Netley, 1986; Nielsen and Pelsen, 1987), and demonstrates no more criminality than observed in XY men when intelligence and parental socioeconomic status are controlled (Schiavi, et al., 1984). There have been, however, deficiencies observed in XXY boys that impact their psychological development. XXY boys commonly exhibit speech and language delays in early childhood that appear predictive of academic difficulties during the school years (Graham et al., 1988). Verbal deficits are frequently observed in XXY boys as measured by the verbal subtests of the Wechsler Preschool and Primary Scale of Intelligence and Wechsler Intelligence Scale for Children-Revised, with a resulting decreased verbal IQ (Nielsen et al., 1979; Stewart et al., 1982a), and it has been reported that verbal deficits continue to be exhibited by XXY adults as measured by the verbal subtests of the WAIS (Porter et al., 1988). The problems XXY males experience in language production, processing, and structuring are thought to interfere not only with the ability to communicate, but also with the acquisition of reading skills and spelling. This has certainly been the case in XXY boys, in that these children demonstrate educational difficulties at a highly significant level especially in the areas of reading and spelling (Stewart et al., 1982a). XXY boys have also been observed to have poor fine and gross motor skills as compared with matched controls that may interfere with school performance in the areas of writing, timed activities, and athletic activities with peers (Robinson et al., 1982, 1986).

The precise relationship between an additional X chromosome and the cognitive development (intelligence, learning, language, and neuromotor skills) of the XXY male is currently speculative. Stewart et al. (1986) postulate that impairments in the cognitive development of XXY males are due to prenatally occurring disturbances in growth. Stewart et al. cite the research of Waber (1977) who found that physical growth and certain cognitive skills are related. She demonstrated that slow maturers are more skilled spatially than verbally, whereas fast maturers demonstrate the opposite pattern of skills. In keeping with Waber's theory, XXY boys demonstrate delayed bone age maturation and are verbally weak. In further support of the relationship of physical growth and cognitive development, Netley and Rovet (1982) report that individual differences in bone age maturation in XXY males are related to their degree of verbal deficit. Waber (1977) also found that maturation rates influence hemispheric organization, with slow development being associated with a greater left versus right hemisphere asymmetry for verbal processing than fast development. XXY males demonstrate lower than normal degrees of left hemisphere specialization for language and greater than normal degrees of right hemisphere specialization for nonverbal processing (Netley and Rovet, 1982). Stewart et al. (1986) postulate that slow rates of prenatal growth retard the development of the left hemisphere, which in turn allows the right to develop free of inhibitory influences from the left. The authors suggest that XXY boys with the slower rates of growth are those whose right hemispheres are more functionally active. Stewart and his colleagues (1986) have found that XXY males demonstrating elevated right hemisphere scores also demonstrate the greatest deficit in verbal IQ relative to performance IQ.

In an effort to understand why XXY males experience similar temperament styles and maladjustment, Stewart et al. (1986) studied hormonal functioning, quality of parenting, and hemispheric specialization of adolescent XXY boys. Each of the three factors studied were found to influence temperament and adjustment. Stewart and his colleagues cite the work of Tucker and Williamson (1984) to explain the relationship between hemispheric functioning and social-emotional development.

The left hemisphere has been identified as playing a role in controlling tonic activation levels, internally focused serial attentional and motor mechanisms, and motivation. The right hemisphere facilitates habituation to repetitive stimuli, responds to novelty, and is considered important in regulating emotion. Stewart et al. (1986) theorize that the hormonal effects on temperament and adjustment emerge during adolescence and act upon qualities of temperament already influenced by hemispheric organization and environmental factors, such as family functioning.

The combination of poor language skills, academic difficulties, and a tendency to poor fine and gross motor coordination would seen to set the stage for social and psychological difficulties. The child may have poor social skills related to language/verbal deficits (Stewart et al., 1986) and diminished self-esteem related to school failure and impaired motor functioning that interferes with athletic abilities and normal adaptive processes (Robinson et al., 1986). The XXY boy's sense of identity and self-concept may be tested during adolescence as he experiences problems in sexual development that may include gynecomastia and decreased testicular volume (Stewart et al., 1982b, 1986).

The early identification of boys with KS is recommended (Nielsen et al., 1982, 1988) in an effort to provide parents with information and counseling regarding the development of KS, particularly the importance of addressing delays in neuromuscular development, language, and learning at an early age.

The diagnosis of KS should be considered in boys with language difficulties, learning problems, behavioral difficulties, lack of coordination, long limbs with upper to lower segment ratio, increased height, and small penis and testes for their age (Jones, 1988). Testosterone treatment at the age of approximately 12 years is recommended in order to bring about a more normal adolescent development and to possibly serve as a prophylactic against deviations in behavior and learning abilities (Nielsen et al., 1979, 1982; Nielsen and Pelsen, 1987; Nielsen et al., 1988).

REFERENCES

Annell, A. L., Gustavson, K. H. & Tenstam, J. (1970), Symptomatology, in schoolboys with positive sex chromatin (the Klinefelter syndrome). *Acta Psychiatr. Scand.*, 46:71–80.

Bancroft, J., Axworthy, D. & Ratcliffe, S. G. (1982), The personality and psycho-sexual development of boys with 47,XXY chromosome constitution. *J. Child Psycho. Psychiatry*, 23:169–180.

Bem, S. L. (1974), The measurement of psychological androgyny. *J. Consult. Clin. Psychol.*, 42:155–162.

Boisen, E. (1979), Testicular size and shape of 47,XYY and 47,XXY men in a double-blind, double-matched population survey. *Am. J. Human Genet.*, 31:697–703.

Bradbury, J. T., Bunge, R. G. & Boccabella, R. A. (1956), Chromatin test in Klinefelter's syndrome. *J. Clin. Endocr. Metab.*, 16:689.

Caldwell, P. D. & Smith, D. W. (1972), The XXY (Klinefelter's) syndrome in childhood: detection and treatment. *J. Pediatr.*, 80:250–258.

Carothers, A. D. & Fillippi, G. (1988), Klinefelter's syndrome in Sardinia and Scotland: comparative studies of parental age and other aetiological factors in 47,XXY. *Hum. Gen.*, 81:71–75.

DeBehar, B. R., Mendilaharzu, H., Rivarola, M. A. & Bergada, C. (1975), Gonadotropin secretion in prepubertal and pubertal primary hypogonadism: response to LHRH. *J. Clin. Endocr. Metab.*, 41:1070–1075.

Evans, J. A., de von Flindt, R., Greenberg, C. et al. (1982), A cytogenetic survey of 14,069 newborn infants, IV, further follow-up on the children with sex chromosome anomalies. In: *Birth Defects: Original Article Series*, ed. D. Stewart. New York: Alan R. Liss, Inc., 18:(4),169–184.

———————————et al. (1986), Physical and psychologic parameters in children with sex chromosome anomalies: further follow-up from the Winnipeg cytogenetic study of 14,069 newborn infants. In: *Birth Defects: Original Articles Series*, eds. S. G. Ratcliffe & N. Paul. New York: Alan R. Liss, Inc., 22:(3),183–207.

Ferguson-Smith, M. A. (1959), The prepubertal testicular lesion in chromatine—positive Klinefelter's syndrome as seen in mentally handicapped children. *Lancet*, i:219–222.

Forssman, H. (1970), The mental implications of sex chromosome aberrations. *Br. J. Psychiatry*, 117:353–363.

———Hambert, G. (1963), Incident of Klinefelter's syndrome among mental patients. *Lancet*, i:1327.

Garbrilove, J. L., Freiberg, E. K. & Nicolis, G. L. (1980), Testicular function in Klinefelter's syndrome. *J. Urol.*, 124:825–826.

Graham, J. M., Bashir, A. S., Stark, R. E., Silbert, A. & Walzer, S. (1988), Oral and written language abilities of XXY boys: implications for anticipatory guidance. *Pediatrics*, 81:795–806.

Hamerton, J. L., Canning, N., Ray, M. & Smith, S. (1975), A cytogenetic survey of 14,069 newborn infants. I. incidence of chromosome abnormalities. *Clin. Genet.*, 8:223–243.

Hook E. B. (1973), Behavioral implications of the human XXY genotype. *Science*, 179:139–179.

Johnson, H. R., Myhre, S. A., Ruvalcaba, R. H. A. et al. (1970), Effects of testosterone on body image and behavior in Klinefelter's syndrome: pilot study. *Dev. Med. Child Neurol.*, 454:460.

Jones, K. L. (1988), *Smith's Recognizable Patterns of Human Malformation*, Fourth Edition. Philadelphia: W. B. Saunders Co.

Klinefelter, H. F., Reifenstein, E. C. & Albright, F. (1942), Syndrome characterized by gynecomastia aspermatogenes without A-Leydigism and increased excretion of follicle stimulating hormone. *J. Clin. Endocr. Metabl.*, 2:615–627.

Klinefelter's Syndrome. (1988), *Lancet*, pp. 316–317.

Leonard, M. F. & Sparrow, S. (1986), Prospective study of development of children with sex chromosome anomalies: New Haven study IV. adolescence. In: *Birth Defects:*

Original Article Series, eds. S. G. Ratcliffe & N. Paul. New York: Alan R. Liss, Inc., 22:(3),221–249.

———Landy, G., Ruddle, F. H. & Lubs, H. A. (1974), Early development of children with abnormalities of the sex chromosomes: a prospective study. *Pediatrics*, 54:208–212.

———Schowalter, J. E., Landy, G., Ruddle, F. H. & Lubs, H. A. (1979), Chromosomal abnormalities in the New Haven newborn study: a prospective study of development of children with sex chromosome anomalies. In: *Birth Defects: Original Article Series*, eds. A. Robinson, H. A. Lubs & D. Bergsma. New York: Alan R. Liss, Inc., XV:(1),115–159.

———Landy, G. & Schowalter, J. E. (1982), A prospective study of development of children with sex chromosome anomalies: New Haven study III. The middle years. In: *Birth Defects: Original Article Series*, ed. D. A. Stewart. New York: Alan R. Liss, Inc., 18:(4),193–218.

MacLean, N., Mitchell, J. M. et al. (1962), A survey of sex chromosome abnormalities among 4514 mental defectives. *Lancet*, i:293–296.

———Court-Brown, W. M. & Jacobs, P. A. (1968), A survey of sex chromatin anomalies in mental hospital patients. *J. Med. Genet.*, 5:165–172.

Netley, C. T. (1986), Summary overview of behavioral development in individuals with neonatally identified X and Y aneuploidy. In: *Birth Defects: Original Article Series*, eds. S. G. Ratcliffe & N. Paul. New York: Alan R. Liss, Inc., 22:(3),293–306.

———(1987), Predicting intellectual functioning in 47,XXY boys from characteristics of sibs. *Clin. Genet.*, 32:24–27.

———Rovet, J. (1982), Verbal deficits in children with 47,XXY and 47,XXX karyotypes: a descriptive and experimental study. *Brain Lang.*, 17:58–73.

Nielsen, J. (1970), Criminality among patients with Klinefelter's syndrome. *Br. J. Psychiatry*, 117:365–369.

———Pelsen, B. (1987), Follow-up 20 years later of 34 Klinefelter males with karyotype 47,XXY and 16 hypogonadal males with karyotype 46,XY. *Hum. Genet.*, 77:188–192.

———Sillesen, I., Sorensen, A. M. & Sorensen, K. (1979), Follow-up until age 4 to 8 of 25 unselected children with sex chromosome abnormalities, compared with sibs and controls. In: *Birth Defects: Original Article Series*, eds. A. Robinson, H. A. Lubs, & D. Bergsma. New York: Alan R. Liss, Inc., XV:15–73.

———Sorensen, A. M. & Sorensen, K. (1982), Follow-up until age 7 to 11 of 25 children with sex chromosome abnormalities. In: *Birth Defects: Original Article Series*, ed. D. A. Stewart. New York: Alan R. Liss, Inc., 18:(4),61–97.

———Wohlert, M., Faaborg-Andersen, J. et al. (1986), Chromosome examination of 20,222 newborn children: results from a 7.5 year study in Arhus, Denmark. In: *Birth Defects: Original Article Series*, eds. S. G. Ratcliffe & N. Paul. New York: Alan R. Liss, Inc., 22:(3),209–219.

———————Sorensen, K. (1988), Follow-up of 30 Klinefelter males treated with testosterone. *Clin. Genet.*, 33:262–269.

Pennington, B. F., Bender, B., Puck, M., Salbenblatt, J. & Robinson, A. (1982), Learning disabilities in children with sex chromosome abnormalities. *Child Dev.*, 53:1182–1192.

Polani, P. E. (1967), Chromosome anomalies and the brain. *Guy's Hospital Reports*, 116:365–396.

Porter, M. E., Gardner, H. A., DeFeudis, P. & Endler, N. S. (1988), Verbal deficits in Klinefelter (XXY) adults living in the community. *Clin. Genet.*, 33:246–253.

Ratcliffe, S. G., Axworthy, D. & Ginsburg, A. (1979), The Edinburgh study of growth and development in children with sex chromosome abnormalities. In: *Birth Defects: Original Article Series*, eds. A. Robinson, H. A. Lubs & D. Bergsma. New York: Alan R. Liss, Inc., XV:(1),243–260.

———Bancroft, J., Axworthy, D. & McLaren, W. (1982a), Klinefelter's syndrome in adolescence. *Arch. Dis. Child.*, 57:13–17.

———Tierney, I., Nshaho, J. et al. (1982b), The Edinburgh study of growth and development of children with sex chromosome abnormalities. In: *Birth Defects: Original Article Series*, ed. D. A. Stewart. New York: Alan R. Liss, Inc., 18:(4),41–60.

———Murray, L. & Teague, P. (1986), Edinburgh study of growth and development of children with sex chromosome abnormalities III. In: *Birth Defects: Original Article Series*, eds. S. G. Ratcliffe & N. Paul. New York: Alan R. Liss, Inc., 22:(3),73–118.

Robinson, A., Lubs, H. A., Nielsen, J. & Sorensen, K. (1979a), Summary of clinical findings: profiles of children with 47,XXY, 47,XXX and 47,XYY karyotypes. In: *Birth Defects: Original Article Series*, eds. A. Robinson, H. A. Lubs & D. Bergsma. New York: Alan R. Liss, Inc., XV:(1),261–266.

———Puck, M., Pennington, B., Borelli, J. & Hudson, M. (1979b), Abnormalities of the sex chromosomes: a prospective study on randomly identified new borns. In: *Birth Defects: Original Article Series*, eds. A. Robinson, H. A. Lubs & D. Bergsma. New York: Alan R. Liss, Inc., XV:(1),203–241.

———Bender, B., Borelli, J., Puck, M., Salbenblatt, J. & Webber, M. L. (1982), Sex chromosome abnormalities (SCA): a prospective and longitudinal study of newborns identified in an unbiased manner. In: *Birth Defects: Original Article Series*, ed. D. A. Stewart. New York: Alan R. Liss, Inc., 18:(4),7–39.

———————Winter, J. S. (1986), Sex chromosome aneuploidy: prospective and longitudinal studies. In: *Birth Defects: Original Article Series*, eds. S. G. Ratcliffe & N. Paul. New York: Alan R. Liss, Inc., 22:(3),23–71.

Samaan, N. A., Stepanas, A. V., Danzinger, J. & Trujillo, J. (1979), Reactive pituitary abnormalities in patients with Klinefelter's and Turner's syndrome. *Arch. Intern. Med.*, 139:198–201.

Sanger, R., Tippett, P., Gavin, J., Teesdale, P. & Daniels, G. L. (1977), Xg groups and sex chromosome abnormalities in people of northern european ancestry: an addendum. *J. Med. Genet.*, 14:210–213.

Schiavi, R. C., Owen, D., Fogel, M. et al. (1978), Pituitarygonadal function in XYY and XXY men identified in a population study. *Clin. Endocrinol.*, 9:233–239.

———Theilgaard, A., Owen, D. R. & White, D. (1984), Sex chromosome anomalies, hormones, and aggressivity. *Arch. Gen. Psychiatry*, 41:93–99.

Sorensen, K., Sorensen, A. M. & Nielsen, J. (1981), Social and psychological development of adolescents with Klinefelter's syndrome. In: *Human Behavior and Genetics*, eds. W. Schmid & J. Nielsen. New York: Biomedical Press, pp. 45–64.

Stewart, D. A., Netley, C. T., Bailey, J. D. et al. (1979), Growth and development of children with X and Y chromosome aneuploidy: a prospective study. In: *Birth Defects: Original Article Series*, eds. A. Robinson, H. A. Lubs & D. Bergsma. New York: Alan R. Liss, Inc., XV:(1):75–114.

————————Park, E. (1982a), Summary of clinical findings of children with 47,XXY, 47,XYY, and 47,XXX karyotypes. In: *Birth Defects: Original Article Series*, ed. D. A. Stewart. New York: Alan R. Liss, Inc., 18(4),1–5.

————Bailey, J. D., Netley, C. T. et al. (1982b), Growth and development of children with X and Y chromosome abnormalities. In: *Birth Defects: Original Article Series*, ed. D. A. Stewart. New York: Alan R. Liss, Inc., 18:(4),99–154.

————————————————Park, E. (1986), Growth and development from early to midadolescence of children with X and Y chromosome aneuploidy: The Toronto study. In: *Birth Defects: Original Article Series*, eds. S. G. Ratcliffe & N. Paul. New York: Alan R. Liss, Inc., 22:(3),119–182.

Theilgaard, A. (1984), A psychological study of the personalities of XYY and XXY men. *Acta Psychiatr. Scand.*, 315:1–133.

————Nielsen, J., Sorensen, A. et al. (1971), A psychological-psychiatric study of patients with Klinefelter's syndrome 47,XXY. *Acta Jutlandica*, 43:1–148.

Tucker, D. M. & Williamson, P. A. (1984), Asymmetric neural control systems in human self-regulation. *Psychol. Rev.*, 91:185–215.

Waber, D. (1977), Sex differences and the rate of physical growth. *Developmental Psychology*, 13:29–38.

Walzer, S., Graham, J. M., Bashir, A. S. & Silbert, A. R. (1982), Preliminary observations on language and learning in XXY boys. In: *Birth Defects: Original Article Series*, ed. D. A. Stewart. New York: Alan R. Liss, Inc., 18:(4),185–192.

————Bashir, A. S., Graham, J. M. et al. (1986), Behavioral development of boys with X chromosome aneuploidy: impact of reactive style on educational intervention for learning deficits. In: *Birth Defects: Original Article Series*, eds. S. G. Ratcliffe & N. Paul. New York: Alan R. Liss, Inc., 22:(3),1–21.

Witkin, H. A., Mednick, S. A., Schulsinger, F. et al. (1976), Criminality in XYY and XXY men. *Science*, 193:547–555.

18

Psychiatric Aspects of Epileptic Children and Adolescents

Wun Jung Kim

Medical College of Ohio at Toledo

Epilepsy is the most prevalent neurological disorder of childhood and adolescence and a very heterogeneous disease with a diverse course of illness. It may be a benign disease for the majority of children and adolescents, who recover spontaneously, or are managed well medically; however, a sizable group of children and adolescents with epilepsy, at least one-third, do manifest various difficulties—seizure control, academic, emotional, behavioral, and family problems. As a group, they have a much higher rate of psychiatric disorder than healthy children and children with other chronic illnesses. This review is undertaken to summarize the literature on epilepsy in children and adolescents, especially with respect to epidemiology, developmental and psychiatric problems, and psychiatric treatment issues.

Epilepsy is primarily a childhood and adolescent disorder. Several epidemiological studies of the general population have reported that at least 75% of epilepsy begins before the age of 20, and 50% of childhood onset epilepsy occurs during the first 5 years of life. (Cowan et al., 1989; Gudmundsson, 1966; Silanpää, 1973).

A general practitioner of child and adolescent psychiatry sees a significant number of children and adolescents with epilepsy who have been referred by physicians, mental health professionals, and families for various reasons, such as behavioral, school problems, and the use of psychotropic drugs. Because the disease involves the central nervous system (CNS), it produces behavioral symptoms. It is also accompanied by adjustment problems because of the chronic nature of the disease.

Reprinted with permission from the *Journal of the American Academy of Child and Adolescent Psychiatry*, 1991, Vol. 30, No. 6, 874–886. Copyright © 1991 by the American Academy of Child and Adolescent Psychiatry.

The author thanks Drs. Joel Zrull and Un Jung Kang for their thoughtful and critical comments.

These behavioral aspects are particularly important in understanding and treating children and adolescents with epilepsy and need to be examined from a developmental vantage point.

There is an abundance of literature on epilepsy and psychiatry, including two books (Blumer, 1984; Reynolds and Trimble, 1981) published on both sides of the Atlantic in the 1980s, reflecting the increasing knowledge of and re-emerging interest in neuropsychiatry. However, the majority of the literature concerns the psychiatric aspects of epilepsy in adults. A survey of child psychiatry textbooks also reveals the cursory attention paid to this issue, which is usually included in a chapter on psychosocial aspects of the chronic childhood illness.

This review was undertaken to summarize the literature on epilepsy in children and adolescents, especially with respect to epidemiology, developmental and psychiatric problems, and psychiatric treatment issues. A computerized bibliographical search was conducted on different subtopics for this review. For example, the keywords of "emotions," "behavioral," "children," "adolescents," "human development," and "epilepsy" through the Medline produced 125 references. In addition, references from relevant review articles, monographs, and books were cross-checked. The references were selected from the studies that specifically deal with developmental issues, although adult studies were also cited for the continuity of and the relevance to the topic of discussion. Findings from the studies that employed scientifically sound methodology, such as the use of representative samples, control groups, or operationalized definitions of variables, will be highlighted.

There are inherent pitfalls in conducting a broad review on a heterogeneous disease like epilepsy with its multiple causes and multiple types. This review focuses on *idiopathic* epilepsy, not a symptomatic epilepsy resulting from other primary medical conditions. Confounding factors associated with epilepsy, such as intellectual, neurodevelopmental deficits, and seizure types, will be discussed while an attempt is made to draw broad, generalized conclusions. There are only a few studies that have incorporated confounding variables and employed scientifically sound research methodology. Therefore, descriptive and case reports in the areas where research is scarce are also incorporated to enhance understanding of the current status of knowledge. However, discrepant findings from different studies will be discussed in relation to methodological issues. The aim of this review is to provide a clinically useful, up-to-date summary of epilepsy, its psychosocial complications, and management issues.

EPIDEMIOLOGY

Epidemiological studies of school children in the United States (Baumann et al., 1977; Haerer et al., 1986; Meighan et al., 1976; Rose et al., 1973; Shamansky and Glaser, 1979) have shown somewhat higher prevalence rates, up to 20 per 1,000 than the rates of 4 to 6 per 1,000 in the general population. This variability of prevalence rates is related to the kinds of populations, the ages of samples, the case definitions, the methods of case ascertainment, and the methods of estimation that different studies have employed. Rutter et al. (1970) and Cowan et al. (1989) have performed methodologically sound epidemiological studies on school children. The Rutter's Isle of Wight study reported an overall 7.2 per 1,000 prevalence rate of epilepsy and a 5.4 per 1,000 prevalence rate of "uncomplicated" epilepsy (i.e., epilepsy without structural brain disorder). The most recent U.S. study by Cowan et al. (1989), using strict criteria for case definition, reported a 5.2 per 1,000 rate for children aged 0 to 4 and a 4.6 per 1,000 rate for children and adolescents, aged 5 to 19. A conservative estimation indicates that at least 500,000 U.S. children and adolescents suffer from nonfebrile recurrent seizures, the majority of which are idiopathic.

Prognosis

The discrepancy in reported prevalence rates between children and the general population may be accounted for by a high remission rate, by a declining incidence in older ages, and possibly by a high mortality rate of epileptic children. Thus, the outlook for an epileptic condition at its onset varies more widely than any other medical illness, setting the scene for interesting psychological ramifications for epileptic children and their families. For instance, the benign epilepsy of childhood with rolandic (centrotemporal) foci, the most common variety of partial epilepsy in childhood, has almost a 100% remission rate after 12 years of age, although it begins with quite remarkable attacks of seizure during sleep or wakefulness (Loiseau et al., 1983).

The reported remission rates range from one-third to three-quarters, depending on the type of seizure studied and on the number of years of follow-up (Annegers et al., 1980; Boulloche et al., 1989; Brorson and Wranne, 1987; Ehrhardt and Forsythe, 1989; Lindsay et al., 1980; Rodin, 1972). The absence seizures appear to have the best prognosis, followed by the generalized tonic-clonic seizures and others. More recent studies of different types of stable seizures (at least two seizure-free years while on medication) have demonstrated a very high remission rate, on the average about 75% during 6-month to 6-year follow-up periods, after withdrawal of antiepileptic drugs (Arts et al., 1988; Callaghan et al., 1988; Matricardi et al., 1989; Shinnar et al., 1985). Factors favoring remission included the absence of a definable cause, a normal neurological examination, normal intelligence, a less abnormal electroencephalogram (EEG), and a low rate of seizure occurrence.

At the opposite end of the spectrum, the mortality rates during childhood and early adult life range from about 20% in children with neonatal seizures and infantile spasms (Dennis, 1979) to about 6% to 10% in children with different childhood epilepsies (Callaghan et al., 1988; Harrison and Taylor, 1976; Silanpää, 1973). A review of these long-term follow-up studies reveals the "one-third" rule, which is, in general, similar to the prognosis of many psychiatric disorders: at least one-third of epileptic children recover fully; about one-third grow up to be functional to varying degrees with good seizure control by medication; and the rest, a little less than one-third, either die prematurely or suffer from a severe handicap.

PSYCHIATRIC MORBIDITY

Because epilepsy involves the CNS, it not only results in psychosocial problems of adjusting to a chronic illness but also in increased cognitive and behavioral problems associated with CNS dysfunction. In addition, the family's adjustment problems, social prejudice, and the cognitive/behavioral toxicity of antiepileptic drugs also complicate the epileptic child's psychosocial adjustments. It is, therefore, not difficult to anticipate increased psychiatric morbidity in epileptic children. There are several up-to-date comprehensive review articles on the psychiatric aspects of epilepsy or epilepsy in relation to psychiatry, covering broad issues of both children and adults (Lesser et al., 1986; Levin et al., 1988; Neppe and Tucker, 1988a, b). The literature reveals a rather grim picture of epileptics in whatever outcome variables are examined—emotional, behavioral, cognitive, academic, interpersonal, family, marital, vocational, etc.

In terms of the psychiatric morbidity of children and adolescents with epilepsy, Whitehouse (1971) and Hinton and Knights (1969) reported that 36% to 56% of epileptic children attending a pediatric neurology clinic in the United States and in Canada, respectively, showed "behavioral problems" or "abnormal psychological diagnosis." Difficulties of interpreting such data arose from the use of selective referred samples of epilepsy with different causes, unstandardized measurement, and lack of control groups. When a community sample or a sample attending a regular school was examined, the rate of behavior problems was only about 20% (Cavazzuti, 1980; Holdsworth and Whitmore, 1974a).

The Rutter's Isle of Wight Study (Rutter et al., 1970) managed to combat the drawbacks of many other studies. The study examined the 5- to 14-year-old child population of 11,865 with findings as follows: In comparison to a 6.6% rate of psychiatric disorder for the general population and an 11.6% rate for children with chronic physical disorders not involving the brain, the rate for children with neuroepileptic disorders was 34.3%. Among neuroepileptic disorders, the rate of psychiatric disorder was 28.6% for uncomplicated epilepsy, 37.5% for a CNS lesion without epilepsy, and 58.3% for epilepsy with a CNS lesion. These figures are comparable with the reports of population studies including both children and adults in which about one-third of epileptic subjects were found to have psychiatric disturbances (Gudmundsson, 1966; Pond and Bidwell, 1959/1960). A higher rate of psychiatric disorder in children with neuroepileptic disorder compared with children with other types of chronic medical illness has been substantiated by other studies, too (Cadman, et al., 1987; Hoare, 1984a).

The degree of psychiatric complication among different types of seizures has been also studied (Hoare, 1984a; Hodgman et al., 1979; Loiseau et al., 1983; Shukla and Katiyar, 1981; Silanpaa, 1973; Stores, 1977). It appears that children with focal EEG abnormalities and temporal lobe epilepsy (TLE), especially with left temporal lobe spikes, show a higher rate of psychiatric disorder. The effect of seizure frequency is somewhat intriguing, as some studies indicated better emotional adjustment with more frequent seizures (e.g., Hodgman et al., 1979). Perhaps the patient accepts the disease and is resigned to it more readily when the disease is severe rather than mild or borderline. However, in general, as in the prognosis of epilepsy, many agree that the severity of epilepsy (duration and frequency of seizure and chronicity) influences the psychosocial adjustments. Family, environmental factors, and anticonvulsants also contribute to the genesis of psychiatric disorder in epileptic children and will be discussed below under separate headings.

SPECIFIC PSYCHIATRIC SYNDROME

Diagnostic Profile Do epileptic children have *unique* psychopathology? Epileptic children have been generally described as dependent, withdrawn, tense, socially isolated, and having low self-esteem (Hartlage and Green, 1972; Hoare, 1984c; Long and Moore, 1979; Stores, 1978). Although relevant and plausible, these general descriptions hardly differentiate epileptic children from children with other chronic medical illnesses. In the Isle of Wight study (Rutter et al., 1970) among children with uncomplicated epilepsy, 12.7% had emotional disorder; 7.5% had conduct disorder; 4.8% had mixed disorder; and 1.6% had hyperkinetic syndrome. These rates were all higher than the rates in the general population. Like the studies of other types of chronic medical illness (Cadman et al., 1987; Eiser, 1990; Offord et al., 1989), that study did not find an association between epilepsy and a specific psychiatric syndrome. As in the general population, the majority of the neuroepileptic children with psychiatric disorder suffered from emotional and conduct disorders.

However, when all epileptic children regardless of underlying brain disorder or mental retardation are included, a different psychiatric profile emerges. Silanpää (1973) documented that in a community sample of southwestern Finland, 29% of children and adolescents with epilepsy had neurosis; 11% had autistic or symbiotic psychosis; and 33.5% had hyperkinetic syndrome. A high prevalence of psychotic and hyperkinetic syndrome reflects a compounding effect of the high prevalence of brain dysfunction and the mental retardation found in epileptic children. Thus, in addition to the extent of psychiatric disorder, the types of psychiatric disorder observed in epileptic children are also influenced by a sampling effect. In the Isle of Wight Study (Rutter et al., 1970), psychosis was found in none of the children with uncomplicated epilepsy, in one of 16 children of normal intelligence with brain disorder, and in five of 38 children of subnormal intelligence with neuroepileptic disorders. In fact, an association between a schizophrenia-like psychosis and epilepsy, especially a left temporal lobe type, has been intensely investigated and fairly well established in the adult literature (Parnas and Korsgaard, 1982; Sherwin, 1984; Slater and Beart, 1963). However, there has been no systematic study on psychosis in epileptic children, except a few case studies (Shah and Kaplan, 1980; Shukla and Katiyar, 1981). A psychotic disorder in a child with epilepsy is rare before puberty (Lindsay, 1972) and may manifest in a minority of brain damaged and mentally retarded epileptic children (Corbett and Trimble, 1983).

Developmental Problems

Certain distinctive personality characteristics of adults with TLE, such as hyperemotionality, viscosity, religiosity, hyposexuality, dissociation, etc., continue to attract research interest (Bear et al., 1982; Schenk and Bear, 1981; Tucker et al., 1987). Much has been written about the so-called "epileptic personality" in children and adolescents, but its validity has been seriously questioned (Gudmundsson, 1966; Nuffield, 1961; Tizard, 1962). During the early period of evolving personality formation, children with neuroepileptic disorders may show the characteristics of *difficult* temperament, which is a predictable variable for later personality and psychosocial function (Hertzig, 1983). A high rate of regressive behaviors in school children with epilepsy, such as nail biting, thumb sucking, stuttering, enuresis, encopresis, etc., has been reported (Rutter et al., 1970; Silanpää, 1973). These behaviors may be viewed as regression in relation to increasing stresses associated with schooling during latency and/or a continuation of earlier neurodevelopmental immaturity. Adolescent adjustment problems, especially with sexual identity, body image, and self-image have been noted (Viberg et al., 1987). In general, there are few studies that have examined problems of epileptic children in relation to specific tasks of psychosocial and biological development.

Aggression and Disruptive Behavioral Disorders

One of the most stereotypical perceptions of the mental problems of epileptic children is the children's inability to control unpredictable and aggressive behaviors. These behaviors symbolically fit the unpredictable and uncontrolled nature of seizure itself. Research has also been heavily focused on the spectrum of the disruptive behavior or impulse control disorders. Pond and Bidwell (1959/1960) found that the majority of epileptic children with psychiatric disorder had conduct disorders.

Aggression and rage attacks are prevalent in epileptic children. These behavioral symptoms were particularly more evident in children with TLE than with other types of epilepsy (Hermann et al., 1981; Keating, 1961; Nuffield, 1961; Williams, 1969). Ounsted and Lindsay (1981) observed that rages were a major problem for over one-third of children with TLE, and many of these aggressive children grew up to be antisocial in adult life. Inattentiveness and overactivity, symptoms of attention-deficit hyperactivity disorder (ADHD), have been often described in both controlled and uncontrolled studies of epileptic children (Hoare, 1984a; Holdsworth and Whitmore, 1974a; Ounsted, 1955; Ounsted and Lindsay, 1981; Stores, 1977, 1978; Stores et al., 1978) especially in boys with TLE. These psychiatric disturbances were viewed as inherently associated with epilepsy and not solely attributable to anticonvulsant effects or a secondary adjustment reaction of chronic illness (Hoare, 1984a; Stores et al., 1978).

Suicide and Depression

A review of suicide risk in adult epileptics points to a four to fives times higher risk than that of the general population (Mathews and Barabas, 1981). There is no such data available for children and adolescents, although there was a report of overrepresentation of epileptics in children and adolescents who attempted suicide (Brent, 1986). TLE and treatment by phenobartital were viewed as an added risk for suicidal behavior. In view of this high suicide risk, a high prevalence of underlying affective disorder may be suspected. In some studies of adults (Betts, 1981; Kogeorgos et al., 1982), depressive disorders, including endogenous depression, were reported to be the most prevalent psychopathology. However, there is no evidence of such a trend in children and adolescents with epilepsy. This may have to do with the difficulty of diagnosing childhood affective disorders in general and the only recently developing interest in childhood affective disorders in the field. It should be noted that many earlier studies relying on a broad diagnostic classification system reported a high incidence of "neurotic" or "emotional" disorders that included anxiety and depressive disorders.

COGNITION, LEARNING, AND EPILEPSY

Subnormal intelligence has been found in as high as one-third of epileptic children, if one includes borderline intelligence (Ellenberg et al., 1984, 1985; Gudmundsson, 1966; Ounsted and Lindsay, 1981; Rutter et al., 1970; Silanpää, 1973). Conversely, the incidence of epilepsy in mentally retarded children range from 3% to 32%, depending on the degree of mental retardation (Corbett et al., 1975; Rutter et al., 1970), the incidence increasing with the degree of mental retardation. As to the fallacy of intellectual degenerative processes found in both the child and adult literature (Dodrill, 1986; Lesser et al., 1986; Pedersen and Dam, 1986; Silanpää, 1973), carefully designed prospective studies demonstrated that intelligence did not deteriorate in the majority of children with epilepsy (Bourgeois et al., 1983; Ellenberg et al., 1985). Early onset epilepsy, brain damage, severity of seizure, and anticonvulsant toxicity, all of which are somewhat interrelated, have been reported to contribute to intellectual deterioration in about 10% of children with epilepsy. Nevertheless, the common association with subnormal intelligence certainly reinforces the stereotypic perception of mental degeneracy in epileptic children.

This stereotype is worsened by the frequent educational underachievement of epileptic children with even normal intelligence. Some reports (Hinton and Knights, 1969; Stedman et al., 1983; Whitehouse, 1971) based on referred samples indicated that 50% of epileptic children had school problems and were in need of a remedial educational program. Although children with uncomplicated epilepsy showed a normal distribution of intelligence scores, there was a greater variability of intelligence in epileptic children than in normal children (Rutter et al., 1970). Many epileptic children of normal intelligence do experience various learning problems—reading, spelling, and arithmetic backwardness (Hinton and Knights, 1969; Holdsworth and Whitmore, 1974a; Rutter et al., 1970; Stedman et al., 1982) especially in boys and in children with left TLE (Stores and Hart, 1976; Stores, 1978). These academic deficits are probably mediated by one or more of the following problems: overactivity and inattentiveness (Stores, 1977; Stores et al., 1978), perceptual and motor coordination problems (Cowan et al., 1989; Hinton and Knights, 1969; Rutter et al., 1970; Silanpää, 1973) type and severity of seizure (Holdsworth and Whitmore, 1974a; Stores and Hart, 1976; Stores, 1977), and the toxicity of anticonvulsants (Addy, 1987; Reynolds, 1975; Trimble and Cull, 1988). Lower expectations caused by child dependency or overprotectiveness and pessimism of both parents and teachers have also been reported to contribute to educational underachievement (Hartlage and Green, 1972; Holdsworth and Whitmore, 1974b; Long and Moore, 1979).

BEHAVIOR, COGNITION, AND ANTICONVULSANTS

Since the earlier observation by Ounsted (1955) on the relation of hyperkinetic syndrome and phenobarbital treatment numerous studies have demonstrated behavioral and cognitive side effects of anticonvulsants. There has been a series of recent review articles, both general (Reynolds, 1975, 1983; Trimble and Thompson, 1983) and in relation to epileptic children (Addy, 1987; Stores, 1975; Trimble and Cull, 1988). Epilepsy itself is accompanied by an increase of behavior and cognitive impairments, which are complicated by the adverse influence of anticonvulsants. Studies have consistently pointed to a greater frequency of behavioral and cognitive side effects with the older class of drugs, such as phenobarbital and phenytoin, than the newer class of drugs, such as carbamazepine and valproate. In a large sample of epileptic children receiving long-term monotherapy, Herranz et al. (1988) reported the rates of clinical side effects with each drug in the following order: phenytoin (71%), phenobarbital (64%), carbamazepine (43%), and valproate (43%). Phenytoin has been associated with "pseudodegenerative disease" (Logan and Freeman, 1969) and clinical or subclinical "encephalopathy" (Vallarta et al., 1974), even under a therapeutic range of blood level, manifested in cerebral (confusion, delirium, psychosis) and cerebellar signs. Phenytoin has also been reported to cause cognitive deterioration (Corbett et al., 1985; Reynolds, 1975; Stores, 1978).

Phenobarbital's adverse cognitive effects have proved to be unequivocal. In a well-designed, placebo-controlled, prospective study on the prophylactic use of phenobarbital on young children who had febrile seizures and were prone to develop recurring seizures. Farwell et al. (1990) reported that after 2 years, the mean IQ was 8.4 points lower in the group assigned to phenobarbital than in the placebo group. Six months later, after medication had been tapered off and discontinued, the mean IQ was 5.2 points lower in the group assigned to phenobarbital. Phenobarbital is also known for its excitable side effects, causing hyperactivity, irritability, insomnia, tantrums, etc. (Wolf and Forsythe, 1978). In addition, a higher incidence of conduct disorder after long-term treatment was reported with phenobarbital than with any other drug (Corbett et al., 1985). Although it is difficult to disengage the effects of primidone from those of its metabolite, primidone by its own right as well as by the effects of its metabolite, phenobarbital, causes serious behavioral and cognitive side effects (Stores, 1975; Trimble and Cull, 1988), similar to the side effects of phenobarbital. In the same manner as for phenobarbital, there were reports of varying degrees of behavioral disturbance with benzodiazepine therapy, more so in children than in adults, in up to 50% of benzodiazepine therapy cases (Reynolds, 1983).

Valproate, which is increasingly becoming one of the popular anticonvulsants used for psychiatric patients, is not without mental effects. Herranz et al. (1988) reported that a significant number of epileptic children receiving valproate monotherapy exhibited irritability, hyperactivity, and labile mood. In the summary of research on carbamazepine, Trimble and Cull (1988) noted many favorable behavioral and cognitive effects in contrast to well-documented adverse effects of other anticonvulsants. In fact, carbamazepine has become one of the new favorite psychotropic drugs in adult psychiatry and somewhat in child psychiatry as well for a wide range of clinical syndromes, from aggressive behavior disorders to affective and schizophrenic disorders (Evans et al., 1987; Neppe, 1983). The effects of brain neurotransmitters, serotonin and dopamine, may account for psychotropic properties, especially in the affective disorders (Elphick, et al., 1990).

At the same time, the adverse behavioral effects of anticonvulsants have been attributed to altered brain monoamine metabolism, especially serotonin function (Reynolds, 1983). In addition, neuropathological damage, altered hormone metabolism, and folate deficiency have also been cited as possible mechanisms for the adverse behavioral and cognitive effects of anticonvulsants. Folate deficiency is an interesting theory in view of its implication in primary psychiatric disorders and findings from epileptic children, in particular, receiving long-term phenytoin therapy (Corbett and Trimble, 1983; Corbett et al., 1985, Reynolds, 1983). However, more data on these effects in epileptic children should be sought through well-designed prospective studies to validate and incorporate the very complex mechanisms hypothesized thus far.

The risk of behavioral toxicity from anticonvulsants is related to earlier onset of epilepsy, brain damage, long-term use of a drug and use of multiple drugs, medical negligence, and metabolic variation (as a result of genetic, developmental, medical, and environmental factors, etc.) (Reynolds, 1975). Needless to say, a toxic blood level of any anticonvulsant and a combination drug therapy are more likely to produce behavioral and cognitive toxicity. Two or more antiepileptic drugs in combination with psychotropic drugs are often prescribed for institutionalized epileptic children and epileptic children who are difficult to manage (Beghi et al., 1987). Difficulties in interpreting the therapeutic range of blood levels and in evaluating the efficacy and side effects and complex pharmacokinetic interactions result in both an increased incidence of toxic blood levels and an increased incidence of behavioral and cognitive toxicity (Bourgeois, 1988). There are also interesting findings from blood level studies, such as a report of excited behavioral problems occurring more commonly at low plasma levels of phenobarbital and primidone (Herranz et al., 1988). It is also of significance that behavioral and cognitive side effects have been observed under *normal* circumstances (Addy, 1987) i.e., in healthy volunteers, within a therapeutic range of anticonvulsant blood levels or in epileptic children who do not have known risk factors, such as mental retardation, brain damage, etc.

FAMILY ISSUES

It is reasonable to assume that a chronic illness, such as epilepsy, causes severe psychosocial reactions on the part of the family, not to mention a financial burden and social embarrassment. Earlier psychoanalytic views focused on the mourning process of loss (Hoare, 1987), denial, anger, depression, and guilt. This kind of neurotic response gives rise to a wide range of parental attitudes, ranging from overprotection and overindulgency to rejection (Ford et al., 1983; Green and Solnit, 1964; Hoare, 1987). The high mortality and complications of early childhood epilepsies perhaps justify the overprotectiveness of parents. The lose of a *healthy* child or the fear of loss by death is very real to the parents who have to helplessly watch their seizing child. The fear evoked by the first seizure may reverberate for a long time (Lindsay, 1972), even if the seizure is well controlled or remits. Hoare (1987) proposed that the family of an epileptic child may be studied from the Minuchin's "psychosomatic family" model, which is characterized by overprotectiveness, enmeshment, rigidity, and lack of conflict resolution (Minuchin et al., 1975). It has been well documented that the overprotective attitudes in the parents of epileptic children compromise the normal development of children, resulting in emotional and social regression, and educational underachievement (Green and Solnit, 1964; Hartlage and Green, 1972).

On the opposite end of the spectrum, parents' poor compliance is not unheard of. The diversity in the course that childhood epilepsy takes is a fertile ground for confusion and misunderstanding. Denial of a severe epileptic condition and the parent's failure to administer medication—because of practical concerns about side effects, cost, unconscious or conscious rejection or whatever reasons—seriously complicate the management of epilepsy (Ford et al., 1983). The literature regarding child maltreatment has implied that the child with physical disability has an increased risk of abuse or neglect (White et al., 1987). Although epilepsy has been mentioned in such literature, there is no reliable information about the extent of abuse and neglect in epileptic children.

Poor marital adjustment in the parents of children with chronic illness in general is a controversial issue and perhaps a myth (Sabbeth and Leventhal, 1984), although there have been reports of a high divorce or separation rate in the parents of epileptic children (Silanpää, 1973). Other studies have examined the impact of epilepsy on the family by ascertaining psychiatric morbidity of parents and siblings (Ferrari et al., 1983; Hoare, 1984b; Rutter et al., 1970). The findings indicated an increase of psychiatric morbidity compared with the general population and the families of children with a different chronic illness (e.g., juvenile diabetes). A higher rate of psychiatric disorder in the siblings of children with chronic epilepsy compared with the siblings of children with newly diagnosed epilepsy was also reported (Hoare, 1984b). Thus, there is evidence for a specific toll from epilepsy. However, genetic and other confounding factors, more than a simple stress reaction, may also play a part in the higher psychiatric morbidity of the families with epileptic children. There is a close association between the psychiatric disturbance of children with chronic epilepsy and the increased psychiatric morbidity of their mothers (Hoare, 1984b), and there is a close association between the psychopathology of the children and their mothers (Rutter et al., 1970). The psychiatric disturbances of families with psychiatrically disturbed epileptic children resembled those of families with psychiatrically disturbed nonepileptic children more than those of families with psychiatrically normal epileptic children (Grunberg and Pond, 1957).

The psychological adjustment in the siblings of chronically ill children and sibling influences on child development in general are beginning to attract a great deal of research interest (Drotar and Crawford, 1985; Dunn, 1988). It is becoming clear that sibling relationship is a very important variable in the normal development of a child and in the genesis of certain behavioral problems, especially aggression, which is the most frequently cited behavioral problem of epileptic children. The siblings of children with chronic illness are known to be another population at risk. It is of note that siblings of epileptic children have a higher risk of developing seizures, too (Lindsay et al., 1980). Research has also suggested that siblings of epileptic children had an increased rate of psychiatric morbidity as a result of chronic stresses (Hoare, 1984b). However, sibling influences cannot be examined by the sibling relationship alone without considering the family context, such as the parent-child relationship and the marital harmony of parents, etc. Instead of unidirectional, monodimensional approaches, interactive and systems approaches would be more useful in understanding dynamic interplays within the family of the epileptic child (Hoare, 1987; Ritchie, 1981).

DEVELOPMENTAL PERSPECTIVE

Infancy and Early Childhood

Among the different types of epilepsies, neonatal seizures, infantile spasms, and myoclonic epilepsies of early childhood have the worse prognosis, with a higher mortality and complications (Hrachovy and Frost, 1989; O'Donohoe, 1985). There are often underlying perinatal trauma, brain damage, and gross mental and physical handicaps. Exposure to antiepileptic drugs during the vulnerable periods of early life may increase the risk for physiological adversity, such as hepatoxicity with valproate and cognitive impairment with phenobartital, etc. (Farwell et al., 1990; Herskowitz, 1987). Such an ominous picture is more likely to foster negative and neurotic reactions on the part of parents. Consequently, during this early critical period of life, the development of attachment and bonding between the child and the mother would be influenced negatively by both the child's neuromaturational deficits and by the mother's anxiety. The dynamics of overprotective, inconsistent parenting, and dependency of the child emerge in the early parent-child relationship, as described in "The Vulnerable Child Syndrome" by Green and Solnit (1964). A child with a myoclonic seizure falling to the ground best illustrates this dilemma (O'Donohoe, 1985, p. 143). The fear and anxiety of both the child and the parent, which are so real, would inhibit normal exploring and learning activities. Additional developmental and physical handicap often associated with early onset epilepsies would compound the problems, further.

Later Childhood

New cases of epilepsy may decline, and the severity of epilepsy may improve during school years (Holdsworth and Whitmore, 1974a; Silanpää, 1973). Entering school is an anxiety provoking event for both parents and children. The task of academic learning and socialization with peers adds stresses to epileptic children, as does the fear of unexpected loss of *self-control* in public. Research has also demonstrated that a significant number of epileptic children suffer from learning deficits to begin with. Some of them may have to attend a special school or a special class, adding another label. Children with epilepsy experience prejudice and rejection (Bagley, 1972; King et al., 1989; Taylor, 1973). Teachers do not help much, as they too are generally ignorant about epilepsy (Holdsworth and Whitmore, 1974b). During this period of early school years, defenses of acting out and withdrawal may become evident along with regression and dependency within the family context (Hartlage and Green, 1972; Hoare, 1984c). Ferrari et al. (1983) reported that epileptic children between 6 and 12 years of age, in comparison to matched diabetic and normal children, tended to be followers rather than leaders, to lack initiative, and to show frequent complaints and periodic irritability.

Adolescence

What influences would puberty and the ensuing physical, psychological and social upheavals of adolescence have on the course of epilepsy and vice versa? On the physical side, research has indicated some influences both ways. Investigators reported an increased seizure frequency in generalized seizures but not in partial seizures during growth spurts (Nijima and Wallace, 1989) and fewer seizures in female adolescents during the postmenarche phase of puberty (Diamantopoulus and Crumrine, 1986). Epilepsy itself or influences of anticonvulsants may delay puberty (Reynolds, 1975) or accelerate puberty in girls, as evidenced by earlier menarche (Silanpää, 1973). Gum hyperplasia and hirsutism caused by phenytoin (Corbett et al, 1985; Herranz et al., 1988) are certain to raise esthetic problems in epileptic adolescents.

On the psychosocial side, increasing drives, peer pressure, and search for one's identity are all said to be demanding forces with which the normal adolescent must cope. Must epileptic teenagers forego all the exciting adolescent activities, such as playing sports, driving, dating, smoking, and drinking, etc.? Psychophysiological excitements disrupt CNS homeostasis and may precipitate seizures (Aird, 1988; Verduyn et al., 1988). These include some common teenage activities, such as exercise, dieting or irregular eating, sleep deprivation, and the many anxiety provoking *first* experiences of adolescence. In may respects, during adolescence, epileptics need closer medical monitoring and more medical counseling than ever. For instance, the diminished effectiveness of oral contraceptives because of interaction with anticonvulsants and many other reproductive issues (Commission on Genetics, Pregnancy, and the Child, International League Against Epilepsy, 1989) must be addressed with sexually active epileptic adolescents. However, adolescents, in general, are the least compliant group, because of their willingness to take risks and their need for *freedom*.

Indeed, their identity formation would be a difficult task for epileptic adolescents who have not been able to build up competencies in the earlier developmental stages. Studies of adults have followed up the outcome of these dilemmas and have demonstrated a lower rate of marriage and employment and, in general, more troubled psychosocial adjustments than the general population (Levin et al., 1988).

SEIZURES AND CHILDHOOD PSYCHIATRIC DISORDERS

To varying degrees, most childhood psychiatric disorders have an *episodic* or *paroxysmal* flavor in their symptom manifestation and course of problems. The child psychiatrist, upon completing an initial evaluation of a child, is often queried by the parent, child-care workers, teachers, or juvenile authorities as to whether the child has a *brain disorder* and whether an EEG should be ordered to investigate this question. As mentioned before, a high proportion of epileptic children develop different kinds of psychiatric disorders, too. Thus, it is natural to find in the psychiatric literature about children some discussion of abnormal EEG findings and antiepileptic drugs for almost all childhood psychiatric disorders.

Historically, minimal brain dysfunction and childhood psychosis have attracted the most attention. There have been reports of specific and nonspecific EEG abnormalities in hyperactivity, conduct disorder, and learning disability (Dykman et al., 1982; Satterfield et al., 1974)—what used to constitute minimal brain dysfunction and childhood psychosis (James and Barry, 1980). A surprisingly high number, 18% of incarcerated, aggressive, delinquent adolescents were found to probably have psychomotor seizures too (Lewis et al., 1982). There is also evidence of an increased incidence of epilepsy—up to one-third of autistic children and adolescents (Gillberg, 1984; Volkmar and Nelson, 1990). Ruling out epilepsy, therefore, is often a high priority in the differential diagnosis of children's behavioral problems.

Electroencephalogram

Although psychiatric research has attempted to find differential diagnostic patterns of the EGG in different childhood psychiatric disorders, studies employing double-bind, case-controlled designs did not find any correlation between EEG patterns and specific diagnostic groups (Fenton et al., 1974; Ritvo et al., 1970). At this point, it is fair to say that the EEG has a specific utility in the diagnosis of epilepsy and in a minority of childhood psychiatric disorders. However, it is only an adjunctive diagnostic tool, even in the investigation of epilepsy. A single routine, normal EEG is not evidence against epilepsy, nor is the finding of paroxysmal EEG discharges evidence for epilepsy. The range of a false negative rate by a single routine EEG is 30% to 70% depending on the type of seizure (Ajmone Marsan and Zivin, 1970; Hopkins and Scambler, 1977; Lee, 1983). Repeated EEG recordings, use of provocation by sleep deprivation or other methods, and long-term and telemetric monitoring reduce the false negative rate to 15% to 30% (Binnie, 1983; Duchowny, 1985; Stores, 1985). Through intensive telemetric EEG monitoring, Duchowny et al. (1988) uncovered nine seizure cases out of 60 children less than 10 years old, with episodic signs and symptoms-believed to be seizures despite the normal routine EEG.

Conversely, a false positive rate is also high, especially in young children, which may have to do with a high prevalence rate of the abnormal EEG in the normal population and problems with the validity and reliability of EEG interpretation. In a Swedish study of a large normal population which was carefully screened against any known risk factors of epilepsy, using well-defined narrow criteria for paroxysmal EEG abnormality, Eeg-Olofsson (1970) found that 15% of 1- to 15-year-old children and 4.9% of 16- to 21-year-old adolescents had abnormal EEGs. Another study of a large sample of a Japanese community (Iida et al., 1985) also reported an 8.1% incidence of spike abnormalities in a nonepileptic population, of whom the majority (90%) were under the age of 19. Besides the age factor, medical illness, drugs, and artifacts may also cause difficulties in interpreting EEG tracings (Lee, 1983). Indeed, epilepsy is primarily a clinical diagnosis, not an EEG diagnosis.

Pseudoseizure

Pseudoseizure is one of the most vexing problems with which the neurologist and psychiatrist must contend. Pseudoseizure has been called "psychogenic seizure," "hysterical seizure," "conversion seizure," "pseudoepileptic seizure," "nonepileptic seizure," etc., each of which has a different connotation (Gummit and Gates, 1986). The once favorite label of "hysterical seizure" may be misleading. A study of adolescents and young adults reported that the psychopathology of patients with hysterical seizure was largely a depressive, suicidal, and borderline symptoms rather than histrionic symptoms (Stewart et al., 1982). In children, anxiety symptoms were reported to be more prevalent than depressive symptomatology (Goodyer, 1985).

Although classical hysterical seizures are said to be a clinical rarity in modern psychiatric practice, pseudoseizurs are not uncommon in epileptic and nonepileptic subjects (Gummit and Gates, 1986; Pierelli, et al., 1989; Ramani et al., 1980; Williams et al., 1978). Prevalence estimates reported for psychogenic seizures range from 5% to 50% of an outpatient population (Gumnit and Gates, 1986). Hysterical seizures in children and adolescents are also believed to be not uncommon and occur at all ages, although more commonly in adolescents and in girls (Goodyer, 1985; Lesser, 1985). The literature on hysterical seizures of children and adolescents is largely filled with case reports emphasizing a stress reaction to various life problems (Goodyer, 1985; Williams et al., 1978), such as incest (Gross, 1979), learning disability (Silver, 1982), etc. Systematic research in children and adolescents has been lacking, although readers will find excellent general information from two books (Gross, 1983; Riley and Roy, 1982) and two review articles (Gumnit and Gates, 1986; Lesser, 1985).

Despite advances in clinical understanding, differential diagnosis is still very difficult, because misdiagnosis of epilepsy as pseudoepilepsy and vice versa is not unusual (Goodyer, 1985; Stores, 1985). Patients with mixed epileptic seizures and pseudoseizures and nonepileptic patients who are misdiagnosed as epileptics are very difficult groups to manage and are often recipients of an inappropriate use of antiepileptic drugs. Intensive EEG monitoring is particularly useful for these groups of patients. Monitoring the level of serum prolactin in adult subjects have also been useful, which showed a post ictal rise of prolactin (greater than $1,000\mu U/ml$ in 15 to 20 minutes) in generalized and complex partial seizures but no such rise after pseudoseizures (Sperling et al., 1986; Trimble, 1978). Replications of such studies involving different types of epileptic seizures and pseudoseizures of children and adolescents would shed light on the rather perplexing problems often encountered in dealing with these difficult groups of youngsters.

PEDIATRIC PSYCHOPHARMACOLOGY AND EPILEPSY

In view of a high prevalence of psychiatric comorbidity, the use of psychotropic drugs may sometimes be considered for children and adolescents with epilepsy. Epileptogenic side effects of psychotropic drugs and drug interactions between psychotropic and antiepileptic drugs have been summarized by Itil and Soldatos (1980) and Trimble (1981), but this knowledge, too, has been derived mostly from psychopharmacology studies of adults. A summary of adult studies will be described below for application to children and adolescents, assuming the pharmacokinetic interaction with antiepileptic drugs and the epileptogenic side effects of psychotropic drugs in children are similar to those of adults.

Epileptogenic side effects of psychotropic drugs are rather rare in psychiatric patients without underlying risk for epilepsy. However, psychotropic drugs invariably produce EEG changes and may induce subclinical or clinical seizures in nonepileptic patients who are vulnerable to seizure. Psychotropic drugs may also aggravate pre-existing epileptic conditions. Risk factors for seizure precipitation by psychotropic drugs include a family history of seizure, pretreatment EEG irregularities, a history of epilepsy, the presence of organic brain disease, a history of brain damage, polypharmacy, a sudden rapid change of dose and/or a high dose regimen, and individual hypersensitivity (Itil and Soldatos, 1980; Trimble, 1981). For instance, the occurrence of seizures was reported in about 0.5% of patients receiving low to moderate dose of phenothiazines and in about 10% of patients receiving large amounts of phenothiazines (Itil and Soldatos, 1980). The use of psychotropic drugs in epileptic children as well as in nonepileptic children with neuromaturational deficits and abnormal EEGs, etc., poses dilemmas for and challenges to the psychiatrist.

Drug interaction studies are rather scarce, and the clinical significance of these drug interactions is uncertain (Reynolds, 1982). Phenobarbital and carbamazepine influence the metabolism of antidepressants, and neuroleptics through hepatic enzymatic induction as well as their own metabolisms through autoinduction of enzymatic systems, (Jatlow, 1987; Reynolds, 1982). Polypharmacy with high-dose regimens is not an uncommon problem in mentally retarded or institutionalized epileptics. Appropriate reduction of the number and the dose of both antiepileptic and psychotropic drugs has been reported to produce improvement of both seizures and behavioral symptoms (Beghi et al., 1987).

Neuroleptics

Roughly speaking, epileptogenic side effects of neuroleptics are related linearly with their sedative properties and inversely with their extrapyramidal side effects. However, piperazine phenothiazines, such as thioridazine and mesoridazine, are an exception and have been used effectively in the treatment of behavioral disorders of epileptics (Pauig et al.. 1961). Several investigators noted the epileptogenic side effects of neuroleptics in the following order of magnitude: aliphatic phenothiazines, piperazine phenothiazines, thioxanthenes, butyrophenones, indole derivatives, and pimozide being the least epileptogenic (Itil and Soldatos, 1980; Trimble, 1981). Chlorpromazine may inhibit the metabolism of phenytoin, and, at the same time, the metabolism of chlorpromazine may be stimulated by phenytoin (Reynolds, 1982), raising the possibility of complex pharmacodynamic interactions. This author's experience with the drug interactions between anticonvulsants and neuroleptics in a small number of child and adolescent cases has been rather unpredictable in the direction of an increase or decrease of the blood levels of either class of drugs.

Antidepressants and Lithium

In general, antidepressants are less epileptogenic than neuroleptics. Although there is little data available, it is presumed that monoamine oxidase inhibitors (MAOIs) have no significant epileptogenic side effects. Trimble (1981) cited studies reported that the incidence of seizures for non-MAOI, antidepressants was 3.0%

for clomipramine, 0.7% for imipramine, 0.2% for maprotiline, and none for 1-tryptophan and nomifensine. A higher dose of antidepressant may be required when concomitantly used with antiepileptic drugs because of the activation of antidepressant's metabolism by many antiepileptic drugs. The withdrawal of either class of drug under the presence of the other class of drug will have to be carried out cautiously for rebound phenomenon (Trimble, 1981).

Lithium may produce reversible paroxysmal and nonparoxysmal EEG changes and may also cause an increase of seizure frequency in epileptic patients (Ghadirian and Lehmann, 1980). But the safe and effective use of lithium in epileptic patients has also been reported (Erwin et al., 1973). In addition, Campbell et al. (1984a, b) reported the effective use of lithium in hospitalized children with aggressive conduct disorder, most of whom had abnormal baseline EEGs, although lithium caused a significant increase of paroxysmal and focal abnormalities. Reynolds (1982) cited case reports of lithium toxicity in the presence of phenytoin despite therapeutic levels of the former, implying that the clinical interpretation of lithium levels may be unreliable in the presence of phenytoin.

Stimulants

In summarizing human and animal research, Trimble(1977) postulated that dopamine antagonists are antipsychotic and mildly epileptogenic, and dopamine agonists such as L-dopa, apomorphine, and amphetamine, are psychotogenic and mildly antiepileptic. Theoretically, stimulant drugs used for ADHD should therefore have some antiepileptic property. As hyperactivity and attentional problems are the most common psychiatric symptoms of epileptic children, this is an interesting proposition. However, there has been no clinical research data supporting such a proposition. More than 3 decades ago, Ounsted (1955) reported that amphetamine produced a behavioral improvement in a quarter of cases and a depressive reaction in two-thirds of cases, but his report did not mention any specific effect on the frequency of seizure. The *Physicians' Desk Reference* (1990) does not list epileptogenic side effects for dextroamphetamine, whereas it lists such side effects for methylphenidate and pemoline, especially in children with pre-existing EEG abnormalities.

Other Drugs

The influence of benzodiazepines on phenytoin has proved variable or contradictory, with reports of both elevation and depression of phenytoin blood level (Reynolds, 1982). In view of y-aminobutyric acid's role in epilepsy (Gale, 1989) and anxiety disorders, a benzodiazepine, such as clonazepam, would be a good choice of drug for anxious and tense epileptic patients (Trimble, 1981). A similar rationale is seen in the use of carbamazepine for epileptic children with behavioral problems.

Commonly used illicit psychotropic drugs by adolescents include alcohol, marijuana, and cocaine, etc. Alcohol is clearly epileptogenic, dose dependent, and independent of withdrawal (Ng et al., 1988). Although intoxication may be epileptogenic at any age (Rivkin and Gilmore, 1989), there is no substantive evidence on the epileptogenic effects of illicit psychostimulants.

SUMMARY AND PSYCHIATRIC MANAGEMENT

In sum, epilepsy is the most prevalent neurological disorder of childhood and adolescence and a very heterogeneous disease with a diverse course of illness; it may be a benign disease for the majority of children and adolescents, who recover spontaneously or are managed well medically. However, a sizable group of children and adolescents with epilepsy, at least one-third, do manifest various difficulties— seizure control, academic, emotional, behavioral, and family problems. As a group, they have a much higher rate of psychiatric disorder than healthy children and children with other chronic illnesses (Hoare, 1987). Even when groups of children with the same psychiatric diagnosis, much as ADHD, are examined across the different neurodevelopmental indices, problems with epileptic youths are much more extensive and severe than with the other groups of children (Harcherik et al., 1982). There is ample evidence that children and adolescents with epilepsy are a population at risk. This increased vulnerability is associated with several factors, including the type of neurological lesion (brain damage, site of origin, type of epilepsy, chronicity, seizure frequency, etc.), the individual characteristics of the child (age, gender, temperament, cognitive ability, etc.), psychiatric disturbance in other family members, and the adverse effects of anticonvulsants (Hoare, 1987). Some of these vulnerability factors are interrelated and mediate various outcomes of epilepsy— seizure control, learning problems, and a host of psychosocial adjustment areas in addition to psychopathology.

The association between epilepsy and schizophrenia-like psychosis has long fascinated neurologists and psychiatrists. Rather than the unique causal relationship found in adult epileptics, psychiatric disorders of epileptic children, as with any childhood psychiatric disorder, appear to be multifactorially determined, with neurological factors, intellectual and educational factors, and sociofamilial influences all playing a part in causation. Similarly, the type of psychiatric disorder manifested in epileptic youths is not uniquely different from the range of psychiatric disorder found in the general population or children with chronic medical illnesses. However, disruptive behavioral disorders, such as ADHD, conduct, and aggressive behavioral disorders, tend to occur more often, especially in boys.

On the basis of such overwhelming empirical data, it would not be an overstatement to say that *all* epileptic children and adolescents deserve interdisciplinary team assessments and interventions, if necessary, including psychiatric input. This is much like the team approach in child psychiatry, but the primary physician takes a much more active role in this case. It may be costly, but, in the long run, it would be economically sensible considering the enormous monetary and nonmonetary burdens placed on the child, the family, and society by less than satisfactory diagnostic accuracy and management of epilepsy (Cadman et al., 1987; Hopkins and Scambler, 1977; Rodin, 1972). Indeed, 3 decades ago, Pond (1961), noting the multihandicapping nature of epilepsy in children, emphatically stated that "the management of the brain-damaged child requires the fullest and deepest psychiatric approach." Many others have also advocated the need for psychiatric input for the treatment of epilepsy itself and emotional/behavioral problems associated with epilepsy in children (Hermann et al., 1981; Holdsworth and Whitmore, 1974a; Keating, 1961; Ounsted and Lindsay, 1981).

What can a psychiatric interdisciplinary team do? Developmental assessments of intellectual, academic, and psychosocial progress should be a routine part of the management of epilepsy in the young population (Lindsay, 1972). Arrangement of a special educational program for some or counseling for teachers and parents of epileptic children attending normal schools is often indicated for their gross or subtle learning handicap as well as for the lack of understanding and appropriate expectations by the teachers and parents (Holdsworth and Whitmore, 1974b; Long and Moore, 1979). How the epileptic youth is making progress in terms of disease, illness, and predicaments (Taylor, 1979) should be periodically assessed. Impairments of control and competency in epileptic children and their families is the major long-term complication (Ziegler, 1981). The mastery of developmental tasks in both the child and the family may be interrupted or lag behind. A cognitive coping strategy model, proposed originally by Lazarus and Folkman (1984) and later applied by Compas (1987) to chronic sickness of children, would be useful in enhancing the mastery and competency of various developmental tasks and, thus, in promoting overall successful adaptation.

Educational and supportive counseling for the child and family members in regard to immediate and long-term prognosis of epilepsy, family coping, and practical management issues should be as important as anticonvulsant therapy. They may be apprised of the stigma and social prejudice about epilepsy from the beginning (Bagley, 1972; Taylor, 1973). Psychotherapeutic skills would be of great value here—to allow them to express their concerns and conflict, to reassure them of their anxiety and worry, and to clarify myths and misinformation (Ford et al., 1983). Of course, these processes may have to be repeated many times, depending on the level of adaptation of the child and the family. Not only the child's maladjustment but also the family members' maladjustment need to be watched for to provide timely evaluation and treatment.

The psychiatrist can also play an important role in detecting behavioral and cognitive side effects of anticonvulsants and work closely with the neurologist. From their own experiences with psychotropic drugs, psychiatrists are all too familiar with the evils of CNS drugs and polypharmacy, which are fairly common in the management of epileptic children and adolescents (Beghi et al., 1987; Bourgeois, 1988; Trimble and Cull, 1988). Their expertise may be rendered useful especially when epilepsy is treated by the general physician rather than the epileptogogist, which is probably the rule rather than the exception in general community medical practice. One should also be familiar with the unnecessary, even harmful, use of antiepileptic drugs and the indications for the withdrawal of them, (Callaghan et al., 1988; Farwell et al., 1990; Loiseau et al., 1983; Taylor and McKinley, 1984). Reynolds (1983) asserted that there is very little difference in anticonvulsant properties between the major antiepileptic drugs. He argued that the relative influence of each drug on mental functions may prove to be the most important factor in the child of an antiepileptic drug for the treatment of epilepsy. This may account for the increasing popularity of carbamazepine. As previously discussed, psychotropic drugs can be used judiciously and effectively for the psychiatric disorders of epileptic youth. These children and adolescents should not be deprived of the benefits of modern pediatric psychopharmacotherapy for the reason of epilepsy alone.

There are also psychosocial interventions directly aimed at the improvement of intractable or difficult-to-treat seizures, which are often stress precipitated or of psychogenic origin. Of 40 known epileptogenic mechanisms, some eight involve transient psychophysiological stress conditions, and there can be therapeutically averted with the help of both the child and the family (Aird, 1988; Verduyn et al., 1988). Effects of a broad-spectrum behavior modification treatment program (Dahl et al., 1985) and EEG operant conditioning (Luba et al., 1981), reflect the recent progress of *behavior medicine* in contributing to the treatment of epilepsy. Although it must be validated, one should not ignore that potential value of psychodynamically oriented psychotherapy for the improvement of epileptic conditions in children and adolescents (Sperling, 1978).

FUTURE DIRECTIONS

The magnitude and extent of problems in epileptic youth are well suited for study by psychiatrists who are biopsychosocially and developmentally oriented. Areas of interest for future research include: 1) differential effects of different types and causes of epilepsy on emotional, cognitive, and social function; 2) effects of epilepsy on different developmental tasks of children in elations to the timing of onset and if remitted, its residual effect; 3) effects of psychotropic drugs on seizure and behavior in children and pharmacokinetic interactions with antiepileptic drugs; and

4) effects of preventive and therapeutic psychosocial interventions on epilepsy and its complications.

REFERENCES

Addy, D.P. (1987), Cognitive function in children with epilepsy. *Dev. Med. Child Neurol.*, 29:394–396.

Aird, R.B. (1988), The importance of seizure-inducing factors in youth. *Brain Dev.*, 10:73–76.

Ajmone Marsan, C. & Zivin, L.S. (1970). Factors related to the occurrence of typical paroxysmal abnormalities in the EEG records of epileptic patients. *Epilepsia*, 11:361–381.

Annegers, J.F., Hauser, W.A., Elveback, L.K. et al. (1980), Remission and relapses of seizures in epilepsy. In: *Advances in Epileptology: The Tenth International Epilepsy Symposim*, eds. J. Wada & J. Penry. New York: Raven Press, pp. 145–147.

Arts, W.F.M., Visser L.H., Loonen M.C.B. et al. (1988), Follow-up of 146 children with epilepsy after withdrawal of antiepileptic therapy. *Epilepsia*, 29:244–250.

Bagley, C. (1972), Social prejudice and the adjustment of people with epilepsy. *Epilepsia*, 29:244–250.

Baumann, R.J., Marx, M.B. & Leonidakis, M.G. (1977), An estimate of the prevalence of epilepsy in a rural Appalachian population. *Am. J. Epidemiology*, 106:42–52.

Bear, D., Levin, K., Blumer, D. et al. (1982), Interictal behavior in hospitalized temporal lobe epileptics—relationship to idiopathic psychiatric syndromes. *J. Neurol. Neurosurg. Psychiatry*, 45:481–488.

Beghi, E., Paola, B., DiMascio, R. et al. (1987), Effects of rationalizing drug treatment of patients with epilepsy and mental retardation. *Dev. Med. Child Neurol.*, 29:363–369.

Betts, T.A. (1981). Depression, anxiety and epilepsy. In: *Epilepsy and Psychiatry*, eds. E. Reynolds & Mr. Trimble. London: Churchill Livingstone, pp.60–71.

Binnie, C.D. (1983), Telemetric EEG monitoring in epilepsy, In: *Recent Advances in Epilepsy*, No. 1, eds. T. Pedley & B. Meldrum. London: Churchill Livingstone, pp. 155–178.

Blumer, D. (1984), *Psychiatric Aspects of Epilepsy*. Washington. DC: American Psychiatric Press, Inc.

Boulloche, J., Leloup, P., Mallet, E. et al. (1989), Risk of recurrence after a single unprovoked, generalized tonic–clonic seizure. *Dev. Med. Child Neurol.*, 31:626–632.

Bourgeois, B.F.D., Prensky, A.C., Palkes, H.S. et al. (1983), Intelligence in epilepsy: a prospective study in children. *Ann. Neurol.*, 14:438–444.

—————————et al. (1988), Problems of combination drug therapy in children. *Epilepsia*, 29(Suppl. 3):S20–S24.

Brent, D.A. (1986). Overrepresentation of epileptics in a consecutive series of suicide attempters seen at a children's hospital, 1978–1983. *J. Am. Acad. Child Psychiatry*, 25:242–246.

Brorson, L.A. & Wranne, L. (1987), Long-term prognosis in childhood epilepsy: survival and seizure prognosis. *Epilepsia*, 28:324–330.

Cadman, D., Boyle, M., Szatmari, P. et al. (1987), Chronic illness, disability and mental and social well-being; findings of the Ontario Child Health Study. *Pediatrics*, 79:805–812.

Callaghan, N., Garrett, A. & Goggin, T. (1988), Withdrawal of anticonvulsant drugs in patients free of seizures for two years. *N. Engl. J. Med.*, 318:942–946.

Campbell, M., Small, A.M., Green, W.H. et al. (1984a), Behavioral efficacy of haloperidol and lithium carbonate. *Arch. Gen. Psychiatry*, 41:650–656.

——Perry, R. & Green, W.H. (1984b), Use of lithium in children and adolescents. *Psychosomatics*, 25:95–106.

Cavazzuti, G.B. (1980), Epidemiology of different types of epilepsy in school age children of Modena, Italy. *Epilepsia*, 21:57–62.

Commission on Genetics, Pregnancy, and the Child, International League Against Epilepsy (1989), Guidelines for the care of epileptic women of childbearing age. *Epilepsia*, 30:409–410.

Compas, B.E. (1987), Coping with stress during childhood and adolescence. *Psychol. Bull.*, 98:310–357.

Corbett, J.A. & Trimble, M.R. (1983), Epilepsy and anticonvulsant medication. In: *Developmental Neuropsychiatry*, ed. M. Rutter. Chap. 6, New York: The Guilford Press, pp. 112–129.

——Harris, R., & Robinson, R.G. (1975) Epilepsy. In: *Mental Retardation and Developmental Disabilities*, vol. VII, ed. J. Wortis. New York: Bruner Mazel, pp. 81–111.

——Trimble, M.R. & Nichol, T.C. (1985), Behavioral and cognitive impairments in children with epilepsy: the long-term effects of anticonvulsant therapy. *J. Am. Acad. Child Psychiatry*, 24:17–23.

Cowan, L.D., Bodensteiner, J.B., Leviton, A. & Doherty, L. (1989) Prevalence of the epilepsies in children and adolescents. *Epilepsia*, 30:94–106.

Dahl, J., Melin, L., Broson, L. et al. (1985), Effects of a broad-spectrum behavior modification treatment program on children with refractory epileptic seizures. *Epilepsia*, 26:303–309.

Dennis, J. (1979), The implications of neonatal seizures. In: *Advances in Perinatal Neurology*, eds. R. Korobkin & C. Guilleninault. New York: Spectrum Publications, pp. 205–224.

Diamantopoulus, N. & Crumrine, P.K. (1986), The effect of puberty on the course of epilepsy. *Arch. Neurol.*, 43:873–876.

Dodrill, C.B. (1986), Correlates of generalized tonic-clonic seizures with intellectual, neuropsychological, emotional, and social function in patients with epilepsy. *Epilepsia*, 27:399–411.

Drotar, D. & Crawford, P. (1985). Psychological adaptation of siblings of chronically ill children: research and practice implications. *Developmental and Behavioral Pediatrics*, 6:355–362.

Duchowny, M.S. (1985), Intensive monitoring in the epileptic child. *J. Clin. Neurophysiol.*, 2(3):203–219.

——Resnick, T.J., Deray, M.J. et al. (1988), Video EEG diagnosis of repetitive behavior in early childhood and its relationship to seizures. *Pediatr. Neurol.*, 4:162–164.

Dunn, J. (1988), Sibling influences on childhood development. *J. Child Psychol. Psychiatry,* 29:119–127.

Dykman, R.A., Holcomb, P.J., Oglesby, D.M. et al. (1982), Electrocortical frequencies in hyperactive, learning disabled, mixed and normal children. *Biol. Psychiatry,* 17:675–685.

Eeg-Olofsson, O. (1970), The development of the electroencephalogram in normal children and adolescents from the age of 1 through 21 years. *Acta. Paediat. Scand.,* Suppl. 208.

Ehrhardt, P. & Forsythe, W.I. (1989), Prognosis after grand mal seizures: a study of 187 children with three-year remissions. *Dev. Med. Child Neurol.,* 31:633–639.

Eiser, C. (1990), Psychological effects of chronic disease. *J. Child Psychol. Psychiatry,* 31:(1):85–98.

Ellenberg, J.H., Hirtz, D.G. & Nelson, K.B. (1984), Age at onset of seizures in young children. *Ann. Neurol.,* 15:127–134.

——————————(1985), Do seizures in children cause intellectual deterioration? *Ann. Neurol.* 18:389.

Elphick, M., Yang, J. & Cowen, P.J. (1990), Effects of carbamazepine on dopamine- and serotonin-mediated neuroendocrine responses. *Arch. Gen. Psychiatry,* 47:135–140.

Erwin, C.W., Gerber, C.H., Morrison, S.D., et al. (1973), Lithium carbonate and convulsive disorders. *Arch. Gen. Psychiatry,* 28:646–648.

Evans, R.W., Clay, T.H. & Gualtieri, C.T. (1987), Carbamazepine in pediatric psychiatry. *J. Am. Acad. Child Adolesc. Psychiatry,* 26:2–8.

Farwell, J.R., Lee, Y.J., Hirtz, D.G. et al. (1990), Phenobarbital for febrile seizures—effects on intelligence and on seizure recurrence. *N. Engl. J. Med.,* 322:364–369.

Fenton, G.W., Fenwick, P.B.C., Dollimore, J. et al. (1974). An introduction to the Isle of Wight EEG study. *Electroencephalogr. Clin. Neurophysiol.,* 37:325.

Ferrari, M., Matthews, W.S. & Barabas, G. (1983), The family and the child with epilepsy. *Family Process,* 22:53–59.

Ford, C.A., Gibson, P. & Dreifuss, F.E. (1983), Psychosocial considerations in childhood epilepsy. In: *Pediatric Epileptology,* ed. F. Dreifuss. Boston, MA: John Wright PSG Inc., pp. 277–295.

Gale, K. (1989), GABA in epilepsy: the pharmacologic basis. *Epilepsia,* 30(Suppl. 3):S1–S11.

Ghadirian, A.M. & Lehmann, H.E. (1980), Neurological side effects of lithium: organic syndrome, seizures, extrapyramidal side effects and EEG changes. *Compr. Psychiatry,* 21:327–335.

Gillberg, C. (1984), Autistic children growing up: problems during puberty and adolescence. *Dev. Med. Child Neurol.,* 26:125–129.

Goodyer, I.M. (1985), Epileptic and pseudo-epileptic seizures in childhood and adolescence. *J. Am. Acad. Child Psychiatry,* 24:3–9.

Green, M. & Solnit, A.J. (1964), Reaction to the threatened loss of child: a vulnerable child syndrome. *Pediatrics,* 34:58–66.

Gross, M. (1979), Incestuous rape: a cause for hysterical seizures in four adolescent girls. *Am. J. Orthopsychiatry,* 49:704–708.

————ed. (1983). *Pseudoepilepsy*, Lexington, MA: Lexington Books.

Grunberg, F. & Pond, D.A. (1957), Conduct disorders in epileptic children. *J. Neurol. Neurosurg. Psychiatry*, 20:65–68.

Gudmundsson, G. (1966), Epilepsy in Iceland. *Acta. Neurol. Scand.*, 43(Suppl. 25):1–124.

Gumnit, R.J. & Gates, J.R. (1986), Psychogenic seizures. *Epilepsia*, 27(Suppl. 2):S124-S129.

Haerer, A.F., Anderson, D.W. & Schoenberg, B.S. (1986), Prevalence and clinical features of epilepsy in a biracial United States population. *Epilepsia*, 27:66–75.

Harcherik, D.F., Carbonari, C.M., Shaywitz, S.E. et al. (1982), Attentional and perceptual disturbances in children with Tourette's syndrome, attention deficit disorder and epilepsy. *Schizophr. Bull.*, 8:356–359.

Harrison, R.M. & Taylor, D.C. (1976), Childhood seizure: a 25-year follow-up. *Lancet*, 1:948–951.

Hartlage, L.C. & Green, J.B. (1972), The relation of parental attitudes to academic and social achievement in epileptic children. *Epilepsia*, 13:21–26.

Hermann, B.P., Black, R.B. & Chhabria, S. (1981), Behavioral problems and social competence in children with epilepsy. Epilepsia, 22:703–710.

Herranz, J.L., Armijo, J.A. & Arteaga, T. (1988), Clinical side effects of phenobarbital, primidone, phenytoin, carbamazepine, and valproate during monotherapy in children. *Epilepsia*, 29(4):794–804.

Herskowitz, J. (1987), Developmental neurotoxicity. In: *Psychiatric Pharmacosciences of Children and Adolescents*, ed. C. Popper. Washington, DC: American Psychiatric Press, pp. 81–124.

Hertzig, M.E. (1983), Temperament and neurological status. In: *Developmental Neuropsychiatry*, ed. M. Rutter. New York: The Guilford Press, pp. 164–180.

Hinton, G.G. & Knights, R.M. (1969), Neurological and psychological characteristics of 100 children with seizures. In: *Proceedings of the First Congress for the International Association for the Scientific Study of Mental Deficiency*, ed. B. Richard. London: Michael Jackson Publishing, pp. 351–356.

Hoare, P. (1984a), The development of psychiatric disorders in school children with epilepsy. *Dev. Med. Child Neurol.*, 26:3–13.

————(1984b), Psychiatric disturbance in the families of epileptic children. *Dev. Med. Child Neurol.*, 26:14–19.

————(1984c), Does illness foster dependency? A study of epileptic and diabetic children. *Dev. Med. Child Neurol.* 26:20–24.

————(1987), Children with epilepsy and their families. *J. Child Psychol. Psychiatry*, 28:651–655.

Hodgman, C., McAnarney, R. & Myers, G. (1979), Emotional complications of adolescent grand mal epilepsy. *J. Pediatr.*, 95:309–312.

Holdsworth, L. & Whitmore, K. (1974a), A study of children with epilepsy attending normal schools. 1:Their seizures patterns, progress, and behavior in school. *Dev. Med. Child Neurol.*, 16:746–758.

————(1974b), A study of children with epilepsy attending normal schools II: information and attitudes held by their teachers. *Dev. Med. Child Neurol.*, 16:759–765.

Hopkins, A. & Scambler, G. (1977), How doctors deal with epilepsy. *Lancet*, 1:183–186.

Hrachovy, R.A. & Frost, J.D. (1989), Infantile spasms. *Pediatr Clin. North Am.*, 36:311–329.

Iida, N., Okada, S. & Tsuboi, T. (1985), EEG abnormalities in non-epileptic patients. *Folia Psychiatrica Neurologica Japonica*, 39:43–58.

Itil, T.M. & Soldatos, C. (1980), Epileptogenic side effects of psychotropic drugs: practical recommendations. *J.A.M.A.*, 244:1460–1463.

James, A.L. & Barry, R.J. (1980), A review of psychophysiology in early onset psychosis. *Schizophr. Bull.*, 6:506–525.

Jatlow, P.I. (1987), Psychotropic drug disposition during development. In: *Psychiatric Pharmacosciences of Children and Adolescents,* ed. C. Popper, Washington, DC: American Psychiatric Press, pp. 29–44.

Keating, L.E. (1961), Epilepsy and behavior disorder in school children. *Journal of Mental Science*, 107:161–180.

King, S.M., Rosenbaum, P., Armstrong, R.W. et al. (1989), An epidemiological study of children's attitudes toward disability. *Dev. Med. Child Neurol.*, 31:237–245.

Kogeorgos, J., Fongay, P. & Scott, D.F. (1982), Psychiatric symptoms patterns of chronic epileptics attending a neurologic clinic: a controlled investigation. *Br. J. Psychiatry*, 140:236–243.

Lazarus, R.S. & Folkman, S. (1984), *Stress, Appraisal and Coping*. New York: Springer.

Lee, S.I. (1983), Electroencephalography in infantile and childhood epilepsy. In: *Pediatric Epileptology*, ed. F. Dreifuss. Boston, MA: John Wright PSG Inc., pp. 33–64.

Lesser, R.P. (1985), Psychogenic seizures. In: *Recent Advances in Epilepsy*, No. 2, eds. T. Pedley & B. Meldrum. London: Churchill Livingstone, pp. 273–296.

————Lüders, H., Wyllie, E. et al. (1986), Mental deterioration in epilepsy. *Epilepsia*, 27(Suppl. 2):S105–S123.

Levin, R., Banks, S. & Berg, B. (1988), Psychosocial dimensions of epilepsy: a review of the literature. *Epilepsia*, 29:805–916.

Lewis, D.O., Pincus, J.H., Shanok, S.S. et al. (1982), Psychomotor epilepsy and violence in a group of incarcerated adolescent boys. *Am. J. Psychiatry*, 139:882–887.

Lindsay, J. (1972), The difficult epileptic child. *Br. Med. J.*, 3:283–285.

————Ounsted, C. & Richards, P. (1980), Long-term outcome in children with temporal lobe seizures, 4. Genetic factors, febrile convulsion and the remission of seizures. *Dev. Med. Child Neurol.*, 22:429–440.

Logan, W.J. & Freeman, J.M. (1969), Pseudodegenerative disease due to diphenyhydantoin intoxication. *Arch. Neurol.*, 21:631–637.

Loiseau, P., Pestre, M., Dartigues, J.F. et al. (1983), Long-term prognosis in two forms of childhood epilepsy: typical absence seizures and epilepsy with Rolandic (centrotemporal) EEG foci. *Ann. Neurol.*, 13:642–648.

Long, C.G. & Moore, J.R. (1979), Parental expectations for their epileptic children. *J. Child Psychol. Psychiatry*, 20:299–312.

Lubar, J.F., Shabsin, H.S., Natelson, S.E. et al. (1981), EEG operant conditioning in intractable epileptics. *Arch. Neurol.*, 38:700–704.

Mathews, W. & Barabas, G. (1981), Suicide and epilepsy: a review of the literature. *Psychosomatics*, 22:515–524.

Matricardi, M., Brinciotti, M. & Benedetti, P. (1989), Outcome after discontinuation of antiepileptic drug therapy in children with epilepsy. *Epilepsia, 30:582–589*.

Meighan, S.S., Queener, L., Weitman, M. (1976), Prevalence of epilepsy in children of Multnomah County, Oregon. *Epilepsia*, 17:245–256.

Minuchin, S., Baker, L., Rosman, B.L. et al. (1975), A conceptual modal of psychosomatic illness in children. *Arch. Gen. Psychiatry*, 32:1031–1038.

Neppe, V.M. (1983), Carbamazepine as adjunctive treatment in nonepileptic chronic inpatients with EEG temporal lobe abnormalities. *J. Clin. Psychiatry*, 44:326–331.

————Tucker, G.J. (1988a), Modern perspectives on epilepsy in relation to psychiatry: classification and evaluation. *Hosp. Community Psychiatry*, 39:262–271.

——————(1988b), Modern perspectives on epilepsy in relation to psychiatry: behavioral disturbances of epilepsy. *Hops. Community Psychiatry*, 38:389–396.

Ng, S.K.C., Hauser, W.A., Brust, J.C.M., et al. (1988), Alcohol consumption and withdrawal in new-onset seizures. *N. Engl. J. Med.*, 319:666–673.

Niijima, S-i. & Wallace, S.J. (1989), Effects of puberty on seizure frequency. *Dev. Med. Child Neurol.*, 31:174–180.

Nuffield, E.J. (1961), Neurophysiology and behavior disorders in epileptic children. *Journal of Mental Science*, 107:438–458.

O'Donohoe, N.V. (1985), *Epilepsies of Childhood*, 2nd ed. London: Butterworths.

Offord, D.R., Boyle, M.H. & Racine, Y. (1989), Ontario child health study: correlates of disorder. *J. Am. Acad. Child Adolesc. Psychiatry*, 28:856–860.

Ounsted, C. (1955), The hyperkinetic syndrome in epileptic children. *Lancet*, 2:303–311.

————Lindsay, J. (1981), The long-term outcome of temporal lobe epilepsy in childhood. In: *Epilepsy and Psychiatry*, eds. E. Reynolds & M. Trimble. London: Churchill Livingstone, pp. 185–215.

Parnas, J. & Korsgaard, (1982), Epilepsy and psychosis. *Acta. Psychiatr. Scand.*, 66:89–99.

Pauig, P.M., Deluca, M.A. & Osterheld, R.G. (1961), Thioridazine hydrochloride in the treatment of behavior disorders in epileptics. *Am. J. Psychiatry*, 117:832–833.

Pedersen, B. & Dam, M. (1986), Memory disturbances in epileptic patients. *Acta Neurol. Scand.*, 74(Suppl. 109):11–14.

Physicians' Desk Reference (1990), Oradell, NJ Medical Economics Company.

Pierelli, F., Chartian, G., Erdly, W.W. et al. (1989), Long-term EEG-video-audio monitoring: detection of partial epileptic seizures and psychogenic episodes by 24 hour EEG record review. *Epilepsia*, 30:513–523.

Pond, D.A. & Bidwell, B.H. (1959, 1960). A survey of epilepsy in 14 general practices. II: social and psychological aspects. *Epilepsia*, 1:285–299.

——————(1961), Psychiatric aspects of epileptic and brain-damaged children. *Br. Med. J.*, 2:1454–1459.

Ramani, S.V., Quesney, L.F., Olson, D. et al. (1980), Diagnosis of hysterical seizures in epileptic patients. *Am. J. Psychiatry*, 137:705–709.

Reynolds, E.H. (1975), Chronic antiepileptic toxicity: a review. *Epilepsia*, 16:319–352.
——————(1982) The pharmacologic management of epilepsy associated with psychological disorders. *Br. J. Psychiatry*, 141:549–557.
——————(1983), Mental effects of antiepileptic medication: a review. *Epilepsia*, 24(Suppl. 2):S85–S95.

Riley, J. & Roy, A., eds. (1982) *Pseudoseizures*. Baltimore: Williams & Wilkins.

Ritchie, K. (1981). Research note: interaction in the families of epileptic children. *J. Child Psychol. Psychiatry*, 22:65–71.

Ritvo, E.R., Ornitz, E.M., Walter, R.D. et al. (1970), Correlation of psychiatric diagnosis and EEG findings—a double blind study of 184 hospitalized children. *Am. J. Psychiatry*, 126:988–996.

Rivkin, M. & Gilmore, H.E. (1989), Generalized seizures in an infant due to environmentally acquired cocaine. *Pediatrics*, 84:1100–1102.

Rodin, E.A. (1972), Medical and social prognosis in epilepsy. *Epilepsia*, 13:121–131.

Rose, S.W., Penry, J.K., Maarkush, R.E. et al. (1973), Prevalence of epilepsy in children. *Epilepsia*, 14:133–152.

Rutter, M., Graham, P. & Yule, W. (1970), A neuropsychiatric study in childhood. *Clinics in Developmental Medicine Nos. 35/36*. London: Heinemann/Spastics International Medical Publications.

Sabbeth, B.F. & Leventhal, J.M. (1984), Marital adjustment to chronic childhood illness: a critique of the literature. *Pediatrics*, 73:762–768.

Satterfield, J.H., Cantwell, D.P. & Satterfield, B.T. (1974), Pathophysiology of the hyperactive child syndrome. *Arch. Gen. Psychiatry*, 31:839–844.

Schenk, L. & Bear, D. (1981), Multiple personality and related dissociative phenomena in patients with temporal lobe epilepsy. *Am. J. Psychiatry*, 138:1311–1326.

Shah, P. & Kaplan, S.L. (1980), Catatonic symptoms in a child with epilepsy. *Am. J. Psychiatry*, 137:738–739.

Shamansky, S.L. & Glaser, G.H. (1979), Socioeconomic characteristics of childhood seizure disorders in the New Haven area: an epidemiologic study. *Epilepsia*, 20:457–474.

Sherwin, I. (1984), Differential psychiatric features in epilepsy: relationship to lesion laterality. *Acta. Psychiatr. Scand.*, 69(Suppl. 313):92–103.

Shinnar, S., Vining, E.P.G., Mellits, E.D. et al. (1985), Discontinuing antiepileptic medication in children with epilepsy after two years without seizures. *N. Engl. J. Med.*, 313:976–980.

Shukla, G.D. & Katiyar, S.C. (1981), Psychiatric disorders in children with temporal lobe epilepsy: a controlled investigation. *Indian Journal of Psychology*, 23:62.

Silanpää, M. (1973), Medico-social prognosis of children with epilepsy: epidemiological study and analysis of 245 patients. *Acta. Paediat. Scand.*, 62(Suppl. 237):3–104.

Silver, L.B. (1982), Conversion disorder with pseudoseizures in adolescence: A stress reaction to unrecognized and untreated learning disabilities. *J. Am. Acad. Child Psychiatry*, 21:508–512.

Slater, E. & Beard, A.W. (1963), The schizophrenia-like psychoses of epilepsy: I. psychiatric aspects. *Br. J. Psychiatry*, 109:95–112.

Slater, E. & Beard, A.W. (1963), The schizophrenia-like psychoses of epilepsy: I. psychiatric aspects. *Br. J. Psychiatry*, 109:95–112.

Sperling, E. (1978), Epilepsy, psychodynamics and therapy. In: *Psychosomatic Disorders in Childhood*, ed. E. Sperling. New York: Jason Aronson, pp. 285–307.

Stedman, J., Van Heyningen, R. & Lindsay, J. (1982), Educational underachievement and epilepsy: a study of children from normal school admitted to a special hospital for epilepsy. *Early Child Development and Care*, 9:65–82.

Stewart, R.S., Lovitt, R. & Stewart, M.S. (1982), Psychopathology associated with hysterical seizures. *Am. J. Psychiatry*, 139:926–929.

Stores, G. (1975), Behavioral effects on anti-epileptic drugs. *Dev. Med. Child Neurol.*, 17:647–658.

———(1977), Behavioral disturbance and type of epilepsy in children attending ordinary school. In: *Epilepsy: The Eighth International Symposium*, ed. J. Penry. New York: Raven Press, pp. 245–249.

———(1978), School children with epilepsy at risk for learning and behavior problems. *Dev. Med. Child Neurol.*, 20:502–508.

———(1985), Clinical and EEG evaluation of seizures and seizure-like disorders. *J. Am. Acad. Child Adolesc. Psychiatry*, 24:10–16.

———Hart, J. (1976), Reading skills of children with generalized or focal epilepsy attending ordinary school. *Dev. Med. Child Neurol.*, 18:705–716.

Taylor, D.C. (1973), Aspects of seizure disorders: II. On prejudice. *Dev. Med. Child Neurol.*, 15:91–94.

———(1979), The components of sickness: diseases, illnesses and predicaments. *Lancet*, 2:1008–1010.

———McKinlay, I. (1984), When not to treat epilepsy with drugs. *Dev. Med Child Neurol.*, 26:822–827.

Tizard, B. (1962), The personality of epileptics: a discussion of the evidence. *Psychol. Bull.*, 59:196–210.

Trimble, M.R. (1977), The relationship between epilepsy and schizophrenia: a biochemical hypothesis. *Biol. Psychiatry*, 12:299–304.

———(1978), Serum prolactin in epilepsy and hysteria. *Br. Med. J.*, 2:1682.

———(1981), Psychotropic drugs in the management of epilepsy. In: *Epilepsy and Psychiatry*, eds. E. Reynolds & M. Trimble. London: Churchill Livingstone, pp. 337–346.

———Thompson, P.J. (1983),, Anticonvulsant drugs, cognitive function and behavior. *Epilepsia*, 24(Suppl. 1):S55–S63.

———Cull, C. (1988). Children of school age: the influence of antiepileptic drugs on behavior and intellect. *Epilepsia*, 29(Suppl. 3):S15–S19.

Tucker, D.M., Novelly, R.A. & Walker, P.J. (1987), Hyperreligiosity in temporal lobe epilepsy: redefining the relationship. *J. Nerv. Ment. Dis.*, 175:181–184.

Vallarta, J.M., Bell, D.B. & Reichert, A. (1974), Progressive encephalopathy due to chronic hydantoin intoxication. *Am. J. Dis. Child*, 128:27–34.

Verduyn, C.M., Stores, G. & Missen, A. (1988), A survey of mothers' impressions of seizure precipitants in children with epilepsy. *Epilepsia*, 29:251–255.

Viberg, M., Blennow, G. & Polski, B., (1987), Epilepsy in adolescence: implications for the development of personality. *Epilepsia*, 28:542–546.

Volkmar, F.R. & Nelson, D.S. (1990), Seizure disorders in autism. *J. Am. Acad. Child Adolesc. Psychiatry*, 29:127–129.

White, R., Benedict, M.I., Wulff, L. et al. (1987), Physical disabilities as risk factors for child maltreatment: a selected review. *Am. J. Orthopsychiatry*, 57:93–101.

Whitehouse, D. (1971), Psychological and neurological correlates of seizure disorders. *The Johns Hopkins Medical Journal*, 129:36–42.

Williams, D. (1969), Man's temporal lobe. *Brain*, 91:639–654.

Williams, D.T., Speigal, H. & Mostofsky, D.I. (1978), Neurogenic and hysterical seizures in children and adolescents: differential diagnostic and therapeutic considerations. *Am. J. Psychiatry*, 135:82–86.

Wolf, S.M. & Forsythe, A. (1978), Behavioral disturbance, phenobarbital and febrile seizures. *Pediatrics*, 61:728–731.

Ziegler, R.G. (1981), Impairments of control and competence in epileptic children and their families. *Epilepsia*, 22:339–346.

19

Early Asthma Onset: Consideration of Parenting Issues

David A. Mrazek and Mary D. Klinnert

University of Colorado at Denver

Patricia Mrazek

*National Jewish Center for Immunology and
Respiratory Medicine, Denver, Colorado*

Terri Macey

University of Colorado at Denver

This report examines the relationship between early parental behavior and the later onset of asthma in a cohort of 150 children who were genetically at risk for developing asthma. Judgments of both parenting problems and maternal coping were made during a home visit when the infant was 3 weeks old. A clinical interview with the mother was developed and reliably coded. The sample was divided into two groups based on the presence or absence of concerns about coping and parenting. During the following 2 years, the respiratory status of the children was monitored. Four categories of respiratory status were defined: (1) asthma; (2) recurrent infectious wheezing; (3) a single isolated wheezing episode; or (4) no wheezing. Early problems in coping and parenting were associated with the later onset of asthma (p < 0.001). Furthermore, parents of children who developed asthma were more likely to have been

Reprinted with permission from the *Journal of The American Academy of Child and Adolescent Psychiatry*, 30:2, March 1991. Copyright © 1991 by the American Academy of Child and Adolescent Psychiatry.

This work was supported through grant No. 88–1013–85 from the W.T. Grant Foundation, grant No. 2K02–MH00430 from the National Institute of Mental Health, and a grant from the Developmental Psychobiology Research Group.

The authors wish to thank Irene Anderson, Amy Brower, Florence Garyet, and David McCormick for their help in the preparation of the data, data analysis, and preparation of the manuscript.

having difficulties at the 3-week visit than those whose children developed infectious wheezing (p < 0.005).

Many studies have examined a wide range of psychological factors that influence the expression of asthmatic symptoms (Mrazek, 1988). However, difficulties in the early parenting of children at genetic risk for developing asthma have not been linked to the *initial* onset of asthma. This is in large part because of the problems associated with collecting unbiased data designed to examine the association between a wide range of potential emotional stressors and the onset of the disease. To avoid the natural inclination to make retrospective judgments that provide an explanation for the onset of the illness, a prospective design is required. This report documents the results of such a prospective study of a sample of infants at increased genetic risk for developing asthma. A highly significant statistical association was demonstrated between two ratings of parental behavior and the later onset of asthma.

It has become increasingly evident that some degree of genetic predisposition is a necessary condition for developing asthma. However, simply having a genotypic vulnerability does not result in phenotypic expression. Family studies have convincingly shown that there is an increased risk for the development of asthma for individuals who have affected relatives (Sibbald et al., 1980; Mrazek et al., 1990). There is also an elevated risk for increased airway reactivity among these family members even in the absence of disease. A methacholine challenge is the current method of choice for the identification of hyperactivity of the airways. Increasingly, large doses of methacholine are inhaled sequentially until a 20% drop in pulmonary function is produced. This technique provides an objective means of confirming a clinical diagnosis of asthma as well as identifying subclinically affected relatives. Using this technique, Longo et al. (1987) demonstrated that there was an elevated risk for increased methacholine sensitivity in nonsymptomatic relatives of asthmatic probands.

Nowhere is the critical interaction between nature and nurture more obvious than in the results of twin studies. These reports show both a high heritability of airway reactivity and a considerable degree of discordance between identical twins (Hopp et al., 1984). Given that the genomes of monozygotic twins are by definition identical, variation in the nonshared environment of monozygotic twins must necessarily be responsible for differential expression of a gene or set of genes that is ultimately involved in the onset of reactive airway disease.

Four classes of environmental risk factors have been hypothesized to affect gene activation. An enduring speculation has been that *respiratory viral infections* play a role in the pathogenesis of asthma (Busse, 1989). Evidence for this view includes clinical studies demonstrating that asthmatic children frequently experience attacks exacerbated by respiratory syncytial virus (RSV) and parainfluenza viral infections (McIntosh et al., 1973), and that RSV infection has been demonstrated to precede the onset of asthma in a small sample of children at genetic risk for the development of asthma (Frick et al., 1979). Furthermore, an intriguing model for the "switching on" of a putative set of genes exists as it is plausible that viral DNA could become incorporated into host cell nuclei and subsequently activate genes linked to expression of airway reactivity.

A second class of potential environmental activators is the wide range of *specific antigens* that can come in contact with the immunoregulatory components of the immune system. These allergens would include antigens derived from a small number of foods (e.g., milk, eggs, peanuts), dust mites, molds, animal danders, and animal saliva. A possible mechanism for the pathogenic effects of environmental antigens is that they may stimulate a classic antibody response involving immunoglobulin E antibodies that could result in a persistent increase in the reactivity of this system. Activated antibody molecules attach to the surfaces of mast cells and basophiles, which leads ultimately to their degranulation. This results in the release of a wide array of mediators from these cells that have been demonstrated to have an influence on the regulation of airway reactivity.

A third class of hypothesized environmental activators are *nonantigenic irritants*. The most widely considered substance in this category is smoke, although a wide range of air pollutants are plausible pathogenic activators. Irritants could directly affect the bronchial receptor systems or act through potentiating allergic mechanisms, resulting in greater reactivity to the antigens.

The fourth class of potential environmental risk factors is *emotional stressors*. The mechanism for the impact of stressors on gene expression has not been demonstrated. One possibility is that stressors could result in a shift in the balance of autonomic tone leading to increased bronchial sensitivity. Another hypothesis is that stressors could have a regulatory effect on the modulation of the immune response. A wide range of potential neuropeptides including substance P and vasointestinal protein have been shown to influence the immune response.

No prospective longitudinal study has conclusively demonstrated the etiological role of any of these factors for asthma onset. However, associations between the first three classes of risk factors and the development of asthma have been demonstrated. This report presents empirical evidence of a statistical association between early parental behavior and a later increase in the incidence of asthma in a cohort of genetically vulnerable infants. The implications of this link have not been determined, and this relationship should not be considered to be a causal one.

THE ASTHMA RISK STUDY

The W.T. Grant/National Jewish Center Asthma Risk Study was designed to identify possible associations between early environmental factors and subsequent asthma expression. Pregnant asthmatic women were recruited with the intention of measuring and monitoring possible risk factors for the onset of asthma in their infants. The development of their infants was subsequently carefully documented. A comparison sample of pregnant nonasthmatic women was also recruited with the expectation that few of their infants would develop asthma. The study is truly prospective as the index infants were still in utero at the time that the data collection with their parents was initiated.

METHOD

Sample

The index risk sample is the focus of this report and consists of 150 families who were living in the Metropolitan Denver area within 2 hours of the National Jewish Center for Immunology and Respiratory Medicine. All 150 mothers in the index risk sample were pregnant. Fourteen of the mothers (9.3%) had a documented history of asthma but had been symptom free for at least 2 years at the time of their entry into the study. Of the 136 mothers who were experiencing symptoms, 68 (45.3%) of the mothers required only intermittent medication to control their wheezing, while 68 (45.3%) were taking medication on a regular basis to control symptoms. Although the mothers in the study had a full range of severity of asthmatic symptoms, this sample does have a larger percentage of more severely asthmatic women than one would expect from an epidemiological study designed to include a representative sample of all the individuals within a catchment area who had asthma. Furthermore, at the 3-week visit, 82% of the mothers reported that their asthma was either in control or that their symptoms were easily resolved with a small modification of their medication dosage. In summary, this was not a severely impaired cohort of asthmatic women. Thirty-two of the fathers in the index sample had a first-degree relative with asthma. An additional 28 of the fathers in the index sample had asthma themselves.

Families who were planning to leave the Denver Metropolitan Area within 2 years of the birth of their infant were not included in this study. Additionally, families in which either parents had a severe psychiatric disturbance were excluded from the study. Only one family was actually not included in the study because of parental psychopathology. The mean scores of the standard clinical scales of the Minnesota Multiphasic Personality Inventory (MMPI) for the mothers and fathers in the sample varied from 49.72 (social introversion) to 57.60 (mania), which is a range that is typical of a nonclinical sample.

The index sample was 92% Caucasian and predominantly middle class (Hollingshead: I = 26%, II–43.3%, III = 22%, IV = 8.7%; Hollingshead, 1975). At the time of the birth of the index child, the mean age of the mothers was 29.3, and the mean age of the fathers was 31.1. Determination of the respiratory status of the children at 2 years of age was possible for all 150 index children as no families were lost to follow-up.

The comparison sample consisted of 30 families in which neither parent had asthma. No significant differences in ethnic background, socioeconomic status (SES), or parental age existed between the comparison and index samples. Similarly, the means of the MMPI scales did not vary between comparison and index samples on any of the clinical scales except for the social introversion scale of the mothers. While the mean score of asthmatic mothers was slightly higher than the controls (52.4 versus 48.60), both mean scores were in the normal range.

Method of Assessment

Perinatal Variables. The parental relationship is a critical aspect of the early experience of the infant. In order to quantify maternal coping and parenting during the first weeks of life, two scales were developed to measure these variables. A guiding principle in the development of these scales was that emotional stressors for the primary caregiver could have a potential effect on the infant. However, the degree of impact of the stressors on the child would be largely determined by the ability of the caregiver to cope with them and to concurrently modulate the emotional experience of the infant.

An interview-based format was chosen for the purpose of assessing parenting strategies and maternal coping. The mother and child were observed together during a home visit while the mother was interviewed using a newly developed semistructured interview. One objective of this new interview was to provide an opportunity for the clinician to observe the efforts of the parent to modulate the child's experience and to collect data reflecting parental sensitivity and competence. Another objective was to assess how the mother was coping with family stressors that were not related to parenting. The parenting data in this report were derived from this interview with the mother and her infant in the family home 3 weeks after the birth of the baby. Given that this sample is not a psychiatrically disturbed cohort, measures were needed to focus on the variability of parenting and coping in relation to the issues of adapting to the new infant. The authors were aware of no standardized measure that was available to capture these aspects of early parenting. Thus, while standardized measures of parental personality and the quality of parental marital relationship would be expected to correlate with early measures of parenting, these more general measures of psychopathology and adjustment would be expected to be less adequate predictors of problems in infant development.

Parenting Interview Rating. The first variable was a global rating of concern regarding parenting based on the maternal interview. Essentially, six characteristics of both parents were taken into account in making this judgment. These included:

(1) the attitude of the parents toward the new infant including their enthusiasm for the parenting role; (2) their sensitivity to the needs of the infant; (3) their effectiveness in responding to the infant; (4) the nature of the parents' strategy for sharing parenting responsibilities; (5) any evidence of disturbed emotional adjustment that would impact upon caring for the infant including the presence of postpartum depression; and (6) adequacy of the plan of the parents to continue with their employment while providing adequate child care. Parenting was scored on a three-point scale. The sample was subsequently dichotomized into two categories. The better performing group experienced only minimal subjective problems and was doing well in all spheres. The problematical group was viewed as experiencing either moderate or severe difficulties. Interrater reliability for this categorical rating was greater than 76%.

Coping Interview Rating. The second rating was of "maternal coping." The interview explored three primary areas of coping: (1) the mother's current management of responsibilities within the family; (2) her ability to plan for the continuation of her own career objectives; and (3) a judgment of her degree of satisfaction with her current adjustment. The interview was first coded on a hierarchical five-point scale, and, subsequently, the sample was dichotomized into two groups. The group designated as coping well was functioning adequately in all three areas and experiencing no chronic difficulties. The mothers designated as demonstrating problematical coping were having difficulties in one or more of the three domains of adaptation. The interrater reliability for this dichotomy was greater than 82%. It should be emphasized that this global rating is of a construct of behavior that is an important component of a traditional family assessment. Consequently, the adequate levels of interrater reliability achieved by clinicians after a training period of approximately 10 hours is possible because of the fairly straightforward nature of these clinical judgments.

Temperament. A third global rating was designed to quantify the degree of difficulty of temperament of each of the infants at the 3-week interview. This judgment was based on both the maternal report of the child's rhythmicity and ability to be soothed during the first 3 weeks of life and the direct observation of the infant. Ratings on a five-point hierarchical scale ranged from very difficult to very easy. The reliability of the differentiation of a dichotomy of "relatively difficult" versus "relatively easy" infants was 86%.

Standardized Measures. The MMPI (Hathaway and McKinley, 1970) and the Dyadic Adjustment Scale (DAS)(Spanier, 1976) were administered to the parents during the final trimester of the pregnancy with the index infant. These standardized instruments measure some aspects of the personality and adjustment of the parents that should be associated with parenting. Consequently, examining the association between these scale scores and the newly developed global scales provided an opportunity to demonstrate aspects of the validity of the global scales. The correlation between these standardized instruments and the rating scales are reviewed in the results section.

Subsequent Health Status The health status of the children was carefully monitored over the first 2 years of their lives with the specific objective of documenting the occurrence of wheezing and respiratory illnesses. Three classes of reactive airway disease were defined for the purpose of characterizing respiratory illnesses with bronchoconstriction. Class I reactive airway disease included only children diagnosed as having "asthma" based on conservative diagnostic criteria, which included documentation of recurrent wheezing episodes by the child's pediatrician. Although many of these attacks occurred with a concurrent viral infection, at least one of these wheezing episodes must have been precipitated by an environmental trigger other than a respiratory infection to be classified as asthma. Class II reactive airway disease was labeled "infectious wheezing" and defined as multiple wheezing episodes with every episode having been associated with a respiratory infection. This category would not be differentiated from "asthma" by many American practioners, but it is widely used as a distinct diagnostic category in Britain. In essence, "infectious wheezing," as used in this study, is distinguished from "asthma" by the requirement that all wheezing episodes must have been associated with documented infections. Class III reactive airway disease was a category reserved for children who had only experienced a single isolated episode of wheezing that was identified by the child's physician. This single documented episode could have occurred with or without a respiratory infection. These children were considered to be at an elevated risk for subsequent attacks but would not be classified as having either "infectious wheezing" or "asthma" until a second episode was documented.

Data Analysis

The relationships between early parental behavior and subsequent infant illness were demonstrated by chi-square analyses. Comparisons of characteristics of the sample were done using chi-square and *t*-test analyses for categorical and continuous data, respectively.

Results

Asthma Status Twenty-one of the 150 children at genetic risk for developing reactive airway disease had been diagnosed with asthma (Class I) when they had reached 2 years of age. Fourteen additional children had experienced multiple episodes of bronchoconstriction that had all been associated with viral infections and were consequently diagnosed as having infectious wheezing (Class II). Twenty-one children had experienced only a single wheezing episode (Class III), and 94 children had never wheezed.

Parenting The clinical judgment of "early parenting difficulties" was found to be a predictor of asthma. This rating of the presence of early parenting difficulties was made based on concerns elicited during interview of some aspect of the ability of the parents to deal with the demands of their young infant. Fifty-two of the infants had parents who were rated as having problematical parenting, while 98 infants had parents who were felt to be adjusting well to the parenting role. Thirteen of the 52 infants whose parents were judged to be having some problems with parenting subsequently developed asthma (25%) as compared with only eight of the infants whose parents were perceived as parenting their infant well (8%) ($p <$ 0.005).

Coping The maternal coping variable was designed to quantify the ability of the mother to cope with a broader range of family stressors that extended beyond parenting. It included a judgment of how well the mother had managed a wide range of family relationships, her family's economic realities, and her changing life circumstances. Sixty-seven of the mothers were having some difficulties in coping, and 13 of their infants subsequently developed asthma (19%). Only eight children of the 83 mothers who were judged to be coping well developed asthma (10%). A trend reflecting an association between better coping and less infant disease was demonstrated ($p = 0.087$).

Parental Difficulty The sample was subsequently divided into two categories based on whether either problematical parenting or problematical coping had been coded. Using this method, 76 mothers were classified as having early parenting difficulties. Figure 1 illustrates that 18 (24%) of these 76 infants whose parents were having difficulties developed asthma. Of those 74 infants whose parents were both coping and parenting well, only three (4%) children had developed asthma by 2 years of age. This difference is highly significant ($p < 0.001$).

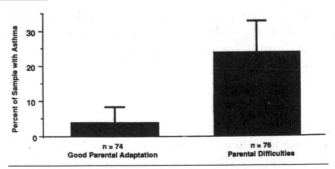

Figure 1. Four percent of the children from families who were coded as having good parental adaptation developed asthma in contrast with 24% of the children whose parents were coded as having parental difficulties. This relationship between the development of asthma and parental adaptation is highly significant ($p < 0.001$).

In contrast to this association between the presence of parenting or coping difficulties and the later onset of *asthma* there was no association between parental difficulties and *infectious wheezing*. Specifically, only 29% of the parents of children who had experienced infectious wheezing, but in whom the problem had not progressed to asthma, were having parenting difficulties during the initial 3 weeks of life of the infant. In contrast, as illustrated in Figure 2, 86% of the parents of children who had developed asthma were having difficulties ($p < 0.005$).

Parenting Difficulties in the Comparison Group The incidence of parenting difficulties as determined by the clinical interview was virtually identical between the control group families and the index families. Fifty-one percent of the asthmatic families were having some parenting difficulties as compared with 53% of the control families.

Comparison of Parents with and without Difficulties A set of analyses was conducted to examine the possible differences in maternal age and SES between infants with parents having difficulties and those doing well based on the parenting and maternal coping codings that had been made when he infants were only 3 weeks old. No differences in maternal age was evident between the two groups, as the mothers having difficulties had a mean age of 28.6 as opposed to the mothers who were doing well who had a mean age of 29.9. Furthermore, no significant differences in SES were shown between the two groups.

A further analysis was conducted to examine whether a possible difference in genetic risk existed between the two groups. Thirty (39%) of the children whose parents were having difficulty had high genetic loading based on the criteria of having asthma documented on the paternal side of the family *and* having a mother with asthma. Similarly, 30 (41%) of the infants whose parents were doing well had a high genetic loading for asthma.

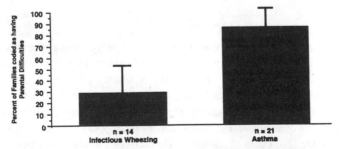

Figure 2. Twenty-nine percent of the children who developed infectious wheezing were from families who were coded as having parental difficulties; whereas 86% of the parents of children who developed asthma were coded as having difficulties. This difference is highly significant ($p < 0.005$).

Correlates of the Clinical Global Ratings A set of analyses to examine correlates with the clinical global ratings judgments was conducted.

Temperament. An association between parenting difficulties and difficult temperament was also noted. Thirty-three infants (43%) of families where parenting difficulties were identified were coded as having difficult temperaments as opposed to 12 (16%) infants of the 74 families in which the parents were doing well ($p < 0.001$). While more children with difficult temperaments did develop asthma, the association between difficult temperament and illness expression was not significant.

Dyadic Adjustment Scale. Families without parenting difficulties were more likely to have higher levels of marital satisfaction as measured by the DAD ($p = 0.05$). However, lower marital satisfaction was not significantly associated with later asthma onset in the children.

MMPI. Mothers who were having parenting difficulties were more likely to have elevated scores on the *F* scale ($p < 0.0001$), depression scale ($p < 0.002$), and the psychopathic deviation scale ($p < 0.02$). Two derived scales were also associated with parenting difficulties. The mothers having problematical parenting and/or coping had elevated scores on the dependency scale ($p < 0.005$) and lower scores on the ego strength scale ($p < 0.02$). They also have a lower score on the K scale ($p < 0.005$). While the means scores of all of the scales of the mothers with parental difficulties were within the normal range, variability within this range was significantly associated with the clinical ratings. These associations provide evidence of the concurrent validity for the clinical interview judgments. Interestingly, no clinical scale and only one derived scale, the dependency scale, of the MMPI was significantly associated with asthma onset in the infants of these women ($p < 0.05$). Given the large number of possible comparisons and the relatively modest level of significance of this association, little interference from the finding of greater maternal dependency and asthma onset should be implied.

DISCUSSION

An association between parenting behavior and later illness expression in genetically at-risk children is in many ways intriguing, but it cannot be considered to be evidence of a causal link. The mechanism by which a particular pattern of parent-children interaction might eventually lead to an increased likelihood for the expression of airway reactivity cannot be elucidated from these analyses. From one perspective, it is quite surprising that a statistical association exists at a single point in time with the later onset of asthma. The fact that such an association does exist suggests, but does not definitely prove, that these judgments capture a more stable aspect of parental behavior. Further exploration of possible mechanisms would be a particularly interesting direction for future research inquiry.

One limitation of this report is that the findings are relevant only to the early onset of asthma. The future clinical course of the respiratory status of these children is as yet unknown. Some children may have a very circumscribed form of the illness and essentially be symptom free for the remainder of their childhood, while other children currently unaffected are likely to develop respiratory symptoms. Following this cohort into the future to examine variations in the pattern of illness expression is yet another direction for future investigation.

The decision to make a home visit when the infant was 3 weeks of age was based on a variety of considerations. One advantage was that a postnatal visit would provide an opportunity to make an assessment of the early adaptation of the mother to the infant at a specific developmental period across the entire sample. All of the mothers were still at home with their infants, and there had been relatively few external factors to complicate the assessment of the mother's parenting. Additionally, a 3-week assessment ruled out the possibility that any of the children would be already demonstrating early airway reactivity, as it is an extremely unusual occurrence for bronchoconstriction to occur within the first month of life. In that regard, this assessment of parenting behavior would, in all likelihood, predate any complications resulting from the impact of the onset of asthma on the behavior of the parents. Finally, doing an assessment in the home had the advantage of maximizing the ability of the interviewer to assess the actual living circumstances of the mother and infant. Despite these advantages for choosing an early postnatal assessment, there is also the clear limitation that this single point does not capture later developments.

Generalizations drawn from these data must be circumspect. It should be emphasized that the characteristics of this sample are not that of a general population cohort. Specifically, the sample is primarily a middle- to upper middle-class white sample, and these results should not be assumed to be valid for disadvantaged cohorts. Additionally, the range of asthmatic symptoms represented in this sample was extensive, ranging from an asymptomatic history of asthma in 9.3% of the index mothers to a requirement of continuous medication in 45.3% of the index mothers. Given the range of medication requirements in epidemiological samples, more seriously asthmatic women were overrepresented. One reason for the somewhat more seriously asthmatic women being referred to the study is that they may well have a greater motivation to participate in a study designed to better understand the expression of an illness that has affected their own lives. It is possible that the frequency of expression of asthma in the infants of more severely asthmatic women may be somewhat greater because the genes associated with more severe illness may be more penetrant. However, this is strictly a speculation, as genetic risk studies of asthma have not demonstrated an association between the severity of the parental disease and a higher incidence of affected offspring. Similarly, in this study, there was no association between the severity of asthma in the parents and an increased risk for asthma expression in the infants.

Interestingly, the association between parenting difficulties and the subsequent development of asthma by 2 years of age in these infants would have been considerably obscured if a less rigorous definition of asthma had been chosen. It was striking that the mothers of children with infectious wheezing were actually doing very well. There is good evidence to suggest that all 35 children with a diagnosis of either asthma or infectious wheezing have a genetic component to their illness that puts them at increased risk for developing asthma. This is supported by the observation that all of these children responded to viral infections with the characteristic pattern of bronchoconstriction and wheezing that is the hallmark of asthma. However, it may be that in families in which parents are functioning at a highly adaptive level, these early viral infections can be resolved without a change in the subsequent airway reactivity of the child. In contrast, in a caregiving environment where parenting difficulties exist, bronchoconstriction may be conditioned to the emotional distress associated with the attack. While a variety of hypotheses can be put forward to explain the associations between early parenting difficulties and later airway reactivity, definitive conclusions regarding the true nature of underlying mechanisms are not possible without additional research and analyses.

This report provides empirical evidence documenting a link between early parenting behavior and the subsequent expression of asthma. If these findings are confirmed, the implications will be considerable as they would suggest that interventions designed to support the parenting of genetically at-risk children may well result in a decrease in the expression of asthma.

REFERENCES

Busse, W.W. (1989), The relationship between viral infections and onset of allergic diseases in asthma. *Clin. Exp. Allergy*, 19:1–9.

Frick, O.L., German, D.F., & Mills, J. (1979), Development of allergy in children. I. Association with virus infections. *J. Allergy Clin. Immunol.* 63:228–241.

Hathaway, S.R. & McKinley, J.C. (1970), *Minnesota Multiphasic Personality Inventory*. Minneapolis: The University of Minnesota Press.

Hollingshead, A.B. (1975), *Four Factor Index of Social Status*. New Haven, CT: Available from Yale University Sociology Department.

Hopp, D.O., Bewtra, A.K., Watt, G.D., Nair, N.M. & Townley, R.G. (1984), Genetic analysis of allergic disease in twins. *J. Allergy Clin. Immunol.*, 73:265–270.

Longo, G., Strinati, R., Poli, F. & Fumi, F. (1987), Genetic factors in nonspecific bronchial hyperreactivity. *Am. J. Dis. Child.*, 41:331–334.

McIntosh, K., Ellis, E.F., Hoffman, L.S., Lybass, T.G., Eller, J.J. & Fulginniti, V.A. (1973), The association of viral and bacterial respiratory infections with exacerbations of wheezing in young asthmatic children. *Pediatrics*, 82:578–590.

Mrazek, D.A. (1988), Asthma: psychiatric considerations, evaluation, and management.

In: *Allergy: Principles and Practice*, 3rd edition, eds. E. Middleton, C.E. Reed & E.F. Ellis. St. Louis: C.V. Mosby, pp. 1176–1196.

Sibbald, B., Horn, M.E.C. & Gregg, I. (1980), A family study of the genetic basis of asthma and wheezy bronchitis. *Arch. Dis. Child.*, 55:354–357.

Spanier, G.B. (1976), Measuring dyadic adjustment: New scales for assessing the quality of marriage and similar dyads. *Journal of Marriage and the Family.* 38:15–28.

20

Adolescent Suicidality: A Clinical-Developmental Approach

Sophie R. Borst, Gil G. Noam, and John A. Bartok
Harvard Medical School, Boston, Massachusetts

This study investigates the relation of ego development, age, gender, and diagnosis to suicidality among 219 adolescent psychiatric inpatients. Using the Diagnostic Interview Schedule for Children, adolescents were classified as suicide attempters or as nonsuicidal and were categorized into three diagnostic groups: affective disorder, conduct disorder, or mixed conduct-affective disorder. Ego development measurement was used to assess developmental maturity. Chi-square analyses demonstrated a relation between suicide attempts and developmental complexity. Attempters were more likely to be diagnosed with affective or mixed conduct-affective disorders and to be girls. Suicidality was not associated with age in this sample. Log-linear analyses demonstrated the interplay of known suicide risk factors with the important new dimension of developmental level.

Over the past few decades, rates of both completed and attempted suicide have rapidly increased among adolescents (Diekstra and Moritz, 1987; Holinger, 1978; Pfeffer, 1986). Although suicidal behaviors are relatively rare under the age of 12, the prevalence increases considerably during middle and late adolescence, constituting the third leading cause of death among 15- to 24-year-olds (Hawton, 1986; Shaffer and Fisher, 1981). The incidence of suicide attempts also increases with

Reprinted with permission from the *Journal of the American Academy of Child and Adolescent Psychiatry*, 1991, Vol. 30, No. 5, 796–803. Copyright ©1991 by the American Academy of Child and Adolescent Psychiatry.

The authors gratefully acknowledge the assistance of Ken Kleinman for data analyses, Dr. Kurt Kreppner, and Dr. Rainer Silbereisen for statistical consultation, Jennifer Stevens, and Dr. Virginia Youngren for editorial assistance, Christopher Recklitis for comments on earlier versions of this manuscript, and Dr. Silvio Onesti and Dr. Rene Diekstra for their administrative and intellectual support.

age, with a sharp rise at ages 13 to 14 (Carlson and Cantwell, 1982; Rutter and Garmezy, 1983).

These statistics have contributed to increased interest in the antecedents and cause of adolescent suicide. Despite recent research efforts to explain what shields children from becoming suicidal (Carlson et al., 1987; Shaffer and Fisher, 1981), little progress has been made in demonstrating specific developmental risk and protective factors. Some investigators have suggested that formal operational levels of cognitive maturation are required to experience the feelings of despair, self-hate, and hopelessness that are necessary to suicidal ideation or suicidal behavior (Carlson, et al., 1987; Shaffer and Fisher, 1981). Similarly, Rutter (1986) hypothesized that the rise in depression and suicidality in adolescence might be due to such cognitive advances as self-observation and future orientation. In addition, it has been suggested that children may lack the psychological sophistication required to make the *decision* to end life (Shaffer and Fisher, 1981). The only empirical study investigating this relationship, using school performance as a measure of cognitive development, found that adolescents below grade level were significantly less often suicidal and less realistic about how to commit suicide than their grade-level peers (Carlson et al., 1987).

Given the lack of systematic studies, the authors began a line of research investigating the relationship of suicide to social-cognitive development and other known suicide risk factors, such as age, gender, and diagnosis. Although many developmental approaches to psychopathology have focused on the description of age-based chronologies of symptoms and disorders (e.g., Rutter and Garmezy, 1983), the need to move beyond age as the principal developmental variable has been gaining acceptance. Kazdin (1989), for example, has argued that developmental psychopathology research must go beyond chronological age alone and assess the cognitive organization of children. Similarly, Achenbach (1982) has noted that many approaches to developmental psychopathology "neglect children's capacities for constructive cognitive adaptation and reorganization" (p. 654).

This study's clinical-developmental orientation (e.g., Noam, 1988; Werner, 1948) builds on the assumption that age by itself is insufficient to clarify the risk and preconditions of suicide. Dimensions of personality, such as the degree of impulsivity and the capacity for delay of gratification, are also closely linked to psychopathology and suicidality. In the clinical-developmental tradition, it is assumed that persons systematically organize meanings about themselves and their lives, and that these perspectives on self and significant others develop across the life-span. In addition, these meaning systems are seen as related to expressions and outcomes of psychopathology. Given this orientation, it was hypothesized that Loevinger's theory of ego development (Loevinger, 1976), with its emphasis on impulse control, complexity of self-reflection, and emotional experience, would lend itself well to the study of suicidality. Combining Eriksonian and Sullivanian concepts of ego functioning with character psychology and cognitive-developmental principles, Loevinger's model encompasses major ego functions of concern in the study of adolescent suicidality.

The ego, as defined by Loevinger, is the master trait around which personality is constructed. Her theory posits that each person has a customary orientation to self and to the world, and that there are stages and transitions along which these "frames of reference" may be grouped. Individuals at Loevinger's earliest positions of ego development are impulsive, have stereotyped cognitive styles, and are dependent or exploitative. The three stages that share there characteristics I–2, Delta, and Delta/3, are referred to as "preconformist" (Browning, 1986). Individuals at the "conformist" stages (I–3 and I–3/4) are particularly concerned with interpersonal acceptance and often express their views in cliches and stereotypes. By contrast, individuals who have reached the "postcomformist" stages of ego development (I–4, I–4/5, I–5, I–6) generally cope with inner conflict through a high degree of self-awareness. They typically show more cognitive complexity and have interpersonal styles that emphasize mutuality and respect for individual differences. These later stages tend to occur only during late adolescence and adulthood.

Although evidence has accumulated that ego development and psychopathology are significantly related, no studies have examined this construct in relation to suicidal behavior. Findings from earlier studies indicate that there are important relationships between ego development, symptomatology, defenses, and treatment requests and an important clinical use for developmental information (Browning, 1986; Dill and Noam, 1990; Noam and Houlihan, 1990; Noam et al., in press). Studies on the relationship between ego development and psychopathology have shown that delinquency, conduct disorders, and externalizing behaviors are associated with preconformist levels of ego development (Frank and Quinlan, 1976; Noam et al., 1984; Paget et al., 1990). Two studies have also suggested a greater degree of maladjustment and psychiatric impairment among adolescents at the preconformist stages, as compared to adolescents at conformist stages (Browning, 1986; Frank and Quinlan, 1976). This is further supported by the finding that the majority of disturbed adolescents are developmentally delayed as compared with nonclinical adolescents (Noam and Houlihan, 1990; Noam et al., 1984). In normative samples, the shift from preconformist to conformist ego levels generally occurs between the ages of 12 and 15 (e.g., Redmore and Loevinger, 1979). However, in previous studies, the majority of adolescent inpatients have been found to be functioning at preconformist developmental levels. This phenomenon was called "age-stage dysynchrony" to point to the difficulties of solving adolescent tasks with a delayed developmental organization (Noam and Houlihan, 1990; Noam et al., 1984).

Research investigating a link between higher levels of ego development and internalizing symptomatology has been less conclusive. However, some findings indicate an association between ego maturity and emotional disorders (Gold, 1980; Paget et al., 1990), supporting the hypothesis that with increasing developmental complexity, psychopathology becomes more internalized, more experienced in psychological than in physical terms, and less action oriented. Because suicidality is, in part, a turning against the self (e.g., Recklitis et al., 1990) the authors pursued the hypothesis that maturation of developmental capacities does not necessarily lead to better adjustment but may in fact lead to a greater vulnerability for suicidality. Although suicidal behavior was not hypothesized to be exclusively a phenomenon of conformist stages, the authors expected to find a higher percentage of suicide attempters within the conformist group than within the group of preconformist adolescents. It was hypothesized that adolescents at conformist levels of ego development are more prone to self-rejection, feelings of depression, guilt, and despair, and more likely to see causes of intrapsychic and interpersonal problems within themselves then preconformist adolescents, who are more likely to externalize and to blame others for their problems.

The complex nature of suicidality suggests, however, a more sophisticated model than a single link between developmental level and suicidal behavior. For that reason, this study also investigates the relation between suicide attempts and three other variables known to affect suicidal risk: type of psychopathology, age, and gender.

Previous research found that psychiatric disorders constitute some of the most important risk factors for adolescent suicide. Kovacs and Puig-Antich (1989) state that "using very global and 'rough' estimates, psychiatrically disturbed youths may be running a risk of suicide about 200-fold (or more) the rate of their general population counterparts" (p. 154). A study of adolescent suicide by Shaffi et al. (1985) found that 95% of the suicide completers were suffering from a *DSM-III* psychiatric disorder. Most completers were diagnosed with a major affective disorder. Depression also has been found present in many young suicide attempters (Pfeffer et al., 1988; Robbins and Alessi, 1985). More recently, studies have found a significant percentage of suicidal adolescents who were not depressed but sought treatment with either a conduct disorder or antisocial behaviors (e.g., Apter et al., 1988; Borst and Noam, 1989). In particular, it has been suggested that the comorbidity of depressive symptoms and aggressive symptoms may be a "lethal combination" (Blumenthal and Kupfer, 1988; Shaffer, 1974).

Because conduct disorders and affective disorders represent the major psychiatric disturbances of childhood and adolescence in inpatient settings, the authors decided to investigate suicidal behavior in relation to these diagnostic groups. A number of studies have found that depression and conduct disorder show a considerable overlap (Carlson and Cantwell, 1980; Chiles et al., 1980; Edelbrock and Achenbach, 1980). This overlap was found in this sample as well and, therefore, a mixed group of patients diagnosed with both conduct and affective disorder was also included. Based on the findings of previous studies, it was hypothesized that the incidence of suicide attempts would be higher in the affective-disorder or mixed-disorder groups than among patients with a conduct disorder alone.

In virtually all studies of attempted suicide, girls outnumber boys with a ratio of 3:1 to 9:1 (Hawton, 1986; Pfeffer, 1986; Rutter and Garmezy, 1983). It was therefore hypothesized that suicidality would be more prevalent among the girls than among the boys of the sample. In addition, girls have been found to be slightly developmentally ahead of boys in both nonclinical (e.g., Redmore and Loevinger, (1979) and psychiatric adolescent samples (Noam et al., 1984; Paget et al., 1990).

This study takes the logical next step of studying adolescent psychopathology and suicidality by adopting a developmental approach to these known suicide risk factors, an approach that has received little or no attention so far. The attempt to understand suicide as a form of psychopathology, while attending to the philosophical and clinical insights of its ties to complex meanings about self and relationships, continues to pose a challenge. The goal of this research is to explore both adolescent suicide as a sign of a serious disorder and the underlying maturational forces that contribute to the emergence of suicidality.

METHOD

Subjects

The sample consisted of 219 adolescent patients, 96 boys and 123 girls, ages 12 to 16 years (to the nearest year). The mean age of the sample was 14.08 (SD = 1.02). The adolescents in the sample were drawn from 480 consecutive admissions to a child and adolescent unit of a private psychiatric hospital between 1983 and 1989. Inclusion criteria were age greater than 11.5 and a *DSM-III* diagnosis of affective disorder and/or conduct disorder. Some subjects ($N = 37$) were excluded because they were prematurely discharged, or they were unable or refused to complete the testing. Furthermore, eight patients who attempted suicide more than 6 months before admission were excluded from the analyses, as their diagnostic status or developmental level might have changed since the time of their attempt. To keep the groups in this study as homogeneous as possible, patients who reported serious ideation ($N = 36$) but had not made any suicidal attempts were excluded from both the suicidal and the nonsuicidal group. This strategy was pursued to have two clearly distinguishable groups to compare.

The majority of the sample (92%) was white and came predominantly from middle- and upper-middle-class families (78% from class 1, 2, and 3), as classified by Hollingshead (1957, unpublished manuscript). The suicide attempters and nonsuicidal adolescents had similar socioeconomic backgrounds (chi-square = 4.28; $df = 4; p = 0.37$). Mean Wechsler Full Scale IQ for the sample was 102.28 (SD

$= 13.82$; $N = 212$). No IQ differences were found between suicidal and non-suicidal adolescents, $F(1,215) = 0.01$; $p = 0.91$.

Instruments and Procedures

Diagnostic Interview Schedule for Children-Child Version (DISC-C). The DISC is a standardized diagnostic interview developed for the National Institute of Mental Health by Costello et al. (1984) for use in epidemiological studies of children and adolescents, ages 6 to 18 years. The DISC-C contains 264 items that inquire about behaviors and emotions, both past and current. Symptoms correspond to *DSM-III* diagnostic criteria for childhood and adolescent disorders and generate a *DSM-III* Axis I diagnosis. Reliability and validity of the DISC has been found to be as good or better than other structured diagnostic interviews (Costello et al., 1985). Trained child psychologists and child psychiatrists interviewed all adolescents within the first 4 weeks of admission.

Included in the sample were adolescents with an affective disorder (18%), conduct disorder (44%), or a mixed conduct-affective disorder (38%). These diagnostic groups contained 75% of the consecutive admissions of age 11.5 and above. The remaining 25% of the sample were assigned to a variety of other diagnoses, the number in each category being too small to allow for appropriate statistical analyses.

Given that the same instrument was used to assess both suicide attempts and affective disorders, a possible measurement confound could not be ruled out. For that reason, the relation between suicidality and diagnosis was also analyzed, using the intake psychiatrist's *DSM-III* diagnosis made during an in-depth admission interview at the authors' psychiatric center. The admission diagnoses were divided into four diagnostic categories: affective disorders, conduct disorders, mixed-conduct affective disorders, and an "other" category that mainly consisted of oppositional disorder, anxiety disorder, and attention deficit disorder.

Suicidality measurement. Adolescents were classified as suicide attempters on the basis of self-report, using the DISC-C. Included in the attempters group were patients who answered "yes" to the following DISC question: "Have you ever tried to kill yourself?" Half of the suicidal adolescents attempted suicide within 2 weeks of admission (76% within 2 months).

The adolescent's self-report was chosen because a number of studies have indicated that adolescents are reliable reporters of suicidality (Robbins and Alessi, 1985; Walker et al., 1990). To check these findings against this data set, two reliability studies were conducted comparing the adolescent's self-report on attempts with information obtained from the parents or from the medical charts. These studies demonstrated high agreement. In the first study, 91 parents were interviewed with the parent version of the DISC (DISC-P) and parent and adolescent reports were compared on the question concerning suicidal attempts. A high percentage of agreement (84.6%) was found on attempts (chi-square $= 34.30$; $df = 1$; $p < 0.0001$). The second study, using a subsample of 65 adolescents, investigated the agreement between self-report on the DISC-C and information about attempts abstracted from the adolescent's medical charts. Again, a high agreement (75.4%) was found on suicide attempts (chi-square $= 14.98$; $df = 1$; $p = 0.0001$). Given the generally low agreement between parent, clinician, and adolescent symptomatology report as suggested by the literature (e.g., Weinstein et al., 1989), the levels of agreement are quite strong.

Loevinger's Washington University Sentence Completion Test (SCT). The SCT consists of 36 incomplete sentence stems, with slightly different versions used for boys and girls. Subjects are asked to complete the sentence stems, such as "When I am with a man . . . ", "The thing I like about myself is . . ."etc. The responses to these stems are rated for manifestation of ego development through the use of a complex scoring manual (Loevinger et al., 1970). Evidence for the construct validity of the SCT measure is favorable (for a review, see Loevinger, 1979). Test-retest studies using the SCT suggest that ego development is a relatively stable construct. High test-retest stability has been found using the SCT with psychiatric outpatients (0.71 for total protocol ratings and 0.90 for item sum scores)(Weiss et al., 1989) and nonclinical adolescents ($r = 0.79$ for total protocol ratings and $r = 0.91$ for item sum scores) (Redmore and Waldman, 1975). Previous studies also support the interrater reliability of Loevinger's measure of ego development with a variety of nonclinical and psychiatric populations, with interrater agreement on ego level score ranging from 0.80 (Weiss et al., 1989) to 0.85 (Redmore and Waldman, 1975).

The SCT was administered by training research assistants within the first 2 weeks of admission. An ego stage score (total protocol rating) and a continuous numerical score (item sum score) were derived for each protocol. The scoring of protocols was performed by trained raters whose reliability was greater than $r = 0.85$. The raters were blind to the diagnostic and suicidal status of the adolescents.

On the basis of the Loevinger score, the sample was divided into two groups: pre-conformist (I–2, delta and delta/3) and conformist (I–3 and above). The majority (88%) of the sample functioned at a preconformist developmental level, with only 12% at conformist or postcomformist levels.

RESULTS

Chi-square comparisons analyzing the relationships between suicidality and age, gender, developmental level, and diagnosis are presented in Table 1.

Age. No relationship was found between age at admission and suicide attempts (chi-square $= 3.66$; $df = 2$; $p = 0.16$).

Gender. Suicide attempts were significantly more common among girls than among

TABLE 1.
Suicidal Status by Age, Gender, Diagnostic Categories, and Ego
Level (N = 219)

Variables	Nonsuicidal Adolescents (N = 141)		Suicide Attempters (N = 78)	
	N	%	N	%
Age				
12 and 13 years	41	67	19	33
14 years	45	54	35	46
15 and 16 years	55	68	29	32
Gender[a]				
Male	78	81	18	19
Female	63	51	60	49
Diagnostic Categories[b] (DISC)				
Conduct disorder	85	88	12	12
Affective disorder	19	49	20	51
Mixed conduct/affective	37	45	46	55
Diagnostic categories[c] (Clinician)				
Conduct disorder	77	81	18	19
Affective disorder	20	35	34	63
Mixed conduct/affective	16	60	10	38
"Other"	28	62	16	36
Ego development[d]				
Preconformist	131	68	62	32
Conformist	10	38	16	62

[a] Chi-square = 21.21; $df = 1$; $p < 0.0001$.
[b] Chi-square = 41.23; $df = 2$; $p < 0.0001$.
[c] Chi-square = 29.22; $df = 3$; $p < 0.0001$.
[d] Chi-square = 8.65; $df = 1$; $p < 0.003$.

boys (chi-square = 21.21; $df = 1$; $p < 0.0001$). Half of the girls had attempted suicide (49%; $N = 60$), compared with only one-fifty of the boys (19%; $N = 18$). *Diagnostic group using DISC-C diagnoses.* Adolescent attempters were diagnosed significantly more often as having affective disorders or mixed conduct-affective disorders than conduct disorders (chi-square = 41.23; $df = 2$; $p < 0.0001$). Of the conduct-disordered adolescents, only 12% ($N = 12$) had attempted suicide, compared with 51% ($N = 20$) of the adolescents with an affective disorder and 55% ($N = 46$) of the adolescents with a mixed disorder. The majority of suicidal adolescents (59%) were diagnosed as having a mixed conduct-affective disorder. *Diagnostic group using clinician's DMS-III diagnoses.* At the time of admission, clinicians diagnosed suicidal adolescents as having affective disorders significantly more often than conduct disorders, mixed conduct-affective disorders, or other disorders (chi-square = 29.22; $df = 3$; $p < 0.0001$). Of the adolescents diagnosed with an affective disorder, 63%(N = 34) were suicidal, compared with only 19% (N = 18) of adolescents diagnosed as having a conduct disorder, 38% (N = 10) of adolescents diagnosed as having a mixed conduct-affective disorder, and 36% (N = 16) of adolescents diagnosed in the "other" category.

Ego development. Chi-square analyses showed that suicide attempts related significantly to conformist levels of ego development (chi-square = 8.65; df = 1; p = 0.003). Of the conformist adolescents, 62% (N = 16) were suicidal compared with 32% (N = 62) of the preconformist adolescents.

Logistic Regression and Log-linear Analyses

Although chi-square analyses demonstrated important associations between pairs of variables, step-wise logistic regression analyses enabled the investigation of the relative strength of each of the variables in predicting suicide attempts. The step-wise logistic regression showed that gender, diagnosis, and ego development each contributed significantly in predicting suicide attempts (chi-square = 33.507; df = 3; p = 0..0001). Ego development was still a significant predictor of suicide attempts even when the variance due to gender and diagnoses had been accounted for. The model including gender, developmental level, and diagnostic status predicted the suicidal status of 78.1% of the sample correctly.

In addition, log-linear analyses were performed to investigate interactions among the independent variables. Log-linear is used to model relationships among categorical variables in multidimensional contingency tables. By building a hierarchical system of models, multiple models can be compared on the basis of theory, goodness of fit, and parsimony.

The hierarchical log-linear models included the variables of ego development, gender, diagnostic group (as measured by the DISC), and suicide. The baseline model included the main effects of these four variables. Models were generated by systematically adding one new term (an interaction between the variables) to the model at a time. The final or saturated model thus contained all possible interactions among these variables. Models were compared using the decrement-to-chi-square test (Kennedy, 1983).

Results show that the best fitting model contains all main effects (suicide, ego, gender, diagnostic group), all two-way interactions between these variables, and one three-way interaction (suicide by gender by diagnostic group), which together are the best predictors of the cell frequencies (residual chi-square = 1.03; df = 1; p = 0.310). The log-linear analyses demonstrated the complex interplay of suicide risk factors. In the present sample, an adolescent attempter was more likely to be a girl, diagnosed as having an affective or mixed conduct-affective disorder and functioning at a more mature, conformist developmental level. Another important finding, resulting from the two-way interactions involving ego development, is that suicidal adolescents, girls, and those diagnosed as having either mixed conduct-affective or affective disorder have a higher level of ego development. Specifically, they are more likely to have reached conformist developmental levels, as compared to nonsuicidal adolescents, boys, and adolescents diagnosed as having conduct disorder.

DISCUSSION

This study demonstrates the relevance of a clinical-developmental approach to the study of adolescent suicide attempts. In addition to the established risk factors of gender and diagnosis, it was found that with increasing ego development, adolescents diagnosed with a conduct and/or affective disorder become more vulnerable to suicidal behaviors. The study further supports the importance of going beyond age as the key developmental variable, as the authors did not find any association between age (12–16) and suicidal attempts in this adolescent sample. Instead, the adolescent's "frame of reference" proved to be a useful concept for understanding the developmental dimensions of suicidality.

In line with the ego development construct, it was hypothesized that with the social-cognitive reorganization that generally occurs in puberty, the unhappiness that was formerly attributed to external sources and dealt with behaviorally becomes increasingly part of inner evaluations of the self. Such transformations are likely to lead to more self-blame and overtly self-destructive symptomatology as typical reactions to interpersonal disappointments (e.g., Noam, 1988). This idea has been influential among clinical theorists (e.g., Blos, 1962; Erikson, 1968) but has not been systematically studied before from a developmental perspective.

In contrast to those investigators of normal development who have stated that higher stages are more adaptive than lower stages (Kohlberg, 1969; Piaget, 1952), the authors' findings suggest that more mature ego stages can be associated with very maladaptive and personally injurious behaviors. In fact, paradoxically, the present study shows that delay in development can function as a protective factor for suicide rather than as an additional suicide risk factor. The self-protective and externalizing qualities of the earlier developmental positions put a person at greater risk for impulsivity, acting-out problems or delinquency (Frank and Quinlan, 1976; Noam et al., 1984) but may shield the adolescent from directing the aggression against the self because the problem is viewed as mainly external.

An additional developmental hypothesis was introduced in the suicide literature by Shaffer and Fisher (1981), who suggested that younger children are missing the cognitive capacity to plan ahead and, therefore, are less likely to kill themselves. Interestingly, comparing children and adolescents who have major depressive disorders, Ryan et al. (1987) found that adolescents attempted suicide using methods of significantly greater lethality, even though there was no significant difference between children and adolescents in the rates of suicide attempts, in the severity of suicidal ideation, or the seriousness of the intent. However, these results may be balanced by the fact that a full realization of the consequences of suicide achieved at more mature developmental levels might also function as a buffer against the impulsive self-destructive acts at earlier developmental positions.

Future research should focus on examining the specific influence of developmental processes on suicidality. It has been suggested that there may be multiple subtypes of suicidal adolescents. For example, Shaffer (1974) delineated two personality types of adolescent suicide completers: an aggressive, antisocial type and a depressed type. Pfeffer and her colleagues (1989) demonstrated important differences between adolescents with both suicidal and assaultive behavior and adolescents who were suicidal but not assaultive. Two similar subtypes suggested are an aggressive, impulsive attempter versus a depressed attempter who also demonstrates significant suicidal ideation (e.g., King et al., 1990). The authors hypothesize that developmental level may account for some of the differences between these subtypes. A study of suicidal adolescents currently underway uses a clinical-research interview to produce insights into these important questions. Preliminary results have yielded two suicidal types: the "preconformist" adolescent attempters who are explicitly angry, impulsive, concrete, and who blame others and have great difficulty taking the perspectives of other people; and the "conformist" attempters who are more self-blaming and depressed and are often overly concerned with being accepted and liked. These distinctions parallel the authors' earlier work defining different developmental topologies of borderline psychopathology in adolescence (Noam, 1986). Whereas all borderline patients share in severe separation anxiety, loss of self, and identity diffusion, three different symptom types based on cognitive and emotional complexity were uncovered. The differences among these developmental subtypes point to a need to combine *DSM-III* diagnostic criteria with research-based methods of assessing developmental organization.

Additional research may help refine the links between development and suicide by exploring developmental subdomains, for example, cognition, morality, emotion, self, etc. By tracing developmental subdomains related to ego development, it may be possible to uncover specific developmental vulnerabilities in suicidal adolescents. For example, a number of studies have suggested that a pattern of cognitive distortions, causing persons to negatively evaluate their experiences and abilities, contribute significantly to suicidal behavior (Beck et al., 1975; Brent et al., 1990; Recklitis et al., 1990). Other work has stressed the importance of moral and epistemological conflict (Dobert and Nunner-Winkler, 1985; Durkheim, 1951) or a lack of self-continuity (Ball and Chandler, 1989) in decisions about suicide. Given the early stages of developmental suicide research, the use of a global indicator, ego development, which incorporates a number of subprocesses, has proven to be useful in uncovering basic associations between development and suicidality.

The authors' findings have a number of clinical implications: First, the overall developmental delay of this and other inpatient populations requires strategies for supporting development in the context of symptom reduction. A number of intervention studies in schools, prisons, and residential settings have shown that group work focusing on perspective taking and on the advancement of group norms is quite effective in fostering development and prosocial behavior (for a review, see Jennings, et al., 1983). However, these interventions have not addressed the increased vulnerability for depression and suicidality, which can be associated with increasing development. For that reason, a clinical-developmental approach requires a great deal of attention to the emergence of new symptomatology with development. Furthermore, assessing the developmental level of the suicidal adolescent brings to attention the need to tailor treatment modalities to the cognitive and social abilities of patients.

The authors' research with adults, using the ego development model, has yielded valuable clinical information. Outpatients at earlier developmental levels requested significantly more direct intervention, whereas patients at more mature levels requested insight-oriented treatments (Dill and Noam, 1990). Although treatment interventions specifically appropriate to suicidal adolescents at different developmental levels have not been delineated in the literature, there are a number of potential applications emerging. Work with patients at earlier developmental positions, for example, requires a great deal of focus on impulse control because the greatest danger for suicide at this position is unreflected, impulsive action where the consequences are not fully anticipated or comprehended. Treatment at this level has to focus on concrete behavioral management as the self-reflective capacities required for insight-oriented therapy are not yet present. Self-esteem is built by supporting impulse control and by introducing more adaptive negotiation strategies with peers and parents.

With the emergence of more mature ego development, the adolescent is capable of understanding interpersonal conflict in a psychological frame; at this level, insight-oriented treatments are appropriate. The treatment of conformist suicidal adolescents can then focus on the psychological ability of the adolescent to gain insight into the origins and dynamics of suicidality. Adolescents at the conformist level usually describe with some detail the source of their suicidality as interpersonal disappointment and resulting pain. These adolescents are usually quite eager to engage in an intense relationship with a supportive adult. The necessary building of self-esteem in these patients occurs through the establishment of a trusting relationship in which feelings of disappointment and anger can be discussed and explored. A great deal more work is necessary to specify the relationships between developmental level and other risk and protective factors to produce differential treatment strategies with adolescent suicidal patients.

Now the issue of mixed affective and conduct disordered adolescents is turned to because it was found that the majority of suicidal adolescents (56%) were diagnosed in this category. Although many studies have found considerable overlap between conduct disorder and affective disorder, their relationship is still poorly understood and the subject of much research and debate in the literature (Alessi et al., 1983; Carlson and Cantwell, 1980; Kashani et al., 1980; Kovacs et al., 1984; Puig-Antich, 1982; Ryan et al., 1987). Whereas, traditionally, the role of depression in suicide has been stressed, more recently a significant number of suicidal adolescents were found to have aggression and conduct problems (e.g., Borst and Noam, 1989). Farberow (1989), reviewing the literature on the relation between aggression and suicide, concludes that "anti-social behavior, especially assaultiveness, when expressed along with suicidal behavior, seems to be an excellent risk factor for suicide potential" (p. 46).

This study found that the presence of aggression and conduct problems alone was an insufficient predictor of suicidal behavior. Only 12% of the adolescents diagnosed with conduct disorder had attempted suicide, as compared with 55% of the adolescents diagnosed with mixed disorder. However, in those adolescents diagnosed with an affective disorder, the presence or absence of a conduct disorder did not increase the risk of suicide attempts. Nevertheless, because the mixed conduct-affective group was twice the size of the affective group, suicide attempters were most likely to be adolescents who had depression combined with a tendency to more impulsive acting-out behavior.

One limitation in the investigation of the relation of suicidality and psychiatric diagnosis is the partial overlap between suicidal ideation and attempts and the *DSM-III* criteria for affective disorder. This overlap might have contributed to the strong relationship that was found between suicidality and affective disorders. To ensure that this relationship was not further confounded by measurement issues, as both classifications were based on responses to the DISC-C, another source of diagnostic information was used that also supported the association between affective disorders and suicide attempts. However, using clinician-identified disorder, it was found that comorbidity actually significantly decreased the likelihood of suicide attempt as compared with a "pure" affective disorder. Clearly, the contribution of comorbidity in understanding adolescent suicide attempts warrants further careful study.

The ability to generalize these findings might be limited to inpatient adolescents with serious psychiatric disorders. Future studies should investigate the relationship between development, age, gender, diagnosis, and suicide among nonclinical adolescent samples and outpatient samples. Given the rapid increase in the incidence of suicidal behavior with the onset of puberty (Rutter and Garmezy, 1983), it is expected that in nonclinical samples as well the developmental move to the conformist level, which normally occurs at that time (e.g., Loevinger et al., 1970), will be accompanied by an increased vulnerability to depressive feelings, suicidal thoughts, and attempts.

The authors have begun to retest adolescents during their hospitalization as well as at 2 years after discharge. These longitudinal designs will provide opportunities for observing continuities and changes in suicidal thought and action in relation to development, psychopathology, and clinical outcome.

REFERENCES

Achenbach, T.M. (1982), *Developmental Psychopathology, Second Edition*, New York: Wiley.

Alessi, N.E., McManus, M., Grapentine, W.L. & Brickman, A. (1983), The characterization of depressive disorders in serious juvenile offenders. *J. Affective Disord.*, 6:9–17.

Apter, A., Bleich, A., Plutchik, R., Mendelsohn, S. & Tyano, S. (1988), Suicidal behavior, depression, and conduct disorder in hospitalized adolescents. *J. Am. Acad. Child Adolesc. Psychiatry*, 27:696–699.

Ball, L. & Chandler, M. (1989), Identity formation in suicidal and non-suicidal youth: the role of self-continuity. *Development and Psychopathology*, 1:257–275.

Beck, A.T., Kovacs, M. & Weissman, A. (1974), Hopelessness and suicidal behavior: an overview. *JAMA*, 234:1146–1149.

Blos, P. (1962), *On Adolescence.* New York: Free Press.

Blumenthal, S.J. & Kupfer, D.J. (1988), Overview of early detection and treatment strategies for suicidal behavior in young people. *Journal of Youth and Adolescence*, 1–22.

Borst, S.R. & Noam, G.G. (1989), Suicidality and psychopathology in hospitalized children and adolescents. *Acta Paedopsychiatrica*, 52:165–175.

Brent, D.A., Kolko, D.J., Allan, M.J. & Brown, R.V. (1990), Suicidality in affectively disordered adolescent inpatients. *J. Am. Acad. Child Adolesc. Psychiatry*, 29:586–589.

Browning, D.L. (1986), Psychiatric ward behavior and length of stay in adolescent and young adult inpatients: a developmental approach in prediction. *J. Consult. Clin. Psychol.*, 54:227–230.

Carlson, G.A. & Cantwell, D.P. (1980), Unmasking masked depression in children and adolescents. *Am. J. Psychiatry*, 137:445–449.

—————(1982), Suicidal behavior and depression in children and adolescents. *J. Am. Acad. Child Adolesc. Psychiatry*, 21:361–368.

———Asarnow, J.R. & Orbach, I. (1987), Developmental aspects of suicidal behavior in children: I. *J. Am. Acad. Child Adolesc. Psychiatry*, 26:186–192.

Chiles, J.A., Miller, M.L. & Cox, G.B. (1980), Depression in an adolescent delinquent population. *Arch. Gen. Psychiatry*, 37:1179–1184.

Costello, A.J., Edelbrock, C.S., Dulcan, M.K., Kalas, R. & Klaric, S.H. (1984), *Development and Testing of the NIMH Diagnostic Interview Schedule for Children on a Clinical Population: Final Report.* (Contract RFP-DB-81-0027). Rockville, MD: Center for Epidemiologic Studies, National Institute for Mental Health.

Costello, E.J., Edelbrock, C.S. & Costello, A.J. (1985), Validity of the NIMH Diagnostic Interview Schedule for Children: a comparison between psychiatric and pediatric referrals. *J. Abnorm. Child Psychol.*, 13:579–595.

Diekstra, R.F.W. & Moritz, B.J.M. (1987), Suicidal behavior among adolescents: an overview. In: *Suicide in Adolescence*, ed. R.F.W. Diekstra. The Hague: Martinus Nijhoff Publishers, pp. 7–24.

Dill, D.L. & Noam, G.G. (1990), Ego development and treatment request. *Psychiatry*, 53:85–91.

Dobert, R. & Nunner-Winkler, G. (1985), Interplay of formal and material role-taking in the understanding of suicide among adolescents and young adults. *Human Development*, 28:313–330.

Durkheim, E. (1951), *Suicide. A Study in Sociology*. New York: The Free Press.

Edelbrock, C.S., & Achenbach, T.M. (1980), A typology of child behavior profile patterns: distribution and correlates for disturbed children aged 6–16. *J. Abnorm. Child Psychol.*, 8:441–470.

Erikson, E. (1968), *Identify, Youth and Crisis*. New York: Norton.

Farberow, N.L. (1989), Preparatory and prior suicidal behavior factors. In: *Report of the Secretary's Task Force on Youth Suicide. Volume 2: Risk Factors for Youth Suicide*. (DHHS Pub. No. ADM 89–1622). Washington, D.C.: Superintendent of Documents, U.S. Government Printing Office.

Frank, S. & Quinlan, D. (1976), Ego development and adjustment patterns in adolescence. *J. Abnorm. Psychol.*, 85:505–510.

Gold, S.N. (1980), Relations between level of ego development and adjustment patterns in adolescents. *J. Pers. Assess.*, 44:630–638.

Hawton, K. (1986), Suicide and Suicide Attempts among Children and Adolescents, In: *Developmental Clinical Psychology and Psychiatry*, Vol. 5, San Mateo, CA: Sage Publications.

Holinger, P.C. (1978), Adolescent suicide: an epidemiological study of recent trends. *Am. J. Psychiatry*, 135:754–756.

Jennings, W., Kilkenny, R. & Kohlberg, L. (1983), Moral developmental theory and practice for youthful and adult offenders. In: *Personality Theory, Moral Development and Criminal Behavior*, eds. W.W. Laufer & J.M. Day. Lexington, MA: Lexington Books.

Kashani, J.H., Manning, G.W., McKnew, D.H., Cytryn, L., Simonds, J.F. & Wooderson, P.C. (1980), Depression among incarcerated delinquents. *Psychiatry Res.*, 3:185–191.

Kazdin, A.E. (1989), Developmental psychopathology. *Am. Psychol.*, 44:180–187.

Kennedy, J.J. (1983), *Analyzing Qualitative Data: Introductory Loglinear Analysis for Behavioral Research*. New York: Praeger Publisher.

King, C.A., Raskin, A., Gdowski, C.L., Butkus, M. & Opipari, L. (1990), Psychosocial factors associated with urban adolescent female suicide attempts. *J. Am. Acad. Child Adolesc. Psychiatry*, 29:289–294.

Kohlberg, L. (1969), Stage and sequence: the cognitive developmental approach to socialization. In: *Handbook of Socialization, Theory and Research*, ed. D. Goslin, New York: Rand McNally, pp. 347–480.

Kovacs, M. & Puig-Antich, J. (1989), Major psychiatric disorders as risk factors in youth suicide. In: *Report of the Secretary's Task Force on Youth Suicide, Volume 2: Risk Factors for Youth Suicide*. (DHHS Pub. No. ADM 89–1622). Washington, DC: Superintendent of Documents, U.S. Government Printing Office.

————Feinberg, T.L., Crouse-Novak, M.A., Paulauskas, S.L. & Finkelstein, R. (1984), Depressive disorders in childhood. *Arch. Gen. Psychiatry*, 41:229–237.

Loevinger, J. (1976), *Ego Development*. San Francisco: Jossey-Bass.

————(1979), Construct validity of the Sentence Completion Test of ego development. *Applied Psychological Measurement*, 3:281–311.

————Wessler, R. & Redmore, C. (1970), *Measuring Ego Development. Vol. 2: Scoring Manual for Women and Girls*. San Francisco: Jossey-Bass.

Noam, G. (1986), The theory of biography and transformation and the Borderline Personality Disorders: a developmental typology. *McLean Hospital Journal*, 11:79–105.

————(1988), A constructivist approach to developmental psychopathology. In: *Developmental Psychopathology and its Treatment. New Directions for Child Development*, Vol. 39, eds. E.D. Nannis & P.A. Cowan. San Francisco: Jossey-Bass, pp. 91–121.

————Houlihan, J. (1990), Ego development and DSM-III diagnoses in adolescent psychiatric patients. *Am. J. Orthopsychiattry*, 60:371–378.

————Hauser, T., Santostefano, S., Garrison, W., Jacobson, A., Powers, S.I. & Mead, M. (1984), Ego development and psychopathology: a study of hospitalized adolescents. *Child Dev.*, 55:184–194.

————Recklitis, C.J. & Paget, K. (in press), Pathways of ego development: contributions to maladaptation and adjustment. *Development and Psychopathology*.

Paget, K.F., Noam, G.G., Borst, S.R. & Bartok, J. (1990, June), *Ego Development, Psychiatric Diagnoses, and Gender in Adolescence: A developmental Psychopathology Study*. Paper presented at the meeting of the American Psychological Society, Dallas.

Pfeffer, C.R. (1986), *The Suicidal Child*. New York: The Guilford Press.

————Newcorn, J., Kaplan, G., Mizruchi, M.S. & Plutchik, R. (1988), Suicidal behavior in adolescent psychiatric patients. *J. Am. Acad. Child Adolesc. Psychiatry*, 27:357–361.

————Newcorn, J., Kaplan, G., Mizrucchi, M.S., & Plutchik, R. (1989), Subtypes of suicidal and assaultive behaviors in adolescent psychiatric patients: a research note. *J. Child Psychol. Psychiatry*, 30:151–163.

Piaget, J. (1952), *The Origins of Intelligence in Children*. New York: International Universities Press.

Puig-Antich, J. (1982), Major depression and conduct disorder in prepuberty. *J. Am. Acad. Child Adolesc. Psychiatry*, 21:118–128.

Recklitis, C.J., Noam, G.G. & Borst, S.R. (1990, March), *Adolescent Suicide and Defense Mechanisms: Differentiating Attempters from Ideators and Non-attempters*. Paper presented at the Society for Research in Adolescence Biannual Meeting, Atlanta, Georgia.

Redmore, C. & Waldman, K. (1975), Reliability of a sentence completion measure of ego development. *J. Pers. Assess.*, 39:236–243.

————Loevinger, J. (19979), Ego development in adolescence: longitudinal studies. *Journal of Youth and Adolescence*, 8:1–20.

Robbins, D.R. & Alessi, N.E. (1985), Depressive symptoms and suicidal behavior in adolescents. *Am. J. Psychiatry*, 142:588–592.

Rutter, M. (1986). The developmental psychopathology of depression: issues and perspectives. In: *Depression in Young People: Developmental and Clinical Perspectives*, eds. M. Rutter, C.E. Izard & P.B. Read. New York: The Guilford Press, pp. 3–30.

——Garmezy, N. (1983), Developmental psychopathology. In: *Socialization, Personality and Social Development*, ed. E.M. Hetherington. Mussen's Handbook of Child Psychology, Vol. 4. New York: Wiley.

Ryan, N.D., Puig-Antich, J., Ambrosini, P. et al. (1987), The clinical picture of major depression in children and adolescents. *Arch. Gen. Psychiatry*, 44:854–861.

Shaffer, D. (1974), Suicide in childhood and early adolescence. *J. Child Psychol. Psychiatry*, 15:275–291.

——Fisher, P. (1981), The epidemiology of suicide in children and adolescents. *J. Am. Acad. Child Adolesc. Psychiatry*, 20:545–565.

Shafii, M., Carrigan, S., Whittinghill, J.R. & Derrick, A. (1985), Psychological autopsy of completed suicide in children and adolescents. *Am. J. Psychiatry*, 142:1061–1064.

Walker, M., Moreau, D. & Weissman, M.M. (1990), Parents' awareness of children's suicide attempts. *Am. J. Psychiatry*, 147:1364–1366.

Weinstein, S.R., Stone, K., Noam, G.G., Grimes, K. & Schwab-Stone, M. (1989), Comparison of DISC with clinicians' DSM-III diagnoses in psychiatric inpatients. *J. Am. Acad. Child Adolesc. Psychiatry*, 28:53–60.

Weiss, D.S., Zilberg, N.J. & Genevro, J.L. (1989), Psychometric properties of Loevinger's Sentence Completion Test in an adult psychiatric outpatient sample. *J. Pers. Assess.*, 53:478–486.

Werner, H. (1948), *Comparative Psychology of Mental Development*. New York: International University Press.

Part V

DIAGNOSIS AND TREATMENT

The papers in this section examine a range of issues of importance in the diagnosis and treatment of psychiatric disorder in children and adolescents. Caron and Rutter begin their thoughtful and thorough discussion of comorbidity in child psychopathology by pointing out that every medical student is taught parsimony with regard to diagnosis. Yet in psychiatry and child psychiatry, particularly in the years following the introduction of DSM-III-R, multiple diagnoses have become exceedingly common. The authors contrast the DSM-III-R and IDC 9 approaches to multiple diagnosis, noting that whereas the WHO system tends to discourage them, and DSM-III-R works the other way around, with neither system providing an optimal solution to the problem. Artifacts introduced by biases in referral practices or screening procedures may contribute to the high frequency of occurrence of comorbid conditions. In addition, apparent comorbidity may arise as a consequence of nosological considerations, including the use of categories in instances when dimensions might be more appropriate, overlapping criteria, artificial subdivision of syndromes, and inadequate attention to longitudinal course. Lest "the baby be thrown out with the bath water," factors that may contribute to the occurrence of true comorbidity are also considered, including the possibility of shared and overlapping risk factors, the comorbid conditions actually constituting a meaningful clinical entity, and the presence of one condition increasing the risk that a second may also occur. Attention to these issues is of great importance, not only to the clinician in the course of the evaluation of individual patients, but also to the researcher planning a clinical investigation.

Utilizing a longitudinal design, the second paper in this section examines links between depression and conduct disorder. Harrington and colleagues report on the adult status of the following groups of child and adolescent psychiatric patients: depressed with no conduct problems ($N = 34$), depressed with comorbid conduct disorder ($N = 13$), and conduct disorder without depression ($N = 17$). From the perspective of adult antisocial outcome, it appears that comorbidity between depression and conduct disorder during childhood does indeed represent the co-occurrence of separate conditions. The antisocial outcomes of depressed children with conduct disorder were very similar to those of nondepressed children with conduct disorder, suggesting that the presence of depression during the index episode had little effect on the long-term course of conduct disorder. However, a different picture emerged when depressive outcomes were considered. There was a strong tendency for children with depression and conduct disorder to have lower rates of depression in adulthood than depressed children without conduct problems. Depressed children with comorbid conduct disorder did not differ from depressed children without conduct problems in depressive symptomatology or demographic characteristics during the index episode. However, depressives with conduct disorder had a higher incidence of adult criminality than depressed children without conduct problems, and there was a strong tendency for depressives with conduct disorder to have a lower risk of depression in adulthood than depressed children without conduct problems. The relatively small sample size suggests the need for replication. Nevertheless, the results of this study demonstrate the power of a longitudinal strategy in assessing the meaning and significance of comorbidity.

Bernstein and Borchardt introduce their timely review of anxiety disorders in children and adolescents with the observation that in the DSM-III-R classification, anxiety disorders are separated into two different sections: the "anxiety disorders" proper and "anxiety disorders of childhood or adolescence." This separation has had an impact on research in two ways. In contrast to the study of depressive disorders in children, studies of anxiety in children have proceeded without the constraints of adult criteria. However, childhood anxiety disorders have often been studied to the exclusion of the disorders, leaving a developmental gap. Nevertheless, epidemiologically based studies have demonstrated the high prevalence rate of anxiety disorders in the general population of children and adolescents. Patterns of comorbidity among the various anxiety disorders and between anxiety and depression, as well as between anxiety and attention deficit hyperactivity disorder, have been identified, and risk factors, environmental and familial, increasingly well described. Less is known about the longitudinal course of anxiety disorders with onset during childhood or adolescence, although developmental differences in the expression of both separation and overanxious disorder at various ages have been described. To date, intervention studies have been limited in scope, indicating a clear need for well-controlled studies of both behavioral and pharmacologic treatments.

Despite the wide recognition of the movement disorders associated with neuroleptic use in adults, including Parkinson's-disease–like symptoms, akathisia, tardive dyskinesia, and tardive dystonia, there has been little systematic examination of side effects in children and adolescents. Moreover, although in adult psychiatry, indications for neuroleptic use are increasingly coming to be restricted to psychotic conditions, pharmacotherapy in child and adolescent psychiatry is largely based on a "drug-to-symptom" approach. Consequently, neuroleptics are frequently prescribed for children and adolescents not only for psychotic disorders, but also for such nonpsychotic conditions as pervasive developmental disorder, conduct disorder, and attention-deficit hyperactivity disorder (ADHD). Richardson and colleagues have conducted a much-needed study of the prevalence and risk factors for neuroleptic-induced movement disorders in 104 children and adolescents who were hospitalized in a state psychiatric facility during a six-month period. Two over-lapping risk groups were identified: 61 patients who were receiving neuroleptics at the time of evaluation were considered at risk for parkinsonism, and 41 patients whose neuroleptic treatment histories revealed at least one period of 90 continuous days of treatment were considered at risk for tardive dyskinesia. The prevalence of parkinsonism was 34% and was significantly associated with longer neuroleptic treatment periods immediately before evaluation. The prevalence of treatment emergent dyskinesia was 12% and showed no association with quantitative neuroleptic treatment variables. The findings highlight the particular vulnerability of the neuroleptic-treated child or adolescent to the development of parkinsonism, and they underscore the importance of the regular and systematic assessment of a full range of neurologic side effects in all children and adolescents who receive neuroleptic medication, even if the duration of treatment is brief.

In a carefully designed and conducted study, Barkley, DuPaul, and McMurray address two issues of considerable concern to those who diagnose and treat children with ADHD: (1) Which children are most likely to respond to stimulant medication? (2) At what dose level? Twenty-three children whose symptoms of ADHD included hyperactivity and 17 children with ADHD who were not hyperactive received three doses of methylphenidate (5, 10, and 15 mg) in a triple-blind, placebo-controlled crossover study. Parent and teacher ratings of behavior, laboratory tests, and behavioral observations during academic performance were used to assess medication response. Results indicated that children with both attentional and activity symptoms were rated as having more pervasive behavioral problems at home and at school. These children were found to be impaired in tests of behavioral inhibition and vigilance, whereas children with attentional symptoms who were not hyperactive were more impaired in the consistent retrieval of verbally learned material. Drug effects were noted on parent and teacher ratings and on performance according to most laboratory measures at all three dose levels in both groups of children. However, analysis of the pattern of response across measures suggests that the greatest effect of medication on those children who were not hyperactive occurred at low doses, with little further improvement obtained from larger doses. In contrast, among children who were hyperactive, improvement appeared to occur with each dose increase. Therefore, in clinical practice low doses of stimulant medication may well be sufficient to address the attentional problems of children whose difficulties are not complicated by hyperactivity, and moderate and high doses may provide greater benefit to those children who are both attentionally impaired and hyperactive.

The final paper in this section tests the hypothesis that infant–parent psychotherapy designed to enhance maternal empathy for the child's developmental needs and affective experience can improve quality of attachment and social–emotional functioning. Lieberman and colleagues randomly assigned anxiously attached, low-SES 12-month-olds and their mothers as assessed in the Ainsworth Strange

Situation to intervention and control groups. Securely attached dyads composed a second control group. Intervention lasted one year and consisted of unstructured 90-minute weekly sessions with mother and baby, which occurred in the home. Monthly contact was maintained with control group mothers via telephone. Outcome measures are carefully described. Results indicate that intervention group toddlers scored significantly lower than anxious controls in avoidance, resistance, and anger, and had significantly higher scores on measures assessing partnership with the mother. Intervention mothers scored higher than anxious controls in empathy and interactiveness with their children. There were no differences on the outcome measures between the intervention and the secure control groups, and within the intervention group, a measure of level of therapeutic process was positively correlated with adaptive scores in child and mother outcome measures. The findings are of considerable interest in that they are consistent with other research findings, which indicate that anxious attachment stems from affective dyssynchronies between mother and infant. As anxious attachment in infancy has been shown to be associated with decreased competence in social–emotional functional during the toddler and early childhood years, the demonstration of an effective intervention, albeit a time-consuming and costly one, is of clinical importance.

21

Comorbidity in Child Psychopathology: Concepts, Issues and Research Strategies

Chantal Caron

Institute of Psychiatry, London, England

Michael Rutter

Institute of Psychiatry, London, England

Epidemiological data show that the co-occurrence of two or more supposedly separate child (and adult) psychiatric conditions far exceeds that expected by chance (clinic data cannot be used for this determination). The importance of comorbidity is shown and it is noted that it is not dealt with optimally in either DSM-III-R or ICD-9. Artifacts in the detection of comorbidity are considered in terms of referral and screening/surveillance biases. Apparent comorbidity may also arise from various nosological considerations; these include the use of categories where dimensions might be more appropriate, overlapping diagnostic criteria, artificial subdivision of syndromes, one disorder representing an early manifestation of the other, and one disorder being part of the other. Possible explanations of true comorbidity are discussed with respect to shared and overlapping risk factors, the comorbid pattern constituting a distinct meaningful syndrome, and one disorder creating an increased risk for the other. Some possible means of investigating each of these possibilities are noted.

INTRODUCTION

Every medical student is taught that, whenever possible, a single diagnosis should be made (Jaspers, 1963; Kendell, 1975). Patients may present with mul-

Reprinted with permission from the *Journal of Child Psychology and Psychiatry*, 1991, Vol. 32, No. 7, 1063–1080. Copyright ©1991 by the Association for Child Psychology and Psychiatry.

Dr. Caron was supported by fellowship No. 891069 from Fonds de la Recherche en Santé du Québec.

tiple diseases but, when there is complex mixed symptomatology, an unusual presentation of a single disorder is more likely that the simultaneous occurrence of two or more unrelated conditions (comorbidity). Yet in child psychiatry, all epidemiological studies that have examined the issues have shown that comorbidity is extremely common (Anderson, Williams, McGee & Silva, 1987; Kashani *et al.*, 1987; Flament *et al.*, 1988; Szatmari, Boyle & Offord, 1989; Weissman *et al.*, 1987). The same has been found in adult psychiatry (Boyd *et al.*, 1984). In this paper, we consider the empirical findings, concepts, and research implications of this important issue.

FREQUENCY OF COMORBIDITY

The first question is whether the observed rate of comorbidity in epidemiological surveys exceeds that expected by chance alone. The expected rate is obtained by multiplying the base rates of each of the separate conditions involved in the comorbidity patterns studied. The epidemiological studies undertaken by Anderson *et al.* (1987) and Kashani *et al.* (1987) both presented their findings in a manner that allows this calculation. The data are summarized in Tables 1a and 1b.

Thus, in the Anderson *et al.* (1987) survey, 7.5% of 11-year-olds showed an anxiety disorder and 6.7% an attention deficit disorder; the expected comorbidity between these two disorders therefore is the product of 7.5% and 6.7%, namely 0.5%. By summing all possible combinations, the overall expected comorbidity rate for different numbers of conditions can be obtained (Table 1b). It is evident that the observed comorbidity rate was more than double that expected by chance; in the Kashani *et al.* (1987) study the excess was even greater. The data used in these calculations (as presented in the original papers) were based on pooled diagnostic groupings. For example, all the various anxiety disorders were combined to form one grouping; the same applied to depressive disorders and to oppositional/conduct disorders. This means that comorbidity within these pooled categories was not taken into account. Accordingly, the true observed comorbidity rate must have been considerably higher, so that the calculated two- to three-fold excess over chance expectation constitutes a gross *under*estimate of the frequency of comorbidity. These two reports were chosen because they presented their findings in a fashion that made it easy to calculate observed and expected comorbidity rates. However, other epidemiological studies are agreed in showing a very high comorbidity rate and it may be concluded that the observed co-occurrence of supposedly separate child psychiatric disorders far exceeds that expected by chance alone.

The fact that the pooling of diagnoses greatly underestimates the true rate of comorbidity is evident in the adult epidemiological data presented by Boyd *et al.* (1984). For example, the population base rate for panic disorder was 67 out of

TABLE 1a.

Base rates of disorders in three community studies that serve to calculate
the expected number of comorbid cases

Author	n	Age	Disorders	Base rates
Anderson	785	11	Oppos/Conduct d.	9.2%
et al.			Anxiety d.	7.5%
(1987)			Attention deficit d.	6.7%
			Depressive d.	1.8%
Kashani	150	14-16	Oppos/Conduct d.	14.7%
et al.			Anxiety d.	8.7%
(1987)			Depressive d.	8.0%

d. = disorder.

TABLE 1b.

Expected and observed number of comorbid cases in two
community studies

Author	Number of disorders	Expected cases (E)	Observed cases (O)	O/E	95% C.I.
Anderson	1	—	100		
et al.	2	17.5	27		
(1987)	3	0.62	4		
	4	0.007	8		
	Total > 1	18.43	39	2.1	1.5-2.9
Kashani	1	—	12		
et al.	2	4.74	7		
(1987)	3	0.17	7		
	Total > 1	4.91	14	2.85	1.7-4.8

95% C.I. = 95% confidence interval.

11,176, 0.6%. However, out of 266 individuals with major depression, 30 had a panic disorder, a rate of 11%, representing a huge increase over chance expectation.

In drawing this conclusion, we have restricted our attention to epidemiological data because general population base rates are essential for the calculation of expected comorbidity rates. Because much of the discussion of comorbidity in the literature is based on the findings of studies of clinic samples, it is necessary to note that clinic data alone cannot provide information on whether or not the observed comorbidity rate exceeds that expected by chance. A simple example serves to illustrate the point. Suppose that disorders A and B are both present in

10% of the general population and that there is a 5% rate for 'pure' A, 5% for 'pure' B, and 5% for the comorbidity pattern of A + B. As the comorbidity expected by chance is 1% (i.e. 10% × 10%), this means that the observed comorbidity rate is five times the chance expectation.

Let us also suppose that all children with these disorders are referred to clinics without any referral bias (and that there are no other disorders). The clinic pattern will, therefore, be the same as that in affected members of the general population; namely 33% with disorder A, 33% with disorder B and 33% with A + B. If the clinic base rate (instead of the general population rate) is used to calculate the comorbidity expected by chance, the expectation is 67% × 67%, i.e. 45%. That is, instead of the true five-fold excess, the clinic data misleadingly appear to indicate that the observed rate is *less* than that expected by chance. Clinic data can be used to assess comorbidity only if the general population rates for each disorder are known *and* if data are available on the clinic referral rate and biases for each disorder.

In that connection, it should be noted that, whenever less than all subjects with disorder are referred, clinic samples will always contain a disproportionately large proportion of patients showing comorbidity (Berkson, 1946). That is because the referral likelihood for subjects with disorders A and B will be a function of the *combined* likelihood of referral for each disorder separately. That is so irrespective of referral biases. However, it is known that in practice there *are* various referral biases and these also need to be taken into account. For example, Shepherd, Oppenheim and Mitchell (1971) found that children were more likely to be referred if there were also parental psychopathology or family problems.

For all these reasons, clinic data need to be used with considerable caution in studying comorbidity. However, provided that epidemiological data have already shown that there is a significantly raised comorbidity, and provided that enough is known on referral influences to consider their possible effects, clinic data may be used to examine possible explanations for comorbidity patterns.

DOES COMORBIDITY MATTER

Comorbidity has been largely ignored in the research literature for years and it is necessary to ask whether it matters sufficiently for detailed attention to be paid to it now. There are two main reasons why a failure to pay attention to comorbidity may lead researchers to draw quite misleading conclusions. First, a study of condition X may produce findings that in fact are largely a consequence of the ignored comorbid condition Y. For example, Anderson *et al.* (1987) found that of the 14 children with depressive disorders, no less than 11 had at least one other psychiatric condition as well. Indeed eight out of the 14 children showed depression *and* an anxiety disorder *and* a conduct disorder *and* an attention deficit disorder! It follows that the correlates, outcome or genetic features reported for childhood depression could in reality be those of attention deficit or conduct disorders.

The second reason is that, when comorbidity is ignored, the implicit assumption is made that the meaning of condition A is the same regardless of the presence or absence of condition B. As shown below, that is an unsafe assumption and in some circumstances it appears to be mistaken.

It might be thought that the solution would be to exclude comorbid cases in order to focus on "pure" groups. However, the extent of comorbidity is such that often this would result in the investigation of tiny atypical samples. For example, as already noted, only three out of 14 cases of depression were "pure" in the Anderson *et al.* (1987) study, and among the 12 cases of depression in the Kashani *et al.* (1987) investigation none was pure. Clearly, that cannot constitute a general solution; moreover, necessarily it involves a loss of the opportunity to determine the reasons for comorbidity, a search that could throw important light on aetiological mechanisms (see below).

DSM-III-R AND ICD-9

The two major psychiatric classification systems, the American Psychiatric Association's (1987) DSM-III-R and the World Health Organization's (1978) ICD-9 (soon to be superseded by ICD-10—W.H.O., 1990), follow quite different approaches to diagnosis (Rutter & Gould, 1985; Rutter, 1988). While the W.H.O. system allows multiple diagnoses, it tends to discourage them by its adoption of a pattern approach to diagnosis. The clinician is expected to review the overall clinical picture made up of history, signs, symptoms, and laboratory findings; and then to match this picture with the prototypical diagnostic pattern that fits best, using a process of pattern recognition. It follows the long-standing medical tradition of recognizing that most disorders involve a complex admixture of specific and nonspecific symptomatology and that, in ordinary circumstances, it is more likely in practice that a patient will have one disease, rather than several. It provides the unifying explanation of protean symptomatology. Thus, there is an appreciation that there are many nonspecific symptoms—such as fever, tachycardia, fatigue, headache and skin rashes—that occur in many quite different somatic diseases. In much the same way, psychiatry has many nonspecific symptoms such as anxiety, depressed mood, poor concentration and restlessness. Of course, a dilemma arises from the fact that many of the nonspecific symptoms also constitute the hallmarks of specific diagnostic entities. The problem lies in the difficulty of deciding when, say, depression is an indicator of a major depressive disorder and when it is just an indication that psychopathologically something is the matter.

The strength of the W.H.O. approach is that the underlying concept is probably correct in many, perhaps most, instances. Thus, in reality, it is unlikely that a high proportion of patients truly have three, four or five entirely separate conditions. The outstanding weakness, however, is that, for many symptom patterns, the data are not available to determine when and how to give precedence to one diagnosis over another (Rutter, 1988). In some instances, this is dealt with by having a combination code. For example, it has long been recognized that there is a need to code schizoaffective disorder (that applies to DSM-III-R as well, although the details of criteria are not quite the same). More controversially, ICD-10 (W.H.O., 1989) has a code for depression combined with conduct disorder. A further limitation of the W.H.O. approach (at least as exemplified in ICD-9; ICD-10 has come closer to DSM-III-R) is that true patterns of comorbidity may be concealed and, therefore, neglected or that an incorrect hierarchical principle may lead to invalid diagnoses.

The APA classification DSM-III-R works the other way round (although its predecessor, DSM-III, included more exclusionary hierarchies). Diagnoses are made on algorithms based on specified symptom constellations without regard to the presence or absence of accompanying symptomatology of a different kind (apart from a few exceptions). The consequence, perhaps the inevitable consequence, of this convention is that when a patient has any one diagnosis, there is usually at least one other diagnosis as well. The first obvious disadvantage of this system is that it contravenes common sense. Indeed, Weinstein, Stone, Noam, Grimes and Schwab-Stone (1989) found that, in a child psychiatric in-patient unit sample, strict adherence to DSM-III rules (freed of hierarchies) led to 78% of the patients showing comorbidity, but this fell to 20% when clinicians were allowed to use their own judgment. However, there are two other disadvantages. Although, in theory, a statistical system could be devised to present data on all possible patterns of comorbidity, no system has been used that way to date. Moreover, even if such data were produced their complexity would make it extremely difficult, if not impossible, to make sense of the huge number of possible double, treble, and quadruple combinations.

The second disadvantage is that although DSM-III-R is supposedly free of diagnostic hierarchies that conceal comorbidity, in fact it includes a bewildering mix of inconsistencies on which combinations are, and which are not, allowed. For example, in adults it is not allowed to diagnose overanxious disorder in the presence of generalized anxiety disorder, but it is allowed to diagnose both separation anxiety disorder and overanxious disorder in children. Or again, it is not allowed to diagnose both social phobia and avoidant disorder but it is possible to diagnose both social phobia and agoraphobia. Similarly, oppositional disorder cannot be diagnosed with conduct disorder but it can be diagnosed with attention deficit disorder. Evidently, there are more diagnostic hierarchies in DSM-III-R than is usually appreciated.

DETECTION ARTIFACTS

Referral Factors

Before considering possible reasons for different patterns of comorbidity, it is necessary to note the variety of ways in which it can be produced artifactually. As already discussed, there is the Berkson (1946) effect by which, for statistical reasons separate from referral biases, the comorbidity rate in clinic samples will always be greater than that in the general population whenever only a small proportion of the conditions making up the comorbidity pattern are refereed to clinics—the state of affairs with the majority of child psychiatric disorders other than the most severe (Rutter, Tizard & Whitmore, 1970). In addition, of course, referral biases may further distort clinic data on comorbidity. For example, when a clinician is known to have a special interest in a particular pattern of comorbidity such cases are more likely to be referred to him or her. Similarly, tertiary referral centers seeing difficult and complicated cases are likely to have a disproportionately high level of comorbidity.

Screening and Surveillance Factors

It is important also to recognize that any general population epidemiological study that relies on screening or surveillance procedures is also open to possible detection artifacts. Thus, it is a common practice to use high scores on questionnaires designed to tap a broad range of behaviour as a means of picking out subjects with a high probability of disorder, who may then be studied individually in greater detail (Newman, Shrout & Bland, 1990; Rutter, 1989a,b). The procedure works well for many purposes but it will tend to miss monosymptomatic disorders and oversample children whose psychopathology includes symptoms of many different types. A similar detection bias will apply whenever the diagnosis of a second disorder is dependent in part on subjects with one diagnosis being subjected to a closer degree of surveillance. This is particularly likely to operate in longitudinal studies investigating patterns of comorbidity over time (rather than concurrently).

These detection artifacts are all open to systematic quantified investigation by means of comparisons with total population unscreened samples.

NOSOLOGICAL CONSIDERATIONS

The usual concept of comorbidity implies the co-occurrence of two independent conditions or disorders. Even if the statistical data have not been distorted by detection artifacts, the apparent overlap between supposedly different disorders may not represent comorbidity as usually conceptualized. This possibility arises because the basic nosological concepts may themselves be mistaken. As Bukstein, Brent and Kamliner (1989) pointed out, one of the major difficulties in studying psychiatric comorbidity is the lack of well validated diagnostic criteria.

Categories or Dimensions?

The first possibility is that the concept of disorder (or disease) categories may itself be misconceived. Instead, as many psychologists have argued, it could be that psychopathology is best thought of as the end product of an admixture of extremes of personality dimensions. According to this view, disorders involve no qualitative discontinuity between abnormality and normality but rather a pattern resulting from quantitative variations on a range of behavioural dimensions. In so far as that is the case, apparent comorbidity is bound to arise from the inevitability of individuals with high scores on two or more dimensions; however, the extent of such apparent comorbidity will be much affected by the particular cut-off points used to define "disorder" and by the extent to which the definitions of disorder involve truncation of dimensions. The same circumstances will arise if the behavioural dimensions operate as risk factors for disorder. For example, numerous studies have shown the strong overlap between attention deficit (hyperactivity) and conduct disorders (Szatmari *et al.*, 1989; Taylor, 1988). Does this imply comorbidity between two different disorders or rather does it mean that both inattention/overactivity and aggressivity are risk factors for disruptive behaviour?

There has been surprisingly little research that has set out to contrast and compare the validity of dimensional and categorical approaches. However, one test would be to determine if behavioural dimensions related to one diagnostic category functioned as a risk factor for the second condition at levels below the diagnostic threshold. This conduct problem before the age of 15 years predicted substance abuse. Thin results showed that they did so at all levels of severity, indicating that conduct problems functioned as a dimensional predictor. Thus, of those with no conduct problems, 38% exhibited substance abuse; of those with one conduct disorder problem, 52% did so; of those with two conduct problems 66% did so; and so on. At least in this population, with these two "disorders", a dimensional approach seemed to account for the findings better than comorbidity between two separate disorders. This research strategy warrants greater usage.

Overlapping Diagnostic Criteria

A second type of nosological confusion arrives from the fact that the *same* item of behaviour appears in the list of diagnostic criteria for several *different* diagnostic categories—a problem highlighted in previous considerations of comorbidity (Pfeffer & Plutchik, 1989) and by the DSM-III Child and Adolescent Psychiatry Working

Party (Shaffer *et al*., 1989). For example, not surprisingly, anxiety/worrying appears in some form in the lists of criteria for all the various supposedly separate anxiety disorders; just as depressed mood forms part of the criteria for dysthymia as well as major depressive disorder. In addition, agitation is one of the criteria for anxiety, depression, and attention deficit/hyperactivity disorder. This is not unreasonable as so many of the behaviours that define specific disorders are also nonspecific indicators of psychopathology. Nevertheless, the fact that this is so will lead to a degree of artifactual comorbidity. A related problem arises from the fact that so many mood states involve mixed emotions. Thus, it is well known that anxiety and depression very commonly occur together regardless of the diagnosis (Grayson, Bridges, Cook & Goldberg, 1990). In so far as an increasing severity of disorder is likely often to involve an increasing number of nonspecific indices of psychopathology (Costello *et al*., 1988; Bird *et al*., 1988; Weissman, Warner & Fendrich, 1990), and in so far as these form part of the sets of criteria for different disorders, there is some danger that there will be an artifactual association between severity and extent of comorbidity. This is simply because severe disorders with many symptoms are likely to have a greater chance of fulfilling the criteria for more than one disorder. It is possible to provide a partial check on whether any severity—comorbidity association is real or artifactual by determining whether the association holds when severity is defined in terms of degree of social impairment rather than number of symptoms. A partial test of the influence on comorbidity of nonspecific indices of psychopathology is also afforded by determining whether the correlates (with respect to features such as family history, prognosis, treatment response etc.) of the behavioural item (e.g., depression or anxiety or restlessness) are similar when it occurs as part of a mixed clinical picture to when it occurs as part of the pure syndrome it defines.

Artificial Subdivision of Syndromes

A somewhat similar problem may arise from the tendency to subdivide disorders defined in terms of one main symptom complex into various subcategories according to particular elements or facets of that complex. For example, anxiety disorders are subdivided into some dozen different syndromes characterized by the generality of the anxiety (e.g., "overanxious disorder" or "generalized anxiety disorder") or its specific focus (e.g., "separation anxiety disorder" or "social phobia") or the presence/absence of some particular feature (e.g. agoraphobia with or without panic), or its association with some stresses (e.g. "post-traumatic stress disorder" or "adjustment disorder with anxious mood"). So far as children are concerned, there is the additional problem that sometimes there are two disorders defined in clearly similar terms, one of which is intended to apply to all age groups and one of which is supposedly particular to childhood, but which are *not* mutually exclusive under the age of 18 years (e.g. "overanxious disorder" and "generalized anxiety disorder"). Not surprisingly, numerous studies (see Barlow, 1988) have shown extensive comorbidity between these various anxiety disorders. Most published investigations have concerned adult patients but the same situation seems to apply in childhood (Last, Hersen, Kazdin, Finkelstein & Strauss, 1987). Thus, in the study cited, half the children with separation anxiety disorder also had overanxious disorder and 95% of this comorbid group had at least one other diagnosis as well! There have been some attempts to test the discriminant validity of these different anxiety disorders (see Barlow, 1988) with some modest success with respect to at least some of the differentiations. For example, Mannuzza, Fyer, Liebowitz and Klein (1990) have reviewed the evidence suggesting that social phobia is meaningfully distinctive from panic disorder and agoraphobia in adults. However, they also point out that the meaningful interpretation of symptoms requires that they can be considered in the individual context (something that is difficult with a symptom check list approach to diagnosis). Less is known about the validity of differentiations among anxiety disorders in childhood. Last *et al.* (1987) found that children with separation anxiety disorders tended to be somewhat younger than those with overanxious disorders but this could reflect age effects on patterns of manifestation rather than a difference between two distinct disorders. Nothing is known on whether there is any meaningful distinction between "overanxious disorder" and "generalized anxiety disorder" and the comorbidity between them seems to have received no attention, perhaps because child psychiatrists tend to choose the category in the children's section of DSM-III-R without checking to see whether the all-ages diagnosis might equally apply.

However, the issue of comorbidity cannot be dealt with merely by testing the discriminant validity of the separate anxiety categories; it is necessary to go on to examine the characteristics of the comorbid groups as they relate to the "pure" diagnoses. For example, it could be that it is useful to separate simple phobias that arise in the absence of generalized anxiety from generalized anxiety disorder but, equally, it might well be the case that high levels of general anxiety tend also to lead to various focused phobias as well. At least, the possibility needs testing. The very high level of comorbidity between different anxiety disorders suggests that some of it represents nosological confusion.

It may well be clinically useful to be able to note that an anxiety disorder has several different facets but, if these do indeed represent varied aspects of the same basic disorder, it seems misleading to view them as examples of comorbidity. Clearly, further research is needed to bring better order into the confusing nosological territory of anxiety disorders.

One Disorder Represents an Early Manifestation of the Other

A further possibility is that one disorder constitutes an early manifestation of the other. When that is the explanation, it may be desirable to code these manifestations separately because the stage of the disorder has important clinical implications. But it would make no sense to regard transitional phases with both early and later manifestations as representing comorbidity. These are well known examples in medicine where distinct stages of a disease are recognized; for example, primary, secondary and tertiary syphilis or the differentiation between cervical carcinoma and precancerous cervical dyskaryosia or dysplasia. In child psychiatry, there are several disorders in which it has been suggested that they represent early manifestations of some other diagnosis. Thus, oppositional disorder is a syndrome mainly diagnosed in younger children and which often seems to be a precursor of conduct disorder (Loeber & Lahey, 1989). Similarly, separation anxiety tends to be diagnosed in younger children and it has been suggested that it may represent an early manifestation of overanxious disorder (Last *et al.*, 1987). Or again, conduct disorder in childhood is an established precursor of antisocial personality disorder in adult life (Robins, 1978).

To test this type of disorder progression hypothesis it is crucial to have longitudinal data (Loeber, 1990). Thus, if condition A is a precursor of B, it must be the case that the presence of A at time 1 increases the likelihood of B at time 2; and that B never precedes A. However, equally, it is to be expected that only some cases of A will develop into B and, if there is more than one precursor of B, there may be instances of B that have not been preceded by A. To date, although there are some data suggesting the plausibility of hypotheses on progression, decisive testing has yet to be undertaken.

One Disorder is Part of the Other

It may also be suggested that one disorder is part of or a secondary manifestation of the other conditions. For example, DSM-III-R specifies that if there is a pervasive developmental disorder, neither attention-deficit hyperactivity disorder, nor pica, nor overanxious disorder can be diagnosed as well. Presumably this is on the basis of the fact that the symptoms characteristic of these other disorders are so very frequently part of the symptomatology of autism. A similar exclusion applies to generalized anxiety that occurs only during the course of a mood disorder. There are several ways in which this hypothesis may be tested. For example, if the comorbid disorders are episodic in nature, it is possible to determine whether the remission and recurrence of the one are associated in time with those of the other and, especially, if the administration of a treatment that is specific to the one leads to the loss of the symptoms of the other disorder. This approach has been followed in the case of the co-occurrence of nocturnal enuresis and other child psychiatric disorders—with largely negative findings (Shaffer, 1973, 1985). It has also been adopted to examine the comorbidity of depression and conduct disorder (Puig-Antich, 1982; Puig-Antich, Lukens, Davies, Goetz & Toddak, 1985), with inconclusive mixed findings. Unfortunately, this strategy is weakened by the weakness and/or nonspecificity of so many treatments; thus, antidepressant medication is not particularly effective in the treatment of depression in children and adolescents (Puig-Antich *et al.*, 1987; Ryan *et al.*, 1986) and tricyclic drugs have a wide range of actions that extend far beyond those on mood. A further limitation is that the two constellations of symptoms may represent *alternative* manifestations of one disorder; variable expression is a well recognized feature of many genetic disorders (as illustrated, for example, by neurofibromatosis). This possibility may be examined through the use of genetic research strategies. There are many examples of the use of family studies for this purpose; for example to examine the association between anorexia nervosa and depression (Strober, Lampert, Morrell, Burroughs & Jacobs, in press) or that between alcoholism and depression (Merikangas *et al.*, 1985, 1988)—in both cases with evidence suggesting independent transmission. However, on their own, family data cannot make a satisfactory differentiation between genetic and environmental mechanisms. Adoptee and twin designs of various kinds (Rutter *et al.*, 1990) are effective for this purpose and may be used to examine comorbidity. For example, Holland, Hall, Murray, Russell and Crisp (1984) found no tendency for affective disorders to occur in the cotwins of subjects with anorexia nervosa and Cadoret, Troughton, Moreno and Whitters (1990) found no direct genetic connection between alcohol and antisocial problems in biological relatives and depressive symptomatology in adopted-away subjects. It would be helpful to make greater use of genetic research strategies in the study of comorbidity in child psychiatry.

POSSIBLE EXPLANATIONS OF TRUE COMORBIDITY

The explanations considered thus far all involve a mechanism by which the apparent comorbidiy represents some type of artifact so that the real situation does not involve the co-occurrence of two or more truly separate and independent conditions. As discussed, that does not mean that the findings should be dismissed; quite often elucidation of the meaning of the apparent comorbidity should throw light on the nature of the disorders involved. However, that is even more the case when there is true comorbidity. Several rather different underlying processes need to be considered.

Shared Risk Factors

One possible reason for overlap between two disorders is that they share the same risk factor or factors. This possibility arises from the fact that many psychiatric disorders are multifactorial in origin and that many causal factors are not diagnosis-specific. For example, there are various extreme temperamental traits or constellations of traits that are associated with a range of psychiatric disorders as well as with learning difficulties (Kohnstamm, Bates & Rothbart, 1990). Thus, it has been suggested that temperamental variables such as overactivity, short attention span and impulsivity might account for the well established comorbidity between conduct disorders and reading difficulties (Yule & Rutter, 1985). Family adversity might also operate in the same way (Offord, Poushinsky & Sullivan 1978; Richman, Stevenson & Graham, 1982), because large family size and social disadvantage carry an increased risk for both conditions (Rutter & Giller, 1983; Sturge, 1982). However, it is not known whether the shared risk factors mechanism does in fact account for this (or any other) pattern of comorbidity. What are needed are investigations in which comorbidity is examined before and after partialling out, or statistically taking account of, shared risk factors.

Overlap Between Risk Factors

A variant of this mechanism is provided by the possibility that, even when the risk factors for two disorders are distinct and different, there may be comorbidity because the risk factors themselves are associated. When that is the case, the individual may be at risk for two separate conditions with the risk mechanisms for each independent, but co-occurring. For example, parental depression constitutes a risk factor for a range of different child psychiatric disorders (Rutter, 1989b). Particular attention has been focused on major depressive disorders in the offspring with the suggestion that they are genetically mediated (Weissman *et al.*, 1987; Weissman, 1988). However, there is also an increased risk of conduct disorder that seems to be a function of family discord, which is much more frequent when one or both parents are depressed (Rutter & Quinton, 1984). Thus, it might be suggested that the comorbidity between depression and conduct disorder could arise, at least in part, because parental depression is associated with a genetic risk for depression in the offspring and an environmental mediated risk(when there is associated discord) for conduct disorders. In order to test this hypothesis, it would be necessary to examine comorbidity after taking account of these two routes to disorder in the child; thus there should be no comorbidity when there is family harmony and cohesion if the postulated mechanisms are operating in the way hypothesized.

Chiles, Miller and Cox (1980) provided data that are consistent with the risk factor overlap concept. Delinquent adolescents with and without comorbid depression were compared. The two groups could not be differentiated on the basis of risk factors for delinquency (a family history of divorce, parental death, child abuse and incest) but the depressed delinquents did differ in being more likely to have factors thought to constitute risk variables for depression (depression or alcoholism in a first degree relative). Thus, it could be argued that depressed delinquents had the risk factors for both disorders whereas the nondepressed delinquents had them for only one. It is of importance to notice here that assortative mating may also be another mechanism by which two disorders are transmitted to the offspring.

The Comorbid Pattern Constitutes a Meaningful Syndrome

The basic assumption that appears to underly the DSM-III-R policy of making diagnoses on the presence of particular constellations of symptoms irrespective of the presence or absence of other constellations is that comorbidity does not alter the meaning of any of the diagnoses involved in the comorbidity pattern. That assumption may be tested by comparing comorbid and "pure" diagnoses on features such as course or family history or responses to treatment that might reflect diagnostic meaning. This strategy has been used relatively infrequently but there are two examples of syndromes where the few available data seem to negate the assumption. There is a large body of data demonstrating that stimulant drugs usually bring about major, sometimes dramatic, short-term benefits in children with attention deficit hyperactivity disorders (ADHD)(Klein, 1987). Taylor *et al.*, (1987) showed that the benefits were *not* evident when the system pattern included marked anxiety; and Pliszka (1989) found that children with ADHD comorbid with anxiety had *no* significant benefit from methylphenidate in a double blind control trial (whereas those without anxiety showed the usual good drug response). The findings from both these studies are striking for two separate reasons. First, as they showed, comorbidity with conduct disorder had no effect on drug response, so that this is not a nonspecific effect of comorbidity of any type. Second, the co-occurrence of anxiety disorder *removed* one of the most characteristic features of one of the two disorders in the comorbid pattern. The implication seems to be either that the comorbid pattern constitutes a variety of anxiety disorder (systematic comparisons with "pure" anxiety disorders are needed to test the hypothesis) or that it constitutes a meaningfully distinctive syndrome in its own right. Either way, the implication is that the comorbidity has altered the meaning to be attached to ADHD and, therefore, that it warrants separate coding in the classification system.

A second example is provided by the comorbid pattern of depression and conduct disorder in childhood. The follow-up into adult life undertaken by Harrington, Fudge, Rutter, Pickles & Hill (in press) showed that the risk of adult criminality associated with conduct disorder was unaffected by the presence or absence of comorbid depression. However, the risk of major depressive disorder in adult life associated with childhood depression *was* affected by comorbid conduct disorder; the low risk in the comorbid group did not differ from that in the group without depression. Puig-Antich *et al.* (1989) also found that the comorbid group differed from children with a "pure" depressive disorder with respect to family history of major depressive disorder. This difference in familiality applied only to the comorbidity with conduct disorder and not to that with separation anxiety. The findings to date are too sparse to warrant firm conclusions and in any case do not differentiate between the alternative hypotheses that comorbid depression and conduct disorder constitute a meaningfully different syndrome and that the depression in the comorbid group is secondary to or part of the conduct disorder. Again, however, it seems that the comorbid pattern may change the meaning of the depressive disorder; it needs to be identified as a separate group and studied further.

One Disorder Creates an Increased Risk for the Other

A further possible explanation for comorbid patterns is that one disorder creates an increased risk for the other. For example, Cadoret *et al.* (1990) using an adoptee deign, showed that an adult diagnosis of antisocial personality or substance abuse was associated with a four-fold increase in risk for depressive symptomatology even though the genetic origins of the two disorders were distinct. Robins and McEvoy (1990), using retrospecitive data from the Epidemiological Catchment Area Study, showed that conduct disorder in childhood was a powerful predictor of later substance abuse. The data were not such as to allow determination of the extent to which these were truly separate disorders. However, the evidence suggested that the mechanisms involved both duration and timing of exposure to illicit drugs, plus, probably, the generation of psychosocial stressors and adversity that serve as risk factors for heavy use of psychoactive substances.

There is an extensive literature on the effects of acute and life stressors as risk factors for psychiatric disorder in both childhood and adult life (Brown & Harris, 1989; Goodyer, 1990). However, less attention has been paid to the origins of these stressors (Champion, 1990; Rutter, 1986). There is increasing evidence that people shape and select their own environments and that various psychiatric disorders play a part in generating stress and adversity. For example, follow-up studies of children with conduct disorder have shown markedly increased rates of unemployment and marital breakdown in adult life (Robins, 1966, 1986), both well established risk factors for depressive disorders. Neuroticism has also been found to be associated with an increased likelihood of marital breakdown (Kelly & Conley, 1987).

It will be appreciated that an adequate testing of this causal chain hypothesis requires several steps. Clearly, a start is provided by longitudinal time sequence data showing that condition A both precedes and is associated with an increased risk for condition B; whereas the reverse does not apply. However, as clearly noted, this could simply mean that A and B constitute different stages in the progression of a single disorder. Data showing that comorbid A + B has correlates that approximate those of "pure" A, but not those of "pure" B, indicate that B cannot have caused A (a strategy used to examine the comorbidity of conduct disorder and reading retardation—Rutter *et al.*, 1970)but, although consistent with the hypothesis that A caused B the findings are open to other interpretations.

In particular, this pattern of results indicates that the meaning of "pure" B and comorbid A + B must be somewhat different. What are needed are data showing that the origins of "pure" B and comorbid A + B involve the same risk factors but that condition A generates those risk factors. In other words, it is necessary to test the several links in the postulated causal chain. This full research strategy has yet to be pursued in the investigation of comorbidity in child psychiatric disorders.

CONCLUSIONS

Many studies document the pervasiveness of patterns of comorbidity in child, as well as adult, psychiatry. However, it is clear that the extent of comorbidity can be assessed only through the use of fully representative epidemiological data. That is primarily because calculation of the chance expectation of comorbidity requires data on the general population base rates of each of the conditions involved in the comorbidity. In addition, the Berkson effect and a variety of referral biases make the use of clinic data hazardous and potentially misleading.

Until relatively recently, comorbidity has received little attention in the research literature and considerations of psychiatric classification issues have generally ignored the extreme frequency with which psychiatric disorders seem to co-occur. This neglect has had two unfortunate consequences. First, the findings of many studies of one specified psychiatric condition are likely to be misleading because the correlates of the disorder being investigated may represent the correlates of some unspecified comorbid condition. Second, there is the unsafe assumption that the meaning of any given disorder is exactly the same regardless of the presence or absence of other disorders. It is sometimes claimed that the DSM-III-R classification system avoids the difficulties associated with diagnostic hierarchies just because it allows any level of comorbidity. However, it is evident that it includes more hierarchies than generally appreciated and that the encouragement of comorbid diagnoses introduces further problems.

In this paper we have outlined some of the detection artifacts that may produce a false picture of comorbidity and have gone on to discuss some of the nosological considerations that apply to comorbidity. These include: the concepts of disorders as categories or dimensions; overlapping diagnostic criteria, artificial subdivisions of syndromes; one disorder representing an early manifestation of the other; and one disorder being part of the other. Finally, we have considered some of the possible explanations of true comorbidity in terms of: shared risk factors; overlapping risk factors; comorbid patterns constituting a meaningful syndrome; and one disorder creating an increased risk for the other. In each case, we have put forward some general guidelines for testing alternative hypothesis. It is evident that it may be quite difficult to differentiate between competing explanations but equally it is clear that an improved understanding of the varied mechanisms underlying comorbidity should shed important light on the processes involved in the genesis and contribution of psychiatric disorders.

REFERENCES

American Psychiatric Association (1987). *Diagnostic and statistical manual of mental disorders* (DSM-III)(3rd edn). Washington, DC: Author.

Anderson, J.C., Williams, S., McGee, R. & Silva, P.A. (1987). DMS-III disorders in preadolescent children. Prevalence in a large sample from the general population. *Archives of General Psychiatry*, 44, 69–78.

Barlow, D.H. (1988), *Anxiety and its disorders. The nature and treatment of anxiety and panic*. New York: Guilford.

Berkson, J. (1946). Limitations of the application of fourfold table analysis to hospital data. *Biometrics*, 2, 47–53.

Bird, H., Canino, G., Rubio-Stipec, M., Gould, M.S., Ribera, J., Sesman, M., Woodbury, M., Huertas-Goldman, S., Pagan, A., Sanchez-Lacay, A. & Moscoso, M. (1988). Estimates of the prevalence of childhood maladjustment in a community survey in Puerto Rico. *Archives of General Psychiatry*, 45, 1120–1126.

Boyd, J.H., Burke, J.D., Gruenberg, E., Holzer, C.E., Rae, D.S., George, L.K., Karno, M., Stoltzman, R., McEvoy, L. & Nestadt, G. (1984). Exclusion criteria of DSM-III. *Archives of General Psychiatry*, 41, 983–989.

Brown, G. & Harris, T. (Eds)(1989). *Life events and illness*. New York: Guilford.

Bukstein, O.G., Brent, D.A. & Kaminer, Y. (1989). Comorbidity of substance abuse and other psychiatric disorders in adolescents. *American Journal of Psychiatry*, 146, 1131–1141.

Cadoret, R., Troughton, F., Moreno, L. & Whitters, A. (1990). Early life psychosocial events and adult affective symptoms. In L. Robins & M. Rutter (Eds), *Straight and devious pathways from childhood to adulthood* (pp. 300–313). New York: Cambridge University Press.

Champion, L. (1990). The relationship between social vulnerability and the occurrence of severely threatening life events. *Psychological Medicine*, 20, 157–161.

Chiles, J.A., Miller, M.L. & Cox, C.B. (1980). Depression in an adolescent delinquent population. *Archives of General Psychiatry*, 37, 1179–1184.

Costello, E.J., Costello, A.J., Edelbrock, C., Burns, B.J., Dulcan, M.K., Brent, D. & Janiszewski, S. (1988). Psychiatric disorders in pediatric primary care. *Archives of General Psychiatry*, 45, 1107–1116.

Flament, M.F., Whitaker, A., Rapaport, J.L., Davies, M., Zaremba Berg, C., Kalikow, K., Sceery, W. & Shafffer, D. (1988). Obsessive compulsive disorder in adolescence: an epidemiological study. *Journal of the American Academy of Child Psychiatry*, 27, 764–771.

Goodyer, I.M. (1990). *Life experiences, development and childhood psychopathology*. Chichester: Wiley.

Grayson, D., Bridges, K., Cook, D. & Goldberg, D. (1990). The validity of diagnostic systems for common mental disorders: a comparison between the ID-CATEGO and the DSM-III systems. *Psychological Medicine*, 20, 209–218.

Harrington, R., Fudge, H., Rutter, M., Pickles, A. & Hill, J. (in press). Adult outcomes of childhood and adolescent depression: II. Links with antisocial disorders. *Journal of the American Academy of Child and Adolescent Psychiatry*.

Holland, A.J., Hall, A., Murray, R., Russell, G.F.M. & Crisp, A.H. (1984). Anorexia nervosa: a study of 34 twin pairs and one set of triplets. *British Journal of Psychiatry*, 145, 414–419.

Jaspers, K. (1963) *General psychopathology*. Manchester: Manchester University Press.

Kashani, J.H., Beck, N.C., Hoeper, E.W., Fallahi, C., Corcoran, C.M., McAllister, J.A., Rosenberg, T.K. & Reid, J.C. (1987). Psychiatric disorders in a community sample of adolescents. *American Journal of Psychiatry*, 144, 584–589.

Kelly, E.L. & Conley, J.J. (1987). Personality and compatibility: a prospective analysis of marital stability and marital satisfaction. *Journal of Personality and Social Psychology*, 52, 27–40.

Kendell, R.E. (1975). *The role of diagnosis in psychiatry*. Oxford: Blackwell Scientific.

Klein, R.G. (1987), Pharmacotherapy of childhood hyperactivity: an update. In H.Y. Meltzer, W. Bunney, J. Coyle, K. Davies, I. Kopin, C.R. Schuster, R.I. Shader & G. Simpson (Eds), *Psychopharmacology: the third generation of progress* (pp. 1215–1224). New York: Raven Press.

Kohnstamm, G.A., Bates, J.E. & Rothbart, M.K. (1990). *Temperament in childhood*. Chichester: Wiley.

Last, C.G., Hersen, M., Kazdin, A.E., Finkelstein, R. & Strauss, C.C. (1987). Comparison of DSM-III separation anxiety and overanxious disorders: demographic characteristics and patterns of comorbidity. *Journal of the American Academy of Child and Adolescent Psychiatry*, 26, 528–531.

Loeber, R. (1990). Development and risk factors of juvenile antisocial behavior and delinquency. *Child Psychology Review*, 10, 1–141.

Loeber, R. & Lahey, B.B. (1989). Recommendations for research on disruptive behavior disorders of childhood and adolescence. In B.B. Lahey & A.E. Kazadin (Eds), *Advances in clinical child psychology* (Vol. 12, pp. 221–257). New York: Plenum Press.

Mannuzza, S., Fyer, A.J., Liebowitz, M.R. & Klein, D.F. (1990). Delineating the boundaries of social phobia: its relationship to panic disorder and agoraphobia. *Journal of Anxiety Disorders*, 4:41–59.

Merikangas, K.R., Leckman, J.F., Prusoff, B.A., Pauls, D.L. & Weissman, M.M. (1985). Familial transmission of depression and alcoholism. *Archives of General Psychiatry*, 42, 367–372.

Merikangas, K.R., Prusoff, B.A. & Weissman, M.M. (1988). Parental concordance for affective disorders: psychopathology in offspring. *Journal of Affective Disorders*, 15, 279–290.

Newman, S.C., Shrout, P.E. & Bland, R.C. (1990). The efficiency of two-phase designs in prevalence surveys of mental disorders. *Psychological Medicine*, 20, 183–193.

Offord, D.R., Poushinsky, M.F. & Sullivan, K. (1978). School performance, IQ and delinquency. *British Journal of Criminology*, 18, 110–127.

Pfeffer, C.R. & Plutchik, R. (1989). Co-occurrence of psychiatric disorders in child psychiatric patients and nonpatients: a circumplex model. *Comprehensive Psychiatry*, 30, 275–282.

Pliszka, S. (1989). Effect of anxiety on cognition, behavior, and stimulant-response to ADHD. *Journal of the American Academy of Child and Adolescent Psychiatry*, 28, 882–887.

Puig-Antich, J. (1982). Major depression and conduct disorder in prepuberty. *Journal of the American Academy of Child Psychiatry*, 21, 118–128.

Puig-Antich, J., Goetz, D., Davies, M., Kaplan, T., Davies, S., Ostrow, L., Asnis, L., Twomey, J., Lyengar, S. & Ryan, N.D. (1989). A controlled family history study of prepubertal major depressive disorder. *Archives of General Psychiatry*, 46, 406–418.

Richman, N., Stevenson, J. & Graham, P.J. (1982). *Pre-school to school: a behavioural study*. London: Academic Press.

Robins, L. (1966), *Deviant children grown up*. Baltimore: Williams & Wilkins.

Robins, L.N. (1978). Sturdy childhood predictors of adult antisocial behavior: replications from longitudinal studies. *Psychological Medicine*, 8, 611–622.

Robins, L.N. (1986). The consequences of conduct disorder in girls. In D. Olweus, J. Block & M. Radke-Yarrow (Eds), *Development of antisocial and prosocial behavior: research, theories and issues* (pp. 385–414). New York: Academic Press.

Robins, L.N. & McEvoy, L. (1990). Conduct problems as predictors of substance abuse. In L. Robins & M. Rutter (Eds). *Straight and devious pathways from childhood to adulthood* (pp. 182–204). New York: Cambridge University Press.

Rutter, M. (1986). Meyersian psychobiology, personality development and the role of life experience. *American Journal of Psychiatry*, 143, 1077–1087.

Rutter, M. (1988). DSM-III-R: a postscript. In M. Rutter, A.H. Tuma, & I.S. Lann (Eds), *Assessment and diagnosis in child psychopathology* (pp. 453–464). New York: Guilford.

Rutter, M. (1989a). Isle of Wight revisited: twenty-five years of child psychiatric epidemiology. *Journal of the American Academy of Child and Adolescent Psychiatry*, 28, 633–653.

Rutter, M. (1989b). Psychiatric disorder in parents as a risk factor for children. In D. Shaffer, J. Phillips, & N.B. Enzer (Eds), with M.M. Silverman & V. Anthony (Associate Eds), *Prevention of mental disorders, alcohol and other drug use in children and adolescents* (pp. 157–189). OSAP Prevention Monograph 2. Rockville, MD: Office for Substance Abuse Prevention, U.S. Department of Health and Human Sciences.

Rutter, M. & Giller, H. (1983). *Juvenile delinquency: trends and perspective*. Harmondsworth: Penguin.

Rutter, M. & Gould, M. (1985). Classification. In M. Rutter & L. Hersov (Eds), *Child and adolescent psychiatry: modern approaches* (pp. 304–321). Oxford: Blackwell Scientific.

Rutter, M. & Quinton, D. (1984). Parental psychiatric disorder: effects on children. *Psychological Medicine*, 14, 853–880.

Rutter, M., Tizard, J. & Whitmore, K. (Eds)(1970). *Education, health and behavior.* London: Longman (reprinted 1981, Melbourne, FL: Krieger).

Ryan, N.D., Puig-Antich, J., Cooper, T., Rabinovich, H., Ambrosini, P., Davies, M., Torres, D. & Fried, J. (1986). Imipramine in adolescent major depression: plasma level and clinical response. *Acta Paediatrica Scandinavica*, 73, 275–288.

Shaffer, D. (1973). The association between enuresis and emotional disorder: a review of the literature. In I. Kolvin, R.C. MacKeith & S.R. Meadow (Eds), *Bladder control and enuresis* (pp. 118–136). London: Heinemann.

Shaffer, D. (1985). Enuresis. In M. Rutter & L. Hersov (Eds), *Child and adolescent psychiatry: modern approaches* (2nd ed.)(pp. 465–481). Oxford: Blackwell Scientific.

Shaffer, D., Campbell, M., Cantwell, D., Bradley, S., Carlson, G., Cohen, D., Denckla, M., Frances, A., Garfinkel, B., Klein, R., Pincus, H., Spitzer, R.L., Volkmar, F. & Widiger, T. (1989). Child and adolescent psychiatric disorders in DSM-IV: issues facing the work group. *Journal of the American Academy of Child and Adolescent Psychiatry*, 28, 830–835.

Shepherd, M., Oppenheim, B. & Mitchell, S. (1971). *Childhood behaviour and mental health.* London: University of London Press.

Strober, M., Lampert, C., Morrell, W., Burroughs, J. & Jacobs, C. (in press). A controlled family study of anorexia nervosa: evidence of familial aggregation and lack of shared transmission with affective disorders. *International Journal of Eating Disorders.*

Sturge, C. (1982). Reading retardation and antisocial behaviour. *Journal of Child Psychology and Psychiatry*, 22, 21–31.

Szatimari, P., Boyle, M. & Offord, D.R. (1989). ADDH and conduct disorder: degree of diagnostic overlap and differences among correlates. *Journal of the American Academy of Child and Adolescent Psychiatry*, 28, 865–872.

Taylor, E. (1988). Attention deficit and conduct disorder syndromes. In M. Rutter, A.H. Tuma & I.S. Lann (Eds), *Assessment and diagnosis in child psychopathology* (pp. 377–407). New York: Guilford.

Taylor, E., Schachar, R., Thorley, G., Wieselberg, H.M., Everitt, B. & Rutter, M. (1987). Which boys respond to stimulant medication? A controlled trial of methylphenidate in boys with disruptive behaviour. *Psychological Medicine*, 17, 121–143.

Weinstein, S.R., Stone, K., Noam, G.G., Grimes, K. & Schwab-Stone, M. (1989). Comparison of DISC with clinicians' DSM-III diagnoses in psychiatric inpatients. *Journal of the American Academy of Child and Adolescent Psychiatry*, 28, 53–60.

Weissman, M.M. (1988). Psychopathology in the children of depressed parents: direct interview studies. In D.L. Dunner, E.S. Gehrson & J.E. Barret (Eds), *Relatives at risk for mental disorders* (pp. 143–159). New York: Raven Press.

Weissman, M.M., Gammon, G.D., John, K., Merikangas, K.R., Warner, V., Prusoff, B.A. & Sholomskas, D. (1987). Children of depressed parents. Increased psychopathology and early onset of major depression. *Archives of General Psychiatry*, 44, 847–853.

Weissman, M.M., Warner, V. & Fendrich, M. (1990). Applying impairment criteria to children's psychiatric diagnosis. *Journal of the American Academy of Child and Adolescent Psychiatry*, 29, 789–795.

22

Adult Outcomes of Childhood and Adolescent Depression: II. Links with Antisocial Disorders

Richard Harrington

Queen Elizabeth Hospital, Birmingham, United Kingdom

Hazel Fudge, Michael Rutter, and Andrew Pickles

The Institute of Psychiatry, London, United Kingdom

Jonathan Hill

Royal Liverpool Children's Hospital, United Kingdom

Sixty-three child and adolescent patients meeting operational criteria for depression and 68 nondepressed child psychiatric controls were followed into adulthood. Twenty-one percent of the depressed group had had conduct disorder (CD) in conjunction with their index depression. Depressed children with comorbid CD did not differ from depressed children without conduct problems with respect to depressive symptom presentation or demographic characteristics. However, depressives with CD had a worse short-term outcome and a higher risk of adult criminality than depressed children without conduct problems. There was a strong trend for depressives with CD to have a lower risk of depression in adulthood than depressed children without conduct problems. The outcomes of depressives with CD were

Reprinted with permission from the *Journal of the American Academy of Child and Adolescent Psychiatry,* 1991, Vol. 30, No. 3, 434–439. Copyright © 1991 by the American Academy of Child and Adolescent Psychiatry.

This research was supported by a grant from the John D. and Catherine R. MacArthur Foundation Research Network on Risk and Protective Factors in the Major Mental Disorders. Thanks are due to the staff at the Home Office who supplied the criminal records data, to Christine Rutter who coded these data, and to Karen John and Myrna Weissman for their help with the training on the SADS-L. The authors gratefully acknowledge the contributions of Christine Groothues and Diana Bredenkamp to this study.

*very similar to those of nondepressed children with CD. The findings
are discussed in the context of current classification schemes.*

One of the most difficult problems arising from recent research into juvenile-
onset affective conditions is a result of the finding that these conditions very often
occur in conjunction with other psychiatric disturbances, such as conduct disorder
(CD) and anxiety. The problem is that the nosological status of these "mixed" or
"comorbid" states is unclear. It is not known, for example, whether these mixed
states should be assigned to a separate diagnostic category, or whether the child
should be given several different, but concurrent, diagnoses. This is an important
issue because, as Puig-Antich et al. pointed out (1989), it seems that the presence
of other psychiatric disorders in juvenile affective conditions is the rule rather than
the exception (Anderson et al., 1987; Fleming et al., 1989; Harrington, 1989). Until
we know how to deal with these mixed clinical pictures in classification schemes,
it will be difficult to identify homogeneous groups with respect to etiology or treatment responsiveness.

The present paper is concerned with the overlap between depression and CD.
This association has been reported in both clinical and community populations
(Rutter et al. 1970; Puig-Antich, 1982; Kashani et al., 1983; Marriage et al. 1986;
Anderson et al., 1987) and has previously been investigated by studying symptom
characteristics (Marriage et al., 1986), short-term outcome (Kovacs et al., 1988;
McGee and Williams, 1988) and family history (Puig-Antich et al., 1989). In this
article, the relationship between depression and conduct problems is examined using
data from a long-term follow-up of depressed children. The aim is to address the
following issues: (1) the prevalence and correlates of CD among a sample of
depressed children referred to a clinic; (2) the diagnostic phenomenology of depression among these children; and (3) the short-term and adult outcomes of depressed
children with CD, depressed children without conduct problems, and nondepressed
children with CD. Using these strategies, the authors hope to clarify the nosological
status of children who have both depression and CD.

METHOD

Childhood Assessments

The full details of childhood assessments, the validity of these assessments, ascertainment of cases and controls, and methods of follow-up into adulthood have been
described elsewhere (Harrington et al., 1990). Briefly, the study was based on the
clinical data records ("item sheets") of children who attended the children's psychiatric department of the Maudsley Hospital during the late 1960s and early 1970s.
The items sheets were completed at the time of the initial contact by a clinically

involved psychiatrist. They contained demographic and background information, standardized ratings on the presence or absence of over 40 psychiatric symptoms, and ratings of the degree of handicap at the time of discharge (see Thorley, 1982, 1987, for a description of the coverage and content validity of the item sheets). Item sheet data have been used in many projects, including studies of hallucinations (Garralda, 1984) and fire setting (Jacobsen, 1985). Goodman and Simonoff (1990) reported that Maudsley psychiatrists' ratings of the item sheets can be of acceptable reliability for research purposes.

In the present study, the symptom ratings were used to identify a group of 80 child patients meeting operational criteria for a depressive syndrome (Pearce, 1974, unpublished manuscript; 1978) and a group of 80 nondepressed controls. Since these criteria for depression differed in several respects from those used in present-day studies, the charts of both the cases and the controls were independently rediagnosed by a child psychiatrist in order to generate Research Diagnostic Criteria (RDC) depressive diagnoses (Spitzer et al., 1978). There was good agreement between the item sheet-derived depressive syndrome and the child psychiatrist's rating of any RDC depression (kappa = 0.71) (Harrington et al., 1990).

Comorbidity between the depressive syndrome and conduct problems was approached from a categorical stance. Accordingly, and in line with other studies that have used a categorical approach to the study of the long-term correlates of conduct disturbances (Robins, 1986), children with three or more of the following conduct symptoms were designated as having CD: disobedience or lying, stealing, destructiveness or malicious damage, fire setting, truancy or staying out late, running away, sexual misbehavior, fighting or bullying, taking drugs, and "other" antisocial behavior. The requirement of at least three out of 10 antisocial symptoms for the diagnosis is similar to the *DSM-III-R* criteria for CD in which three of 13 antisocial symptoms are sufficient. To sharpen up the comparisons between depressed children with and without CD, children with one or two conduct symptoms were omitted from most of the analyses. However, in the final part of the results section, outcome data are presented on depressed children with one or two conduct symptoms.

Adult Assessments

At follow-up, on average 18 years after the initial contact, outcome information was obtained on 63 depressed subjects and 68 controls. Follow-up assessments were made "blind" to childhood symptomatology in all but four cases.

Psychiatric disorders in adulthood were assessed by a modified version of the Schedule for Affective Disorders and Schizophrenia-Lifetime Version (SADS-L) (Spitzer and Endicott, 1975). Data on the reliability and concurrent validity of this schedule in a British sample have been presented elsewhere (Harrington et al., 1988).

In the first publication from this follow-up study (Harrington et al, 1990), the adult psychiatric status of the sample was described. In brief, children with the depressive syndrome were found to be at an increased risk of depressive disorder in adulthood and were more likely than the controls to have had subsequent psychiatric treatment. Moreover, they did not differ from the controls in respect to their risk for nondepressive psychiatric disorders in adulthood. These data provide further support for the validity of the operational definition of childhood depression.

Data on criminal convictions in adulthood were obtained from the central Criminal Records Office in London and coded by a research worker who had not been involved in the interviewing and who was blind to all the other study data. Police cautions and minor crimes, such as less serious traffic offences and drunkenness, are excluded from these records. The most common offences were thefts, burglaries, and unauthorized takings of motor vehicles.

Social dysfunction in adulthood was evaluated by the Adult Personality Functioning Assessment (APFA) (Hill et al., 1989). In the APFA, functioning over a specified period in adulthood (usually from 21 to 30 years of age) is rated in six domains: work, love relationships, friendship, nonintimate social contacts, negotiations, and everyday coping. For each domain, the rating of level of functioning is made on a six-point scale extending from "0" (very effective functioning) to "5" (complete failure of role performance in the domain). In addition, a rating is made of "general social dysfunction," operationally defined as a total APFA score of 16 or greater (Hill et al., 1989).

In a previous study, the two interviewers, who conducted the follow-up (R.H. and H. F.), achieved high interrater reliability on APFA ratings (Hill et al., 1998). To check for interviewer drift during the course of the present study, R.H. and H.F. independently rated 14 case vignettes. The average intraclass correlation coefficient across the six APFA domains was 0.78.

Statistical Methods

Nominal data were analyzed via χ^2 tests (corrected for continuity when appropriate) and quantitative data by t-tests or Mann-Whitney U tests as appropriate. Between group differences on several correlated continuous measures (i.e., APFA scores) were analyzed via multivariate analysis of variance (MANOVA). Time-varying outcome variables (such as time to first criminal conviction in adulthood) were analyzed by survival analyses and the Lee-Desu statistic (Statistical Package for the Social Sciences, 1983).

RESULTS

Overlap with Conduct Symptoms

Within the depressed group, the most common conduct symptoms during the index episode were disobedience or lying (36), destructiveness (17%), stealing (16%), truancy (13%), and fighting (11%). Twenty-nine of the 63 depressed probands (46%) had at least one conduct symptom. Of these, 16 had one or two conduct symptoms, and 13 (21% of the depressed group) had three or more conduct symptoms.

Seventeen of the 68 child psychiatric controls (25%) had three or more conduct problems.

Depressive Phenomenology and Demographic/Clinical Characteristics

To examine whether comorbidity with conduct problems affected depressive phenomenology during the index episode, children with the depressive syndrome who had comorbid CD ($N = 13$) were compared with those who had no conduct problems ($N = 34$), using the item sheet ratings of depressive symptomatology. As Table 1 shows, the difference between the groups was significant at the 5% level in just one of the nine symptoms (irritability); no more than would be expected by chance. There were, however, trends for school refusal, eating problems, and abdominal pain to be more common among depressed children who had no conduct problems,

TABLE 1.
Symptomatology of Children with the Depressive Syndrome
Grouped by Number of Conduct Problems

Symptom	Percentage of Depressed Cases with Symptom in the Presence of		
	No Conduct Problems ($N = 34$)	Conduct Disorder (three or more conduct problems) ($N = 13$)	p
Suicidal idea/threat	41	46	0.76
Hypochondriasis	23	15	0.54
Irritability	44	77	0.04
School refusal	50	23	0.09
Disturbed eating	53	23	0.06
Disturbed sleeping	71	69	0.92
Obsessions	29	15	0.54
Psychotic phenomena	15	38	0.17
Abdominal pain	41	15	0.18

and psychotic phenomena tended to be more common among depressed children with CD.

Next, these two groups were compared using the child psychiatrist's retrospective RDC diagnoses of the charts. Depressed children without conduct problems were more often diagnosed as having RDC major depression during the index episode than depressed children with CD (79% vs. 46%), although the difference just failed to reach significance at the 5% level (χ^2 3.5, $p = 0.06$).

Finally, the authors examined whether there were differences between the groups on demographic and clinical features. As Table 2 indicates, depressed children with comorbid CD did not differ from depressed children with no conduct disturbance in regard to sex distribution, age at index attendance, social class, or pubertal status. However, they were more likely to have had a duration of problem of greater than 3 years at the time of the index attendance (χ^2 4.11, df 1, $p < 0.05$).

Short-Term Outcome

Two ordinal measures of short-term outcome were available: (1) degree of recovery at the time of discharge and (2) degree of handicap at the time of discharge and (2) degree of handicap at the time of discharge. Both of these assessments had been recorded on the item sheet by the clinically involved psychiatrist who had seen the child during the index attendance.

TABLE 2.
Clinical Characteristics of Depressed Children Grouped by
Number of Conduct Problems during Index Childhood Episode

	Depressed children		
	No Conduct Problems	Conduct Disorder	
Characteristic	($N = 34$)	($N = 13$)	p
Male sex, %	50	54	0.81
Mean age at index episode, yr	12.9	13.2	0.69
Prepubertal, %	39	25	0.58
Manual social class, %	71	62	0.84
Duration of disorder, %			
6 mo or less	26	8	
6 mo to 1 yr	9	8	
1 yr to 2 yr	18	23	
2 yr to 3 yr	18	—	
3 yr or more	29	61	0.04*
Not living with two natural parents, %	23	46	0.25

*X^2 test. $p < 0.05$.

TABLE 3.
Degree of Recovery and Degree of Handicap at the End of the
Index Childhood Attendance at the Maudsley in Depressed
Children without Conduct Problems, Depressed Children with
Conduct Disorder, and Nondepressed Children with
Conduct Disorder

	Depressed, No Conduct Problems ($N = 34$) %	Depressed, Conduct Disorder ($N = 13$) %	Nondepressed, Conduct Disorder ($N = 17$) %
Degree of recovery[a]			
No change	21	56	60
Slight improvement	14	—	7
Improved	24	44	13
Much improved	28	—	13
Recovered	14	—	7
Degree of handicap[b]			
Normal	10	—	13
Trivial abnormality	33	—	20
Slight handicap	27	12	27
Moderate handicap	23	50	13
Marked handicap	7	37	27

[a]Degree of recovery: depressed, no conduct problems vs. depressed, conduct disorder; χ^2 8.83, df 4, $p = 0.07$.

[b]Degree of handicap: depressed, no conduct problems vs. depressed, conduct disorder, χ^2 10.12, df 4, $p < 0.05$. Depressed conduct disorder vs. nondepressed conduct disorder, χ^2 6.04, df 4, $p = 0.19$.

Table 3 presents the comparison between depressed children without conduct problems, depressed children with CD, and nondepressed children from the control group with CD. On both measures of short-term outcome, depressed children with CD fared significantly worse than depressed children without conduct problems during their index episode. Indeed, depressed children with comorbid CD were more handicapped at the time of discharge than children with CD alone.

Adult Antisocial Outcomes

As Figure 1 illustrates, the depressed children with comorbid CD exhibited a higher rate of officially recorded criminality in adulthood than the depressed children without conduct problems. Over the follow-up period, the cumulative probabilities of adult criminality were 0.62 and 0.15, respectively, with the estimated relative risk of 6.25 being significantly different from 1 ($p < 0.001$). The nondepressed children with CD shared a similar pattern to that of the comorbid group

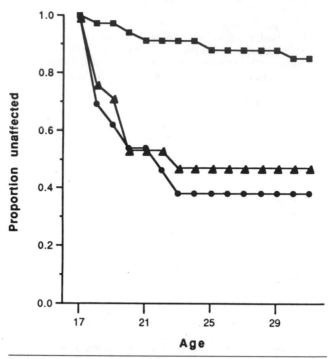

Figure 1. Survival from any adult criminal conviction. Depressed, no conduct problems ■; Depressed, conduct disorder ●; Conduct disorder, not depressed ▲.

with a cumulative probability of 0.53 and an estimated relative risk compared with the comorbid group of 0.70, not significantly different from 1 ($p = 0.5$).

Official criminal records tend to underestimate antisocial activity. Accordingly, the prevalence of antisocial personality disorder in adulthood was examined next, as measured by the SADS-L interview and RDC (adult criteria). Depressed children with CD had a much higher rate of adult antisocial personality disorder than depressed children without conduct problems (61% vs. 6%, χ^2 14.2, $p < 0.001$), similar to that of the children with CD alone (53%, $\chi^2 = 0.22$, $p = 0.64$).

Depressed children with CD were also at higher risk of alcohol abuse/dependence in adulthood than depressed children without conduct disturbance (cumulative probabilities 0.32 and 0.08, respectively, $p < 0.05$).

Adult Depressive Outcomes

Figure 2 shows that the outcomes of depressed children with CD and non-depressed children with CD were also similar when the risk of adult major depres-

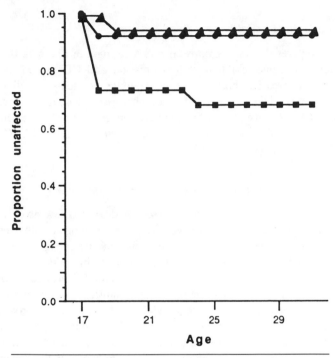

Figure 2. Survival from any adult criminal depression. Depressed, no conduct problems ■; Depressed, conduct disorder ●; Conduct disorder, not depressed ▲.

sive disorder was considered. Both these groups were at low risk for the development of major depression in adulthood (cumulative probabilities 0.08 and 0.06, respectively). Their relative risks of adult major depression compared with the depressed children without CD (cumulative probability of 0.32) were almost identical, 0.22 and 0.18, respectively, and did not differ significantly. However, the difference between depressed children without conduct problems and depressed children with CD failed to reach significance at the 5% level ($p = 0.09$).

Similar findings were obtained when the criterion was broadened so that any type of adult depressive disorder meeting RDC criteria was counted. Depressed children without conduct problems had a cumulative probability of 0.69 for the development of any RDC affective disorder in adulthood; whereas, depressed children with CD had a cumulative probability of 0.47 (relative risk 0.45, $p. = 0.06$).

Since the differential diagnosis of CD and bipolar disorder can be difficult, the relationship between CD in childhood and the subtype of affective disorder occurring in adulthood was examined. None of the five child depressives diagnosed in adulthood as bipolar I or II disorder had had CD as a child.

Social Functioning in Adulthood

Table 4 compares the three groups on APFA ratings. In line with the findings on short-term outcome, children with depression and CD tended to be more impaired than depressed children without conduct problems. In all six APFA domains, depressed children with CD had a higher mean score than depressed children without CD. However, the difference between the groups on the combination of APFA variables failed to reach significance at the 5% level (MANOVA, multivariate F statistic 1.93, $p = 0.10$).

Depressed Children with One to Two Conduct Problems

The analyses so far have compared depressed children who have no conduct problems with depressed children who have CD (three or more conduct problems). Clearly, the question arises as to the outcomes of the intermediate group of depressed children with one or two conduct problems in childhood.

The intermediate group closely resembled the group of depressed children without conduct problems on most of the outcome variables. Thus, on both measures of short-term outcome, depressed children with one to two conduct problems could not be distinguished from depressed children without conduct problems and had significantly better ($p < 0.05$) outcomes than depressed children with CD. Similarly, only 12% of depressed children with one to two conduct problems developed antisocial personality disorders in adulthood, a rate that was significantly lower than that found in depressed children with CD (χ^2 5.6, $p < 0.05$) and similar to the rate in depressed children without conduct problems (6%). The affective outcomes of the intermediate group were also very similar to the affective outcomes of depressed children without conduct problems. The cumulative probability of adult major depression in depressed children with one to two conduct problems was identical to that of depressed children with no conduct problems (0.32).

Comment

The two main systems for classifying child psychiatric disorders, *DSM-III-R* ICD-10 (World Health Organization, 1988), differ in their approach to the overlap between depression and CD. In *DSM-III-R,* there is no separate category for conditions characterized by both problems. Rather it is assumed that comorbidity between depression and CD represents the co-occurrence of separate conditions. The implication is that the presence of comorbidity does not alter the meaning of either of the two disorders. By contrast, in ICD-10, comorbid states showing a mixture of depression and conduct problems are separately coded as "depressive conduct disorder" (Rutter, 1989). Here, the assumption is that a mixed clinical picture

TABLE 4

Adult Personality Functioning Assessment (APFA) Ratings in Depressed Children without Conduct Problems, Depressed Children with Conduct Disorder, and Nondepressed Children with Conduct Disorder

APFA Domain Score	Depressed, No Conduct Problems (N = 34)		Depressed, Conduct Disorder (N = 13)		Nondepressed, Conduct Disorder (N = 16)	
	$\bar{X}$	SD	$\bar{X}$	SD	$\bar{X}$	SD
Work	2.4	1.5**	3.8	0.8	3.1	1.5
Intimate relationships	3.1	1.3	3.5	1.3	3.6	1.1
Friendships	2.1	1.4	2.8	1.6	3.0	1.3
Nonintimate social contacts	2.1	1.2	2.8	1.4	2.9	1.1
Negotiations	1.7	1.3	2.4	1.4	2.6	1.2
Practical coping	2.1	1.5	2.5	1.3	3.4	1.3
General social dysfunction, %	23		54		62	

Note: All APFA data were missing on one nondepressed subject with conduct disorder.
**Depressed no conduct problems vs. depressed conduct disorder $p < 0.01$.

is more likely to mean a single disorder with varied manifestations than several different disorders that happen to occur in the same individual at the same time.

When the "test" of adult antisocial outcomes was applied, the findings seemed to support the position that is implicit in *DSM-III-R*. The presence of depression during the index episode appeared to have little effect on the long-term course of the CD. The antisocial outcomes of depressed children with CD were very similar to those of nondepressed children with CD. These data are consistent with the findings of Kovacs and her colleagues (1988) who reported that depressed children who had ever had a CD were more likely to have had antisocial problems during the follow-up interval than depressed children without CD.

When depressive outcomes were considered, however, a different picture emerged. There was a strong trend for children with depression and CD to have lower rates of depression in adulthood than depressed children without conduct problems. This trend just failed to reach significance at the 5% level, but it should be noted that there was a fourfold difference between these groups in the cumulative probabilities of major adult depression (0.08 and 0.32, respectively). By contrast, the difference between the co-morbid group and the "pure" CD group (cumulative probabilities of 0.08 and 0.06, respectively) was not only a nonsignificant one but also trivial in absolute terms.

It seemed, then, that the negative mood state of children with CD and the depressive syndrome did not have the same prognostic implications as in "pure" cases of childhood depression. These findings suggest either that there is a nosologically distinct comorbid group, as ICD-10 suggests, or that depression is in some sense secondary to the conduct disturbance. The findings are incompatible with the hypothesis, that the conduct disturbance is part of the depression.

It should be borne in mind, nonetheless, that in some of these analyses, the cell sizes were small, and the significance levels were marginal. There is a need, therefore, to turn to other kinds of evidence in order to choose between these competing hypotheses.

Comorbidity with conduct problems did not appear to affect the depressive phenomenology that was recorded on the item sheets. On the other hand, rediagnosis of the charts, using the more restrictive criteria of the RDC, raised the possibility that the depressive conditions of children with CD were slightly atypical when compared with children with "pure" depression. That is, the charts of children with "pure" depression were more often diagnosed as meeting the criteria for RDC major depression than the charts of children with depression and CD, although this difference failed to reach significance.

It will be appreciated, however, that both the phenomenology of a disorder and its course may be influenced by many extraneous factors and should not, therefore, have overwhelming weight in classification. It is necessary to examine other, independent features that might permit differentiation between the groups. In this regard, family history variables are likely to be especially important since there is evidence that depressed juveniles have high familial rates of psychiatric disorders (Strober et al., 1988; Puig-Antich et al., 1989).

To the authors' knowledge, there has been just one published family history study of the links between childhood depression and CD. The findings were consistent with those of the present study in suggesting that there are important differences between children with "pure" depression and children with depression and CD. Puig-Antich et al. (1989) found that children with CD and major depression had lower rates of depression and alcoholism among relatives than depressed children without CD.

It is important to note that the present longitudinal study and the family study of Puig-Antich et al. (1989) were both based on relatively small numbers. A strong case exists, therefore, for replicating these studies with larger samples. Nonetheless, it is striking that these different forms of inquiry, in different places, and using different research methods, gave similar results. Children with depression and CD seem to differ from children with "pure" depression in respect to both longitudinal and familial correlates. If future research should confirm the reality of these differences, then the implication would be that mixed states of depression and CD should either be assigned to a separate diagnostic category or classified together with the conduct disorders. Clearly, the issue of how to deal with these mixed states in classification systems is one that requires further study.

REFERENCES

Anderson, J. C., Williams, S., McGee, R. & Silva, P. A. (1987), DSM-III disorders in preadolescent children: prevalence in a large sample from the general population. *Arch. Gen. Psychiatry,* 44:69–76.

Fleming, J. E., Offord, D. R. & Boyle, M. H. (1989), Prevalence of childhood and adolescent depression in the community. Ontario child health study. *Br. J. Psychiatry,* 155:647–654.

Garralda, M. E. (1984), Hallucinations in child disorders: I. The clinical phenomena. *Psychol. Med.,* 14:589–596.

Goodman, R. & Simonoff, E. (1990), Reliability of clinical ratings by trainee child psychiatrists. *J. Child Psychol. Psychiatry,* (in press).

Harrington, R. C. (1989), Child and adolescent depression: recent developments. *Current Opinion in Psychiatry, 2:480–483.*

———Hill, J., Rutter, M., John, K., Fudge, H., Zoccolillo, M. & Weissman, M. M. (1988), The assessment of lifetime psychopathology: a comparison of two interviewing styles. *Psychol. Med.,* 18:487–493.

———Fudge, H., Rutter, M., Pickles, A. & Hill, J. (1990), Adult outcomes of childhood and adolescent depression: I. psychiatric status. *Arch. Gen. Psychiatry,* 47:465–473.

Hill, J., Harrington, R. C., Fudge, H., Rutter, M. & Pickles, A. (1989), Adult Personality

Functioning Assessment (APFA): an investigator based standardized interview. *Br. J. Psychiatry*, 155:24–35.

Jacobsen, R. R. (1985), Child firesetters: a clinical investigation. *J. Child Psychol. Psychiatry*, 26:759–768.

Kashani, J. H., McGee, R. O., Clarkson, S. E. et al. (1983), Depression in a sample of 9-year-old children. *Arch. Gen. Psychiatry*, 40:1217–1223.

Kovacs, M., Paulauskas, S., Gatsonis, C. & Richards, C. (1988), Depressive disorders in childhood. III. A longitudinal study of comorbidity with and risk for conduct disorders. *J. Affective Disord.*, 15:205–217.

Marriage, K., Fine, S., Moretti, M. & Haley, G. (1986), Relationship between depression and conduct disorder in children and adolescents. *J. Am. Acad. Child Psychiatry*, 27:342–348.

Pearce, J. B. (1978), The recognition of depressive disorder in children. *J. R. Soc. Med.*, 71:494–500.

Puig-Antich, J. (1982), Major depression and conduct disorder in prepuberty. *J. Am. Acad. Child Adolesc. Psychiatry*, 21:118–128.

———Goetz, D., Davies, M. et al. (1989), A controlled family history study of prepubertal major disorder. *Arch. Gen. Psychiatry*, 46:406–418.

Robins, L. N. (1986), The consequences of conduct disorder in girls. In: *Development of Antisocial and Prosocial Behaviour: Research, Theories, and Issues*, eds. D. Olweus, J. Block & M. Radke-Yarrow, Orlando, FL: Academic Press Inc., pp. 385–414.

Rutter, M. (1989), Child psychiatric disorders in ICD-10. *J. Child Psychol. Psychiatry*, 30:499–513.

———Tizard, J. & Whitmore, K., (1970), *Education, Health and Behaviour*, London: Longman.

Spitzer, R. L. & Endicott, J. (1975), *Schedule for Affective Disorders and Schizophrenia-Lifetime Version*, New York: Biometrics Research.

——— ———Robins, E. (1978), Research Diagnostic Criteria: rationale and reliability. *Arch. Gen. Psychiatry*, 35:773–782.

Statistical Package for the Social Sciences (SPSS), Version X (1983), New York: McGraw-Hill.

Strober, M., Morrell, W., Burroughs, J., Lampert, C., Danforth, H. & Freeman, R. (1988), A family study of bipolar I disorder in adolescence: early onset of symptoms linked to increased familial loading and lithium resistance. *J. Affective Disord.*, 15:255–268.

Thorley, G. (1982), The Bethlem Royal and Maudsley Hospitals clinical data register for children and adolescents. *J. Adolesc.*, 5:179–189.

———(1987), Factor study of a psychiatric child rating scale: based on ratings made by clinicians on child and adolescent clinic attenders. *Br. J. Psychiatry*, 150:49–59.

World Health Organization (1988), *ICD-10 1988, draft of Chapter V: categories F00-F99, mental, behavioural and developmental disorders. Clinical descriptions and diagnostic guidelines*. Geneva: World Health Organization.

23

Anxiety Disorders of Childhood and Adolescence: A Critical Review

Gail A. Bernstein

University of Minnesota Medical School at Minneapolis

Carrie M. Borchardt

University of Minnesota Medical School at Minneapolis

The 1980s were a decade of advancement in the knowledge of anxiety disorders in children and adolescents; this sets the stage for research achievements in the 1990s. This review examines the anxiety disorders of childhood and adolescence (separation anxiety disorder, overanxious disorder, and avoidant disorder), including prevalency rates, demographic profiles, comparisons of clinical presentations in different developmental age groups, and panic disorder in children and adolescents are also evaluated. The controversy of whether panic attacks occur in prepubertal children is addressed. A brief review of behavioral and pharmacological treatment studies is included. Future directions for research are suggested.

The last decade brought a mushrooming of investigations and knowledge of anxiety disorders in children and adolescents. With this progress, there has been improvement in methodologies of the research. Recent epidemiological work has demonstrated that anxiety symptoms and disorders are one of the most common psychiatric problems in this age group. For these reasons, a critical review of the theories and research regarding anxiety disorders in childhood is timely.

Before launching into the body of this review, a few comments on the *DSM-III-R* classification of anxiety disorders are in order. In contrast to the classification of affective disorders and psychotic disorders, the anxiety disorders are separated into two different sections of the manual. The "anxiety disorders" section contains cri-

Reprinted with permission from the *Journal of the American Academy of Child and Adolescent Psychiatry,* 1991, Vol. 30, No. 4, 519–532. Copyright ©1991 by the American Academy of Child and Adolescent Psychiatry.

teria for panic disorder, agoraphobia, social phobia, simple phobia, obsessive-compulsive disorder, post-traumatic stress disorder, generalized anxiety disorder, and anxiety disorder not otherwise specified. All of these diagnoses can be used for children and adolescents. Studies of adult anxiety patients have centered around these disorders. The studies of anxiety disorders in childhood, however, have revolved around another section of *DSM-III-R:* "anxiety disorders of childhood or adolescence." These disorders include separation anxiety disorder, overanxious disorder, and avoidant disorder of childhood or adolescence. There is considerable overlap in symptoms between the anxiety disorders of both sections. In fact, at times, it is difficult to decide whether child or adult criteria should be employed (e.g., diagnosis of avoidant disorder versus social phobia or diagnosis of overanxious disorder versus generalized anxiety disorder).

The separation of anxiety disorders into two sections of *DSM-III-R* has produced in some ways an advancement and in other ways a slowing of research. In contrast to the study of depressive disorders in children, investigations of anxiety in children have taken place without the constraints of the adult criteria, providing data that might not otherwise be available. On the other hand, the childhood anxiety disorders have often been studied to the exclusion of the disorders seen in adults, leaving a development gap. This will become more evident as the review unfolds.

EPIDEMIOLOGY

In the past 5 years, there have been a number of epidemiological studies reporting the prevalence rates of anxiety disorders in nonreferred children and adolescents. In general, the methodologies of these studies are sound, and the investigations represent a great advance in knowledge. Overall, the results of these studies indicate that anxiety disorders are probably one of the most common, if not *the* most prevalent category of childhood and adolescent disorders.

In evaluating the results of prevalence studies, several characteristics of the studies must be considered, including whether the sample is derived from a clinical or nonclinical population. Because of referral biases, data from clinical samples may not be representative of the general population. The studies reported here are from general populations. Second, the age range of the subjects needs to be kept in mind, because studies of referred patients indicate that certain anxiety disorders are more common in young children and other anxiety disorders are more common in adolescents (e.g., separation anxiety disorder is more prevalent in prepubertal than postpubertal children) (Geller et al., 1985; Ryan et al., 1987).

A third criterion to evaluate is whether child report, parent report, or both are used in determining prevalence rates. There is low agreement between child and parent reports of prevalence rates of childhood anxiety disorders (Costello, 1989; Kashani and Orvaschel, 1990). In studies that use both child and parent reports

(Costello, 1989; Kashani and Orvaschel, 1990; McGee et al., 1990), the prevalence rates are higher, based on the children's reporting of symptoms compared with parents' reports. Fourth, the use of validated structured interviews for diagnosis should be noted. All the studies presented below employed such interviews with the exception of the Whitaker et al. study (1990) that was initiated before the availability of structured interviews for adolescents and the Bowen et al. study (1990) that used a symptom checklist that was later matched to *DSM-III-R* criteria.

Finally, several of the studies determine rates of disorders with and without the additional criterion of impairment in functioning (Bird et al., 1988; Kashani and Orvaschel, 1988). When a functional impairment criterion is included, the rates of disorders decrease (Bird et al., 1988; Kashani and Orvaschel, 1988). Functional impairment is a criterion necessary when making some *DSM-III-R* diagnoses (e.g., avoidant disorder, simple phobia) and helps clinicians avoid unnecessarily labeling anxiety as a "disorder" when the symptoms are not pathological. Although this technique assures identification of fewer false positive cases (Kashani and Orvaschel, 1990), it "may have the unintended effect of selecting for an unrepresentative subset of persons with a disorder, perhaps those with a more long-term course, thus distorting our picture of the natural history of the disorder and its correlates in the general population" (Whitaker et al., 1990, p. 493).

Two studies investigate rates of anxiety disorders in children (Anderson et al., 1987; Costello, 1989). In both studies, close to 800 children were screened. Anderson and colleagues (1987) evaluated 11-year-olds in New Zealand and found the following rates: 3.5% having separation anxiety disorder, 2.9% with overanxious disorder, 2.4% with simple phobia, and 1.0% with social phobia. Costello (1989) reported an overall rate of 8.9% in a sample of general pediatric patients (ages 7–11) meeting criteria for at least one anxiety disorder. This included 4.1% with separation anxiety disorder, 4.6% with overanxious disorder, 9.2% having simple phobia, 1.0% with social phobia, 1.6% with avoidant disorder, and 1.2% with agoraphobia.

Several epidemiological studies evaluate prevalence rates of anxiety disorders in adolescents. Kashani and Orvaschel (1988) interviewed a representative sample of 150 adolescents. The overall rate of adolescents having at least one anxiety disorder was 17.3%. However, this overall percentage decreased to 8.7% when the added criterion of clinical dysfunction requiring treatment was added, including 7.3% with overanxious disorder, 4.7% with simple phobia, and 0.7% with separation anxiety disorder. Whitaker et al. (1990) screened over 5,000 adolescents, interviewing 356 in the second stage of the study. Weighted prevalence estimates were based on the use of stratified random samples. Of the anxiety disorders, lifetime prevalence rates included 3.7% for generalized anxiety disorder and 0.6% for panic disorder. The weighted prevalence rates for obsessive-compulsive disorder in the same sample included 1.0% for current episode and 1.9% for lifetime disorder (Flament et al., 1988). McGee et al. (1990) evaluated close to 1,000 adolescents in New Zealand. The most prevalent disorder was overanxious disorder (5.9%); the second was nonaggressive conduct disorder (5.7%); and the third most common was simple phobia (3.6%), with the most common fears expressed being phobias related to speaking in front of the class, heights, airplanes, and being in the water.

Bird et al. (1988) in a Puerto Rican sample that included both children and adolescents found that 6.8% met criteria for separation anxiety disorder; this was reduced to 4.7% if a functional impairment criterion was added. In addition, 3.9% had simple phobias, which decreased to 2.6% if the maladjustment criterion was employed (Bird et al., 1988). Bowen et al. (1990) found rates of 3.6% for overanxious disorder and 2.4% for separation anxiety disorder in a sample of over 3,000 children and adolescents. Kashani and Orvaschel (1990) studied 70 subjects each of ages, 8, 12, and 17. Anxiety disorders were the most commonly diagnosed type of disorder across all three age groups. A greater percentage of 8-year-olds met criteria for separation anxiety disorder, whereas a greater percentage of 17-year-olds met criteria for overanxious disorder.

SEPARATION ANXIETY DISORDER

The essential feature of this disorder is excessive anxiety about separation from parents or attachment figures. Empirical reports have described separation from the mother as most problematic (Eisenberg, 1958; Johnson et al., 1941; Waldfogel et al., 1957). The separation reactions are extreme, beyond that expected for the child's developmental level. It should be remembered that separation anxiety is a normal developmental phenomenon from approximately age 7 months to the early preschool years. Three of nine criteria are needed to make the *DSM-III-R* diagnosis. These criteria include unrealistic worry about harm to self or to parents during periods of separation, school refusal, reluctance to sleep alone or to sleep away from home, avoidancy of being alone, recurrent nightmares with themes of separation, physical complaints and signs of distress in anticipation or at the time of separation (American Psychiatric Association, 1987).

In nonreferred prepubertal children, separation anxiety disorder is probably the most common of the childhood anxiety disorders (Anderson et al., 1987). The prevalence rate of separation anxiety disorder is lower in adolescents (Kashani and Orvashel, 1988, 1990) than in children. The adolescents with this disorder usually manifest school refusal and somatic complaints (Francis et al., 1987).

Some information is available about the demographic profile of children with separation anxiety disorder. The mean age of presentation of children with separation anxiety disorder to a clinic setting is significantly younger (9.1 years) than the mean age of presentation of children with overanxious disorder (13.4 years) (Last et al., 1987a). The same study showed a predominance of female children and primarily Caucasian children from lower socioeconomic families (Last et al., 1987a). In a study of 776 children in the general population (Velez et al., 1989), lower socioeconomic status was a significant risk factor for having separation anxiety disorder.

Developmental differences in the expression of separation anxiety symptoms in children and adolescent have been demonstrated. Francis et al. (1987) evaluated 45 children and adolescents with separation anxiety disorder. There were no differences between the responses of boys and girls to each of the nine criteria. However, there were differences among age groups with regard to which criteria were most frequently endorsed. Young children (ages 5–8) were most likely to report worries about unrealistic harm to attachment figures and school refusal, whereas children aged 9 to 12 more frequently endorsed excessive distress at times of separation. Adolescents (ages 13–16) most frequently reported school refusal and physical complaints. Nightmares about separation were commonly described by the young children but rarely reported by subjects aged 9 to 16. Diagnoses of separation anxiety disorder in young children were based on endorsement of a large number of symptoms, with the adolescents generally reporting the minimum of three symptoms (Francis et al., 1987). A recent study suggests that the separation anxiety fears of harm to self or to attachment figures are common in nonreferred children (Bell-Dolan et al., 1990). The extent to which children in the general population report separation anxiety symptoms has not been fully established; additional data are needed to support the required number of three symptoms now needed for a clinical diagnosis.

Specific types of fears expressed by children with separation anxiety disorder are different from those reported by children with other anxiety disorders. Last and colleagues (1989) administered the Fear Survey Schedule for Children—Revised (FSSC-R) (Ollendick, 1983) to children with separation anxiety disorder, to those with overanxious disorder, and to children with a phobia of school. Although the total fear score on the instrument did not differentiate the three groups, the specific types of fears differentiated the groups. Children with separation anxiety disorder most commonly endorsed a fear of getting lost. They also reported fears of germs/illness and bee stings. Overanxious children most often reported social and performance concerns (e.g., being criticized, being teased, and making mistakes). These fears reported by children with separation anxiety and overanxious disorders are not commonly reported by children in the general population (Ollendick et al., 1985).

Somatic complaints are not specific to children and adolescents with separation anxiety disorder. Children with psychosis and children with separation anxiety disorder reported a significantly greater number of physical symptoms than those with other diagnoses (Livingston et al., 1988). Regarding specific somatic symptoms, abdominal pain was significantly associated with depressive disorder, psychosis, and separation anxiety disorder. Palpitations were significantly more common in psychotic children and those with separation anxiety disorder compared with children with other psychiatric disorders.

Cantwell and Baker (1989) followed children an average of 4 years after initial evaluation in a speech and language clinic. Nine children (average age 3.6 years) initially were diagnosed with separation anxiety disorder. At follow-up, four were well, showing a recovery rate of 44%, and only one (11%) still met criteria for separation anxiety disorder. The remaining four subjects were diagnosed at follow-up with overanxious disorder and/or disruptive behavior disorders. The children with separation anxiety disorder had the youngest average age of all subjects at baseline presentation. Perhaps some of the children had normal separation anxiety rather than the disorder, explaining the high remission rate. Additionally, "it remains to be demonstrated whether diagnoses rendered in middle or later childhood are equally applicable during the preschool years" (Beitchman et al., 1987, p. 694).

Several authors (Ayauso et al., 1989; Gittelman and Klein, 1984; Klein, 1964; Zitrin and Ross, 1988) have commented on the relationship between separation anxiety disorder and agoraphobia or panic disorder. Many adults with agoraphobia report histories of separation anxiety in childhood (Berg et al., 1974; Klein, 1964; Zitrin and Ross, 1988). Similarly, children who exhibit severe distress upon separation from their parents may look panicky. However, there are no longitudinal studies extending into adulthood of children with separation anxiety disorder that can definitively answer the question as to whether separation anxiety disorder is a precursor to agoraphobia or panic disorder.

OVERANXIOUS DISORDER

In this anxiety disorder of childhood or adolescence, there is excessive anxiety that is not focused on a specific object or situation, and the anxiety is not a result of a recent stressor. These children are worriers. Four of the following seven criteria are needed: worry about future events, worry about past behavior, concern about competence, physical complaints, marked self-consciousness, continual need for reassurance, feelings of tension, and the inability to relax (American Psychiatric Association, 1987). A key criterion is the first one listed. All but two subjects in a sample of 55 children and adolescents with overanxious disorder endorsed having unrealistic worries about future events (Strauss et al., 1988b).

Demographic characteristics of referred children with this disorder include an older age at presentation than children with separation anxiety disorder (Last et al., 1987a) (see the section on separation anxiety disorder). In this study, approximately the same number of girls and boys met criteria for overanxious disorder. In addition, the sample of overanxious children included only Caucasians, although 35% of the children referred to the institution in which the study was conducted were black. There was an overrepresentation of children from middle- and upper-class families (Last et al., 1987a). On the other hand, the epidemiological study by Bowen and colleagues (1990) reported a female predominance in this disorder.

In contrast to separation anxiety disorder, older children and adolescents with overanxious disorder endorse significantly more symptoms than younger children (McGee, 1990; Strauss et al., 1988b). In the Strauss et al. study (1988b), the subjects were divided into a younger group of children (ages 5–11) and an older group of children and adolescents (ages 12–19). Sixty-six percent of the older group reported greater than five symptoms compared with 35% of the younger group reporting greater than five symptoms. The criterion of worry about past behavior was significantly more common in the older group (Strauss et al., 1988b).

Comorbid diagnoses included attention deficit hyperactivity disorder (in 35%) and separation anxiety disorder (in 70%) of the younger children and simple phobia (in 41%) and major depressive episode (in 47%) of the older group. The older group had elevated anxiety scores on the State Trait Anxiety Inventory for Children (Spielberger, 1973) and Revised Children's Manifest Anxiety Scale (Reynolds and Richman, 1978) and elevated depression scores on the Children's Depression Inventory (Kovacs and Beck, 1987), whereas the younger children with overanxious disorder did not show elevation on these scales compared with a normative sample (Strauss et al., 1988b).

Overanxious disorder symptoms are common in children in the general population (Achenbach et al., 1989; Bell-Dolan et al., 1990). Based on the finding that 66% of teenagers with this disorder in a clinic sample endorsed six or seven of the possible seven symptoms (Strauss et al., 1988b), perhaps more than five symptoms should be required for a diagnosis.

Regarding stability of the disorder, the follow-up study of young children referred to a speech and language clinic (Cantwell and Baker, 1989) included eight children (mean age of 7.3 years) with overanxious disorder. This anxiety disorder had the lowest recovery rate, with only two children (25%) completely well at a 4-year follow-up. Two were diagnosed with overanxious disorder at follow-up (25% stability). The remaining subjects were rediagnosed with avoidant disorder ($N = 21$), major depression ($N = 1$) and disruptive behavior disorders ($N = 3$). One of the above children met criteria for both avoidant disorder and attention deficit hyperactivity disorder. Because the mean age of presentation of overanxious disorder in Last and colleagues' study was 13.4 years (1987a), the young sample studied by Cantwell and Baker (1989) may not be representative of referred overanxious children.

AVOIDANT DISORDER

The essential feature of this disorder is avoidance of contact with unfamiliar persons that is severe enough to interfere with social relationships; yet there is a desire for social contact with family members and other familiar persons (American

Psychiatric Association, 1987). The diagnosis is not made before age 2-1/2 years because stranger anxiety is a normal developmental phenomenon up to this age. There is some overlap in symptoms with children who meet the criteria for social phobia.

There has been little research on this disorder compared with separation anxiety disorder and overanxious disorder. This disorder has been cited as comorbid with other anxiety disorders. In a clinical sample, 4.5% of the children and adolescents with separation anxiety disorder also met criteria for avoidant disorder, and 27.3% of those with overanxious disorder also were diagnosed with avoidant disorder (Last et al., 1989). It has been suggested that children with avoidant disorder almost invariably have an additional concurrent anxiety disorder—commonly, overanxious disorder (Klein and Last, 1989).

In the Cantwell and Baker study (1989), 14 children (mean age of 5.0 years) were diagnosed has having avoidant disorder. At follow-up, four (29%) met criteria for the same diagnosis, and five (36%) were completely well. The most common other follow-up diagnoses were overanxious disorder ($N = 4$), dysthymia ($N = 2$), and disruptive behavior disorders ($N = 3$). Of the six children who were ill at follow-up with other diagnoses, three had multiple diagnoses. Beitchman's follow-up study (1987) of 98 children in a therapeutic nursery school identified four children at baseline with avoidant disorder. Overall, the children with emotional disorders (anxiety and depressive disorders) had the lowest diagnostic stability rates of all categories studied (Beitchman et al., 1987).

FEARS AND SIMPLE PHOBIAS

The essential feature of a simple phobia is the specific, isolated, persistent fear of a circumscribed stimulus, not specifically fear of separation (as in separation anxiety disorder), fear of strangers (as in avoidant disorder), fear of humiliation or embarrassment in social settings (social phobia), or fear of having a panic attack. The diagnosis is made only if the associated avoidance behavior interferes with the normal functioning of the child (American Psychiatric Association, 1987). Because of their cognitive level of development, children, in contrast to adults, may not recognize the irrational nature of their phobias (Silverman and Nelles, 1990). There are a limited number of studies employing *DSM-III-R* criteria for assessment of simple phobias in children and adolescents (Anderson et al., 1987; Bird et al., 1988; McGee et al., 1990). However, there are a moderate number of studies evaluating fears in children. Conclusions from reviewing these studies are that mild fears are quite common in children of all ages (Silverman and Nelles, 1990). In addition, girls report more fears than boys (Ollendick et al, 1985; Silverman and Nelles, 1989) and the influence of age and socioeconomic class is inconclusive (Silverman and Nelles, 1990).

When the FSSC-R (Ollendick, 1983) has been used, it has been demonstrated that girls report significantly more fears ($N = 18$) than boys ($N = 10$) (Ollendick et al., 1989). Children aged 7 to 10 endorsed significantly more specific fears than 11- to 13-year-olds or 14- to 16-year-olds (Ollendick et al., 1989). Both American and Australian children reported the same average number of fears. Girls scored significantly higher on their total fear score compared with boys on the FSSC-R, with 7- to 10-year-olds scoring significantly higher than 11- to 13- and 14- to 16-year-olds (Ollendick et al., 1989).

The 10 most common fears endorsed were being hit by a car, not being able to breathe, a bombing attack, getting burned by fire, falling from a high place, burglar breaking into the house, earthquake, death, getting poor grades, and snakes. These common fears were similar to those reported by Scherer and Nakamura (1968), using the nonrevised version of the FSSC. These common fears were remarkably consistent throughout the different age, gender, and cultural groups studied (Ollendick et al., 1989). Because the types of fears are similar across different age groups, it appears that some childhood fears may not be transitory (Ollendick et al., 1985).

Although mild fears are quite common, phobias are more unusual. Agras et al. (1969) evaluated 325 children and adults, using data from multiple sources. The rate of "mild" phobias was 7.5%, and the rate of "severe" phobias was 0.2%. The prevalence rates of simple phobias in epidemiological studies are similar with rates of 2.4% in children (Anderson et al., 1987), 3.6% in adolescents (McGee et al., 1990), and 2.6% in a sample of children and adolescents (Bird et al., 1988).

The age of onset of phobias may vary depending on the type of phobia (Marks and Gelder, 1966). A retrospective study reported that specific animal phobias started before five, whereas social phobias (e.g., eating in public, being the center of attention) had an onset after puberty. Other specific situational phobias (e.g., heights, darkness, storms) had a variable age of onset.

Regarding the natural courses of childhood fears and phobias, mild fears and phobias often represent transient developmental phenomena (Silverman and Nelles, 1990). However, a subset of children with simple phobias have persistent symptoms. In following 30 untreated children and adults with simple phobias, Agras et al. (1972) reported that 100% of those under 20 improved, whereas only 43% of the adults improved. When Ollendick (1979) reinterpreted the data, it was determined that only 40% of those under 20 were truly free of symptoms. Thus some simple phobias appear to continue from childhood into the adult years.

OBSESSIVE-COMPULSIVE DISORDER

Obsessions are recurrent, persistent thoughts that are experienced as intrusive and senseless. Compulsions are repetitive, purposeful behaviors, or rituals. To meet criteria for obsessive-compulsive disorder, either obsessions or compulsions and their associated features are present (American Psychiatric Association, 1987). The symptoms of obsessive-compulsive disorder are practically identical in children and adults (Berg et al., 1989). From one-third to one-half of adults with obsessive-compulsive disorder report the onset in childhood or adolescence.

Several studies indicate a male predominance in this disorder in referred children and adolescents (Hollingsworth, 1980; Last and Strauss, 1989a; Rapoport, 1986; Swedo et al., 1989). However, in the epidemiological study of adolescent obsessive-compulsive disorder (Flament et al., 1988) and in a recent study of referred children and adolescent with this disorder (Riddle et al., 1990), the male predominance was not replicated, with approximately equal numbers of males and females with the disorder in each sample.

Flament and colleagues (1988) reported a mean age of 16.2 years in their nonreferred sample of high school students with obsessive-compulsive disorder, with average age of onset at 12.8 years. Although onset was usually gradual, in some cases it was sudden. Rapoport (1986) previously described the disorder occurring in children with no premorbid obsessive-compulsive traits. Only four of 20 teenagers in the sample (Flament et al., 1988) had received any psychiatric treatment, including three for associated anxiety and/or depressive symptoms who did not reveal any of their obsessive-compulsive symptoms.

The most commonly reported obsessions were fear of contamination in 35% and thoughts of harm to self and familiar figures in 30% (Flament et al., 1988). The most frequent compulsions were washing and cleaning rituals in 75%, checking behavior in 40%, and straightening in 35%. Obsessions without rituals were rare, occurring in only one of the 20 adolescents. Teenagers with multiple obsessions and compulsions were common (Flament et al., 1988). A follow-up of the sample showed that a previous diagnosis of obsessive-compulsive disorder or of another psychiatric disorder with obsessive-compulsive features predicted obsessive-compulsive disorder 2 years later (Berg et al., 1989).

Last and Strauss (1989a) evaluated 20 referred children with obsessive-compulsive disorder, with a mean age at evaluation of 12.7 years and a mean age at onset of 10.7 years. Boys in their sample reported a significantly earlier age of onset than girls (9.5 versus 12.6 years). Sixteen of 20 reported rituals. Four had obsessions only. The most common rituals were washing, arranging objects, checking, and counting. Half of the children with compulsions reported multiple rituals.

Riddle and colleagues (1990) studied 21 referred children with a mean age at evaluation of 12.2 years; the mean age at onset was 90.0 years. Nineteen reported obsessions and compulsions. Two subjects had only compulsions. The most common obsessions were thoughts of contamination in 52%, aggressive or violent images in 38%, and somatic concerns in 38%, The most prevalent rituals included repeating in 76%, washing in 67%, ordering in 62%, and checking in 57%.

Please refer to the risk factors section for discussion of the association of obsessive-compulsive disorder with Tourette's disorder and reports of subtle neurological findings in children and adolescents with obsessive-compulsive disorder.

PANIC DISORDER

In panic disorder, the essential feature is discrete panic attacks. At least some of the panic attacks are not precipitated by events and occur unexpectedly, and they must be associated with at least four out of 13 characteristic symptoms. Ten of these symptoms are somatic, and three are psychological (American Psychiatric Association, 1987).

In the Environmental Catchment Area studies, the prevalence of panic disorder was found to be 0.6% to 1.0% in the community adult samples (Von Korff et al., 1985). About 3% of the entire sample reported having a panic attack within the previous 6 months. Age of onset of the first panic attack peaked at 15 to 19 years.

Relatives of patients with panic disorder have a higher risk of panic disorder and panic attacks than relatives of controls (Crowe et al., 1983). A twin study also provides evidence for the heritability of panic attacks (Torgersen, 1983). Monozygotic twins are five times more likely to be concordant for anxiety disorders with panic attacks than dizygotic twins.

Does panic disorder exist in prepubertal children? This is a controversial question. Some psychiatric disorders are rare before puberty, presumably because of developmental, structural, and neuroendocrine changes in the brain that occur at puberty. Such disorders include bipolar disorder schizophrenia, substance abuse, and behaviors, such as suicide attempts. On the other hand, perhaps panic disorder in children is missed because of the separation in our classification system between childhood and adult anxiety disorders. Most of the instruments for measuring anxiety disorders in childhood do not adequately screen for panic disorder, including two of the most commonly used structured interviews, the Diagnostic Interview for Children and Adolescents-Revised (Reich and Welner, unpublished instrument, 1990) and the Kiddie-Schedule for Affective Disorders and Schizophrenia for School-Age Children (Chambers et al., 1985).

Panic disorder occurs in adolescence (Alessi et al., 1987; Black and Robbins, 1990; Last and Strauss, 1989b; Moreau et al., 1989). Last and Strauss (1989b) found a prevalence of 9.6% for panic disorder in 177 consecutive admissions to their outpatient child and adolescent anxiety disorder clinic. All but one of the 17 panic disordered patients were postpubertal (Tanner 3 or 4).

The occurrence of panic attacks and panic-like symptoms in "prepubertal" children has been reported (Alessi and Magen, 1988; Ballenger et al., 1989; Enzer and Walker, 1967; Garland and Smith, 1990; Last and Strauss, 1989b: Moreau et al.,

1989). Because none of these studies reported pubertal status, this is an assumption based upon subject age. This assumption must be maintained with caution, however, because girls as young as 9 years can experience menarche, and adrenarche (early pubertal changes in the adrenal gland associated with secretion of adrenal hormones) precedes obvious secondary sex characteristics by 1 to 2 years. The studies cited above report on only nine children with panic disorder who were evaluated under the age of 11. A recent study (Vitiello et al., 1990) describes six prepubertal children (Tanner 1 or 2) with panic disorder. Age at diagnosis ranged from 8 to 13 years, with an average of 3 years from onset of the disorder to diagnosis. There was a positive family history of panic disorder in all patients.

Perhaps panic disorder in childhood is rare because, although children have symptoms of panic, they do not have spontaneous panic attacks. *DSM-III-R* criteria for panic disorder specify that at least some panic attacks must be spontaneous in order to have panic disorder. This criterion may be justified since there is some evidence that people who have uncued panic attacks have more severe symptoms than those who have only cued attacks. A self-report survey of 660 high school and college students found that those who endorsed spontaneous attacks reported greater severity of attacks, more depression, and greater lifestyle change as a result of the attacks (Macaulay and Kelinknecht, 1989). Another survey of college students found similar results. Those with spontaneous panic attacks had more attacks and more severe feelings of unreality and tachycardia (Norton et al., 1986). However, both of these studies found much higher rates of panic attacks than were found in the Environmental Catchment Area studies, where subjects were actually interviewed, raising doubt about the validity of what the students were rating as panic attacks.

Nelles and Barlow (1988) speculated that children are not capable of spontaneous panic attacks because they lack necessary cognitive development. They divided panic into a somatic component, which children do experience, and a cognitive-attributional component, which they do not. They take a Piagetian developmental perspective to explain how attributions of internal causality, which they believe to be necessary for the cognitive component of panic, are not present until the more abstract cognitive stages of development are reached in adolescence. Therefore, children will attribute their somatic symptoms of panic to external events or objects, whereas adolescents will begin to attribute such symptoms to internal sensations and feelings, thereby setting the stage for spontaneous attacks.

Similarly, some have divided anxiety disorders into "exogeneous" and "endogenous" disorders (Sheehan et al., 1981; Thyer et al., 1985). The exogenous disorders are phobic disorders without spontaneous panic attacks. The endogenous disorders are those with spontaneous panic attacks. Both of these studies showed the exogenous disorders to have a younger age of onset, predominantly preadolescent, whereas onset for the endogenous disorders was primarily in adolescence and young adulthood. The authors theorize that the exogenous disorders are a result of traumatic exposures whereas endogenous anxiety disorders are biological in their pathogenesis.

POST-TRAUMATIC STRESS DISORDER

Post-traumatic stress disorder is a disorder that has been more extensively studied in adults than in children (e.g., adult males who have been exposed to combat stress). Most of the research has been done on Vietnam war veterans. The *DSM-III-R* criteria for post-traumatic stress disorder include some symptoms that are typical of depression (insomnia, poor concentration, diminished interest in activities, restricted range of affect, irritability), anxiety (nightmares, avoidance, hypervigilance, exaggerated startle response, autonomic reactivity), and dissociation (flashbacks).

In childhood, there are situations in which individuals are exposed to a single traumatic event and also situations in which children are exposed to repeated trauma over a period of time, such as with child physical and sexual abuse. These two types of trauma will be examined separately.

In studying the victims of the Chowchilla school-bus kidnapping, Terr (1981, 1983, 1985) described differences between post-traumatic stress symptoms caused by a one-time traumatic event in childhood and post-traumatic stress in adults. In general, children over the age of 3 to 4 do not become amnesic for the traumatic events, and they do not demonstrate psychic numbing; nor do they experience sudden intrusive visual flashbacks or suffer prolonged effects on school or work performance, as adults do. However, unlike adults, they commonly engage in post-traumatic play and reenactment behavior. They also show more distortion in sense of time and a particularly striking foreshortened view of the future.

A study of the children exposed to a single violent event, a sniper attack on an elementary school playground, validated the existence of post-traumatic stress disorder in childhood (Pynoos et al., 1987). This incident resulted in the deaths of one child and a passerby and injuries in 13 children. Results of the evaluations of 159 randomly selected children were analyzed by degree of proximity to the event. Proximity was significantly correlated with severity of symptomatology, and the most severely symptomatic children reported the full range of *DSM-III* post-traumatic stress disorder symptoms. The symptoms that best differentiated children with moderate to severe reactions from those with little to no reactions were intrusiveness, emotional constriction and avoidance of reminders of the trauma. The symptoms that most differentiated severe from moderate reactions were disturbances of sleep and concentration.

Childhood physical and sexual abuse is a more complicated trauma to study. These types of trauma may occur over long periods of time and in families with other disadvantages, such as poverty, child neglect, parent alcoholism, and drug abuse (Lynch et al., 1975; Oliver, 1985, 1988; Widom, 1989). Because abuse commonly occurs over time, the normal development of the child would be expected to be more disrupted than in the case of a single traumatic event where the child was presumably normal before the experience.

Studies of child abuse victims have shown that they may develop typical symptoms of post-traumatic stress disorder (Adams-Tucker, 1982; Kiser et al., 1988; McLeer et al., 1988). McLeer et al. found 48% of sexually abused children in their sample of 31 met *DSM-III-R* criteria for post-traumatic stress disorder. In this sample, 75% of those abused by biological fathers, 25% of those abused by trusted adults, and none of the children abused by an older child met criteria for post-traumatic stress disorder. In a study of young children sexually abused at a day-care center, Kiser et al. (1988) reported subsequent sexual acting-out in day-care settings and the development of typical childhood fears and specific trauma-related fears.

Finally, it appears that there may be a familial predisposition for developing post-traumatic stress disorder. Studies of the offspring of Holocaust survivors have indicated that these individuals are more prone to symptoms and post-traumatic stress disorder when exposed to stress or trauma than people who are not the offspring of severe trauma victims (Solomon et al., 1988). In a study of young adults, risk factors for developing post-traumatic stress disorder after exposure included early separation from parents, neuroticism, preexisting anxiety and depression, and a family history of anxiety disorder (Breslau et al., 1991).

COMORBIDITY

The association of children and adolescents having concurrent anxiety and depressive disorders has been reported in the general population (Anderson et al., 1987; Kashani and Orvaschel, 1988; McGee et al., 1990) and in clinic samples (Bernstein, 1991; Bernstein and Garfinkel, 1986; Geller et al., 1985; Mitchell et al., 1988; Puig-Antich and Rabinovich, 1986; Ryan et al., 1987; Strauss et al., 1988a; Weissman et al., 1987).

Two large epidemiological studies show similar findings. In the survey involving children, 17% of the children with anxiety disorders also met criteria for major depression. The Kashani and Orvaschel (1988) study of 150 adolescents reported a much higher comorbidity rate, with 69% (9/13) of those with an anxiety disorder associated with functional impairment also having a major depression.

Greater than 40% of referred children and adolescents with a major depressive episode have concurrent anxiety disorders, with separation anxiety disorder being the most common anxiety disorder associated with major depression (Kovacs et al., 1989; Mitchell et al., 1988; Ryan et al., 1987). Strauss and associates (1988a) identified 28% of their anxiety disorder patients as having major depression. The anxiety disorder patients with a concurrent diagnosis of major depression were more

likely to meet criteria for multiple anxiety diagnoses (Strauss et al., 1988a). In referrals to a school refusal clinic, 47% of those with anxiety disorders also had major
depression (Bernstein, 1991).

Children with concurrent anxiety and depressive disorders are significantly older
at presentation than those with anxiety disorders only (Bernstein, 1991; Strauss
et al., 1988a). In addition, the comorbidity of anxiety and depressive disorders in
children and adolescents is associated with increased severity of both anxiety
(Bernstein, 1991; Strauss et al., 1988a) and depressive symptomatology (Bernstein,
1991; Mitchell et al., 1988), compared with children with pure anxiety or pure
depressive disorders. Kovacs and colleagues (1989) found that psychopathology
and poor physical health were significantly more common in mothers of children
with comorbid anxiety and depressive disorders compared with mothers of children
with depression only.

The association of anxiety disorders and attention deficit hyperactivity disorder
has been reported in epidemiological studies (Anderson et al., 1987; Bird et al.,
1988) and in clinic samples of children with anxiety disorders (Last et al., 1987a;
Strauss et al., 1988b). In addition, it has been reported that children of parents with
panic disorder or major depression are significantly more likely to meet criteria
for attention deficit disorder than children of parents with no diagnosis (McClellan
et al., 1990).

Last and colleagues (1987d) have examined patterns of comorbidity of anxiety
disorders in children. Children and adolescents with primary overanxious disorder
compared with those with primary separation anxiety disorder are more likely to
have another disorder, especially simple phobia, panic disorder (Last et al., 1987a),
social phobia, or avoidant disorder (Last et al., 1987d). Approximately a third of
the children with a primary diagnosis of separation anxiety disorder have a concurrent diagnosis of overanxious disorder (Last et al., 1987d). In these studies, the
primary diagnosis is defined as the disorder causing the greatest functional impairment and the disorder that was targeted first for intervention. Thirty-six percent
($N = 16$) of the 44 children with anxiety disorders in the recent study by Kashani
and Orvaschel (1990) met criteria for two or more anxiety disorders.

What explains the comorbidity patterns: Three hypotheses are offered by Kashani
and Orvaschel (1990) regarding comorbidity patterns among children with anxiety
disorders. These explanations include the following: 1) having one type of anxiety
serves as a risk factor for other types of anxiety, 2) different types of anxiety have
the same underlying pathogenesis or nonspecific risk factors, and 3) symptoms
of different anxiety disorders overlap, and therefore children meet criteria for more
than one diagnosis.

Similar hypotheses could be presented to explain the comorbidity of anxiety and
depressive disorders. In fact, some researchers believe that anxiety and depressive
disorders are on a continuum and represent different manifestations of the same

underlying abnormality. This is referred to as the "unitary model" (Stavrakaki and Vargo, 1986) or the "dimensional approach" (Kovacs et al., 1989).

RISK FACTORS

The cause of childhood anxiety disorders is still poorly understood. However, there are preliminary data to guide future investigations. Environmental stress appears to be associated with the manifestation of anxiety symptoms. A significantly higher number of environmental stressors, as measured on the Life Events Checklist (Johnson and McCutcheon, 1980), have been reported by children (Kashani et al., 1990) and adolescents (Bernstein et al., 1989) with high levels of anxiety compared with those having low levels of anxiety. In fact, researchers have suggested that conditioning by environmental stress is prominent in the development of simple phobias (Sheehan et al., 1981; Thyer et al., 1985). Severe, extraordinary trauma is the event that precedes the development of post-traumatic stress disorder.

There is a growing body of literature documenting the familiar patterns in anxiety disorders. Studies of offspring of adults with anxiety disorders as well as studies of the first-degree relatives of children with anxiety disorders, have been completed. Controlled studies of adult anxiety disorder patients show an increased prevalence rate of anxiety disorders in the offspring (Turner et al., 1987; Weissman et al., 1984). Weissman and colleagues (1984) demonstrated an elevated rate of separation anxiety disorder in children of mothers with major depression plus panic disorder or agoraphobia compared with children of normals or children of mothers with major depression only. A limitation of this investigation is that diagnoses in children were made by family history data rather than by direct child interviews.

Offspring of adults with anxiety disorder (obsessive-compulsive disorder or agoraphobia), of adults with dysthymia, and of adults with no diagnoses were compared with normal school children, using structured interviews (Turner et al., 1987). Children of parents with anxiety disorders were seven times as likely to be diagnosed with a *DSM-III-R* anxiety disorder as children in the two normal groups and twice as likely to meet criteria for an anxiety disorder as children of dysthymics.

An intriguing study showed that the children of adults with panic disorder or agoraphobia are more likely to have "behavioral inhibition to the unfamiliar" (Kagan et al., 1984) than the offspring of parents without these anxiety disorders (Rosenbaum et al., 1988). Behavioral inhibition in 2- to 7-year-olds was measured by parameters, such as a long latency to start to speak spontaneously to an examiner and low frequency of spontaneous verbalizations. These extremely cautious children with a tendency to withdrawal and autonomic arousal in unfamiliar situations appear to be at risk for the development of anxiety disorders in childhood (Biederman et al., 1990).

Last and colleagues (1987b,c) have evaluated the mothers of children with anxiety disorders. There were significantly higher rates of current and lifetime anxiety disorders in mothers of anxiety disorder children ($N = 58$) compared with the mothers of psychiatric controls ($N = 58$) compared with the mothers of psychiatric controls ($N = 15$), using a semistructured interview (Last et al., 1987b). In comparing mothers of children with separation anxiety disorder, mothers of children with overanxious disorder, and mothers of psychiatric controls, a specific relationship was found between overanxious disorder in children and their mothers (Last et al., 1987c). A higher prevalence rate of overanxious disorder in childhood (42%) was reported by mothers of children with overanxious disorder compared with the other two groups of mothers. However, the mothers of children with separation anxiety disorder did not show a higher rate of separation anxiety disorder than the other two groups.

In a pedigree study of a small group of school refusers with both major depression and anxiety disorder, structured interviews of parents and siblings showed high rates of anxiety and depressive disorders compared with the families of children in the psychiatric control group (Bernstein and Garfinkel, 1988).

The above studies document the familial pattern in anxiety disorders but do not address the question of biological versus environmental factors and their contribution to anxiety disorders in children. Family studies show that "if a higher frequency of a disorder is not observed among biological relatives, then genetic factors can not be involved" (Klein and Last, 1989, p. 97). Answers regarding hereditary contribution will come through twin studies, adoption studies, segregation analyses, and genetic linkage studies.

Studies of the genetics of Tourette's disorder suggest a biological relationship between some cases of obsessive-compulsive disorder and Tourette's disorder (Pauls and Leckman, 1986). Researchers have described an increased rate of obsessive-compulsive disorder in children with Tourette's disorder (Grad et al., 1987) and in their first-degree relatives (Pauls et al., 1986), compared with the controls and in the families of controls. Segregation analyses of data collected by direct family interviews of all first-degree relatives of probands with Tourette's syndrome (Pauls and Leckman, 1986) suggest that obsessive-compulsive disorder is part of the genetically mediated spectrum of Tourette's syndrome, and Tourette's syndrome is transmitted as a sex-influenced, autosomal dominant trait.

The role of neurological differences in children with anxiety disorders has been examined in children and adolescents with obsessive-compulsive disorder. Behar et al. (1984) found a significantly higher mean ventricular-brain ratio on CAT scans in 16 obsessive-compulsive disorder children and adolescents compared with the matched control group. The experimental group also displayed spatial-perceptual deficits on neuropsychological testing compared with controls. However, the patients' neuropsychological results did not correlate with the CAT scan findings. Subsequent studies in children and adolescents with obsessive-compulsive disorder showed subtle impairment of right hemispheric functions on neuropsychological tests (Cox et al., 1989) and abnormalities on neurological examination, including left hemisyndrome, chroieform syndrome, and neurodevelopmental differences (Denckla, 1989).

Lastly, there are developmental differences in the expression of the anxiety disorders. Children and adolescents with overanxious disorder and separation anxiety disorder show specific characteristics in different age groups, and certain fears and phobias are more common at different ages. Furthermore, panic disorder generally develops after puberty. These observations indicate that there may be certain "at risk" times for the expression of specific anxiety symptoms (Lein and Last, 1989).

BEHAVIORAL TREATMENT

School Refusal

Up to 75% to 80% of school refusers may manifest separation anxiety (Berney et al, 1981; Gittelman and Klein, 1984). School refusers may present with separation anxiety disorder and/or overanxious disorder, with or without major depression (Bernstein, 1991). A number of case reports and two comparative studies evaluate behavioral treatments for school refusal.

The behavioral conceptualization of school refusal is based on classical and operant conditioning models (Trueman, 1984). Theorists using the classical conditioning model describe anxiety as a learned conditioned response to either stimuli in the school environment or separation from caregivers (Garvey and Hegrenes, 1966; Patterson, 1965; Yates, 1970). Classical conditioning based interventions include systematic desensitization and exposure and flooding procedures (Wolpe, 1982). Case studies report success with classical conditioning treatment procedures for school refusal (Croghan, 1981; McNamara, 1988; Miller, 1972).

Theorists supporting the operant conditioning model hypothesize that the school refusing child receives positive and negative reinforcement for not attending school (Doleys and Williams, 1977). The operant conditioning treatment strategies involve rearranging contingencies in the family and school environments to facilitate the child's attendance at school (e.g., child is positively reinforced for school attendance or receives negative consequences for nonattendance). Case studies employing operant behavioral techniques describe success with school refusal children (Asyllon et al., 1970; Brown et al., 1974; Doleys and Williams, 1977; Hersen, 1970; Kolko, 1987; McNamara, 1988; Patterson, 1965). A combination of cognitive and operant behavioral therapy was reported to be efficacious in the treatment of two children with separation anxiety (Mansdorf and Lukens, 1987). The cognitive therapy included the teaching of coping self-statements to the children and also included cognitive restructuring of the parents' distorted perceptions about their children.

Two comparative studies suggest the efficacy of behavioral methods in treating school refusers. Blagg and Yule (1984) compared a combination of classical and operant methods *(N* = 30), hospitalization (*N* = 16), and home tutoring and psychotherapy (*N* = 20). The average duration of treatment was 2.5 weeks for the behavioral treatment group, 45 weeks for the inpatient group, and 72 weeks for the home tutoring. Children in the behavioral treatment group showed more improvement than the other two groups on measures of self-esteem and extroversion. At follow-up, about 1 year later, 83%, 31%, and 0%, respectively, of the children in the three treatment groups were attending school regularly. Miller et al. (1972) compared systematic desensitization, psychotherapy, and waiting list for childhood phobias (69% had "school phobia"). Parental ratings showed both active treatments to be superior to waiting list in reducing fears in the children. However, clinician ratings showed no differences among the three groups after treatment. In the Miller et al. study (1972), subjects were randomized to the three treatments, but subjects in the Blagg and Yule study (1984) were not randomly assigned.

Kearney and Silverman (1990a) are the first to examine prescriptive cognitive and behavioral treatment for school refusal. Seven children and adolescents were evaluated with the School Refusal Assessment Scale, an instrument designed to identify variables maintaining the school refusal behavior, including fearfulness/general overanxiousness, escape from aversive social situations, attention getting or separation anxiety, and tangible reinforcement. Based on this functional assessment, one of the above variables was identified as predominant, and the subjects' symptoms were treated with one of the following methods: relaxation therapy/systematic desensitization, modeling and cognitive restructuring, shaping and differential reinforcement of other behavior, and contingency contracting for each of the above variables, respectively. Six of the seven subjects maintained full-time attendance after treatment and at 6-month followup.

Overanxious Disorder

Strauss (1988) has suggested that relaxation techniques and cognitive therapy be evaluated for treatment of overanxious disorder. Kim and Kendall (1989) treated four children with overanxious disorder with cognitive-behavioral therapy and all showed improvement on clinician, parent, and self-report rating scales. In general, gains were maintained at follow-up, 3 to 6 months later.

Fears and Phobias

The treatment studies of fears have focused on nighttime fears, fear of medical or dental procedures, and anxiety about public speaking. Most studies have included anxious children without documented anxiety disorders.

The techniques used to treat fears include the classical conditioning procedures of systematic desensitization, implosion, flooding, and modeling. Also, operant procedures of contingency management (including positive/negative reinforcement, shaping and extinction) have been employed (Silverman and Kearney, in press). Cognitive behavioral interventions have also been used to treat fears. Cognitive techniques for fear reduction focus on teaching children to employ certain thinking strategies when confronted with the fear-producing stimulus (Morris and Kratochwill, 1983). Because of design limitations in the available studies, strong conclusions about the efficacy of cognitive behavioral techniques in children with fears would be premature (Kendall et al., 1988). Nevertheless, this approach appears promising in treating children's fears, and additional research is underway.

Obsessive-Compulsive Disorder

Response prevention is a successful behavioral intervention for treatment of rituals associated with obsessive-compulsive disorder in children and adolescents as described in case reports (Stanley, 1980; Zikis, 1983) and in an uncontrolled multiple case series (Bolton et al., 1983). Response prevention involves blocking the ritualistic behavior (e.g., preventing the washing or checking behavior). Fifteen adolescents with cleaning and/or checking rituals were treated with response prevention and family therapy by Bolton and associates (1983). Rituals were eliminated completely or were reduced to a mild level in 87% (13 of 15). Treatment gains were maintained at follow-up, 9 to 48 months later. A recent case report (Kearney and Silverman, 1990b) described successful treatment of an adolescent with obsessive-compulsive disorder, using a treatment design that alternated response prevention and cognitive therapy.

Family participation in the treatment of youth with obsessive-compulsive disorder is considered to be integral. "A typical factor which distinguishes the presentation of obsessive compulsive disorder in the adolescent from that in the adult is the adolescent's tendency to involve parents in rituals" (Bolton et al., 1983, p. 456). Thus, parents are often encouraged to participate in the response prevention program for their children.

Shortcomings

Silverman and Kearney (in press) identify a number of shortcomings in the current reports of behavioral interventions for anxiety disorders in children as described below. These studies are composed primarily of case reports, many of which are uncontrolled and without systematic followup. In addition, some studies (e.g., Blagg and Yule, 1984) combine treatment procedures so that it is unclear which components explain the treatment outcomes. Furthermore, children with anxiety symptoms exhibit comorbid symptoms (e.g., depression, attentional difficulties), and these associated symptoms often are not described at baseline or after treatment. Failure to include checks of whether the treatment techniques are being used is another limitation (Kendall et al., 1988). Clearly, the treatment of childhood anxiety disorders with behavioral interventions requires additional systematic investigation.

PHARMACOLOGICAL TREATMENT

Three double-blind, placebo-controlled pharmacological treatment studies of anxiety disorders in children and adolescents have been with school refusal subjects. Sample sizes have been small, and results overall are inconclusive, although promising. These studies have examined the use of tricyclic antidepressants for school refusal and associated symptoms of anxiety and depression (Berney et al., 1981; Bernstein et al., 1990; Gittelman-Klein and Klein, 1987, 1973). In the first study, 35 subjects, ages 6 to 14, with separation anxiety disorder were treated with imipramine, 100 to 200 mg/d or placebo (Gittelman-Klein and Klein, 1971, 1973). Children receiving imipramine were significantly more successful in returning to school than those receiving placebo. In addition, children receiving imipramine had a significant improvement in symptoms. The second study, a double-blind, placebo controlled trial, failed to show a significant treatment effect for clomipramine (Berney et al., 1981). This study had 51 subjects, ages 9 to 14, and used 40 to 75 mg/d clomipramine.

Bernstein et al. (1990) compared imipramine to alprazolam and failed to find significant differences between active medications and placebo, although on almost all of the dependent measures, there were trends for both alprazolam and imipramine to produce greater improvement. It was unclear whether the trends were explained by baseline differences in symptom severity between treatment groups or medication effects. This study included 24 subjects, ages 7 to 17. Imipramine dosages ranged from 150 to 200 mg/d, and plasma levels were monitored. Alprazolam dosages were 1.0 to 3.0 mg/d.

These three studies differ in several ways. In the second and third studies, subjects were older, and they displayed more depressive symptoms, whereas the first study was of subjects with primary separation and anxiety disorder. The Berney et al. study (1981) used clomipramine, which is a serotonergic tricyclic antidepressant with different properties from other antidepressants in that it is particularly useful in treating obsessive-compulsive disorder (Insel et al., 1985).

The Gittelman-Klein and Klein (1971, 1973) and the Vernstein et al. (1990) studies used higher doses of tricyclic antidepressants than the Berney et al. study (1981).

There are several small studies of the use of benzodiazepines for childhood anxiety disorders. These studies have used chlordiazepoxide for the treatment of school refusal in an open trial (D'Amato, 1962), chlordiazepoxide in the treatment of mixed psychiatric disorders in an open trial (Kraft et al., 1965), and chlordiazepoxide plus phenelzine in the treatment of phobic and school phobic disorders in a double-blind, crossover comparison with phenobarbitone plus placebo (Frommer, 1967). Alprazolam has been studied in cancer patients with anticipatory and acute situational anxiety associated with bone marrow aspirations in an open trial (Pfefferbaum et al, 1987), in children with avoidance and/or overanxious disorders in a single-blind uncontrolled study (Simeon and Ferguson, 1987), and for treatment of school refusal (Bernstein et al., 1990). Clonazepam was reported to be beneficial in two cases of separation anxiety disorder and one case of overanxious disorder (Biederman, 1987). Overall, these small, diverse studies indicate that benzodiazepines are useful in alleviating severe anxiety symptoms in children.

Clomipramine has been reported to be effective in treating obsessive-compulsive disorder in children and adolescents in controlled trials (Flament et al., 1985a,b; Leonard et al., 1988). Clomipramine is a potent inhibitor of serotonin receptacle (Insel, 1990). The efficacy of this drug is likely mediated through its effect on serotonin. Improvement while receiving clomipramine has been correlated with reduction in platelet serotonin level during clomipramine treatment (Flament et al., 1987).

A glaring absence in the pharmacological studies of anxiety disorders in children and adolescents is the lack of systematic, placebo-controlled study of medications for panic disorder in adolescents. There are case reports that suggest the benefit of treatment with tricyclic antidepressants and benzodiazepines (Ballenger et al., 1989; Biederman, 1987; Black and Robbins, 1990; Garland and Smith, 1990). This is reminiscent of where pharmacological treatment of child and adolescent depression was 10 years ago. Although controlled studies have not demonstrated tricyclic antidepressants and benzodiazepines (Ballenger et al., 1989; Biederman, 1987; Black and Robbins, 1990; Garland and Smith, 190). This is reminiscent of where pharmacological treatment of child and adolescent depression was 10 years ago. Although controlled studies have not demonstrated tricyclic antidepressants to be significantly more efficacious than placebo for children and adolescents with major depression (Geller et al., 1989; Kramer and Feiguine, 1981; Puig-Antich et al., 1987; Ryan, 1990), tricyclics for panic disorder and other anxiety disorders are in need of additional study. Similarly, the use of monoamine oxidase inhibitors for panic disorder should be investigated.

FUTURE DIRECTIONS

The work of the past decade has produced a number of well-designed research studies in the area of childhood anxiety disorders. The high prevalence rate of these disorders in the general population has been demonstrated. Distinct demographic profiles and patterns of comorbidity of children and adolescents with overanxious disorder and those with separation anxiety disorder have been demonstrated in samples of referred children. For each of these two childhood anxiety disorders, there are developmental differences in the expression of the disorder at various ages.

Further investigations of the demographics of referred children and analyses of their symptoms, using the current *DSM-III-R* criteria for the childhood anxiety diagnoses, are needed. Community samples of children will determine how clinically referred anxious children differ from those who are not referred. In addition, study of the prevalence of these anxiety symptoms in normal subjects in the general population will help determine what threshold number of symptoms should be used to define the presence of a disorder. This knowledge will help clinicians avoid unnecessarily labeling children as having psychopathology when it is not present. Comprehensive assessment of children, using the criteria for the adult anxiety disorders, is important. This will indicate which of these disorders are prevalent in children and adolescents and will provide data about age of onset and vulnerability factors.

Panic attacks and panic disorder need more investigation. Panic disorder may serve as a key disorder to study in order to answer questions about cognitive, neuroendocrine, and physiological changes around puberty that set the stage for vulnerability to psychiatric illness. Research should progress from description of prevalence rates and types of childhood fears to assessment of avoidant behavior and functional impairment leading to phobias.

Longitudinal studies of children and adolescents with anxiety disorders are essential. These studies will address the unresolved issues of stability of the childhood diagnoses and remission rates. Follow-up studies will help answer questions regarding which childhood diagnoses persist into adolescence and then into adulthood. Do specific childhood anxiety disorders have continuity with specific adults disorders? For example, it has been postulated that separation anxiety disorder may be a precursor to panic disorder or agoraphobia.

Investigation of physiological correlates and biological markers for anxiety in children should be pursued (e.g., physiological arousal measures, dexamethasone suppression test, association of panic disorder with mitral valve prolapse, sleep studies). If biological markers are identified, this information may shed light on the etiological factors in anxiety disorders. In addition, well-controlled behavioral and pharmacological treatment studies are needed.

Finally, early identification and intervention for at-risk children and adolescents are important priorities. The high comorbidity rates with mood disorders, association of high levels of anxiety with histories of physical and sexual abuse (Bernstein et al., 1989) and with the use of street drugs (Bernstein et al., 1989) and the use of alcohol and over-the-counter medications to self-medicate anxiety symptoms (McGee et al., 1990) indicate that a prevention approach should be pursued.

REFERENCES

Achenbach, T. M., Conners, C. K., Quay, H. C., Verhulst, F. C. & Howell, C. T. (1989), Replications of empirically derived syndromes as a basis for taxonomy of child/adolescent psychopathology. *J. Abnorm. Child Psychol.,* 17:299–323.

Adams-Tucker, C. (1982), Proximate effects of sexual abuse in childhood: a report on 28 children. *Am. J. Psychiatry,* 139:1252–1256.

Agras, S., Sylvester, D. & Oliveau, D. (1969), The epidemiology of common fears and phobia. *Compr. Psychiatry,* 10:151–156.

———Chapin, H. N. & Oliveau, D. C. (1972), The natural history of phobia: course and prognosis. *Arch. Gen. Psychiatry,* 26:315–317.

Alessi, N. E. & Magen, J. (1988), Panic disorder in psychiatrically hospitalized children. *Am. J. Psychiatry,* 145:1450–1452.

———Robbins, D. R. & Dilsaver, S. C. (1987), Panic and depressive disorders among psychiatrically hospitalized adolescents. *Psychiatry Res.,* 20:275–283.

American Psychiatric Association (1987), *Diagnostic and Statistical Manual of Mental Disorders (Third Edition-Revised),* Washington, DC: American Psychiatric Association.

Anderson, J. C., Williams, S., McGee, R. & Silva, P.A. (1987), DSM-III disorders in preadolescent children: prevalence in a large sample from the general population. *Arch. Gen. Psychiatry,* 44:69–76.

Ayllon, T., Smith, D. & Rogers, M. (1970), Behavioral management of school phobia. *J. Behav., Ther. Exp. Psychiatry,* 1:125–138.

Ayuso, J. L., Alfonso, S. & Rivera, A. (1989), Childhood separation anxiety and panic disorder: a comparative study. *Prog. Neuropsychopharmacol. Biol. Psychiatry,* 13:665–671.

Ballenger, J. C., Carek, D. J., Steele, J. J. & Cornish-McTighe, D. (1989), Three cases of panic disorder with agoraphobia in children. *Am. J. Psychiatry,* 146:922–924.

Behar, D., Rapoport, J. L., Berg, C. J. et al. (184), Computerized tomography and neuropsychological test measures in adolescents with obsessive-compulsive disorder. *Am. J. Psychiatry,* 141:363–369.

Beitchman, J. H., Wekerle, C. & Hood, J. (1987), Diagnostic continuity from preschool to middle childhood. *J. Am. Acad. Child Adolesc. Psychiatry,* 26:694–699.

Bell-Dolan, D. J., Last, C. G. & Strauss, C. C. (1990), Symptoms of anxiety disorders in normal children. *J. Am. Acad. Child Adolesc. Psychiatry,* 29:759–765.

Berg, C. Z., Rapoport, J. L., Whitaker, A. et al. (1989). Childhood obsessive compulsive disorder: a two-year prospective follow-up of a community sample. *J. Am. Acad. Child Adolesc. Psychiatry,* 28:528–533.

Berg, I., Marks, I., McGuire, R. & Lipsedge, M. (1974). School phobia and agoraphobia. *Psychol. Med.,* 4:428–434.

Berney, T., Kolvin, I., Bhate, S. R., Garside, R. F., Jeans, J., Kay, B. & Scarth, L. (1981), School phobia: a therapeutic trial with clomipramine and short-term outcome. *Br. J. Psychiatry,* 138:110–118.

Bernstein, G. A. (1991), Comorbidity and severity of anxiety and depressive disorders in a clinic sample. *J. Am. Acad. Child Adolesc. Psychiatry,* 30:43–50.

———Garfinkel, B. D. (1986), School phobia: the overlap of affective and depressive disorders. *J. Am. Acad. Child Psychiatry,* 25:235–241.

——————(1988), Pedigrees, functioning and psychopathology in families of school phobic children. *Am. J. Psychiatry,* 145:70–74.

——————Hoberman, H. M. (1989), Self-reported anxiety in adolescents. *Am. J. Psychiatry,* 146:384–386.

——————Borchardt, C. M. (1990), Comparative studies of pharmacotherapy for school refusal. *J. Am. Acad. Child Adolesc. Psychiatry,* 29:773–781.

———Biederman, J. (1987), Clonazepam in the treatment of prepubertal children with panic-like symptoms. *J. Clin. Psychiatry,* 48[Suppl]:38–41

———Rosenbaum, J. F., Hirschfeld, D. R., Bolduc, E. A., Faraone, S. V. & Kagan, J. (1990), Further evidence of an association between behavioral inhibition and anxiety disorders: results from a family study of children from a non-clinical sample. *Scientific Proceedings of the Annual Meeting of the American Academy of Child and Adolescent Psychiatry,* 6:56.

Bird, H. R., Canino, G., Rubio-Stipec, M. et al. (1988). Estimates of the prevalence of childhood maladjustment in a community survey in Puerto Rico. *Arch. Gen. Psychiatry,* 45:1120–1126.

Black, B. & Robbins, D. R. (1990), Panic disorder in children and adolescents. *J. Am. Acad. Child Adolesc. Psychiatry,* 29:36–44.

Blagg, N. R. & Yule, W. (1984), The behavioural treatment of school refusal—a comparative study. *Behav. Res. Ther.,* 22:119–127.

Bolton, D., Collins, S. & Steinberg, D. (1983), The treatment of obsessive-compulsive disorder in adolescence: a report of fifteen cases. *Br. J. Psychiatry,* 142:456–464.

Bowen, R. C., Offord, D. R. & Boyle, M. H. (1990), The prevalence of overanxious disorder and separation anxiety disorder: results from the Ontario child health study. *J. Am. Acad. Child Adolec. Psychiatry,* 29:753–758.

Breslau, N., Davis, G. C., Andreski, P. & Peterson, E. (1991), Traumatic events and post-traumatic stress disorder in an urban population of young adults. *Arch. Gen. Psychiatry,* 48:216–222.

Brown, R., Copeland, R. E. & Hall, R. V. (1974), School phobia: effects of behavior modification treatment applied by an elementary school principal. *Child Study J.,* 4:125–133.

Cantwell, D. P. & Baker, L. (1989), Stability and natural history of DSM-III childhood diagnoses. *J. Am. Acad. Child Adolesc. Psychiatry,* 28:691–700.

Chambers, W. J., Puig-Antich, J., Hirsch, M., Paez, P., Ambrosini, P. J., Tabrizi, M. A. & Davies, M. (1985). The assessment of affective disorders in children and adolescents by semistructured interview: test-retest reliability of the Schedule for Affective Disorders and Schizophrenia for School-Age Children. Present Episo Version. *Arch. Gen. Psychiatry,* 42:696–702.

Costello, E. J. (1989), Child psychiatric disorders and their correlates: a primary care pediatric sample. *J. Am. Acad. Child Adolesc. Psychiatry,* 28:851–855.

Cox, C. S., Fedio, P. & Rapoport, J. L. (1989), Neuropsychological testing of obsessive-compulsive adolescents. In: *Obsessive-Compulsive Disorder in Children and Adolescents,* ed. J. L. Rapoport. Washington, D.C.: American Psychiatric Press, Inc., pp. 73–85.

Croghan, L. M. (1981), Conceptualizing the critical elements in rapid desensitization to school anxiety: a case study. *J. Pediatric Psychol.,* 6:165–170.

Crowe, R. R., Noyes, R., Pauls, D. L. & Slymen, D. (1983), A family study of panic disorder. *Arch. Gen. Psychiatry,* 40:1065–1069.

D'Amato, G. (1962), Chlordiazepoxide in the management of school phobia. *Diseases of the Nervous System,* 23:292–295.

Denckla, M. B. (1989), Neurological examination. In: *Obsessive-Compulsive Disorder in Children and Adolescents,* ed. J. L. Rapoport. Washington, D.C.: American Psychiatric Press, Inc., pp. 107–115.

Doleys, D. M. & Williams, S. C. (1977), The use of natural consequences and a make-up period to eliminate school phobic behavior: a case study. *J. Sch. Psychol.,* 15:44–50.

Eisenberg, L. (1958), School phobia: a study in the communication of anxiety. *Am. J. Psychiatry,* 114:712–718.

Enzer, N. B. & Walker, P. A. (1967), Hyperventilation syndrome in childhood. *J. Pediatr.,* 70:521–532.

Flament, M. F., Rapoport, J. L., Berg, C. J. & Kilts, C. (1985a), A controlled trial of clomipramine in childhood obsessive compulsive disorder. *Psychopharmacol. Bull.,* 21:150–152.

———Sceery, W., Kilts, C., Mellström, B. & Linnoila, M. (1985b), Clompiramine treatment of childhood obsessive compulsive disorder. *Arch. Gen. Psychiatry,* 42:977–983.

———Murphy, D. L., Berg, C. J. & Lake, C. R. (1987), Biochemical changes during clomipramine treatment of childhood of obsessive-compulsive disorders. *Arch. Gen. Psychiatry,* 44:219–225.

———Whitaker, A., Rapoport, J. L. et al. (1988), Obsessive compulsive disorder in adolescence: an epidemiological study. *J. Am. Acad. Child Adolesc. Psychiatry,* 27:764–771.

Francis, G., Last, C. G. & Strauss, C. C. (1987), Expression of separation anxiety disorder: the roles of age and gender. *Child Psychiatry Hum. Deve.,* 18:82–89.

Frommer, E. A. (1967), Treatment of childhood depression with antidepressant drugs. *Br. Med. J.,* 1:729–732.

Garland, E. J. & Smith, D. H. (1990), Case study: panic disorder of a child psychiatric consultation service. *J. Am. Acad. Child Adolescent Psychiatry,* 29:785–788.

Garvey, W. P. & Hegrenes, J. R. (1966), Desensitization technique in the treatment of school phobia. *Am. J. Orthopsychiatry,* 36:147–152.

Geller, B., Chestnut, E. C., Miller, M. C., Price, D. T. & Yates, E. (1985), Preliminary data on DSM-III associated features of major depressive disorder in children and adolescents. *Am. J. Psychiatry,* 142:643–644.

————Cooper, T. B., McCombs, H. G., Graham, D. & Wells, J. (1989), Double-blind, placebo-controlled study of nortriptyline in depressed children using a "fixed plasma level" design. *Psychopharm. Bull.,* 25:101–108.

Gittelman, R. & Klein, D. F. (1984), Relationship between separation anxiety and panic and agoraphobic disorders. *Psychopathology.* 17(Suppl. 1); 56–65.

Gittelman-Klein, R. & Klein, D. F. (1971), Controlled imipramine treatment of school phobia. *Arch. Gen. Psychiatry,* 25:204–207.

————(1973), School phobia: diagnostic considerations in the light of imipramine effects. *J. Nerv. Ment. Dis.,* 156:199–215.

Grad, L. R., Pelcovitz, D., Olson, M., Matthews, M. & Grad, G. J. (1987), Obsessive-compulsive symptomatology in children with Tourette's syndrome. *J. Am. Acad. Child Adolesc. Psychiatry,* 26:69–73.

Hersen, M. (1970), Behavior modification approach to a school phobia case. *J. Clin. Psychol.,* 26:128–132.

Hollingsworth, C. E., Tanguay, P. E., Grossman, L. & Pabst, P. (1980), Long-term outcome of obsessive-compulsive disorder in childhood. *J. Am. Acad. Child Psychiatry,* 19:134–144.

Insel, T. R. (1990), Serotonin in obsessive compulsive disorder. *Psychiatr. Ann.,* 20:560–564.

————Murphy, D. L., Cohen, R. M., Alterman, I., Kilts, C. & Linnoila, M. (1983), Obsessive-compulsive disorder: a double-blind trial of clomipramine and clergyline. *Arch. Gen. Psychiatry,* 40:605–612.

Johnson, A. M., Falstein, E. I., Szurek, S. A. & Svendsen, M. (1941), School phobia. *Am. J. Orthopsychiatry,* 11:702–711.

Johnson, J. H. & McCutcheon, S. M. (1980), Assessing life stress in older children and adolescents: preliminary findings with the Life Events Checklist. In: *Stress and Anxiety,* vol. 7, eds. I. G. Sarason & C. D. Spielberger. Washington, D.C.: Hemisphere.

Kagan, J., Reznick, J. S., Clarke, C., Snidman, N. & Garcia-Coll, C. (1984), Behavioral inhibition to the unfamiliar. *Child Dev.,* 55:2212–2225.

Kane, M. T. & Kendall, P. C. (1989), Anxiety disorders in children: a multiple-baseline evaluation of a cognitive-behavioral treatment. *Behavior Therapy,* 20:499–508.

Kashani, J. H. & Orvaschel, H. (1988), Anxiety disorders in midadolescence: a community sample. *Am. J. Psychiatry,* 145:960–964.

———— ————(1990), A community study of anxiety in children and adolescents. *Am. J. Psychiatry,* 147:313–318.

————Vaidya, A. F., Soltys, S. M., Dandoy, A. C., Katz, L. M. & Reid, J. C. (1990), Correlates of anxiety in psychiatrically hospitalized children and their parents. *Am. J. Psychiatry,* 147:319–323.

Kearney, C. A. & Silverman, W. K. (1990a), A preliminary analysis of a functional model of assessment and treatment for school refusal behavior. *Behav. Modif.*, 14:340–366.

———— ————(1990b), Treatment of an adolescent with obsessive-compulsive disorder by alternating response prevention and cognitive therapy: an empirical analysis. *J. Behav. Ther. Exp. Psychiatry*, 21:39–47.

Kendall, P. C., Howard, B. L. & Epps, J. (1988), The anxious child—cognitive-behavioral treatment strategies. *Behav. Modif.*, 12:281–310.

Kiser, L. J., Ackerman, B. J., Brown, E., Edwards, N. B., McColgan, E., Pugh, R. & Pruitt, D.B. (1988), Post-traumatic stress disorder in young children: a reaction to purported sexual abuse. *J. Am. Acad. Child Adolesc. Psychiatry*, 27:645–649.

Klein, D. F. (1964), Delineation of two drug-responsive anxiety syndromes. *Psychopharmacologia*, 5:397–408.

Klein, R. G. & Last, C. G. (1989), *Anxiety Disorders in Children*. Newbury Park, CA: Sage Publications.

Kolko, D. J. (1987), Positive practice routines in overcoming resistance to the treatment of school phobias: a case study with follow-up. *J. Behav. Ther. Exp. Psychiatry*, 18:249–257.

Kovacs, M. & Beck. A. (1977), An empirical-clinical approach toward a definition of child-hood depression. In: *Depression in Childhood*, eds. J. G. Schulterbrandt & A. Raskin. New York: Raven Press, pp. 1–25.

————Gatsonis, C., Paulauskas, S. L. & Richards, C. (1989), Depressive disorders in child-hood: IV. A longitudinal study of comorbidity with and risk for anxiety disorders. *Arch. Gen. Psychiatry*, 46:776–782.

Kraft, I. A., Ardali, C., Duffy, J. H., Hart, J. T. & Pearce, P. (1965), A clinical study of chlordiazepoxide used in psychiatric disorders of children. *Int. J. Neuropsychiatry*, 1:433–437.

Kramer, A. D. & Feiguine, R. J. (1981), Clinical effects of amitriptyline in adolescent depression: a pilot study. *J. Am. Acad. Child Psychiatry*, 20:636–644.

Last, C. G. & Strauss, C. C. (1989a), Obsessive-compulsive disorder in childhood. *Journal of Anxiety Disorders*, 3:295–302.

———— ————(1989b), Panic disorder in children and adolescents. *Journal of Anxiety Disorders*, 3:87–95.

————Hersen, M., Kazdin, A. E., Finkelstein, R. & Strauss, C. C. (1987a) Comparison of DSM-III separation anxiety and overanxious disorders: demographic characteristics and patterns of comorbidity. *J. Am. Acad. Child Adolesc. Psychiatry*, 26:527–531.

———— ———— ————Francis, G. & Grubb, H. J. (1987b), Psychiatric illness in the mothers of anxious children. *Am. J. Psychiatry*, 144:1580–1583.

————Phillips, J. E. & Statfeld, A. (1987c), Childhood anxiety disorders in mothers and their children. *Child Psychiatry Hum. Dev.*, 18:103–112.

————Strauss, C. C. & Francis, G. (1987d), Comorbidity among childhood anxiety disorders. *J. Nerv. Ment. Dis.*, 175:726–730.

————Francis, G. & Strauss, C. C. (1989), Assessing fears in anxiety-disordered children with the revised fear survey schedule for children (FSSC-R). *Journal of Clinical Child Psychology,* 18:137–141.

Leonard, H., Swedo, S., Rapoport, J. L., Coffey, M. & Cheslow, D. (1988), Treatment of childhood obsessive compulsive disorder with clomipramine and desmethylimipramine: a double-blind cross-over comparison. *Psychopharmacol. Bull.,* 24:93–95.

Livingston, R., Taylor, J. L. & Crawford, S. L. (1988), A study of somatic complaints and psychiatric diagnosis in children. *J. Am. Acad. Child Adolesc. Psychiatry,* 27:185–187.

Lynch, M. A., Lindsay, J. & Ounsted, C. (1975), Tranquilizers causing aggression. *Br. Med. J.,* 1:266.

Macaulay, J. L. & Kleinknecht, R. A. (1989), Panic and panic attacks in adolescents. *Journal of Anxiety Disorders,* 3:221–241.

Mansdorf, I. J. & Lukens, E. (1987), Cognitive-behavioral psychotherapy for separation anxious children exhibiting school phobia. *J. Am. Acad. Child Adolesc. Psychiatry,* 26:222–225.

Marks, I. M. & Gelder, M. G. (1966), Different ages of onset in varieties of phobia. *Am. J. Psychiatry,* 123:218–221.

McClellan, J. M., Rubert, M. P., Reichler, R. J. & Sylvester, C. E. (1990), Attention deficit disorder in children at risk for anxiety and depression. *J. Am. Acad. Child Adolesc. Psychiatry,* 29:534–539.

McGee, R., Feehan, M., Williams, S., Partridge, F., Silva, P. A. & Kelly, J. (1990), DSM-III disorders in a large sample of adolescents. *J. Am. Acad. Chld Adolesc. Psychiatry,* 29:534–539.

McGee, R., Feehan, M., Williams, S., Partridge, F., Silva, P. A. & Kelly, J. (1990), DSM-III disorders in a large sample of adolescents. *J. Am. Acad. Child Adolesc. Psychiatry,* 29:534–539.

McLeer, S. V., Dehlinger, E., Atkins, M. S., Foa, E. B. & Ralphe, D. L. (1988), Post-traumatic stress disorder in sexually abused children. *J. Am Acad. Child Adolesc. Psychiatry,* 27:650–654.

McNamara, E. (1988), The self-management of school phobia: a case study. *Behavioural Psychotherapy,* 16:217–229.

Miller, L. C., Barrett, C. L., Hampe, E. & Noble, H. (1972), Comparison of reciprocal inhibition, psychotherapy and waiting list control for phobic chidren. *J. Abnorm. Psychol.,* 79:269–279.

Miller, P. M. (1972), The use of visual imagery and muscle relaxation in the counterconditioning of a phobic child: a case study. *J. Nerv. Ment. Dis.,* 154:457–460.

Mitchell, J., McCauley, E., Burke, P. M. & Moss, S. J. (1988), Phenomenology of depression in children and adolescents. *J. Am. Acad. Child Adolesc. Psychiatry,* 27:12–20.

Moreau, D. L., Weissman, M. & Warner, V. (1989), Panic disorder in children at high risk for depression. *Am. J. Psychiatry,* 146:1059–1060.

Morris, R. J. & Kratochwill, T. R. (1983), *Treating Children's Fears and Phobias: A Behavioral Approach.* New York: Pergamon.

Nelles, W. B. & Barlow, D. H. (1988), Do children panic? *Clinical Psychology Review,* 8:359–372.

Norton, G. R., Dorward, J. & Cox, B. J. (1986), Factors associated with panic attacks in nonclinical subjects. *Behavior Therapy,* 17:239–242.

Oliver, J. E. (1985), Successive generations of child maltreatment: social and medical disorders in the parents. *Br. J. Psychiatry,* 147:484–490.

———(1988), Successive generations of child maltreatment: the children. *Br. J. Psychiatry,* 153–543–553.

Ollendick, T. H. (1979), Fear reduction techniques with children. In: *Progress in Behavior Modification,* Vol. 8, eds. P. Miller & R. Eisler. New York: Academic Press.

———(1983), Reliability and validity of the revised fear survey schedule for children (FSSC-R). *Behav. Res. Ther.,* 21:685–692.

———King, N. J. & Frary, R. B. (1989), Fears in children and adolescents: reliability and generalizabilty across gender, age and nationality. *Behav. Res. Ther.,* 27:19–26.

———Matson, J. L. & Helsel, W. J. (1985), Fears in children and adolescents: normative data. *Behav. Res. Ther.,* 23:465–467.

Patterson, G. R. (1965), A learning theory approach to the problem of the school phobia child. In: *Case Studies in Behavior Modification,* eds. L. P. Ulmann & L. Krasner. New York: Holt, Rinehart and Winston.

Pauls, D. L. & Oleckman, J. F. (1986), The inheritance of Gilles de la Tourette's syndrome and associated behaviors: evidence for autosomal dominant transmission. *N. Engl. J. Med.,* 315:993–997.

———Towbin, K. E, Leckman, J. F., Zahner, G. E. P. & Cohen, D. J. (1986), Gilles de la Tourette's syndrome and obsessive-compulsive disorder: evidence supporting a genetic relationship. *Arch. Gen Psychiatry,* 43:1180–1182.

Pfefferbaum, B., Overall, J. E., Boren, H. A., Frankel, L. S., Sullivan, M. P. & Johnson, K. (1987), Alprazolam in the treatment of anticipatory and acute situational anxiety in children with cancer. *J. Am. Acad. Child Adolesc. Psychiatry,* 26:532–535.

Puig-Antich, J. & Rabinovich, H. (1986), Relationship between affective and anxiety disorders in childhood. In: *Anxiety Disorders of Childhood,* ed. R. Gittelman. New York: Guilford Press, pp. 136–156.

———Perel, J. M., Lupatkin, W. et al. (1987). Imipramine in prepubertal major depressive disorders. *Arch. Gen. Psychiatry,* 44:81–89.

Pynoos, R. S., Frederick, C., Nader, K. et al. (1987), Life threat and post-traumatic stress in school-age children. *Arch. Gen. Psychiatry,* 44:1057–1063.

Rapoport, J. L. (1986), Annotation childhood obsessive compulsive disorder. *J. Child Psychol. Psychiatry,* 27:289–295.

Reynolds, C. R. & Richman, B. O. (1978), What I think and feel: a revised measure of children's manifest anxiety. *J. Abnorm. Child Psychol.,* 6:271–280.

Riddle, M. A., Scahill, L., King, R. et al. (1990), Obsessive compulsive disorder in children and adolescents: phenomenology and family history. *J. Am. Acad. Child Adolesc. Psychiatry,* 29:766–772.

Rosenbaum, J. F, Biederman, J., Gersten, M. et al. (1988), Behavioral inhibition in children of parents with panic disorder and agoraphobia. *Arch. Gen. Psychiatry,* 45:463–470.

Ryan, N. D. (1990), Pharmacotherapy of adolescent major depression: beyond TCAs. *Psychopharmacol. Bull.,* 26:75–79.

———Puig-Antich, J., Ambrosini, P. et al. (1987), The clinical picture of major depression in children and adolescents. *Arch. Gen. Psychiatry,* 44:854–861.

Scherer, M. W. & Nakamura, C. Y. (1968), A fear survey schedule for children (FSS-FC): a factor analytic comparison with manifest anxiety (CMAS). *Behav. Res. Ther.,* 6:173–182.

Sheehan, D. V., Sheehan, K. E. & Minichiello, W. E. (1981), Age of onset of phobic disorders: a reevaluation. *Compr. Psychiatry,* 22:544–553.

Silverman, W. K. & Kearney, C.A., Behavioral treatment of childhood anxiety. In: *Handbook of Behavior Therapy and Pharmacotherapy for Children: A Comparative Analysis,* eds. V. B. Van Hasselt & M. Hersen. New York: Grune and Stratton (in press).

———Nelles, W. B. (1990), Simple phobia in childhood. In: *Handbook of Child and Adult Psychopathology: A Longitudinal Perspective,* ed. M. Hersen & C. G. Last. New York: Pergamon Press pp. 183–196.

——— ———(1988). The influence of gender on children's ratings of fear in self and same-aged peers. *J. Gen. Psychol.,* 148:17–21.

Simeon, J. G. & Ferguson, H. B. (1987), Alprazolam effects in children with anxiety disorders. *Can. J. Psychiatry,* 32:570–574.

Solomon, Z., Kotler, M. & Mikulincer, M. (1988), Combat-related post-traumatic stress disorder among second-generation holocaust survivors: preliminary findings. *Am. J. Psychiatry* 145:865–868.

Spielberger, C. (1973), *Manual for the State-Trait Anxiety Inventory for Children.* Palo Alto: Consulting Psychologists Press.

Stanley, L. (1980), Treatment of ritualistic behavior in an eight-year-old girl by response prevention: a case report. *J. Child Psychology Psychiatry,* 21:85–90.

Stavrakaki, C. & Vargo, B. (1986), The relationship of anxiety and depression: a review of the literature. *Br. J. Psychiatry,* 149:7–16.

Strauss, C. C. (1988). Behavioral assessment and treatment of over anxious disorder in children and adolescents. *Behav. Modif.,* 12:234–251.

———Last, C. G., Hersen, M. & Kazdin, A. E., (1988a), Association between anxiety and depression in children and adolescents with anxiety disorders. *J. Abnorm. Child Psychol.,* 16:57–68.

———Lease, C. A., Last, C. G. & Francis, G. (1988b) Overanxious disorder: an examination of developmental differences. *J. Abnorm. Child Psychol.,* 16:433–443.

Swedo, S. E., Rapoport, J. L., Leonard, H., Lenane, M. & Cheslow D. (1989), Obsessive-compulsive disorder in children and adolescents. *Arch. Gen. Psychiatry,* 46:335–341.

Terr, L. C. (1981), Psychic trauma in children: observations following the Chowchilla school-bus kidnapping. *Am. J. Psychiatry,* 138:14–19.

———(1983), Chowchilla revisited: the effects of psychic trauma four years after a school-bus kidnapping. *Am. J. Psychiatry,* 140:1543–1550.

———(1985), Children traumatized in small groups. In: *Post-Traumatic Stress Disorder in*

Children, eds. S. Eth & R. S. Pynoos. Washington, D.C.: American Psychiatric Press, Inc., pp. 47–70.

Thyer, B. A., Parrish, R. T., Curtis, G. C., Nesse, R. M. & Cameron, O. G. (1985), Ages of onset of DSM-III anxiety disorders. *Compr Psychiatry,* 26:113–122.

Torgersen, S. (1983), Genetic factors in anxiety disorders. *Arch. Gen. Psychiatry,* 40:1085–1089.

Trueman, D. (1984), The behavioral treatment of school phobia: a critical review. *Psychology in the Schools,* 21:215–223.

Turner, S. M., Beidel, D. C. & Costello, A. (1987), Psychopathology in the offspring of anxiety disorders patients. *J. Consult. Clin. Psychol.,* 55:229–235.

Velez, C. N., Johnson, J. & Cohen, P. (1989), A longitudinal analysis of selected risk factors for childhood psychopathology. *J. Am. Acad. Child Adolesc. Psychiatry,* 28:861–864.

Vitiello, B., Behar, D., Wolfson, S. & McLeer, S. V. (1990), Case study: diagnosis of panic disorder in prepubertal children. *J. Am. Acad. Child Adolesc. Psychiatry,* 29:782–784.

Von Korff, M. R., Eaton, W. W. & Keyl, P. M. (1985), The epidemiology of panic attacks and panic disorder: results of three community surveys. *Am. J. Epidemiol.,* 122:970–981.

Waldfogel, S., Coolidge, J. C. & Hahn, P. B. (1957), The development, meaning and management of school phobia. *Am. J. Orthopsychiatry,* 27:754–780.

Weissman, M. M., Leckman, J. F., Merikangas, K. R., Gammon, G. D. & Prusoff, B. A. (1984), Depression and anxiety disorders in parents and children. *Arch. Gen. Psychiatry,* 41:845–852.

————Gammon, G. D., John, K., Merikangas, K. R., Warner, V., Prusoff, B. A. & Sholomskas, D. (1987), Children of depressed parents: increased psychopathology and early onset of major depression. *Arch. Gen. Psychiatry,* 44:847–853.

Whitaker, A., Johnson, J., Shaffer, D. et al. (1990). Uncommon troubles in young people: prevalence estimates of selected psychiatric disorders in a nonreferred adolescent population. *Arch. Gen. Psychiatry,* 47:487–496.

Widom, C. S. (1989), The cycle of violence. *Science,* 244:160–166.

Wolpe, J. (1982), *Psychotherapy by Reciprocal Inhibition.* Stanford, CA: Stanford University Press.

Yates, A. J. (1970) *Behavior Therapy.* New York: Wiley.

Zikis, P. (1983), Treatment of an 11-year-old obsessive-compulsive ritualizer and Tiqueur girl with in vivo exposure and response prevention. *Behavioural Psychotherapy,* 11:75–81.

Zitrin, C. M. & Ross, D. C. (1988), Early separation anxiety and adult agoraphobia. *J. Nerv. Ment. Dis.,* 176:621–625.

24

Neuroleptic Use, Parkinsonian Symptoms, Tardive Dyskinesia, and Associated Factors in Child and Adolescent Psychiatric Patients

Mary Ann Richardson, Gary Haugland, and Thomas J. Craig
Nathan S. Kline Institute for Psychiatric Research,
Orangeburg, New York

Objective: *The authors' goal was to determine the prevalence of and risk factors for neuroleptic-induced movement disorders in a group of psychiatrically hospitalized children and adolescents.* **Method:** *They evaluated the presence or absence of parkinsonism, tardive dyskinesia and akathisia in 104 children and adolescents who were in residence in or admitted over a 6 month period to a state-operated child psychiatric center. They applied a standardized, structured assessment procedure used in research on adult and geriatric psychiatric patients and the mentally retarded.* **Results:** *The prevalence of parkinsonism among the 61 subjects at risk was 34% and was significantly associated with longer neuroleptic treatment periods immediately before evaluation. The prevalence of treatment-emergent tardive dyskinesia among the 41 subjects at risk was 12% and showed no association with quantitive neuroleptic treatment variables. However, patients with tardive dyskinesia were significantly more likely to have a family history of mental illness and significantly less likely to have a history of assaultive behavior. A pattern of complex pharmacological responses for parkinsonism and tardive dyskinesia, some of which are not typical of those most commonly reported in adults, was seen in this group of young patients.* **Conclusions:** *The study data highlight the acute sensitivity of the neuroleptic-treated child and adolescent to the development of parkinsonism, the possible role of certain patient characteristics in the vul-*

Reprinted with permission from the *American Journal of Psychiatry,* 1991, Vol, 148, 1322–1328. Copyright ©1991 by the American Psychiatric Association.

nerability to develop tardive dyskinesia, and the possibility that neuroleptic-induced side effects experienced by children and adolescents differ in some ways from those experienced by adults. The data further strongly support the need for systemic monitoring of neuroleptic-treated child and adolescent patients for a full range of side effects.

Pediatric psychopharmacology is complicated by a lack of diagnostic specificity and important differences in drug effects between children and adolescents and adults [1-4]. Pharmacotherapy in child and adolescent psychiatry, therefore, has largely been based on a "drug to symptom" approach rather than one of "drug to disease"[1,2]. Although in adult psychiatric patients the indications for the use of neuroleptics is being progressively narrowed to conditions characterized by psychotic behavior, these drugs are used for both psychotic and nonpsychotic diagnostic categories in pediatric psychiatric patients (e.g., those with autism and conduct disorders), in hyperkinetic children, and in pediatric neurological patients [5-11].

Despite this broad use of neuroleptics in child and adolescent patients and the widespread recognition in adult psychiatry of the movement disorders associated with neuroleptic use (Parkinson's-disease-like symptoms [parkinsonism], akathisia, tardive dyskinesia, and tardive dystonia), there has been little systematic examination of the prevalence of these side effects across the broad range of child psychiatric patients. Dyskinesias have been the most studied side effect, particularly in autistic children and the mentally retarded [12-17]. The examination of dyskinesias has focused primarily on withdrawal-emergent symptoms (those which occur after discontinuation of neuroleptic medication), which generally spontaneously remit in a matter of weeks or months. The prevalence of withdrawal-emergent dyskinesias has been found to be as high as 51% [13]. Further, there has been relatively little effort to identify risk factors that may increase a child or adolescent patient's likelihood of developing these movement disorders as a first step toward preventive intervention.

The few studies addressing neuroleptic-induced movement disorders are limited in a number of ways. First, virtually all prevalence studies of extrapyramidal side effects and tardive dyskinesia focused on either the mentally retarded or patients with autism or childhood schizophrenia. Second, only one study [18] included a systematic examination of movement disorders in a comparison group of patients from the same clinical environment who had never received neuroleptics, and this study found no difference between these two groups in the prevalence of movement disorders. Finally, the search for risk factors has tended to be limited to demographic and medication-related variables rather than clinical and family data that might suggest greater individual predisposition to these side effects.

The present study is unique in its examination of a broad spectrum of childhood psychiatric disorders, a full range of neuroleptic-induced movement disorders, specific patient-related risk factors, and the presence of nonexposed comparison patients as well as its use of standardized clinical assessments by a research team with extensive experience in rating movement disorders in adult and geriatric psychiatric patients and the mentally retarded.

METHOD

The study pool consisted of all children and adolescents who were residents at a psychiatric center at the beginning of the study or who were admitted during the following 6 months. All residents were evaluated as a clinical procedure, and consent was obtained from parents or guardians for the use of the data. Verbal assent was obtained from all of the patients before they participated in the study. A total of 133 children and adolescents were inpatients during the study period; 20 were discharged before the rating was done, three refused to be evaluated, and six did not have parental consent for inclusion in the study, leaving a study group of 104 (78% of the eligible pool).

The patients were rated for tardive dyskinesia, parkinsonism, and akathisia by using the Simpson Abbreviated Dyskinesia Scale[19], the Abnormal Involuntary Movement Scale (AIMS)[20], and the Simpson-Angus Neurological Rating Scale[21]. A clinical evaluation was also performed for tardive dystonia. Subjects were evaluated by two raters (M.A.R. and G.H.), who used a 23-step movement disorder rating procedure lasting approximately 45 minutes per patient. This procedure was designed to maximize the validity of the differential diagnosis and included tested activities to increase and diminish movement counts. The reliability of the rating procedures has been previously reported.[22]

The criterion measures for tardive dyskinesia were derived from the Abbreviated Dyskinesia Scale and the AIMS. The Abbreviated Dyskinesia Scale criterion for presence of tardive dyskinesia was based on a clinical diagnosis from a consensual rating by the two raters derived from a score of mild to severe on a global scale that has been described previously [21]. For the AIMS, the Schooler-Kane research diagnoses for tardive dyskinesia criterion[29] was used. The presence of parkinsonism was defined by a mean score of 0.4 on items 1–10 of the Simpson-Angus scale[21]. The presence of akathisia was determined by a score of 2 or more on the akathisia item of the Abbreviated Dyskinesia Scale. In addition, a mannerism and stereotypy scale that had been developed for a study in the mentally retarded[22] was applied. Raters were kept blind to the patient's medication status, diagnosis, and psychiatric treatment history.

Subsequent to the rating, neuroleptic treatment histories were collected from a computerized information system at the facility and records were obtained from the patient's first treating facility and from the facility where the patient had been admitted immediately preceding the current admission. Only medication received while an inpatient was analyzed because interviews with the patients revealed a high rate of out-of-hospital noncompliance. The neuroleptic use variables that were tested for association with parkinsonism and tardive dyskinesia status were length of time since first neuroleptic treatment, chlorpromazine-equivalent dose[30] at evaluation, and continuous days of neuroleptic treatment before evaluation. Additionally, review of all of the facility records collected identified other potential risk factors, such as a family history of psychiatric hospitalization in first-degree relatives and a history of assaultive behavior in the patient.

The overall demographics of all 104 patients were studied. Side effect risk subgroups were also constructed: the 61 patients who were receiving neurolentics at the time of evaluation were considered at risk for parkinsonism, and the 41 patients whose neuroleptic treatment histories revealed at least one period of 90 continuous days of treatment were considered at risk for tardive dyskinesia. These two risk categories were not mutually exclusive. Sixteen (26%) of the patients in the parkinsonism risk group received two side effect ratings (approximately 1 month apart), and 11 (27%) of the patients in the tardive dyskinesia risk group did so. All of the patients with tardive dyskinesia received two side effect ratings, with the exception of one adolescent who eloped from the facility after the first rating.

Group differences were tested for significance by application of the Fisher exact test and the Wilcoxon rank sum test. The problem of repeated statistical analyses was handled by using the Holm procedure[31], which is a more powerful technique than the commonly used Bonferroni method. According to the Holm procedure, the statistical test having the smallest computed p value is declared significant at the 0.05 level only if the computed p value of the test statistic is less than 0.05 divided by the number of tests. When performing multiple tests of six independent variables, therefore, a probability level of ≤ 0.0083 ($0.05 \div 6$) is considered significant. If one variable is thereby declared significant, the probability level for significance of the next variable becomes $0.05 \div (N-1)$, or $\leq 0.05 \div 5$. The procedure terminates when no variable attains the required significance level.

RESULTS

Sixty-seven (64%) of the 104 patients included in the overall analyses were boys and 37 (36%) were girls. Their mean$\pm$SD age was 14.9 ± 2.2 years, and they had been in patients at the facility for a mean of 95 ± 146.4 days. According to their charts, 60 (58%) had *DSM-III* diagnoses of conduct or adjustment disorders, 19 (18%) had psychoses and/or affective disorders (15 had schizophrenia, three had major affective disorder, and one had atypical psychosis), 13 (13%) had developmental disorders (primarily attention deficit disorder), and 12 (12%) had dysthymia, drug abuse, or personality disorders. The patients displayed a variety of behavioral problems; the most frequently noted were assaultive behavior (79 patients [76%]), suicidal behavior or ideation (55 patients [53%]), running away (44 patients [42%]), drug abuse (37 patients [36%]), hyperactivity (32 patients [31%]), and alcohol abuse (25 patients [24%]). A family history of psychiatric hospitalization was noted for 19 (18%) of the patients, and 37 (36%) had been physically or sexually abused. Sixty-one (59%) were receiving neuroleptics at evaluation (mean chlorpromazine-equivalent dose of 444.4±S14.3 mg/day) and had been receiving neuroleptics for a mean of 92.4±111.0 continuous days before the rating day, and 11 (11%) were receiving antiparkinsonian agents. Among those with a history of neuroleptic treatment, the mean length of time since their first treatment was 452±495.1 days. Those not receiving neuroleptics on the day of evaluation who had a previous history of receiving neuroleptics had been neuroleptic-drug-free for 189.9±231.3 days.

None of the 104 patients manifested symptoms of tardive dsytonia. Three patients exhibited stereotypic behaviors but did not show signs of parkinsonism, tardive dyskinesia, or akathisia.

Parkinsonism Risk Group

The parkinsonism risk group (N = 61) showed pharmacological stability in that 46 (75%) of them had been receiving neuroleptics continuously for at least 3 weeks before evaluation. Some degree of clinical stability could also be assumed because 27 (44%) of these patients had been inpatients for at least 3 months before evaluation and only seven (12%) had been continuously hospitalized for less than 3 weeks. Twenty-one (34%) of these patients had parkinsonism. Equal numbers of these 21 patients had conduct or adjustment disorders (N = 7[33.3%]) and psychoses or affective disorders (N = 7 [33.3%]) and psychoses or affective disorders (N = 7 [33.3%]). Eighteen (45%) of the 40 patients in the parkinsonism risk group who did not have parkinsonism had conduct or adjustment disorders, and 10 (25%) had psychoses or affective disorders.

As table 1 shows, no significant differences in the median length of time since first neuroleptic treatment, the median chlorpromazine-equivalent dose at evaluation, or median age were found between patients in the parkinsonism risk group who did or did not have parkinsonism. There was a wide range in these values, however. The number of continuous days of neuroleptic treatment before evaluation was significantly higher for the patients with parkinsonism than for those without the disorder. Seventeen (81%) of the 21 patients with parkinsonism in the parkinsonism risk group exhibited assaultive behavior, compared with 31 (78%) of the 40 patients who did not have parkinsonism (p = 1.00, Fisher's exact test, two-tailed). Although also not significantly different (p = 0.21, Fisher's exact test, two-tailed), a larger percentage of the patients with parkinsonism (33% [N = 7]) than without (18% [N = 7]) did reveal positive family histories of psychiatric hospitalization in first-degree relatives.

TABLE 1.
Relationship of Presence or Absence of Parkinsonism and Tardive Dyskinesia to Neuroleptic Use and Age in Psychiatrically Hospitalized Children and Adolescents Taking Neuroleptics

Variable	Condition Present			Condition Absent			Wilcoxon Rank Sum Test	
	N	Median	Range	N	Median	Range	Z	p
Parkinsonism in patients taking neuroleptics at evaluation	21			40				
Neuroleptic use								
Dose								
Milligrams per day[a]		300	50–2500		225	38–2025	0.72	0.47
Significance								
Length of current use								
Days		117	15–297		34	1–704	2.63	0.008[b]
Significance								
Time since first use								
Days		228	15–1479		238	6–1869	0.60	0.55
Significance								
Age								
Years		15.2	10–18		15.3	9–18	-0.60	0.55
Significance								
Tardive dyskinesia in patients taking neuroleptics continuously for 3 months	5			36				
Neuroleptic use								
Dose								
Milligrams per day[a]		750	38–2500		300	50–2025	0.45	0.65
Significance								
Length of current use								
Days		141	18–168		128	11–704	-0.02	0.98
Significance								
Time since first use								
Days		319	160–525		611	135–2252	-1.55	0.12
Significance								
Age								
Years		15.5	14–17		15.4	10–18	0.22	0.83
Significance								

[a] Chlorpromazine equivalents.
[b] p=0.05 by Holm procedure.

Eleven (18%) of the 61 patients in the parkinsonism risk group were receiving antiparkinsonian drugs; three exhibited parkinsonism despite the use of these agents. Eighteen of the patients who were not receiving antiparkinsonian agents exhibited parkinsonism.

Six additional male patients, 13.3 to 16.5 years old, who were not receiving neuroleptics at evaluation also met Simpson-Angus scale criteria for parkinsonism. Thus, the study group as a whole included 27 patients who met Simpson-Angus scale criteria for parkinsonism was substantial: 17 of the 27 patients had Simpson-Angus scale total scores at least double the minimum criterion for a positive case.

Tardive Dyskinesia Risk Group

As in the parkinsonism risk group, pharmacological and clinical stability can be assumed in the tardive dyskinesia risk group. Of the 36 patients who were receiving neuroleptics at evaluation, 32 (89%) had been receiving them for at least 3 weeks. Of the 41 patients considered at risk for tardive dyskinesia, 21 (51%) had been inpatients for 3 months; only four (10%) had been hospitalized for less than 3 weeks. Five (12%) of the 41 patients had tardive dyskinesia according to our primary study criterion (the Abbreviated Dyskinesia Scale). When the quantitative Schooler-Kane research diagnoses for tardive dyskinesia criterion was used, three (7%) of the patients were diagnosed as having the disorder. All of the patients found to have tardive dyskinesia had at least one period of more than 90 days of continuous use of neuroleptic treatment in their history. The dyskinesia was treatment emergent because the tardive dyskinesia occurred while the patients were receiving neuroleptics.

Three patients with tardive dyskinesia had conduct or adjustment disorders, and two had psychoses or affective disorders. Among the 36 patients at risk for tardive dyskinesia who did not have it, however, all four diagnostic categories were represented: 17 (47%) had conduct or adjustment disorders, 10 (28%) had psychoses or affective disorders, and nine (25%) had developmental disorders or dysthymia, drug abuse, or personality disorders.

The comparisons that were tested for significance between the patients in the tardive dyskinesia risk group who did or did not have tardive dyskinesia are the same as those for the patients in the parkinsonism risk group who did or did not have parkinsonism; these are presented in table 1. The median chlorpromazine-equivalent dose at evaluation did not differ between patients with and without tardive dyskinesia, nor did the number of continuous days of neuroleptic administration before evaluation. Although the difference in total neuroleptic treatment durations between the groups with and without tardive dysinesia was not significant, four of the five patients with tardive dyskinesia had durations well below the median for the total risk group (520 days), and the fifth was just above at 525 days. The two groups did not differ in age at evaluation.

There was a significant difference between the groups with and without tardive dyskinesia in family history of psychiatric hospitalization of a first-degree relative. Significantly more of the patients with (80% [N = 4]) than without 17% [N = 6] had such a history (p = 0.003, Fisher's exact test, two-tailed; p = 0.05 by the Holm procedure). Differences were also significant for a patient history of assaultive behavior. Significantly more of the patients without (89%) [N = 32]) than with (20% [N = 1]) tardive dyskinesia had such a history (p = 0.009, Fisher's exact test, two-tailed; p = 0.05 by the Holm procedure). Further strengthening these findings is the fact that no associations were found in the entire study group between either a family history of psychiatric hospitalization (p = 0.206, Fisher's exact test, two-tailed) or assaultive behavior (p = 0.206, Fisher's exact test, two-tailed) or assaultive behavior (p = 0.483, Fisher's exact test, two-tailed) and the neuroleptic treatment history categories of less than 3 months or 3 months or more.

The five patients with tardive dyskinesia were all adolescents; three were girls and two were boys. All five patients manifested oral-facial dyskinesia, and one also showed finger and wrist movements. Two patients had single tardive dyskinesia movements, and three (those who also met the Schooler-Kane criterion on the AIMS scale) had multiple movements and coexisting parkinsonism. Two of the latter patients were being treated with antiparkinsonian agents, which could have contributed to the greater severity of their tardive dyskinesia. There was an atypicality, however, in the medication-to-symptom relationship of these three patients in that higher neuroleptic doses were associated with more severe symptoms, in contrast to the typical finding in adults that higher neuroleptic doses are associated with less severity due to neuroleptic masking.

Atypicality in the relationship of medication to tardive dyskinesia and parkinsonism was also demonstrated by results obtained during follow-up evaluations of four of the five patients with tardive dyskinesia. One patient left the hospital before followup evaluation, and three of the remaining four were identified as having coexisting parkinsonism. One patient, who had two evaluations, had an atypical pharmacological response to his treatment for both tardive dyskinesia and parkinsonism. Tardive dyskinesia symptoms occurred only at the evaluation when he was receiving the lower benztropine dose, and the severity of his parkinsonism was similar at both evaluations despite a doubling of his benztropine dose. A second patient, who had three evaluations over a 3.5-month period, exhibited both typical and atypical tardive dyskinesia. Her tardive dyskinesia was typical in that the most substantial severity was seen when no neuroleptics were being administered (Abbreviated Dyskinesia Scale total score of 11 versus scores of 1 and 6) but atypical in that her second highest tardive dyskinesia score occurred when she was receiving a markedly higher heuroleptic dose than she had been receiving when she achieved her lowest score (1250 versus 300 mg/day of chlorpromazine-equivalents [molindone versus trifluoperazine]). This patient also showed an atypical parkinsonism pattern in that she had markedly more severe parkinsonism while receiving the lower neuroleptic dose (Simpson-Angus scale total score of 14 versus 7) and her parkinsonism persisted beyond neuroleptic discontinuation. A third patient, who was receiving molindone, was evaluated twice over a 5-month period and showed an atypical tardive dyskinesia pattern in that her symptoms were seen only at the evaluation done while she was receiving more neuroleptic agent and less antiparkinsonian agent. Her parkinsonism pattern, however, was typical in that she showed symptoms only while receiving half the antiparkinsonian agent resulted in fewer symptoms of parkinsonism, but never sufficiently severe to be a positive case.

Akathisia symptoms were seen in two adolescent patients (one boy and one girl). The symptoms were mild and there was no coexisting tardive dyskinesia and parkinsonism. Both of these patients had psychotic diagnoses and a history of assaultive behavior.

DISCUSSION

A major strength of this study is its focus on all patients hospitalized during a 6-month period in a children's psychiatric center that serves as the tertiary care facility for a seven-county catchment area having few other inpatient child psychiatric resources. The study group is thus typical of a broad range of hospitalized children and adolescents and permits generalization of the findings beyond the more narrowly defined groups of subjects in previous studies, e.g., the mentally retarded [15-17] and children with autism and childhood schizophrenia.[13,14] Of interest is the high prevalence of neuroleptic use despite the relative rarity of conditions considered specific for such drugs in adult patients: psychoses and major affective disorders represented only 28% of the diagnoses among the child and adolescent patients who were receiving neuroleptics at evaluation.

This study's focus on parkinsonism contributes to the literature the first body of data on this disorder in child and adolescent patients to our knowledge. The significant association between the presence of parkinsonism and the length of neuroleptic treatment can serve as a benchmark for the clinician. The overall study findings regarding parkinsonism, however, demonstrate no easy solutions but, rather, a serious, complex, and troublesome phenomenon that demands monitoring by the clinician and more attention from the research community. The seriousness is attested to by the high prevalence found (34%), which exceeds that found in several other study groups—for instance, 24% in adults 25 to 34 years old[32,33], 3% in developmentally disabled children[18], and 23% in children with autism and childhood schizophrenia[34]—and is comparable to a rate of 36% reported for psychotic adolescent inpatients[35].

The pharmacology of the parkinsonism was complex in that 1) symptoms were seen to remain constant despite a doubling of the benztropine dose, 2) symptoms worsened at a lower neuroleptic dose, and 3) the symptoms of 22% of the patients with parkinsonism persisted beyond neuroleptic discontinuation. Although not the focus of enough attention, this latter phenomenon has been reported in adult and geriatric psychiatric patients and neurology patients whose parkinsonism symptoms persisted up to 18 months beyond neuroleptic discontinuation[32,33,36-38].

The parkinsonism findings are also troublesome because we learned during the course of the study that 1) staff clinicians indicated little expectation that parkinsonism would develop, which would contribute to the underrecognition suggested by the infrequent prescription of antiparkinsonian agents, 2) in some patients the severity of their parkinsonism interfered with age-specific neuromuscular activities, such as running and swimming, and 3) the patients were well aware of these symptoms in themselves and their peers, describing them as "zombie-like" and implicating them as a reason for outpatient treatment noncompliance.

Unlike parkinsonism, the prevalence of treatment-emergent tardive dyskinesia (12%) was lower than in adult patients. This prevalence is not likely to be an underestimate because of the lower probability of neuroleptic masking in children than in adults. Although the prevalence is lower than would be expected among adults, it is higher than that reported for more severely ill children or adolescents—for instance, 4% in children with childhood schizophrenia[34], 6% in autistic children[13], and 7% in mentally retarded children[17]. This suggests a possible clinical risk factor for less severely ill patients.

We found no positive relationship between tardive dyskinesia and either lifetime measures of neuroleptic treatment or neuroleptic status at evaluation. Other studies examining neuroleptic use risk factors have focused primarily on withdrawal-emergent symptoms and are therefore not comparable but did show positive associations with indexes of neuroleptic use[15,17,34,39]. The most recent of these [13] included a few children with treatment-emergent tardive dyskinesia but reported no association between dyskinesia and neuroleptic use. What seemed to be of primary importance for the development of tardive dyskinesia in the present study were markers of patient vulnerability or lack of vulnerability.

The strong statistical association between tardive dyskinesia and assaultive behavior in the face of the small number of patients with tardive dyskinesia and the lack of a similar association for parkinsonism is intriguing. To our knowledge, this has not been reported in other work. It is all the more striking because the prevalence of that behavioral characteristic was markedly lower in the group without tardive dyskinesia than in the other three groups (patients with tardive dyskinesia and those with and without parkinsonism). This finding suggests a possible biologically mediated lack of vulnerability to tardive dyskinesia coexisting with assaultive behavior.

The significant association between the presence of tardive dyskinesia and a family history of psychiatric hospitalization and the substantially (but not significantly) higher rate of a positive family history in the group with parkinsonism than in the group without parkinsonism suggest a predisposition to these disorders occurring along with a familial loading for mental illness. Findings such as these have also been reported in adult schizophrenic patients: a family history of depression was associated with severity of parkinsonism [40] and a family history of affective illness was associated with tardive dyskinesia[40]. It would seem that a knowledge of family psychiatric history can be of utility as a marker in predicting a vulnerability to neuroleptic side effects.

The pharmacological pattern of the tardive dyskinesia symptoms in our study might be interpreted as either an atypicality from adult patterns or an example of pharmacological heterogeneity[42,43], intrapatient variability[44], or initial dyskinesias[45]. A previous finding that the only two children with treatment-emergent dyskinesias showed a reduction in symptoms with neuroleptic reduction[46], plus the present finding from our multiple evaluations of four patients that three of them had atypical pharmacological tardive dyskinesia patterns, suggests that atypicality is more prevalent in children and adolescents than adults. This suggestion, along with the high rates of withdrawal-emergent symptoms seen primarily in children and adolescents, raises the possibility of differing neurochemical substrates in the dyskinesias in children and adolescents compared with those in adults.

Akathisia has already been reported in child psychiatric patients[46] and in nonpsychotic children treated for Tourette's disorder[47]. It has been associated with the worsening of psychosis in adults and the worsening of Tourette's symptoms in children[48,49]. Both of the patients in the present study with akathisia carried a psychotic diagnosis and were therefore at risk for a psychotic worsening or a misinterpretation of akathisia as a psychotic worsening. Either of these conditions could precipitate an increase in neuroleptic dose, which in turn could produce an even further increase in symptoms.

From a clinical perspective, this point prevalence study of neurological side effects of neuroleptics in child and adolescent psychiatric patients demonstrates that these patients are vulnerable to the development of symptoms of tardive dyskinesia, akathisia, and, particularly, parkinsonism. In addition, symptom patterns often go beyond the typical or expected. In attempting to counteract these side effects, the clinician must be aware of the complex response pattern of these disorders to pharmacological interventions. Child and adolescent psychiatric patients who are exposed to even short neuroleptic treatment durations need baseline, continual, and systematic (i.e., using rating scales) monitoring for a full range of neurological side effects. Further, side effects other than the neurological may be heightened in children or in nonpsychotic patients, as seen in children with Tourette's disorder who, although treated with low neuroleptic doses, demonstrated dose-related depression, dysphoria, hostility, aggression, fog states, and frank seizures[47].

To the research community, the presence of a clinical risk factor for treatment-emergent dyskinesia, a possible behavioral marker of reduced vulnerability to tardive dyskinesia, the high frequency of atypical dyskinesia, the high prevalence of parkinsonism, the persistence of parkinsonism beyond neuroleptic discontinuation, and the complex pharmacological pattern of parkinsonism suggest areas for future investigation in an attempt to identify the neurochemical correlates and mechanisms of these disorders. The similarities and differences between the children and adolescents of the present study and the adults reported in the literature can be heuristic for the field of movement disorders research in general. Further, findings across study groups where some neurochemical substrate differences among the groups may be known, such as age differences in monoamine oxidase levels among children, adolescents, adults, and the elderly, can be useful in generating hypotheses not possible in research approaches based on any one of these groups.

REFERENCES

1. Simeon JG: Pediatric psychopharmacology. Can J Psychiatry 1989; 34:115–122
2. Simeon JG: Depressive disorders in children and adolescents. Psychiatr J. Univ Ottawa 1989; 14:356–363
3. Lapierre YD, Raval KJ: Pharmacotherapy of affective disorders in children and adolescents. Psychiatr Clin North Am 1989; 12:951–961
4. Campbell M, Spencer EK: Psychopharmacology in child and adolesent psychiatry: a review of the past five years. J Am Acad Child Adolesc Psychiatry 1988; 27:269–279
5. Campbell M: On the use of neuroleptics in children and adolescents. Psychiatr Annals 1985; 15:101–107
6. Silverstein FS, Johnston MV: Risks of neuroleptic drugs in children. J Child Neurol 1987; 2:41–43
7. Anderson LT, Campbell M, Adadms P, Small AM, Perry R, Shell J: The effects of haloperidol on discrimination learning and behavioral symptoms in autistic children. J. Autism Dev Disord 1989; 19:227–239
8. Bruun RD: Gilles de la Tourette's syndrome. J Am Acad Child Adolesc Psychiatry 1984; 23:126–133
9. Campbell M, Small AM, Green WH, Jennings SJ, Perry R, Bennett WG, Anderson L: Behavioral efficacy of haloperidol and lithium carbonate. Arch Gen Psychiatry 1984; 41:650–656
10. Greenhill LL, Solomon M, Pleak R. Ambrosini P: Molindone hydrochloride treatment of hospitalized children with conduct disorder. J Clin Psychiatry 1985; 46:20–254
11. Gittelman-Klein R, Klein DF, Katz S, Saraf K, Pollack E: Comparative effects of

methylphenidate and thioridazine in hyperkinetic children, I: clinical results. Arch Gen Psychiatry 1976; 33:1217–1231

12. Campbell M, Grega DM, Green WH, Bennett WG: Review: neuroleptic-induced dyskinesias in children. Clin Neuropharmacol 1983; 6:207–222

13. Campbell M, Adams P, Perry R, Spencer EK, Overall JE: Tardive and withdrawal dyskinesia in autistic children: a prospective study. Psychopharmacol Bull 1988; 24:251–255

14. Perry R, Campbell M, Green WH, Small AM, Die-Trill ML, Meiselas K, Golden RR, Deutsch SI: Neuroleptic-related dyskinesias in autistic children: a prospective study. Psychopharmacol Bull 1985; 21;140–143

15. Gualtieri CT, Barnhill J, McGimsey J, Schell D: Tardive dyskinesia and other movement disorders in children treated with psychotropic drugs. J Am Acad Child Psychiatry 1980; 19:491–510

16. Gualtieri CT, Schroeder SR, Hicks RE, Quade D: Tardive dyskinesia in young mentally retarded individuals. Arch Gen Psychiatry 1986; 43:335–340

17. Gualtieri CT, Quade D, Hicks RE, Mayo JP, Schroeder SR: Tardive dyskinesia and other clinical consequences of neuroleptic treatment in children and adolescents. Am J Psychiatry 1984; 141:20–23

18. Stone RK, Alvarez WF, May JE: Dyskinesia, antipsychotic-drug exposure and risk factors in a developmentally-disabled population. Pharmacol Biochem Behav 1988; 29:45–51

19. Simpson GM, Lee JH, Zoubok B, Gardos G: A rating scale for tardive dyskinesia. Psychopharmacology (Berlin) 1979; 64:171–179

20. Guy W (ed): ECDEU Assessment Manual for Psychopharmacology: Publication ADM 76–338. Washington, DC, US Department of Health, Education, and Welfare, 1976, pp 534–537

21. Simpson GM, Angus JWS: Drug induced extra-pyramidal disorders. Acta Psychiatr Scand 1970; 46(suppl 212):1–58

22. Richardson MA, Haugland G, Pass R, Craig TJ: The prevalence of tardive dyskinesia in a mentally retarded population. Psychopharmacol Bull 1986; 22:243–249

23. Richardson MA, Craig TJ: The coexistence of parkinsonism-like symptoms and tardive dyskinesia. Am J Psychiatry 1982; 139:341–343,1382

24. Richardson MA, Pass R, Bregman Z, Craig TJ: Tardive dyskinesia and depressive symptoms in schizophrenics. Psychopharmacol Bull 1985; 21:130–135

25. Richardson MA, Pass R, Craig TJ, Vickers E: Factors contributing to the prevalence and severity of tardive dyskinesia. Psychopharmacol Bull 1984; 20:33–38

26. Richardson MA, Casey DE: Tardive dyskinesia status: stability or change. Psychopharmacol Bull 1988; 24:471–475

27. Richardson MA, Suckow R, Whittaker R, Boggiano W, Sziraki I, Kushner H., Perumal A: The plasma phenylalanine/larger neutral amino acid ratio: a risk factor for tardive dyskinesia. Psychopharmacol Bull 1989; 25:47–51

28. Richardson MA, Pass R, Craig TJ: The coexistence of parkinsonism-like symptoms and tardive dyskinesia, in Biological Psychiatry, 1985: Developments in Psychiatry,

vol 7. Edited by Shagass C, Josiassen RC, Bridger WH, Weiss KJ, Stoff D, Simpson GM. New York, Elsevier, 1986

29. Schooler N, Kane JM: Research diagnoses for tardive dyskinesia (RD-TD). Arch Gen Psychiatry 1982; 39:486–487

30. Davis JM: Organic therapies, in Comprehensive Textbook of Psychiatry, 4th ed, vol 2. Edited by Freedman AM, Kaplan HI, Sadock BJ. Baltimore, Williams & Wilkins, 1985

31. Holm S: A simple sequentially rejective multiple test procedure. Scand J Statistics 1979; 6:65–70

32. Richardson MA: Neuroleptic-induced parkinsonism: current concepts, in Proceedings of the New York State Office of Mental Health Second Annual Research Conference. Albany, New York State Office of Mental Health, 1989, p. 15

33. Richardson MA, Casey D, Bitter I: Elderly psychiatric patients: parkinsonism, sex, and MAO relationships. Biol Psychiatry 1989; 25(suppl 7a): 73A

34. Engelhardt DM, Polizos P: Adverse effects of pharmacotherapy in childhood psychosis, in Psychopharmacology: A Generation of Progress. Edited by Lipton MA, DiMascio A, Killam KF. New York, Raven Press, 1978

35. Chiles JA: Extrapyramidal reactions in adolescents treated with high-potency antipsychotics. Am J Psychiatry 1978; 135:239–240

36. Simpson GM, Amuso D, Blair JH, Farkas T: Phenothiazine-produced extra-pyramidal symptom disturbance. Arch Gen Psychiatry 194; 10:199–208

37. Hershon HI, Kennedy PF, McGuire RJ: Persistence of extrapyramidal disorders and psychiatric relapse after withdrawal of long-term phenothiazine therapy. Br J Psychiatry 1972; 120: 41–50

38. Klawans HL Jr, Bergen D, Bruyn GW: Prolonged drug-induced parkinsonism. Confin Neurol 1973; 35:368–377

39. McAndrew JB, Case Q, Treffert DA: Effects of prolonged phenothiazine intake on psychotic and other hospitalized children. J Autism Child Schizophr 1972; 2:75–91

40. Galdi J, Rieder RO, Silber D, Bonato RR: Genetic factors in the response to neuroleptics in schizophrenia: a psychopharmacogenetic study. Psychol Med 1981; 11:713–728

41. Wegner JT, Catalano F, Gibralter J, Kane JM: Schizophrenics with tardive dyskinesia: neuropsychological deficit and family psychopathology. Arch Gen Psychiatry 1985; 42:860–865

42. Casey D, Denney D: Pharmacological characterization of tardive dyskinesia. Psychopharmacology (Berlin) 1977; 54:1–8

43. Lieberman J, Lessser M, Johns C, Pollack S, Saltz B, Kane J: Pharmacologic studies of tardive dyskinesia. J Clin Psychopharmacol 1988; 8(4, suppl): 57S–63S

44. Richardson MA, Craig TJ, Branchey MH: Intra-patient variability in the measurement of tardive dyskinesia. Psychopharmacology (Berlin) 1982; 76:269–272

45. Gerlach J: Pathophysiological mechanisms underlying tardive dyskinesia, in Dyskinesia: Research and Treatment. Edited by Casey DE, Chase TN, Christensen AV. New York, Springer-Verlag, 1985

46. Polizos P, Engelhardt DM: Dyskinetic phenomena in children treated with psychotropic medications. Psychopharmacol Bull 1978; 14:65–68

47. Bruun RD: Subtle and underrecognized side effects of neuroleptic treatment in children with Tourette's disorder. Am J Psychiatry 1988; 145:621–624

48. van Putten T, Mutalipassi LR, Malkin MD: Phenothiazine-induced decompensation. Arch Gen Psychiatry 1974; 30:102–105

49. Weiden P, Bruun R: Worsening of Tourette's disorder due to neuroleptic-induced akathisia. Am J Psychiatry 1987; 144:504–505

25

Attention Deficit Disorder With and Without Hyperactivity: Clinical Response to Three Dose Levels of Methylphenidate

Russell A. Barkley, George J. DuPaul, and Mary B. McMurray
University of Massachusetts Medical Center, Worcester

The response of 23 children with attention deficit disorder (ADD) with hyperactivity (+H) and 17 children with ADD without hyperactivity (−H) to three doses of methylphenidate (5, 10, and 15 mg twice a day) was evaluated in a triple-blind, placebo-controlled crossover design using parent and teacher ratings of behavior, laboratory tests of ADD symptoms, and behavioral observations during academic performance. Results indicated that the children with ADD + H were rated as having more pervasive behavioral problems at home and more pervasive and severe conduct problems at school than the children with ADD−H. Laboratory tests found the children with ADD + H to be impaired in behavioral inhibition and vigilance whereas children with ADD−H were more impaired in the consistent retrieval of verbally learned material. Drug effects were noted on the parent and teacher ratings and on most laboratory measures, with all three doses typically producing significant changes but rarely differing among themselves in effectiveness. The groups were not found to differ significantly on any measures in their response to methylphenidate. However, more children with ADD−H were clinically judged as having either no clinical response (24%) or responding best to the low dose (35%) of medication. In contrast, most ADD + H (95%) children were judged to be positive

Reprinted with permission from *Pediatrics*, 1991, Vol. 87, No. 4, 519–531. Copyright ©1991 by the American Academy of Pediatrics.

This research was supported by National Institute of Mental Health grant 41464.

We are grateful to Judy Tessier and Ellen Mintz-Lennick for their assistance with the data collection, scoring, and computer entry and to Craig Edelbrock, PhD, for his assistance with selecting and scoring some of the dependent measures.

responders and most were recommended to receive the moderate to high dose (71%).

Attention deficit disorder (ADD) comprises a heterogeneous group of children believed to have in common the characteristics of developmentally inappropriate levels of inattention, impulsivity, and in some cases overactivity.[1,2] However, it is believed that disturbances in sustained attention, particularly vigilance, signify all children with this disorder. Despite these apparent commonalities, children with ADD have a diversity of related psychiatric symptoms, family backgrounds, developmental courses, and responses to treatments.[3,4] In the past decade, increasing attention has been paid to identifying approaches to subtyping this disorder into more homogeneous, clinically meaningful subgroups that may provide important differential predictions of etiologies, developmental courses, outcomes, or responses to therapies.

One subtyping approach of considerable clinical interest is based on the presence and degree of overactivity.[1] This method of creating subtypes of ADD was first proposed in the *Diagnostic and Statistical Manual of Mental Disorders,* 3rd edition (DSM-III). It was later relegated to a minor status in the DSM-III-R because of the lack of research at that time on the utility of this approach.[5] Several early studies found few, if any, important differences between ADD children with hyperactivity (+ H) and those without it (–H).[6,7] Just as many, however, indicated that + H children were more aggressive, more rejected by peers, had lower self-esteem, and may be more impaired in cognitive and motor test performance than –H children.[8,9] Those children with ADD–H were characterized as more anxious, daydreamy, lethargic, and sluggish than children with ADD + H by means of teacher ratings of classroom adjustment.[10-12] These studies have begun to intimate the possibility that ADD–H is a different type of attention disorder and a distinct child psychiatric condition from ADD + H.

Two methodological problems plague most of these prior studies. First, many used teacher ratings to classify their subjects as having ADD + H or ADD–H and then used subscales from the same or a highly related rating scale as their dependent measures. Such a confounding of both the source and type of independent and dependent measures ensures that the study will find differences between these two groups. A second problem occurs where studies relied on the DSM-III criteria for diagnosing these two subtypes. Although these criteria list symptom items under the separate constructs of inattention, impulsivity, and overactivity, empirical analysis of these items, such as by factor or cluster analysis, indicates that they do not cluster in the manner in which they are listed in these criteria.[12,13] Only two dimensions or lists are found. One is an inattention-restless factor and the second is a hyperactive-impulsive factor. DSM-III guidelines state that a child with ADD–H must be significantly deviant on both inattention and impulsivity items but not on the hyperactivity items. Consequently, sorting children by these criteria will confound the −H group with highly impulsive children who are overactive but not sufficiently so to meet the cutoff for hyperactivity. It would be better to sort the children with ADD using a more empirically established set of items for the two behavioral dimensions found in factor analytic studies. A further problem with the DSM-III criteria is that the cutoff scores for clinical significance for each of the three items lists were derived entirely by committee consensus with no effort to empirically validate these cutoff scores. One cannot be certain whether children so selected are in fact deviant for their developmental level.

Recent research in our laboratory[14] has used a more empirical approach to diagnosing children and sorting them into the subgroups of −H and +H by using a rating scale of the two behavioral dimensions of inattention and hyperactive-impulsive items and requiring children to be statistically deviant on one or both, respectively. Our research has shown that children with ADD−H have difficulties with focused attention and cognitive processing speed as manifested in deficiencies in timed perceptual-motor tasks but less so in impulsivity or sustained attention. In contrast, children with ADD+H did not have impaired perceptual-motor speed but, as expected, displayed considerable difficulties with behavioral inhibition (impulse control) and sustained attention on a vigilance test. The children with ADD+H also were impaired in several neuropsychological tests of frontal lobe functions, particularly those sensitive to disinhibition—deficits not seen in the ADD-H group.

These groups also differed significantly in their educational and family psychiatric histories as well as in their current behavioral adjustment. Children with ADD+H were more likely to be placed in special education programs for behavior-disordered children and to have been suspended from school more frequently than children with ADD−H. The family histories of the former children also showed a greater prevalence of hyperactivity and attention problems as well as substance abuse among their relatives compared with ADD−H children whereas children with ADD−H had a higher prevalence of anxiety disorders and learning disabilities among their relatives compared with those with ADD+H. Moreover, those children with ADD+H manifested considerably greater problems with peer relations and were rated by both parents and teachers as more aggressive and antisocial at school and at home than ADD−H children. These findings support the notion that ADD−H probably represents a different child psychiatric and attention disorder than ADD+H rather than being a subtype of the same, shared attention disturbance.

As noted above, a further purpose of subtyping children with ADD may be to indicate a different response to treatment between them. To our knowledge, no studies have examined these two types of ADD for their response to behavioral or psychological interventions, and only two have studied the response of these subtypes to stimulant medication.[15,16] In the study by Famularo and Fenton,[15] the investigators found that the majority of children (80%) responded positively to methylphenidate. This sole drug study is seriously flawed in its methodology, however, in that only 10 children were evaluated, all of whom had a diagnosis of ADD-H. The study involved an open trial of methylphenidate, without placebo control subjects, and a diverse range of doses between 0.4 and 1.2 mg/kg per day with no attempt to systematically evaluate the effect of standard doses on these children or to compare their dose response directly with that of children with ADD + H. The study used only parent and teacher ratings of academic grades across a considerable time period (approximately 27 weeks of school) using ratings taken prior to and then during treatment. Rating scales are highly subject to practice effects, with scores improving significantly between first and second rating without intervening treatment.[17] Treatment effects in this drug study are therefore confounded with practice effects, making it possible to determine change that is specifically due to treatment. The second study, by Ullmann and Sleator,[16] unfortunately collapsed the two subtypes into a single group for the analysis of drug effects, thereby obscuring any differences in treatment response between these two subtypes.

The purpose of our study was to conduct a more comprehensive and systematic evaluation of the responses of children with ADD + H and ADD–H to three different dose levels of methylphenidate (5, 10, and 15 mg twice a day) using a triple-blind, placebo-controlled crossover design. In addition to the traditional parent and teacher ratings of behavior common to stimulant drug studies, we used a battery of objective laboratory tests of sustained attention, impulse control, and verbal learning and memory as well as systematic behavioral observations of inattention and overactivity during performance of an academic task. Side effects were formally assessed across drug conditions to evaluate possible group differences in this aspect of drug responding as well. The subjects were a subset of those children used in our research described above and were empirically defined as developmentally deviant and sorted into groups by using a diagnostic procedure more rigorous than those used in past research.

METHODS

Subjects

A total of 40 children with ADD between 6 and 11 years of age were used in this study. The study was approved by the Institutional Review Board at our medical center and all parents signed statements of informed consent permitting their children's participation in the project. Each subject entering this study (1) had an IQ estimate of 80 or higher on a standardized IQ test given within the past year or on the Wechsler Intelligence Scale for Children-Revised given at the study screening; (2) was the biological child of the current parents or had been adopted by them shortly after birth (within first year); and (3) had no evidence of deafness, blindness, severe language delay, cerebral palsy, epilepsy, autism, or psychosis as established through medical history, parental interview, and child play diagnostic interview.

The 23 children with ADD + H (21 boys, 2 girls) met the following additional criteria: (1) teacher complaints of short attention span, impulsivity, and overactivity as revealed by parent reports; (2) a duration of these problems of 6 months, (3) an age of onset of these problems before 7 years; (4) a score greater than the 93rd percentile on the Inattention *and* Overactivity scales of the Child Attention Problems (CAP) rating scale (This brief 12-item rating scale is derived from the Child Behavior Checklist Teacher Report Form Inattention and Overactivity Scales.[18] An inattention scale was created from 7 items and an overactivity scale was created from 5 items by Edelbrock.[19] Norms were constructed for this scale from the same normative data used in the larger Child Behavior Checklist Teacher Report Form); and (5) no history of treatment with stimulant drugs or, if such a history, physician consent to stop taking medication for 48 hours prior to evaluation in the study.

The children with ADD–H (15 boys, 2 girls) met the same criteria as the children with ADD + H except for criterion 4 above. Instead, the children with ADD–H had to have a score greater than the 93rd percentile on the Inattention scale of the CAP but a score below the 84th percentile on the Overactivity scale of the CAP. This effectively separated the ADD subtypes by at least 0.5 standard deviation on the Overactivity scale.

All children with ADD were recruited from consecutive referrals to the outpatient clinics of the Departments of Psychiatry and Pediatrics. We excluded the following children with ADD from participation in the drug study: (1) children with a history of tics or Tourette syndrome, given the controversy over whether stimulants may create or exacerbate these conditions; (2) those with a history of cardiac surgery, high blood pressure, or cerebral vascular accident given the known cardiac pressor effects of the stimulants; and (3) those with a history of adverse reactions to stimulant medications.

The results for each subject group on various demographic and subject selection measures are displayed in Table 1. These results were analyzed using *t* tests to assess possible differences between the groups. The groups were found to differ significantly on child's IQ score, with the ADD–H group scoring significantly lower than the ADD + H group.

Medication

Children were randomly assigned to one of six possible drug orders within which each drug condition lasted 1 week before crossing over to the next drug condition. There were four drug conditions: placebo (P), 5 mg bid (low dose [L], 10 mg bid (moderate dose [M]), and 15 mg bid (high dose [H]). Although there were four

TABLE 1.
Initial Demographic Information by Group*

Measure	ADD+H (n = 23)		ADD−H (n = 17)		t Test	P
	Mean	SD	Mean	SD		
Child age, y	8.3	1.2	9.0	1.4	−1.61	...
Grade, y	2.4	1.2	2.5	1.2	−0.31	...
Child IQ	106.9	11.6	98.9	12.7	2.04	<.05
Mother's age, y	33.6	4.4	34.4	3.4	−0.35	...
Mother's education, y	13.2	2.1	13.2	2.2	−0.01	...
Father's age, y	35.3	3.3	38.0	4.9	−2.01	<.06
Father's education, y	14.2	2.4	13.6	3.1	0.62	...
Hollingshead 2-factor index	51.8	23.8	58.8	24.5	−0.90	...
No. of children in family	1.5	0.7	1.8	0.8	−1.05	...

* ADD+H, attention deficit disorder with hyperactivity; ADD−H, attention deficit disorder without hyperactivity.

drug conditions, we constructed only six drug orders so that the highest dose (15 mg bid) was never given unless preceded by the moderate dose (10 mg bid). By coupling these two drug conditions, we ensured that our subjects would not experience side effects unnecessarily by starting on the high dose as their first active drug condition, a problem noted in several past studies.[20] Drug orders were PLMH, PMHL, LPMH, LMHP, MHLP, MHPL. Fixed doses of medication were used rather than using a milligram-per-kilogram formula as optimal dose has been found not to depend on body weight[21] and such a formula may overdose heavier children.

The hospital pharmacy prepared the placebo (lactose powder) and methylphenidate by crushing and placing them in no. 6 orange opaque gelatin capsules, with a 10-day supply prepared for each drug condition. Parents were given only one bottle of capsules each week at the beginning of each new drug condition and had to return unused capsules at the end of the week for a check of compliance to the protocol. Children were permitted to miss 1 day of medication during the past 7 days and still remain in the study. No families were removed from the study because of noncompliance as defined in this way. One capsule was given in the morning and a second at noon each day. Children were seen in the clinic for brief testing at the end of each drug condition. Project staff questioned parents carefully to ensure that the medication was taken approximately 1 hour before the psychological testing.

Procedures

Families referred to the project were initially screened by telephone and then were seen for a brief clinical evaluation to determine eligibility. This evaluation included a diagnostic interview with parent, play interview with child, and completion of parent and teacher Child Behavior Checklists. Eligible children and their mothers were then seen on a single day for the 3.5-hour evaluation which served as a pretreatment evaluation. Mothers were interviewed further while the children were tested by a research assistant. The children were given the intelligence and achievement tests, after which the research assistant conducted the psychological tests described below. The behavioral observations from the Restricted Academic Task were then taken. The results of the measures collected at that initial evaluation are reported in a separate paper.[14]

The children with ADD in the present study were then seen briefly by the project pediatrician for a physical examination and medical history review to determine their acceptability for drug treatment. Children were then evaluated in the clinic at the end of each drug condition (weekly) for a 1-hour assessment of drug response. At the end of each week, parents and teachers also completed several rating scales of child behavior and drug side effects. At the end of the drug protocol, parents were provided with feedback on the outcome of the drug trial and a report was sent to the child's pediatrician.

Dependent Measures

Psychological Tests. The following tests were administered at the end of each drug condition. Different yet equivalent versions of the psychological tests were constructed to avoid practice effects.

1. Wisconsin Selective Reminding Test: This is a verbal learning and memory test adapted from Buschke's test used in adult neuropsychology. Children were orally given a list of 12 unrelated words to remember and then immediately asked to name all words. On each trial the subject was reminded only of the words missed and then asked to repeat the entire list again. This continued for 10 trials or until the child recalled the entire list correctly without reminding on two consecutive trials. We calculated the following scores: (1) total recall—the total number of words recalled across all trials (2) long-term storage—the number of words recalled on at least two consecutive trials; and (3) consistent long-term retrieval—the number of words recalled on at least two trials and then consistently on every trial thereafter.

2. Continuous Performance Test[23]: This vigilance first required that the child sit before a small computerized device which administered the test in a machine-paced procedure. The device contained a small display screen on which numbers flashed randomly at the rate of one per second. Each number is displayed for 200 milliseconds with an 800-millisecond interval between each signal. Below the display was a blue button which the child was instructed to press every time he or she observed a number 1 followed by a number 9. The device recorded the number of correctly detected 1/9 sequences, the number of commission errors, and the number of omission errors. The task lasted 12 minutes and 60 target 1/9 sequences were presented during this period. The device has an alternate form on which the correct sequence is 3 followed by 5. Each of these versions was alternated across the four drug conditions.

3. Kagan Matching Familiar Figures Test[24]: In this commonly used measure of impulse control, the child was shown a page containing a sample picture, below which were six very similar pictures. The child was told to point to the picture that was identical with the sample picture. If mistaken, the child was told to try again until the correct picture was identified. Twelve trials were presented. Scores were the mean time to first response across trials and total number of error responses. Four different forms of this test were constructed by rearranging the six possible responses into a different array such that the correct picture appeared in a different position in each version. A different version was used in each drug condition.

4. Attention Deficit Disorder Behaviors During a Restricted Academic

Situation[20]: In this task, designed to measure ADD symptoms during independent academic work, the child was placed alone in a clinic playroom and provided with a packet of math problems to complete. The child was told to complete as many math problems as possible, not to leave his or her chair at the table, and not to touch any toys. Math problems were selected from six available difficulty levels to be below the child's math grade level at school. Toys were provided on a bookshelf in the playroom. The situation lasted 15 minutes and the child's behavior was videotaped. Later, the videotape was scored using five behavioral categories: off-task, fidgets, out of seat, vocalizes, and plays with objects. Every 30 seconds, the coder checked on the coding sheet whether any of the five behavior categories were observed. This yielded 30 possible occurrences for each of the five behavior categories. The scores were the percent occurrence of each category as well as a total percent occurrence for all behavior categories (total ADD behaviors). In addition, the number of math problems completed during the 15-minute period and the percent correctly completed were also scored.

Intercoder agreement in previous studies using this coding system ranged between 0.77 and 0.89.[20,25] The coding system has been found to be quite sensitive to stimulant medication effects.[20,26] Coders in the study were trained to a level of agreement of 0.80 and intercoder reliability was evaluated on 20% of the videotapes. Reliabilities in the present study were as follows: off-task = 74%, fidgets = 67%, vocal = 74%, plays with objects = 87%, and out of seat = 79%.

Parent Rating Scales. Mothers completed the following rating scales at the end of each drug condition:

1. Home Situations Questionnaire (HSQ)[27]: This scale measures the pervasiveness of child behavior problems across 16 home situations. Parents rate each situation on a scale of severity from 1 (mild) to 9 (severe). Scores are obtained for the number of problem settings and mean severity of problems.
2. ADHD Rating Scale[28]: To assess the symptoms used in the diagnosis of attention deficit hyperactivity disorder (ADHD), we used a rating scale of the 14 DSM-III-R symptoms. Parents rated each symptom as follows: not at all, just a little, pretty much, and very much (0, 1, 2, 3). Two scores were calculated: total points and total number of significant symptoms (items rated 2 or higher).
3. Home Side Effects Rating Scale[29]: This rating scale lists 16 possible side effects of methylphenidate. Each is rated on a scale of severity from 0 (not present) to 9 (severe). Two scores were calculated, these being the number of side effects and the mean severity (average severity rating across all endorsed side effects).

Teacher Rating Scale. Teachers completed the following rating scales at the end of each drug condition:

1. School Situations Questionnaire (SSQ)[27]: This scale assesses the pervasiveness of behavior problems across 12 school situations. Like the HSQ above, each situation is rated on a scale of severity from 1 (mild) to 9 (severe). Scores were the number of problem situations and the mean severity of problems.
2. Child Attention Problems (CAP) rating scale[19]: This scale, described above, was used for classifying the children as having ADD and then sorting them into those who were +H and −H based on scores on the separate inattention and overactivity scales. Raw scores for each subscale were used in this study.
3. Teacher Self-Control Rating Scale[30]: This scale was originally developed by Kendall and Wilcox[31] to assess self-control in children. Humphrey[30] slightly modified the scale and reported norms for more than 750 children. The scale was used here to provide a measure of impulse control in children at school. Raw scores were used in this study.
4. School Side Effects Rating Scale: This scale was identical with the Home Side Effects Rating Scale, described under "Parent Rating Scales."

RESULTS

The comparisons of the two groups on the initial selection measures described earlier found that the groups differed significantly in child IQ. To determine whether child IQ should be used as a covariate in the subsequent analyses, child IQ was correlated with all of the dependent measures. These results indicated significant relationships between IQ and only two measures: (1) the behavioral category of out-of-seat from the restricted academic situation and (2) total recall from the Wisconsin Selective Reminding Test. Child IQ was therefore used as a covariate in the analyses of these two dependent measures.

The results for all dependent measures were analyzed using 2 × 4 (group × drug condition) analyses of variance with repeated measures on the second factor. Where a significant main effect for drug condition was found, pairwise comparisons using Newman-Keuls tests were conducted to evaluate the possible differences among the drug conditions.

Parent Ratings

The findings for the parent rating scales for each group in each drug condition, along with the results of the initial statistical tests, are displayed in Table 2. The results indicated a significant main effect for group only on the number

TABLE 2.

Means and Statistical Test Results for Parent Rating Scales Across Each Drug Condition by ADD Subtype*

Measure by Group	Drug Conditions				Results	
	Placebo	5 mg	10 mg	15 mg	Eff.	Cont.
HSQ, no. of settings						
ADD+H	10.4	9.5	9.1	8.3	G, D	c, e
ADD–H	5.9	6.9	5.1	5.4		
HSQ, mean severity						
ADD+H	4.4	3.7	3.4	3.3	D	a, b, c
ADD–H	3.5	2.9	2.5	2.8		
ADHD Scale, total score						
ADD+H	25.5	19.4	18.3	-14.5	D	a, b, c, e
ADD–H	18.4	17.6	12.5	13.4		
ADHD Scale, no. of items ≥2						
ADD+H	9.1	5.9	5.8	3.7	D	a, b, c, e, f
ADD–H	5.6	4.9	3.7	3.2		
Side effects, no.						
ADD+H	5.3	6.3	6.7	6.2	…	
ADD–H	5.4	4.7	4.5	5.8		
Side effects, mean severity						
ADD+H	3.2	3.5	3.8	3.1	…	
ADD–H	3.1	4.0	2.9	3.3		

* Eff.: Effects that reached statistical significance ($P < .05$) from the overall analyses of variance; G = main effect for group, D = main effect for drug condition, and G × D = interaction of group × drug condition. Cont.: Results of pairwise contrasts between drug conditions that reached significance ($P < .05$) in analyzing the significant main effects for drug condition; a = placebo vs 5 mg, b = placebo vs 10 mg, c = placebo vs 15 mg, d = 5 mg vs 10 mg, e = 5 mg vs 15 mg, and f = 10 mg vs 15 mg. HSQ, Home Situations Questionnaire; ADD+H, attention deficit disorder with hyperactivity; ADD–H, attention deficit disorder without hyperactivity; ADHD Scale, Attention Deficit Hyperactivity Disorder Rating Scale.

of problem settings from the HSQ. The ADD + H group scored significantly higher or worse on this scale than the ADD–H group.

A main effect for drug condition was found on four of the six parent rating scales. These indicated statistically significant declines on both the number of problem settings and mean severity scores from the HSQ, and the total score and the number of significant symptoms from the ADHD Rating Scale.

Pairwise comparisons were then conducted on these measures. Results for the number of problem settings on the HSQ indicated that only the high dose was significantly different from placebo condition. It was also significantly different from the low-dose condition. Neither the low nor moderate doses differed from the placebo condition. It appears that only the high dose resulted in a decline in the pervasiveness of the children's behavior problems at home relative to the placebo condition. Dose effects on the mean severity rating from the HSQ were such that all three doses led to significant declines in the severity of home behavior problems compared with placebo but did not differ from each other in this respect. No other comparisons reached significance. The interaction of group by drug condition was also not significant on either HSQ score.

For the ADHD Rating Scale, the pairwise comparisons on the total score revealed that all three doses produced significant declines in the severity of ADHD symptoms relative to the placebo condition. They differed from each other only in that the high dose produced a significantly greater reduction in this score than the low dose. No other comparisons were significant. On the score of the number of significant symptoms (items with ratings ≥ 2), the pairwise comparisons suggested that all three doses were again effective in reducing the number of ADHD symptoms rated by parents. In this case, the high dose was also significantly more effective than the low and moderate doses, which did not differ from each other in effectiveness. Thus, it appears that methylphenidate produces significant declines in both ADD groups in the number and severity of their ADHD symptoms. There was no significant group × drug condition interaction on either score.

No significant main effects for drug condition were noted on either score from the home side effects questionnaire. There was a trend for a group × drug condition interaction (F = 2.49, df = 3/114, $P < 0.07$), but this did not quite reach statistical significance and so further contrasts to evaluate this effect were not conducted.

Teacher Ratings

The results of the analyses of the teacher rating scales are shown in Table 3. They indicated a significant main effect for group on the Overactivity scale from the CAP, on the number of problem settings and mean severity score from the SSQ, and on the Teacher Self-Control Rating Scale. In each case, the ADD + H group scored significantly worse than the ADD–H group. The difference on the CAP

TABLE 3.

Means and Statistical Test Results for Teacher Rating Scales Across Each Drug Condition by ADD Subtype*

Measure by Group	Drug Conditions				Results	
	Placebo	5 mg	10 mg	15 mg	Eff.	Cont.
CAP scale, inattention						
ADD+H	9.2	8.0	6.2	6.8	D	b, c
ADD−H	8.6	6.4	6.5	6.6		
CAP scale, overactivity						
ADD+H	7.0	5.3	4.6	4.5	G, D	a, b, c
ADD−H	3.5	2.0	2.1	2.4		
SSQ, no. of settings						
ADD+H	5.7	4.5	5.0	3.7	G, D	a, b, c
ADD−H	3.6	2.4	1.7	1.8		
SSQ, mean severity						
ADD+H	4.4	3.5	2.8	2.3	G, D	a, b, c
ADD−H	2.6	1.4	1.5	1.8		
Side effects, no.						
ADD+H	4.5	4.0	3.6	4.4	...	
ADD−H	5.0	3.9	3.9	4.1		
Side effects, mean severity						
ADD+H	4.1	3.6	3.2	4.1	...	
ADD−H	3.5	3.2	3.1	3.2		
Teacher SCRS						
ADD+H	36.6	39.7	44.0	45.3	G, D	a, b, c
ADD−H	42.7	51.7	50.8	51.1		

* Eff.: Effects that reached statistical significance ($P < .05$) from the overall analyses of variance; G = main effect for group, D = main effect for drug condition, and G × D = interaction of group × drug condition. Cont.: Results of pairwise contrasts between drug conditions that reached significance ($P < .05$) in analyzing the significant main effects for drug condition; a = placebo vs 5 mg, b = placebo vs 10 mg, c = placebo vs 15 mg, d = 5 mg vs 10 mg, e = 5 mg vs 15 mg, and f = 10 mg vs 15 mg. CAP scale, Child Attention Problems rating scale; SSQ, School Situations Questionnaire; Teacher SCRS, Teacher Self-Control Rating Scale; ADD+H, attention deficit disorder with hyperactivity; ADD−H, attention deficit disorder without hyperactivity.

Overactivity scale was expected in view of its use to sort the subjects into +H and −H subtypes.

A number of significant main effects for drug condition were noted on the teacher rating scales. These were on the CAP Inattention and Overactivity scales, the number of problem settings and mean severity scores from the SSQ, and the Teacher Self-Control Rating Scale.

For the teacher ratings on the CAP scale, the pairwise comparisons evaluating the significant main effect for drug condition indicated that only the moderate and high doses resulted in significant declines in the Inattention score compared with placebo. The doses did not differ significantly from each other in their effects. On the Overactivity scale, all three doses significantly reduced these ratings but again the doses did not differ significantly from each other in this respect. These findings indicate that moderate to high doses were needed to effect change in the teacher ratings of inattentive behavior but all three doses did so on ratings of overactivity. In both cases, no differences between the doses were noted, implying that the moderate to low doses, respectively, were as effective as the higher dose in producing significant change on these ratings. Again, the interaction of group membership with drug condition was not significant.

The pairwise comparisons for the teacher ratings on the SSQ scores across drug conditions indicated that all three doses were significantly effective in reducing the pervasiveness of behavior problems across school situations (number of problem settings). The doses again did not differ among themselves in their effectiveness. The same results were found for the mean severity score on the SSQ, once again showing that all three doses were equally effective in reducing the mean severity of behavior problems across all settings at school. The group × drug interaction was not significant for either score on this scale.

As with the parent ratings of side effects at home, teacher ratings of side effects at school revealed no significant effects of medication at the doses used here. There was also no significant interaction of group membership with drug condition on either score from the rating scale.

Using the Teacher Self-Control Rating Scale, teachers rated the self-control of the children with ADD. Results of the pairwise comparisons on this scale used to evaluate the significant main effect for drug condition revealed that all three doses were effective in significantly improving the self-control of both groups of children. The doses did not differ among themselves in their effectiveness. There was also no significant interaction of group with drug condition on this rating scale.

To summarize, significant improvements in the behavior of both groups of children were noted on all teacher ratings, with all three doses producing equal effectiveness on these measures. All three doses were also effective in improving behavior ratings at home. The high dose, however, produced significantly greater effects than the low dose on parents' ratings of the pervasiveness of their children's behavior problems and in the number and severity of ADHD symptoms at home. No significant increase in the number or severity of drug side effects was found at home or school. Given the absence of any significant interaction of group × drug condition on any of these rating scales, it would appear that methylphenidate produces equivalent effects on teacher ratings in both subtypes of ADD.

Psychological Tests and Behavioral Observations

The results of the psychological tests and behavioral observations are shown in Table 4. There were significant main effects for group membership on several of the various psychological tests and on two of the behavioral observation codes. These indicated that the ADD + H subtype had significantly more commission errors and omission errors on the Continuous Performance Test than the ADD–H group. The former children also were observed to display more total ADD behaviors during the restricted academic situation than the –H children. Finally, the children with ADD–H were significantly more impaired in their consistent long-term retrieval of verbal information across all drug conditions compared with those with ADD + H. These findings suggest that children with ADD + H are more impulsive and less vigilant and are more likely to display ADHD behaviors during their academic work than children with ADD–H. The latter children by contrast appeared to be more impaired in their retrieval of verbal information from memory than those children with ADD + H.

Significant main effects for drug condition were detected on 8 of the 15 measures in Table 4. Methylphenidate produced significant reductions in errors of omission on the vigilance task but not on commission errors. The behaviors of off-task, fidgeting, playing with objects, and total ADHD behavior during the academic task were also significantly reduced by medication. Finally, there was a significant increase in the accuracy of math problems completed during drug treatment. There were no significant interactions of group membership with drug condition on any of the laboratory measures, behavioral observations, or psychological tests.

Subsequently, pairwise comparisons were conducted on those measures on which significant main effects for drug condition were found. For omission errors on the Continuous Performance Test, only the moderate and high doses produced significant reductions in these errors relative to placebo. The high dose produced a greater reduction than the low dose condition as well. No other comparisons reached significance.

For the behavioral observations, both the moderate and high doses produced significant declines in off-task behavior, fidgeting, and playing with objects. On the category of off-task, the moderate and high doses also produced significantly

TABLE 4.

Means and Statistical Test Results for the Laboratory Tests and Behavioral Observations Across Each Drug Condition by ADD Subtype*

Measure by Group	Drug Conditions					Results	
	Placebo	5 mg	10 mg	15 mg	Eff.	Cont.
CPT, omission errors							
ADD+H	21.6	17.6	14.4	12.3	G, D	b, c, e
ADD−H	3.6	8.4	5.6	5.5		
CPT, commission errors							
ADD+H	28.0	21.7	26.5	15.0	G	
ADD−H	13.6	8.2	9.9	11.4		
Kagan MFFT, mean latency (s)							
ADD+H	9.3	8.4	9.9	23.1	...	
ADD−H	11.0	13.7	12.0	12.0		
Kagan MFFT, total errors							
ADD+H	11.5	11.6	12.9	9.7	...	
ADD−H	10.4	11.1	9.6	10.5		
WSRT, total recall							
ADD+H	71.8	71.0	73.5	72.7	...	
ADD−H	68.9	70.7	72.3	75.2		
WSRT, long-term storage							
ADD+H	66.1	68.2	66.2	70.0	...	
ADD−H	62.4	64.5	63.4	70.4		
WSRT, consistent retrieval							
ADD+H	53.8	53.5	56.0	53.2	G	
ADD−H	40.4	40.1	42.1	46.6		

Continued

TABLE 4.

Means and Statistical Test Results for the Laboratory Tests and Behavioral Observations Across Each Drug Condition by ADD Subtype*(continued)

					Eff.	Eff.
RAS, % off-task						
ADD+H	51.1	50.0	33.8	30.0	D	b, c, d, e
ADD–H	33.8	34.8	27.9	29.3		
RAS, % fidgets						
ADD+H	33.5	31.6	23.0	14.7	D	b, c, e
ADD–H	23.5	17.8	14.6	13.1		
RAS, % vocal						
ADD+H	36.8	31.3	39.4	43.0	...	
ADD–H	24.8	26.6	27.4	32.4		
RAS, % plays						
ADD+H	17.7	15.3	7.3	6.0	D	b, c
ADD–H	8.7	4.4	5.1	5.9		
RAS, % out of seat						
ADD+H	27.3	23.0	18.5	17.0	...	
ADD–H	13.1	11.2	8.8	7.4		
RAS, % total ADD behaviors						
ADD+H	33.4	30.0	29.3	21.9	G, D	c
ADD–H	21.1	19.4	16.9	17.8		
RAS, no. of math problems						
ADD+H	82.8	80.3	89.1	95.7	...	
ADD–H	75.0	71.2	82.9	85.9		
RAS, % math correct						
ADD+H	80.7	86.0	93.4	91.7	D	b, c, d
ADD–H	77.1	86.2	92.2	89.4		

* Eff.: Effects that reached statistical significance ($P < .05$) from the overall analyses of, variance; G = main effect for group, D = main effect for drug condition, and G × D = interaction of group × drug condition. Cont.: Results of pairwise contrasts between drug conditions that reached significance ($P < .05$) in analyzing the significant main effects for drug condition; a = placebo vs 5 mg, b= placebo vs 10 mg, c = placebo vs 15 mg, d = 5 mg vs 10 mg, e = 5 mg vs 15 mg, and f = 10 mg vs 15 mg. CPT, Continuous Performance Test; MFFT, Matching Familiar Figures Test; WSRT, Wisconsin Selective Reminding Test; RAS, restricted academic situation; ADD+H, attention deficit disorder with hyperactivity; ADD–H, attention deficit disorder without hyperactivity.

greater declines in this behavior than did the low dose. The high dose also produced a significant reduction in fidgeting relative to the low-dose condition. For the category of total ADHD behavior, only the high dose resulted in a significant decline in this summary score. Finally, pairwise comparisons on the measure of math accuracy (percent correct) indicated that the moderate and high doses resulted in significant increases in this measure over the placebo condition. The high dose also produced significantly greater improvements in this measure than the low dose. No other comparisons reached statistical significance.

Clinical Judgment of Drug Responding

At the conclusion of the drug trial, the psychologist and pediatrician supervising the drug trial reviewed all of the available information on the child's responding during the trial to make a recommendation about whether the child should continue to receive medication and, if so, at what dose. This review included all dependent measures described above as well as comments made by the parent and teacher each week. A summary sheet of all of these results was prepared and measures on which the children changed at least one standard deviation (using available normative data) between placebo and any drug condition were highlighted. In general, judgments of positive responding were primarily based on a child showing changes on the majority of measures taken in at least two of the three assessment settings (home, school, and clinic) with the least degree of side effects. That dose showing the greatest degree of change in the most settings with the least side effects was judged the best dose for subsequent clinical management of the children. The children's referring pediatrician was then provided with this recommendation and its rationale.

The percentage of children in the −H subgroup receiving each dose level was as follows: no response = 24%, low dose (5 mg bid) = 35%, moderate dose (10 mg bid) = 29%, and high dose (15 mg bid) = 12%. The percentage at each dose for the + H subgroup was as follows: no response = 5%, low dose = 24%, moderate dose = 52%, and high dose = 19%. It is obvious from these results that considerably more of the −H children were recommended for either no medication or the low dose after the trials were completed than in the + H group. The latter group was considerably more likely (71%) to receive the moderate or high dose as their recommended therapeutic level than the −H subgroup, of which only 41% were recommended for this dose range. Therefore, even though both groups may show positive responses on the various dependent measures used here, the totality of their drug responses clearly indicates that the −H subtype is likely to do well on lower doses of medication, with a large minority showing little positive response whereas the + H subtype is likely to receive the moderate to high dose range for clinical management.

DISCUSSION

The present study rigorously evaluated the drug responses of two subtypes of children with ADD to three different doses of methylphenidate using multiple types of measures from multiple sources. The findings will be discussed separately as they pertain to overall group differences on some of the measures and to drug effects on the battery of ratings, tests, and behavioral observations.

Differences in ADD Subtypes

Several differences between the ADD subtypes were noted, many of which parallel the differences found between larger samples that included these same subjects at the comprehensive initial assessment.[14] On both parent and teacher ratings, the children with ADD + H displayed behavior problems across significantly more situations in the home and school than did the children with ADD–H. In school, the + H subtype was also rated as having more severe behavior problems in all situations and as displaying considerably less self-control than the –H subtype. These findings continue to support the notion that + H children are not only more active, but with their increased activity level comes the risk of more serious and pervasive conduct problems and less self-control in social situations than is seen in children with ADD who are not overactive. These findings are quite consistent with other previous studies of this subtype which found greater aggression and peer relationship problems in ADD children with hyperactivity compared with those without hyperactivity.[10,12]

The group differences on several psychological tests and behavioral observations were also revealing of unique difficulties to each group. Children with ADD + H displayed considerably more difficulties with both errors of omission, often interpreted as reflecting inattention, and errors of commission, frequently viewed as reflecting impulsivity. These group differences were also found at the initial baseline or pretreatment assessment of these subjects.[14] Scores for the children with ADD–H on both measures were within the range considered normal for this age range, implying that the attentional problem seen in these children is not likely to be one of vigilance (maintenance of set) or impulsivity (disinhibition) but may reside more in a different component of attention. Underscoring this interpretation was the significantly greater impairment in the consistent retrieval of verbal material from memory in the –H group than in the + H group in this study as well as the poorer performance of this group on the Wechsler Intelligence Scale for Children-Revised Coding subtest taken during the initial pretreatment assessment as reported in our other paper. Again, overactive and disinhibited behavior appears characteristic of children with ADD + H but considerably less so of those with ADD–H.

Mirsky[32] has proposed an empirically derived four-factor model of attention that is well suited to understanding the qualitative differences noted between +H and −H children in the nature of their attention deficits. By factor analyzing a large set of attentional measures similar to those we are using, Mirsky derived four separate components of attention: (1) focus execute—measured by Coding (Wechsler Intelligence Scale for Children-Revised), Trail Making Test, Letter Cancellation tests, and the Stroop Test; (2) sustained attention—measured by continuous performance tests or vigilance tasks; (3) encode—measured by mental Arithmetic and Digit Span, from the Wechsler scales; and (4) shift or flexibility—measured by the Wisconsin Card Sort Test. These factors were replicated in a large sample of normal second-grade children. The different types of attention are believed to have different neuroanatomical loci. Sustained attention is more likely a function of the anterior prefrontal lobes and their rich connections with the limbic system. Focused attention is more likely a function of posterior parietal/temporal substrates. In the context of this model, our findings indicate that ADD + H is typically a problem of vigilance or sustained attention whereas ADD−H is characterized by problems with focused attention. If these findings can be replicated, they will strongly suggest that these are not subtypes of a common, shared attention disorder but actually represent different attention disturbances altogether. Certainly the results discussed earlier from our more extensive initial assessment of these groups point in this direction with respect to presenting behavioral and social problems and family histories of psychiatric disorders.[14] Even so, it is still open to question whether −H represents a qualitatively different disorder given that on the majority of measures taken here and in the initial assessment, especially parent and teacher ratings of behavior, −H children presented as deviant along many of the same behavioral dimensions as +H children but not nearly to the same degree. Only on the cognitive tests did qualitative differences emerge.

Drug Effects on the ADD Subtypes

In general, our results indicated that both groups of children with ADD displayed significant, positive improvements in their behavior problems, inattention, self-control, and academic performance on a math task as a result of treatment with methylphenidate. No significant interactions between group membership and drug condition were noted on any measures, indicating that the effects of methylphenidate seem to be identical in these two groups. On most of the behavioral ratings affected by medication, all three doses produced significant effects but were not significantly different from each other in their effectiveness. This was not true on many of the tests and behavioral observations where moderate to high doses were required to achieve significant changes on these measures. Such findings indicate that the low dose was as effective as the moderate or high doses in changing the behavior of these children at school but that moderate to high doses were needed to produce improved behavior at home and better task performance on the clinic assessment battery.

However, inspection of the means for rating scales for each group across the drug conditions suggests that the greatest effect of medication on the −H group occurred at the low dose, with little noticeable improvement obtained from the larger doses. This has to do with an apparent floor effect for this group of children where the low dose was able to bring their scores down within the range seen in the normal control group studied in our companion papers with little further room for improvement. In contrast, on many measures, the drug effect for the + H group was reasonably linear, improving with each dose increase, although not usually to a degree that was statistically significant. This impression was clearly supported when we inspected the clinical recommendations made about the children's subsequent drug treatment following the trial. These results indicated that considerably more −H children were recommended for either no medication (24%), having shown minimal or no positive response, or the low dose (35%). In contrast, only 5% of the + H children showed no response and 71% were recommended for the moderate to high doses for their clinical management. Such an observation suggests that in clinical practice with these groups of children, the lowest dose used here (5 mg bid) may be sufficient for many of the children with ADD−H whereas both the moderate and high doses (10 and 15 mg bid) may provide greater benefit to the children with ADD+H in many cases. This finding is consistent with many other drug studies[20,21,26] that indicate that the greatest effect of methylphenidate occurs on those measures on which children with ADD are farthest from the normal mean. Given that + H children show considerably greater behavioral deviance, disinhibition, and poor vigilance, the drug effects would be greater in them, particularly at higher doses, than in the −H children. In any case, our results do not contraindicate the use of stimulants with either group of children with ADD and suggest a similar, positive behavioral effect of the medication in both groups. However, they do suggest that lower doses may be sufficient to achieve an optimum therapeutic effect with the −H subtype whereas higher doses may be more beneficial for the + H subtype.

The pattern of drug effects on these measures is also consistent with past research on methylphenidate.[20,21,26] Parent and teacher ratings proved to be sensitive to all three doses of medication. In contrast, only moderate to high doses produced significant effects on the omission score while having no effect on the commission score on this vigilance task. Previous studies have also found this version of a vigilance task to be unreliable in sensing medication effects and to be insensitive to changes in behavior being produced at the lower doses used in these studies. The behavioral observations, by contrast, were sensitive to all three doses of medication. The absence of significant side effects at these dose levels is also in keeping with these previous studies and continues to underscore the relatively mild and benign nature of most side effects seen in most children given these doses of methylphenidate.[33] These results must be viewed in the context of several limitations in the methods of the present drug study. First, most of the measures we used have been previously shown to assess positive drug responses to medication. As a result, our study was not able to reveal any information with regard to possible "cognitive toxicity" from any of the doses used here.[34] Although the existence of such toxicities has not been well-established as yet, it may be that these subtypes of ADD show different patterns of adverse reactions to stimulant medication on other cognitive tasks not used here such as flexibility of shifting attention or concept learning. Second, our use of week-long drug conditions may not have been as adequate at revealing the different behavioral responses of these subtypes as might longer-term trials allowing for larger samplings of behavior across a greater array of situations. Finally, our method of separating these subtypes of ADD relied on a relatively simple rating scale of behavior using scores that separated the groups by only 0.5 standard deviation. Such a procedure may create some overlap between the subtypes such that some children who had actually mild forms of the + H subtype may have been erroneously classified as −H in this study, thereby possibly obscuring differences in their initial behavioral presentation and drug response. The finding that at least 30% of the −H subtype met criteria for ADHD at their initial evaluation intimates just such a problem.[14] Future studies might use criteria that separate these groups by at least a standard deviation on this scale to lessen the likelihood of such misclassification.

SUMMARY

In conclusion, children with ADD–H may have a qualitatively different impairment in attention, perhaps in focused or selective attention, than do children with ADD + H, whose deficits are mainly in behavioral disinhibition and poor vigilance or maintenance of effort. Much research remains to be done, however, before this issue can be considered resolved. Yet if such findings continue to appear in systematic replications of this work, evidence will have accumulated to indicate that ADD-H is not in fact a subtype of ADD + H but is a distinctly separate diagnostic label and criteria for its clinical diagnosis. This study also indicates that these two disorders of attention do not show any dramatic differences in their manner of responding to methylphenidate across the three dose levels used here, with both groups displaying generally positive drug responses. However, examination of the total clinical response of the children across all measures revealed a somewhat different pattern such that more −H children had minimal or no response or did best on the low dose of medication whereas the vast majority of + H children showed a positive response, primarily to the moderate to high doses of methylphenidate.

REFERENCES

1. American Psychiatric Association, Committee on Nomenclature and Statistics. *Diagnostic and Statistical Manual of Mental Disorders.* 3rd ed. Washington, DC: American Psychiatric Association; 1980
2. American Psychiatric Association, Committee on Nomenclature and Statistics. *Diagnostic and Statistical Manual of Mental Disorders.* 3rd ed., revised. Washington, DC: American Psychiatric Association, 1987
3. Ross D, Ross S. *Hyperactivity.* 2nd ed. New York, NY: Wiley; 1982
4. Weiss G, Hechtman L. *Hyperactive Children Grown Up.* New York, NY: Guilford; 1986
5. Spitzer RL, Davies M, Barkley RA. The DSM-III-R field trial for the disruptive behavior disorders. *J Am Acad Child Adolesc Psychiatry.* 1990; 29:690–697
6. Maurer RG, Stewart M. Attention deficit disorder without hyperactivity in a child psychiatry clinic. *J Clin Psychiatry.* 1980; 41:232–233
7. Rubinstein RA, Brown RT. An evaluation of the validity of the diagnostic category of attention deficit disorder. *Am J Orthopsychiatry.* 1984; 54:398–414
8. Berry CA, Shaywitz SE, Shaywitz BA. Girls with attention deficit disorder: a silent minority? A report on behavioral and cognitive characteristics. *Pediatrics.* 1985; 76:801–809
9. King C, Young R. Attentional deficits with and without hyperactivity: teacher and peer perceptions. *J Abnorm Child Psychol.* 1982; 10:483–496
10. Edelbrock C, Costello A, Kessler MD. Empirical corroboration of attention deficit disorder. *J Am Acad Child Psychiatry.* 1984; 23:285–290
11. Lahey BB, Shaughency E, Strauss C, Frame C. Are attention deficit disorders with and without hyperactivity similar or dissimilar disorders? *J Am Acad Child Psychiatry.* 1984; 23:302–309
12. Lahey BB, Shaughency E, Hynd G, Carlson C, Nieves N. Attention deficit disorder with and without hyperactivity: comparison of behavioral characteristics of clinic-referred children. *J Am Acad Child Psychiatry.* 1987; 26:718–723
13. Hart EA, Lahey BB, Hern K, Hynd GW, Frick PJ, Hanson K. Dimensions and types of ADD: two replications. Manuscript submitted for publication, University of Georgia, 1989
14. Barkley RA, DuPaul GJ, McMurray MB. A comprehensive evaluation of attention deficit disorder with and without hyperactivity as defined by research criteria. *J Consult Clin Psychol.* 1990; 58:775–789
15. Famularo R, Fenton R. The effect of methylphenidate on school grades in children with attention deficit disorder without hyperactivity: a preliminary report. *J Clin Psychiatry.* 1987; 8:112–114
16. Ullmann RK, Sleator EK. Attention deficit disorder children with and without hyperactivity: which behaviors are helped by stimulants? *Clin Pediatr (Phila).* 1985; 24:547–551
17. Barkley RA. Child behavior rating scales and checklists. In: Rutter M, Hussain AH, Lann IS, eds. *Assessment and Diagnosis in Child Psychopathology.* New York, NY: Guilford; 1988:113–155

18. Achenbach TM, Edelbrock CS. *Manual for the Teacher's Report Form and Teacher Version of the Child Behavior Profile*. Burlington, VT: Thomas Achenbach; 1986

19. Barkley RA. Attention. In: Tramontana M, Hooper S, eds. *Issues in Child Clinical Neuropsychology*. New York, NY: Plenum; 1988: 145–176

20. Barkley RA, Fischer M., Newby R, Breen M. Development of a multi-method clinical protocol for assessing stimulant drug responses in ADHD children. *J Clin Child Psychol.* 1988; 17:14–24

21. Rapport M, Stoner G, DuPaul G, Birmingham B, Tucker S. Methylphenidate in hyperactive children: differential effects of dose on academic, learning, and social behavior. *J Abnorm Child Psychol.* 1985; 13:227–244

22. Newby R. *The Wisconsin Selective Reminding Test*. Milwaukee, WI: Author, 1989

23. Gordon M. *The Gordon Diagnostic System*. DeWitt, NY: Gordon Systems; 1983

24. Kagan J. Reflection-impulsivity: the generality and dynamics of conceptual tempo. *J Abnorm Psychol.* 1966; 71:17–24

25. Fischer M, Barkely RA, Edelbrock CS, Smallish L. The adolescent outcome of hyperactive children diagnosed by research criteria, II: academic, attentional, and neurospsychological status. *J Consult Clin Psychol.* In press

26. Barkley RA, McMurray MB, Edelbrock CS, Robbins K. The response of aggressive and nonaggressive ADHD children to two doses of methylphenidate. *J Am Acad Child Adolesc Psychiatry.* 1989; 28:873–881

27. Barkely RA, Edelbrock CS. Assessing situational variation in children's behavior problems: the Home and School Situations Questionnaires. In: Prinz R, ed. *Advances in Behavioral Assessment of Children and Families*. Greenwich, CT: JAI Press; 1987; 3:157–176

28. DuPaul GJ. Parent and teacher ratings of ADHD symptoms: psychometric properties in a community-based sample. *J Clin Child Psychol.* In press

29. Barkley RA. *Hyperactive Children: A Handbook for Diagnosis and Treatment*. New York, NY: Guliford, 1981

30. Humphrey LL. Children's and teachers perspectives on children's self-control: the development of two rating scales. *J Consult Clin Psychol.* 1982; 54:624–633

31. Kendall PC, Wilcox LE. Self-control in children: development of a rating scale. *J Consult Clin Psychol.* 1979; 47:1029–1029

32. Mirsky AF. Behavioral and psychophysiological markers of disordered attention. *Environ Health Perspect.* 1987; 74:191–199

33. Barkley RA, McMurray MB, Edelbrock CS, Robbins K. The side effects of methylphenidate: a systematic, placebo-controlled evaluation. *Pediatrics.* 1990; 86:184–192

34. Sprague R, Sleator E. Methylphenidate in hyperkinetic children: differences in dose effects on learning and social behavior. *Science.* 1977; 198: 1274–1276

26

Preventive Intervention and Outcome with Anxiously Attached Dyads

Alicia F. Lieberman, Donna R. Weston, and Jeree H. Pawl

University of California, San Francisco

Anxiously attached 12-month-olds and their mothers as assessed in the Strange Situation were randomly assigned to an intervention and a control group to test the hypothesis that infant-parent psychotherapy can improve quality of attachment and social-emotional functioning. Securely attached dyads comprised a second control group. Intervention lasted 1 year and ended when the child was 24 months. ANOVAs were used to compare the research groups at outcome. Intervention group toddlers were significantly lower than anxious controls in avoidance, resistance, and anger. They were significantly higher than anxious controls in partnership with mother. Intervention mothers had higher scores than anxious controls in empathy and interactiveness with their children. There were no differences on the outcome measures between the intervention and the secure control groups. The groups did not differ in maternal child-rearing attitudes. Within the intervention group, level of therapeutic process was positively correlated with adaptive scores in child and mother outcome measures.

Developmental research has documented that anxious attachment in infancy is associated with decreased competency in social-emotional functioning in toddlerhood and early childhood. The finding has been reported both with normative samples (Arend, Gove, & Sroufe, 1979; Lewis, Feiring, McGoffog, & Jaskir, 1984;

Reprinted with permission from *Child Development*, 1991, Vol. 62, 199–209. Copyright ©1991 by the Society for Research in Child Development, Inc.

This research was supported by NIMH Prevention Research Branch grant 5 ROI MH39973 to the first author. We wish to thank Cristina Casero, Marta Martinez, Rut Gubkin, and Maria Alvarez for their contributions as the intervenors. We also want to thank John Martin for his methodological consultation and helpful comments on an earlier version of the manuscript. Finally, we thank the reviewers for their excellent suggestions for revision.

Main, Kaplan, & Cassidy, 1985; Matas, Arend, & Sroufe, 1978) and with families at risk (Erickson, Sroufe, & Egeland, 1985; Sroufe, Fox, & Pancake, 1983). The evidence raises a new question: Can later developmental correlates of anxious attachment be prevented through early intervention?

The present study tests the hypothesis that anxiously attached infant-mother dyads can improve the quality of their relationship through participation in infant-parent psychotherapy, a model of early intervention that aims at removing affective obstacles in the mother-child relationship (Fraiberg, 1980; Fraiberg, Lieberman, Pekarsky, & Pawl, 1981; Lieberman, 1985; Lieberman & Pawl, 1988). In this sense, our study involves an integration of the theoretical framework and research methods of attachment theory with the clinical contributions of infant-parent psychotherapy to infant mental health.

Clinical and research findings indicate that anxious attachment stems from affective dyssynchronies between mother and infant. Anxious attachment can be considered as the outcome of a series of interactions in which the mother has been unable to be adequately responsive to the individual characteristics and specific needs of her infant, creating in the child negative expectations which may in turn exacerbate the mother's conflicts (Ainsworth, Blehar, Waters, & Wall, 1978; Fraiberg, 1980).

As described by Fraiberg (1980), infant-parent psychotherapy seeks to alleviate this pathogenic process through a clinical exploration of the mother's and infant's experience in the context of their actual interaction as it unfolds during the sessions. The assumption is that behavioral improvement will follow from the changes in the internal experience of both mother and child promoted by the intervention. This clinical approach is conceptually compatible with the emphasis of attachment theory on the generational transmission of quality of attachment through the mother's internal working models of attachment and of the self (Bowlby, 1980; Main & Goldwyn, 1984, in press).

The available evidence indicates that improvement is unlikely in the absence of intervention because the psychological factors affecting anxious attachment tend to remain unchanged. The research shows that patterns of attachment are stable between 12 and 18 or 20 months (Main & Weston, 1981; Waters, 1978) unless substantial changes occur in the mother's psychological availability (Thompson, Lamb, & Estes, 1982; Vaugh, Egeland, Sroufe, & Waters, 1979). In untreated maltreatment samples, quality of attachment tends to deteriorate between 12 and 18 months (Egeland & Srouge, 1981a, 1981b; Schneider-Rosen, Braunwald, Carlson, & Cichetti, 1985).

Our goal was to promote secure attachment by using infant-parent psychotherapy to enhance maternal empathy for the child's developmental needs and affective experience. We hypothesized that anxiously attached dyads in the intervention group would have significantly more adaptive scores than similar dyads in a control group on outcome measures of maternal empathy, maternal attitudes, and infant interaction with the mother. We also hypothesized that at outcome the intervention group would not differ significantly from a securely attached control group. We anticipated that the incidence of stressful life events would be similar for all three groups at both entry and outcome, so that any improvement in the intervention group could be attributable to the effectiveness of the intervention rather than to changes in external circumstances.

We also made an effort to identify the therapeutic factors that may contribute to the effectiveness of the intervention. We hypothesized that within the intervention group, the level of maternal involvement in the therapeutic process would be positively associated with adaptive mother and infant functioning at outcome.

Our study began when the infants were 12 months old and ended shortly after their second birthday. This period spans important developmental changes such as the consolidation and expansion of autonomous locomotion and the emerging use of language and symbolic play as means of social communication. These changes are likely to affect the behavioral manifestations of quality of attachment between infancy and toddlerhood.

We selected avoidance and resistance toward the mother as entry and outcome measures because these behaviors are useful indicators of anxious attachment during and after infancy (Main et al., 1985). In addition, we developed outcome measures based on concepts that are theoretically linked to quality of attachment in toddlerhood, such as goal-corrected partnership (Bowlby, 1969/1982; Marvin, 1975), aggression toward the mother (Main, 1973), and range versus restriction of affect vis-à-vis mother (Emde, 1980). We also used Waters and Deane's (1985) Q-sort for security of attachment to assess secure base behavior in the home.

The understanding of anxious attachment and its ramifications is central to the study of infant mental health and calls for an integration between academic and clinical views of the infant (Stern, 1985). This study is an initial effort at such integration.

METHOD AND PROCEDURES

Participants

The sample comprised 100 low-SES, Spanish-speaking mothers recently immigrated from Mexico or Central America and their infants in the second year of life. This groups was considered at risk for disorders of attachment because recent Latino immigrants face a high incidence of depression and anxiety as a result of poverty, unemployment, and cultural uprootedness (Padilla, Carlos, & Keefe, 1976; Valle & Vega, 1980). We surmised that the infants would be at risk for anxious attachment because their mothers might be relatively emotionally unavailable due to their circumstances.

The dyads were recruited from pediatric clinics at a large teaching hospital and neighborhood health clinics.

TABLE 1.
Sample Characteristics at Study Entry

		EXPERIMENTAL GROUPS			
CHARACTERISTIC	Whole Sample	Secure Control	Anxious Control	Anxious Intervention	p^a
Target child:					
Male (%)	44.0	32.4	44.0	52.9	N.S.
Firstborn (%)	52.0	44.1	52.0	55.9	N.S.
Birth complications (%)	29.6	23.5	32.0	32.3	N.S.
In day-care (%)	28.7	36.3	16.7	30.3	N.S.
Father:					
Education (years)	8.41	9.03	7.57	8.65	N.S.
Live in home (%)	80.6	85.3	80.0	76.5	N.S.
Unemployed (%)	35.4	34.5	15.0	53.8	.024
Living arrangement:					
Nuclear family (%)	25.8	23.5	16.0	36.4	N.S.
Mother:					
Mean age	25.08	25.88	25.08	24.84	N.S.
Years in U.S.	3.10	3.10	3.00	3.40	N.S.
N children	1.62	1.82	1.50	1.56	N.S.
Education (years)	9.42	10.03	9.08	9.18	N.S.
Life stress	11.34	11.29	10.16	12.09	N.S.
Unemployed (%)	71.4	64.7	64.0	82.3	N.S.
Prior therapy (%)	4.3	3.1	.0	9.1	N.S.
12-month classifications:					
Secure (B)	36.56	100.0	.0	.0	. . .
Avoidant (A)	32.26	.0	48.0	52.94	. . .
Resistant (C)	6.45	.0	12.0	8.82	. . . .
U/D	24.73	.0	40.0	38.24	. . .

^{a} Chi-squares or ANOVAs were conducted as appropriate. Significance levels are for two-tailed tests.

Characteristics of the sample at entry are summarized in Table 1. The mothers ranged in age from 21 to 39 years, had been in the United States for less than 5 years, had five or fewer children, and showed no flagrant psychological disorders. The infants ranged from 11 to 14 months of age at entry and had no congenital birth defects; 44% were male and 52% were firstborn.

Economic hardship is reflected in living situations and parents' employment. Most families shared living quarters with others (74.2%). Only 44.3% of fathers and 8.2% of mothers worked full-time, mostly in low-paying service jobs.

Procedural Overview

Initial assessment. The 12-month assessment consisted of a home visit followed within a week by the Strange Situation (Ainsworth et al., 1978). During the home visit, the Life Event Inventory (Egeland, Deinard, & Brunquell, 1979) was administered to the mothers to assess stressful circumstances. Maternal child-rearing attitudes were assessed using Egeland et al.'s (1979) abbreviated version of the Maternal Attitude Scale (Cohler, Weiss, & Grunebaum, 1970).[1]

Mother-infant dyads were classified as secure (B), anxious-avoidant (A), or anxious-resistant (C) using the criteria of Ainsworth et al. (1978). Infants not classifiable in the A, B, or C groups were assigned to a U/D category that included the D classification as well as a small number of "unclassifiable" infants (Main & Weston, 1981).

Anxiously attached dyads were assigned to the intervention or the control group by block randomization for infant sex and birth order (first, later). Fifty-nine dyads were randomly assigned (intervention group $N = 34$ and anxious control group $N = 25$). Securely attached dyads formed a second control group ($N = 34$). Seven cases dropped out after the home visit but before the 12-month Strange Situation and could not be assigned. The three research groups do not differ in demographic characteristics or reported life stress (see Table 1).

As anticipated, the incidence of anxious attachment for this sample was high (63.4%) when compared to the 35% incidence of anxious attachment generally reported for normative Anglo-American samples (Ainsworth et al., 1978).

Intervention model. The intervention began immediately after research group assignment. The format was unstructured weekly sessions with mother and baby.[2] Visits took place mostly in the home and lasted 1½ hours. Each dyad had one intervenor during the entire intervention period. The four intervenors were bicultural, bilingual women with master's degrees in psychology or social work and with clinical experience. Each received weekly supervision by senior faculty.

The main focus of the intervention was to respond to the affective experiences of mother and child, both as reported by the mother and as observed through the mother-child interaction. There was no didactic teaching. Instead, the intervenors sought to alleviate the mothers' psychological conflicts about their children and to provide developmental information that was clinically timed and tailored to the child's temperament and individual style. The developmental information focused on areas relevant to quality of attachment, such as contingency to signals, availability of age-appropriate opportunities for exploration, and negotiation of infant-mother conflicts to promote a goal-corrected partnership.

In attachment theory language, this intervention approach intends to provide the mother with a corrective attachment experience. The intervenor spoke for the mother's affective experience, addressing the legitimacy of her longings for protection and safety both when she was a child and currently as an adult, and enabling her to explore unsettling feelings of anger and ambivalence toward others (including the child and the intervenor). The intervenor linked this process to the child through

---

[1]The present report is concerned with outcome and will focus only on the 12- and 24-month assessments. Mothers received $15.00 and transportation costs at the time of each laboratory visit.

[2]Monthly contact was maintained with control group mothers via phone calls.

appropriately timed developmental information to reduce negative attributions and to support a benign perception of the child's motives. When feasible, the intervenor also tried to provide concrete elements of protection by helping to secure needed goods and services.

Outcome assessment. The 24-month assessment consisted of a home visit and a laboratory situation. The Life Event Inventory and the Maternal Attitude Scale were administered as in the initial assessment. The Strange Situation was not used at this age because the attachment system of toddlers is not as consistently mobilized by 3-min episodes as is the case with younger children (Marvin, 1975).

Mother and child were observed in a 1¾-hour videotaped laboratory session designed to assess maternal empathy, mother-child interaction, and the child's social-emotional functioning in relation to the mother. This laboratory session is modeled after the Strange Situation but has longer episodes. The sequence includes an introduction to the procedures (10 min); mother-child free play (20 min); play with a female stranger in mother's presence (20 min); child-directed play, with child being asked to entertain him/herself while the adults talk (20 min); separation from mother, with stranger in the room (10 min); reunion, when mother returns and stranger leaves (5 min); snack shared by mother, child, and the observer conducting the session (10–15 min).

All the mother-toddler dyads completed this laboratory session without difficulty, probably due to the mothers' positive attitude toward our program and the friendliness of the stranger.

Outcome Measures

Free-play measures. These measures were coded from the free-play episode in the 24-month videotaped laboratory session. Maternal *empathic responsiveness* was rated on a 9-point scale using criteria based on body orientation, postural and facial expression, and timing and content of responses.

Concurrent validity of the empathic responsiveness scale was evaluated by computing correlations with two subscales of the HOME (Bradley, Caldwell, & Elardo, 1977) that assess quality of maternal care: maternal responsiveness ($r = .38$, $p<.001$) and maternal involvement ($r = .43$, $p<.0001$). These scales were scored by the home visitor during the 24-month home visit.

Maternal *initiation of interaction* was rated on a 7-point scale for frequency, quality, and persistence of mothers' efforts to initiate interaction with the child. High scores denote consistency without stridency in the mother's efforts. Low scores indicate relative absence of efforts to initiate interaction.

Measures of toddler behavior were developed to assess social-emotional functioning in relation to the mother.

Restriction of affect was rated on a 7-point scale that describes range and contextual appropriateness of affective expression. High scores denote a range of appropriately modulated positive and negative affects. Low scores indicate either inhibited or uncontrolled expression of affect.

Angry behavior was measured as a frequency count of instances when the toddler hit, kicked, bit, or yelled at the mother, or engaged in nonexploratory hitting and banging of toys (a behavior considered a displacement of anger toward the mother in free play).

A second judge rated 12 tapes to establish interrater agreement for 24-month free-play measures. Interjudge agreement using the Spearman rank order correlation coefficient is as follows: maternal empathic responsiveness, $r = .92$; maternal initiation, $r = .82$; restrictions of affect, $r = .83$; toddler's angry behavior, $r = .70$.
Behavior on reunion. These measures were coded from the reunion episode in the 24-month videotaped laboratory session. *Goal-corrected partnership* was rated for each mother-toddler dyad during reunion using a 9-point scale. High scores denote eagerness and reciprocity in both mother and child to resume interaction after the separation. Low scores indicate mutual indifference, awkwardness, hesitancy, or mixed messages, or anger in the process of restoring interaction. Interrater reliability was established in 23 videotapes. The Pearson correlation coefficient is $r = .93$.
Avoidance and resistance were rated using Ainsworth et al.'s (1978) interactive behavior scales. Reliability was established on 18 training tapes. Computing Pearson correlation coefficients, reliability for avoidance is $r = .87$, and for resistance, $r = .87$.
Security of attachment was assessed using the 90-item Attachment Q-sort (Waters & Deane, 1985), which was completed by the home visitor after the 24-month home visit.
Life circumstances. Incidence of stressful events was assessed in the home visit at 12, 18, and 24 months using the 39-item Life Event Inventory (Egeland et al., 1979). The items address socioeconomic problems and family discord, and scores reflect the relative impact of each event. The authors report a normative sample mean core of 4.0 and a high-risk sample mean score of 8.0. A score of 11 or higher places the family in the upper 20% for incidence of stressful events.
Maternal child-rearing attitudes. Egeland et al.'s (1979) abbreviated version of the Maternal Attitude Scale (Cohler et al., 1970) was translated to Spanish using the double-translation method and pilot tested on 15 Latino mothers. The inventory was administered in home visits. Each item is a statement rated on a 6-point Likert scale ranging from "strongly agree" to "strongly disagree." The inventory consists of 27 items, nine for each of three subscales:

1. Encouragement of reciprocity: Adaptive attitudes reflect maternal recognition and acceptance of the infant's cues for social interaction. High scores indicate adaptive attitudes.

2. Control of aggression: Adaptive attitudes indicate acceptance and appropriate

modulation of child aggression. Maladaptive scores reflect punitive restrictiveness or, more rarely, overpermissiveness. High scores are adaptive.

3. Awareness of complexity in child rearing: High scores indicate recognition that raising children is fraught with contradictory feelings that need to be negotiated. Maladaptive (low) scores indicate overidealization of the maternal role.

Assessment of the intervention process. Following the final intervention session with each mother, the intervenor met with the senior author to review the therapeutic process. A consensus score for maternal involvement was given using Greenspan and Wieder's (1987) Level of Therapeutic Process Scale. This 10-point scale, still in the process of validation, describes the mother's use of self-observation to identify and articulate her emotions and to link her current feelings and behavior with her past experiences. A score of 1 indicates that the mother communicates only factual information with no emotional content. A score of 3 denotes that the mother discusses relationships but without addressing the feelings involved. A score of 5 denotes the mother's use of self-observation to describe a variety of unrelated feelings. A score of 7 indicates the mother's efforts to make connections between feelings experienced toward the intervenor, toward important figures in the past, and toward key emotional figures in the present. The highest score of 10 is given when the mother shows a consolidation of the emotional gains made in the course of the intervention, including the capacity to articulate and endure the feelings of loss, anger, and sadness involved in termination of the intervention.

Coding Procedures

The Strange Situation was coded by fully trained and experienced judges. The home and laboratory measures were scored by coders who were blind to the 12-month classification and group assignment of the dyads. Different coders scored the home and laboratory measures. In the 24-month laboratory situation, the free-play measures and reunion measures were scored by different coders. Intervention process raters had no access to other outcome data. These procedures were adopted to protect the independence of the different ratings.

Attrition Rate

Overall attrition was 18% and did not differ for the experimental groups. At the 24-month assessment, the sample consisted of 82 dyads: 29 in the anxious-intervention group, 23 in the anxious-control group, and 30 in the secure-control group.

RESULTS

Hypotheses were tested using one-way ANOVAs with a priori contrasts to (1) test for intervention effects by comparing the intervention and anxious control groups, and (2) compare the intervention and secure control groups to evaluate the hypothesis that these groups would not differ after intervention.

Intervention and Anxious Control Group Comparisons

Table 2 presents the means, standard deviations, and significance levels for the first a priori contrast comparing the experimental and anxious control groups. As predicted, mothers and toddlers in the intervention group have significantly more adaptive scores at outcome than their control group counterparts. Experimental group mothers have higher scores in *empathic responsiveness, F(1,81)* = *6.10, p<.05,* and *initiation, F*(1,80) = 4.06, *p<.05*. Experimental group toddlers have lower scores in *angry behavior, F*(1,81) = 4.19, *p<.05,* and higher scores on *goal-corrected partnership on reunion, F*(1,80) = 21.51, *p<.0001*. There are no group differences on restriction of affect or on the Q-sort of security of attachment.

Repeated-measures ANOVAs were conducted for *proximity avoidance* and *contact resistance* from 12 to 24 months. Here again the differences are significant in the predicted direction. There was no significant difference in *proximity avoidance* between intervention and control groups at 12 months, but there was at 24 months (see Table 2). The 24-month a prior contrast for avoidance shows a significant group effect, *F*(1,80) = 15.44, *p<.0001*. For *contact resistance,* the repeated-measures ANOVA was conducted for the subgroup of subjects whose 12-month scores indicated presence of contact resistance (scores>1). A number of subjects (21%) had scored 1, indicating absence of resistance, and the subgroup analysis allowed us to detect *decreases* in contact resistance from 12 to 24 months. The three experimental groups did not differ at 12 months on frequency of scores greater than 1, χ^2 (2) = .41,N.S. The 24-month a priori contrast between the intervention and anxious control groups shows a strong trend toward significance, *F*(2,48) = 3.76, *p* = .057. There is no effect for age of assessment, but the interaction effect approaches significance, *F*(2,59) = 2.85, *p* = .065.[3]

---

[3]The a priori contrast on the whole sample shows a significant effect for the groups, *F* (1,80) = 5.54, *p<.05,* no effect for age at assessment, and no interaction (*p* = .25). Post hoc Scheffe test results indicated that the group means differed as expected at 12 months. The secure group was significantly lower than both anxious groups and the two anxious groups did not differ. Another post hoc comparison was performed to detect decreases in resistance scores from 12 to 24 months between the anxious control and intervention subgroups with resistance scores greater than 1 at 12 months. The repeated measures ANOVA approaches significance for groups effects, *F* (1,37) = 3.53, *p* = .06 (two-tailed), as does the interaction term (*p* = .06). The overall pattern of results from these exploratory analyses supports the significant results of the original a priori contrast.

TABLE 2.
Outcome Comparisons of Intervention and Control Groups: ANOVAs with a Priori Contrasts

	GROUP MEANS, 24 MONTHS			A PRIORI CONTRASTS: SIGNIFICANCE LEVELS	
	Secure Control (n = 29)	Anxious Control (n = 23)	Anxious Interven (n = 30)	a	b
Maternal behavior:					
Empathy:					
M	5.414	4.152	5.833	p < .05	N.S.
SD	2.428	2.409	2.429		
Initiation:					
M	4.375	3.522	4.483	p < .05	N.S.
SD	1.746	1.780	1.932		
Toddler behavior:					
Angry behavior:					
M	.517	1.609	1.233	p < .05	N.S.
SD	.949	2.017	2.285		
Restrict affect:					
M	2.828	3.130	2.483	N.S.	N.S.
SD	1.055	1.471	1.405		
Avoidance:					
M	2.828	4.044	2.259	p < .001	N.S.
SD	1.713	1.651	1.360		
Resistance:					
M	2.121	2.761	1.983	p < .05	N.S.
SD	1.646	2.241	1.617		
Security (Q-sort)					
M	.414	.299	.252	N.S.	N.S.
SD	.245	.335	.413		
Dyadic behavior:					
Partnership:					
M	5.000	3.239	5.466	p < .05	N.S.
SD	1.082	1.445	1.700		
Maternal attitudes:					
Control aggression:					
M	27.217	23.238	24.885	N.S.	N.S.
SD	6.557	7.028	5.617		
Encourage reciprocity:					
M	36.478	31.238	32.154	N.S.	N.S.
SD	7.767	7.635	6.967		
Complexity:					
M	28.044	26.762	26.500	N.S.	N.S.
SD	6.197	4.867	7.961		

[a] First a priori contrast—test of predicted difference.
[b] Second a priori contrast—test of null hypothesis.

One-way ANOVAs with repeated measures were used to test for intervention effects on maternal child-rearing attitudes between 12 and 24 months. There are no significant differences for *control of aggression. Encouragement of reciprocity* shows no group effects, a significant main effect for time of assessment, $F(2,140)$ = 3.85, $p<.05$, and no interaction, indicating that scores for this measure declined similarly for each experimental group between entry and outcome.[4] *Awareness of complexity in child rearing* shows no effect for groups, a significant main effect for time of assessment, $F(2,140) = 7.39$, $p<.001$, and no interaction effect, indicating that scores became more adaptive for each experimental group between 12 and 24 months.

A one-way ANOVA with repeated measures for life stress between 12 and 24 months shows no significant group effect, a significant effect for time, $F(2,140) = 15.826$, $p<.001$, and no interaction. The scores were comparable to those of high-risk U.S. populations. Reported life stress was very high at entry ($M = 11.3$) and declined similarly for all three experimental groups to an overall sample mean of 7.42.

Intervention and Secure Control Group Comparisons

After determining that the two anxiously attached groups differed significantly at outcome, a second a priori contrast was conducted to see whether the intervention group was now comparable to the secure controls. Since the hypothesis of no difference cannot be tested directly, alpha was set at a high level ($p = .20$) to guard against the Type II error of retaining the null hypothesis when it is false (Blalock, 1979).

There were no significant group differences in any of the outcome measures, indicating that the groups were comparable following intervention. The null hypothesis could not be accepted for the Q-sort of security of attachment because there was a trend toward higher scores in the secure control group, $F(1,69) = 2.42$, $p<.20$ (two tailed).

Relationships between Intervention Process and Outcome

Pearson product-moment correlations were used to determine whether maternal level of involvement in the therapeutic process is related to outcome within the intervention group ($N = 34$). Table 3 shows that there are significant correlations between maternal level of involvement and maternal empathy ($r = .459$, $p<.01$), initiation of interaction ($r = .384$, $p<.04$), and attitudes encouraging reciprocity ($r = .403$, $p<.03$). Maternal involvement is also correlated with child functioning at outcome, specifically with the Q-sort security of attachment ($r = .584$, $p<.001$)

---

[4]To test for effects of father's presence and absence on outcome measures, the intervention group was divided into subgroups and the analyses repeated. Subgroup 1 consisted of dyads where father was present at all assessments. Subgroup 2 consisted of dyads for whom father was present at most for two of the three assessments. Results of one-way ANOVAs with a priori contrasts for the two subgroups were similar to findings for the whole sample on every measure. The number of dyads in the father-absent subgroup is too small to warrant firm conclusions.

TABLE 3.
Intervention Group: Correlation Between Level of Therapeutic Process and
24-Month Outcome Measures

	r	*p*
M empathic response	.459	.014
M initiation to C	.384	.043
C angry behavior	−.275	.157
C restriction of affect	−.238	.223
C proximity avoidance	−.431	.022
C contact resistance	−.262	.178
M-C security (Q-sort in home)	.584	.001
M-C partnership on reunion	.369	.052
M control of aggression	.224	.253
M encourage reciprocity	.403	.034
M complexity in child rearing	.022	.911

NOTE.—All significance levels are for two-tailed tests. M = mother, C = child.

and lowered avoidance ($r = -.431$, $p<.02$) and with the dyadic measure of goal-corrected partnership on reunion ($r = .369$, $p<.052$).

Level of therapeutic process is not related to family demographic characteristics at entry, including child attributes, parents' education, employment or living situation, and life stress. The measure is related to mother's age at entry ($r = .41$, $p<.05$) and to number of children in the family ($r = .35$, $p<.05$).

DISCUSSION

The findings suggest that the intervention was effective in enhancing maternal empathy and interaction with the child; decreasing toddler avoidance, resistance, and anger; and increasing goal-corrected partnership. These data support the hypothesis that the intervention would promote substantial improvement in mother-child interaction and the negotiation of conflict, two parameters of quality of attachment.

The present study attempts to explore and extend the clinical applications of attachment theory and research. Although there have been previous efforts in this direction (Belsky & Nezworski, 1988), this is the first systematic effort to apply attachment theory to a conceptually compatible intervention model, to test the effectiveness of the intervention using an experimental design, and to document clinical outcome employing measures derived from attachment theory.

The pattern of the findings deserves some comment. The outcome measures showing significant differences between the intervention and anxious control groups were maternal empathy, toddler avoidance, resistance, angry behavior, and goal-corrected partnership upon reunion. These measures were based on the videotaped interactions between mother and child. On the other hand, the Q-sort measure, which assesses secure base behavior in the home, showed no differences between the two anxiously attached groups. The secure controls showed a trend toward higher Q-sort scores than the intervention group.

One possible meaning of these findings is that after 1 year of intervention, the progress made by the experimental group was shown clearly in interactive measures of attachment but was not yet consolidated enough to affect scores in the Q-sort, which attempts to provide a measure of internalized security. Another possibility is that our Q-sort data were less sensitive to actual differences between the two anxious groups than the codings of videotaped behavior in the laboratory. Our home visitors expressed doubts about some of their sorts because the home visits did not always yield the observations needed to make confident sorting decisions.

The possibility that the data reflect a gradually consolidating process of therapeutic change is given some support by two sets of observations. One is anecdotal. The coders of the 24-month laboratory data repeatedly made notations that particular dyads had harmonious interactions but seemed a little tentative, as if they were trying out new skills. These invariably turned out to be dyads in the intervention group. More quantitative evidence comes from a preliminary analysis of the 18-month data. Between 12 and 18 months, most of the avoidant (A) infants in the intervention group became either secure (B), anxious-resistant (C), or disorganized/unclassifiable (U/D). In contrast, most of the avoidant infants in the anxious control groups remained avoidant at 18 months.

The different pattern shown by the experimental as compared to the anxious control group between 12 and 18 months may indicate that intervention helped to break down distancing defenses and to replace them by the direct expression of anger and ambivalence midway in the intervention year. Yet at 24 months the intervention infants did not differ from the secure controls in anger to the mother and were significantly less angry than the anxious controls. This suggests that their 18-month anger and disorganization might have been a transitional emotional expression that was superseded as the psychological changes brought about by the intervention became better internalized.

It is possible that this gradual internalization of more adaptive modes of emotional expression is also reflected in the overall pattern of child scores at the 24-month outcome. If this is the case, the intervention helped to significantly reduce toddler avoidance, resistance, and anger and to enhance the dyad's ability to negotiate the stresses of separation and reunion, but had not yet substantially altered the toddler's internalized sense of the mother as a secure base in the home.

It is noteworthy that the intervention had rather specific effects on the mothers. Maternal changes occurred in the areas of empathy and social initiative, which were the focus of the intervention. Contrary to our expectations, the intervention was not related to significant changes in maternal attitudes. This area was not explicitly addressed in the intervention because we believed that taking issue with child-rearing beliefs could easily depart from the therapeutic model of attunement to the mother's affective experience, raising the possibility of disagreements that might make the mother feel defensive and in the wrong. Nevertheless, we had expected maternal attitudes to change as a by-product of the intervention. The absence of such change may mean that attitudes remained compartmentalized throughout the intervention.

Cultural factors may have influenced these findings. An item-by-item review of the data shows that the majority of the mothers (up to 80% of the sample) gave the highest agreement score to items advocating child obedience, the firm suppression of child aggression, the acknowledgment of innate gender differences between boys and girls, the primacy of parental authority in running the household, and the importance of personal sacrifice and self-effacement in raising children. This pattern is different from that considered adaptive by Cohler et al. (1970) in their Anglo samples. However, our findings confirm the literature on prevalent Latino cultural values (Acosta, Yamamoto, & Evans, 1982). The absence of intervention effects on maternal attitudes might well be related to the fact that the scale items tapped strongly held cultural values.

Cultural attitudes are not necessarily rigid. The views sponsored by mothers in our sample changed in the same direction for the three research groups over the course of the year, supporting the view that child-rearing attitudes are influenced by the child's age (Cohler et al., 1970). The fact that mothers in the anxious control group also changed their attitudes over time suggests that these mothers are not necessarily rigidly locked into their perceptions and are capable of responding to developmental changes in their children. Mothers' attitudes shifted toward lesser encouragement of mother-infant reciprocity and a less idealized and self-sacrificing view of motherhood. These findings suggest that as their children moved from infancy to toddlerhood, the mothers in all the research groups became less absorbed in the "primary maternal preoccupation" (Winnicott, 1957) associated with mothering in the first year of life.

It may be argued that the attitude scales may not be sensitive enough to detect maternal change as the result of intervention. It is worth noting, however, that within the intervention group mothers who had higher scores in level of therapeutic process also had more adaptive scores in encouragement of reciprocity. This finding indicates that the scale showed change in mothers who made more effective use of the intervention. The fact that the attitudinal scores for the whole sample are consistent both with developmental expectations and with cultural factors lends additional credibility to the scales.

Stern-Bruschweiler and Stern (1989) raise the question of whether absence of change following intervention stems from the difficulty in changing any one element of the internal representation, or from rigidity in the expected causal sequence of changes. This important question cannot be answered by our study because we did not attempt to change attitudes directly, but it remains an interesting area for future research. What seems clear from our data is that behavioral change does not necessarily bring about attitudinal change, and attitudinal change is not a prerequisite for behavioral change.

Maternal involvement in the therapeutic process appears as a key variable in fostering adaptive change. Within the intervention group, mothers who achieved a higher level in the therapeutic process tend to be more empathic and interactive and to have children who show more security of attachment, more goal-corrected partnership, and less avoidance upon reunion at outcome. These results lend support to Fraiberg's (1980) view that intervention with the mother can have beneficial effects on the child's emotional functioning. The findings suggest that assessing the mother's use of intervention should become an integral part of intervention research in infant mental health.

The present study is a first effort at systematically implementing the clinical applications of attachment theory and research. In this sense, the study is both hypothesis-testing and exploratory in nature. While we tested specific hypotheses regarding outcome, we also explored possible conceptual domains of outcome measures because at present there is no cohesive approach to the measurement of security of attachment in toddlerhood. Although from a strict hypothesis-testing perspective we may have more analyses than is optimal for sample size, the results provide direction regarding useful outcome measures for future research.

Further studies are needed to investigate the parameters of change in other high-risk samples and other age groups, and to elucidate the long-term effects of intervention through sustained follow-up of early intervention research populations. In the meantime, the present study suggests that the second year of life is a ripe period for the clinical application of attachment theory and research.

REFERENCES

Acosta, F. Y., Yamamoto, J., & Evans, L. A. (1982). *Effective psychotherapy for low-income and minority patients.* New York: Plenum.

Ainsworth, M. D. S., Blehar, M. C., Waters, E., & Wall, S. (1978). *Patterns of attachment: a psychological study of the Strange Situation.* Hillsdale, NJ: Erlbaum.

Arend, R., Gove, F., & Sroufe, L. A. (1979). Continuity of individual adaptation from infancy to kindergarten: A predictive study of ego resiliency and curiosity in preschoolers. *Child Development, 50,* 950–959.

Belsky, J., & Nezworski, T. (Eds.). (1988) *Clinical implications of attachment.* Hillsdale, NJ: Erlbaum.

Blalock, H. M., Jr. (1979). *Social statistics* (2d ed.). New York: McGraw-Hill.

Bowlby, J. (1980). *Attachment and loss: Vol. 3. Loss, sadness, and depression.* New York: Basic.

Bowlby, J. (1982). *Attachment and loss: Vol. I. Attachment* (2d ed.). New York: Basic. (Original work published 1969)

Bradley, R. H., Caldwell, B. M., & Elardo, R. (1977). Home environment, social status, and mental test performance. Journal of Educational Psychology, **69**, 647–701.

Cohler, B., Weiss, J., & Grunebaum, H. (1970). Child-care attitudes and emotional disturbance among mothers of young children. *Genetic Psychology Monographs, 82*, 3–47.

Egeland, B., Deinard, A., & Brunquell, D. (179). *A prospective study of the antecedents of child abuse.* Final Report to the National Center on Child Abuse and Neglect (unpublished).

Egeland, B., & Sroufe, L. A. (1981a). Attachment and early maltreatment. *Child Development,* **52**, 44–52.

Egeland, B., & Sroufe, L. A. (1981b). Developmental sequelae of maltreatment in infancy. In R. Rizley & D. Cicchetti (Eds.), *Developmental perspective in child maltreatment* (pp. 77–92). San Francisco: Jossey-Bass.

Emde, R. N. (1980). Emotional availability: A reciprocal reward system for infants and parents with implications for prevention of psychosocial disorders. In P. M. Taylor (Ed.), *Parent-infant relationships* (pp. 87–115). Orlando, FL: Greun & Stratton.

Erickson, M. L., Sroufe, L. A., & Egeland, B. (1985). The relationship between quality of attachment and behavior problems in preschool in a high-risk sample. In I. Bretherton & E. Waters (Eds.), Growing points in attachment theory and research (pp. 147–166). *Monographs of the Society for Research in Child Development,* **50**(1–2, Serial No. 209).

Fraiberg, S. (Ed.). (1980). *Clinical studies in infant mental health.* New York: Basic.

Fraiberg, S., Lieberman, A. F., Pekarsky, J. H., & Pawl, J. H. (1981). Treatment and outcome in an infant psychiatry program: Part I. *Journal of Preventive Psychiatry,* **1**, 89–111.

Greenspan, S., & Wieder, S. (1987). Dimensions and levels of the therapeutic process. In S. Greenspan, S. Wieder, A. F. Lieberman, R. Nover, M. Robinson, & R. Louric (Eds.), *Infants in multirisk families* (pp. 391–431). Madison, CT: International Universities Press.

Lewis, M., Feiring, C., McGoffog, C., & Jaskir, J. (1984). Predicting psychopathology in six-year-olds from early social relations. *Child Development,* **55**, 123–126.

Lieberman, A. F. (1985). Infant mental health: A model for service delivery. *Journal of Clinical Child Psychology,* **14**, 196–201.

Lieberman, A. F., & Pawl, J. H. (1988). Clinical applications of attachment theory. In J. Belsky & T. Nezworski (Eds.), *Clinical implications of attachment* (pp. 327–351). Hillsdale, NJ: Erlbaum.

Main, M. (1973). *Exploration, play and cognitive functioning as related to child-mother attachment.* Unpublished doctoral dissertation, The Johns Hopkins University.

Main, M., & Goldwyn, R. (1984). Predicting rejection of her infant form mother's representation of her own experience: Implications for the abused-abusing intergenerational cycle. *Child Abuse and Neglect,* **8**, 203–217.

Main, M., & Goldwyn, R. (in press). Interview-based adult attachment classification related to infant-mother and infant-father attachment. *Developmental Psychology.*

Main, M., Kaplan, N., & Cassidy, J. (1985). Security in infancy, childhood, and adulthood:

A move to the level of representation. In I. Bretherton & E. Waters (Eds.), Growing points in attachment theory and research (pp. 66–104). *Monographs of the Society for Research in Child Development*, **50,**(1–2, Serial No. 209).

Main, M., & Weston, D. R. (1981). The quality of the toddler's relationship to mother and to father: Related to conflict behavior and the readiness to establish new relationships. *Child Development*, **52,** 932–940.

Marvin, R. (1975). An etiological-cognitive model for the attentuation of mother-child attachment behavior. In T. M. Alloway, I. Krames, & P. Pliner (Eds.), *Advances in the study of communication and affect: Vol. 3. The development of social attachments* (pp. 25–60). New York: Plenum.

Matas, L., Arend, R. A., & Sroufe, L. A. (1978). Continuity of adaptation in the second year: The relationship between quality of attachment and later competence. *Child Development*, **49,** 547–556.

Padilla, A. M., Carlos, M. L., & Keefe, S. E. (1976), Mental health utilization by Mexican Americans. In M. R. Miranda (Ed.), *Psychotherapy with the Spanish speaking: Issues in research and service delivery*. Los Angeles: University of California.

Schneider-Rosen, K., Braunwald, K. G., Carlson, V., & Cicchetti, D. (1985). Current perspectives in attachment theory: Illustration from the study of maltreated infants. In I. Bretherton & E. Waters (Eds.), Growing points in attachment theory and research (pp. 194–210). *Monographs of the Society for Research in Child Development*, **50,**(1–2, Serial No. 209).

Sroufe, L. A., Fox, N. E., & Pancake, V. R. (1983). Attachment and dependency in developmental perspective. *Child Development*, **54,** 1615–1627.

Stern, D. (1985). *The interpersonal world of the infant*. New York: Basic.

Stern-Bruschweiler, N., & Stern, D. (1989). Model for conceptualizing the role of the mother's representational world in various mother-infant therapies. *Infant Mental Health Journal*, **10**, 142–156.

Thompson, R., Lamb, M. E., & Estes, D. (1982). Stability of infant-mother attachment and its relationship to changing life circumstances in an unselected middle-class sample. *Child Development*, **53,** 144–148.

Valle, K., & Vega, W. (1980). *Hispanic natural support systems*. State of California Department of Mental Health.

Vaughn, B., Egeland, B., Sroufe, L. A., & Waters, E. (1979). Individual differences in infant-mother attachment at twelve and eighteen months: Stability and change in families under stress. *Child Development*, **50,** 971–975.

Waters, E. (1978). The reliability and stability of individual differences in infant-mother attachment. *Child Development*, **49,** 483–494.

Waters, E., & Deane, K. E. (1985). Defining and assessing individual differences in attachment relationships: Q-methodology and the organization of behavior in infancy and early childhood. In I. Bretherton & E. Waters (Eds.), Growing points in attachment theory and research (pp. 44–65). *Monographs of the Society for Research in Child Development*, **50**(1–2, Serial No. 209).

Winnicott, D. (1957). *Mother and child*. New York: Basic.

Part VI
Special Issues

The articles in this section are on intrauterine cocaine exposure, homelessness, and the informed consent process. The first two articles address relatively new stressors in the lives of children. Both topics, cocaine exposure and homelessness, have received significant attention in the mass media. With any new social problem, there is a lag between the recognition of the problem and the formation of a research base to inform treatment and policy. The formation of a research base is further delayed when developmental studies are needed to understand the effects of a specific stressor; they often take years to complete.

One example of the delay from the occurrence of a problem to its recognition and subsequent study is the impact of cocaine on the developing fetus. Children prenatally exposed to cocaine during a use surge in the 1980's are now entering the school system in large numbers. Children have been described as having a variety of problems, often contradictory, such as passivity and hyperactivity. Thus, the educational and behavioral needs of these children are unclear, and inner-city school administrators are concerned about cocaine-exposed children overwhelming already burdened school systems. Results of studies now in progress will not be available to help the first groups of children. However, some studies are available to explain some of the contradictory behavioral descriptions.

Lester and his colleagues account for the conflicting evidence on the effects of cocaine on newborn behavior by proposing two neurobehavioral syndromes. With a cocaine-exposed group and a control group, they analyzed the cries of 2-day-old infants. Using a path model, they found that the direct neurotoxic effects of cocaine led to an excitable response system, and that the indirect effects of cocaine secondary to intrauterine growth retardation led to a depressed behavioral syndrome. In their conclusion, the authors describe the importance of "goodness of fit" between the individual and the environment in predicting subsequent outcomes for these children. In this case, the biological compromise is the result of social factors. Unless there is some type of intervention with the biological parent or with a foster care system, these babies may not receive the environmental support they need to maximize their capabilities.

Although there have always been homeless children, in the past decade there has been a proliferation of homeless families as a result of economic, political, and social factors. Rafferty and Shinn review the new literature on homeless children. They cover a range of problems, including health and nutrition, academic and developmental delays, and emotional and behavioral problems. They have tried to find

589

studies that compare homeless children not just with the population at large, but with economically impoverished children with homes. As detailed in Section II, any study of a risk factor should examine the unique contribution of that risk (e.g., homelessness) over the effects of the more global problem (e.g., abject poverty).

The last article in this section is on research ethics and the informed consent process. In recent years, investigators and research centers have become increasingly concerned about protecting subjects' rights. Abramovitch, Freedman, Thoden and Nikolich examine children's understanding of the process of informed consent in a series of innovative studies. The standard procedure in developmental research is to obtain parental consent and to give children the opportunity to assent or dissent if they have some capacity for understanding what is involved. The investigators describe the capacities of 5- to 12-year-olds to assent. Children understood what the studies involved, but they did not believe their performance would be confidential. In studies designed to gather sensitive personal information, data can be affected substantially if children believe that their parents will see their responses. In addition, children expressed reluctance to dissent once their parents had given permission for them to participate. Findings are discussed as they relate to children's understanding of consent for medical research and treatment and of their participation in legal proceedings.

27

Neurobehavioral Syndromes in Cocaine-Exposed Newborn Infants

Barry M. Lester

Brown University Program in Medicine, Providence, Rhode Island

Michael J. Corwin

Boston University School of Medicine, Massachusetts

Carol Sepkoski

Cry Research, Inc.

Ronald Seifer

Brown University Program in Medicine, Providence, Rhode Island

Mark Peucker

Women & Infants' Hospital, Providence, Rhode Island

Sarah McLaughlin and Howard L. Golub

Cry Research, Inc.

The effects of fetal cocaine exposure on newborn cry characteristics were studied in 80 cocaine-exposed and 80 control infants. The groups were stratified to be similar on maternal demographic characteristics and maternal use of other illegal substances and alcohol during pregnancy. The hypothesis was that excitable cry characteristics were related to the direct effects of cocaine, while depressed cry characteristics were related to the indirect effects of cocaine secondary to low birthweight. Structural equation modeling (EQS) showed direct effects of cocaine on cries with a longer duration, higher fundamental frequency, and a higher and more variable first formant frequency. Indirect effects of cocaine secondary to low birthweight resulted in cries with

Reprinted with permission from *Child Development*, 1991, Vol. 62, 694–705. Copyright ©1991 by the Society for Research in Child Development, Inc.

This work was supported by NICHD grant R44-HD-20737 and by NICHD contract N01-HD-6-2930.

a longer latency, fewer utterances, lower amplitude, and more dysphonation. Cocaine-exposed infants had a lower birthweight, shorter length, and smaller head circumference than the unexposed controls. Findings were consistent with the notion that 2 neurobehavioral syndromes, excitable and depressed, can be described in cocaine-exposed infants, and that these 2 syndromes are due, respectively, to direct neurotoxic effects and indirect effects secondary to intrauterine growth retardation.

The alarming rise in the use of cocaine by pregnant women has led to increased concern about the potential deleterious effects of in utero cocaine exposure on the infant (Clayton, 1985). Cocaine use during pregnancy has been related to medical complications in the mother and infant, including reductions in infant birthweight, length, and head circumference (Bingol, Fuchs, Diaz, Stone, & Gromish, 1987; Chasnoff & MacGregor, 1987; Cherukuri, Minkoff, Feldman, Parekh, & Glass, 1988; Fulroth, Phillips, & Durant, 1989; Hadeed & Siegel, 1989; Livesay, Ehrlich, & Finnegan, 1987; Oro & Dixon, 1987; Ryan, Ehrlich, & Finnegan, 1987; Zuckerman et al., 1989).

Neurological and behavioral abnormalities have been documented in neonates exposed to cocaine; there are inconsistencies in the literature, however, and the pathogenesis of these observations is not clear. Neurological findings include tremors, irritability, high-pitched and excessive crying, jitteriness, hyperactivity, rigidity, hypertonicity, hypotonia, coarse and choreiform movements, vigorous sucking, and abnormal neuromuscular signs (Bingol et al., 1987; Cherukuri et al., 1988; Doberczak, Shanzer, Senie, & Kandall, 1988; Fulroth et al., 1989; LeBlanc, Parekh, Naso, & Glass, 1987; Madden, Payne, & Miller, 1986; Oro & Dixon, 1987). Other reports include feeding difficulties and poor sleep-wake organization (Chasnoff & Griffith, in press; Oro & Dixon, 1987), abnormal electroencephalographic and visual evoked responses (Dixon, Coen, & Crutchfield, 1987; Doberczak et al., 1988; Oro & Dixon, 1987), and an increase in brainstem conduction time (Anday, Cohen, Schwartz, & Hoffman, 1989; Shih, Cone-Wesson, Reddix, & Wu, 1989). In studies using the Brazelton Scale, diminished interactive abilities (Chasnoff, Burns, Schnoll, & Burns, 1985, 1986; Dixon et al., 1987) and poor state organization (Chasnoff et al., 1985, 1986) suggest impaired responses to environmental stimuli.

Several studies have attempted to determine if cocaine-exposed infants show a true abstinence syndrome analogous to opiate withdrawal. Bingol (Bingol et al., 1987) reported signs of mild withdrawal (irritability, crying, and vigorous suck) in 10% of exposed infants. These findings are supported by three studies showing higher scores on abstinence scales indicative of withdrawal in exposed infants (Doberczak et al., 1988; Fulroth et al., 1989; Oro & Dixon, 1987). However, no evidence of symptomatology was reported in five studies (Dixon & Behar, 1989;

Hadeed & Siegel, 1989; Livesay et al., 1987; Madden et al., 1986; Ryan et al., 1987). In fact, Livesay et al. (1987) reported significantly lower total abstinence scores for cocaine-exposed infants, including individual item effects for cry, tremors, and tone. Ryan et al. (1987) reported no statistically significant differences in abstinence scores between cocaine-exposed infants and controls, but noted that the cocaine infants had lower scores on 19 of the 21 items on the abstinence scale. Low abstinence scores indicative of hyporesponsiveness were found in a study of infants with echoencephalographic findings of cranial abnormalities (Dixon & Behar, 1989).

Neurobehavioral Syndromes

These studies have not established a consistent pattern of findings that may be due, in part, to methodological problems in sample selection and in the identification of confounding variables (Bauchner, Zuckerman, Amaro, Frank, & Parker, 1987; Frank et al., 1988; Zuckerman et al., 1989). It is also possible that some of the apparently discrepant findings may be due to different physiological effects of cocaine on the infant. Based on the literature, two neurobehavioral patterns or syndromes, which we have labeled "excitable" and "depressed," can be described in cocaine-exposed infants. Excitable infants are easily aroused infants who show signs of withdrawal such as irritability, excessive and high-pitched cry, tremors, jitteriness, and hypertonicity. "Depressed" is used in the medical sense, referring to a decrease in functional activity. Depressed infants are underaroused, show lower abstinence scores, are difficult to wake, and have fleeting attention and low orientation and state scores. The hypothesis of this study was that the excitable pattern of behavior is due to the direct neurotoxic effects of cocaine, and that the depressed behavior is due to the indirect effects of cocaine secondary to fetal hypoxia and intrauterine growth retardation (IUGR).

Direct and Indirect Effects

We know from preclinical studies that the teratogenic effect of a drug can be produced by an action on the maternal animal, directly on the fetus, or by alteration of normal maternal-fetal metabolic pathways (Inglass, Curley, & Prindle, 1952). Cocaine has both direct and indirect effects on the fetus and infant (Jones & Lopez, 1988). Direct effects include the action of cocaine on the fetus consequent to transfer of the drug through the placenta. These systemic effects of cocaine on the nervous system are probably mediated by alterations in synaptic transmission (Cregler & Mark, 1986). Cocaine blocks the presynaptic reuptake of the neurotransmitters norepinephrine and dopamine, producing an excess of transmitter at the postsynaptic receptor sites (Ritchie & Greene, 1985). This mechanism effects the sympathetic nervous system and produces vasoconstriction, an acute rise in arterial blood pressure, tachycardia, and a predisposition to ventricular arrhythmias and seizures (Cregler & Mark, 1986; Tarr & Macklin, 1987).

Indirect effects can be attributable to changes in the fetal environment and effects on the mother's central nervous system (CNS) that place the infant at risk. Studies with ewes (Woods, Plessinger, & Clark, 1987) and mice (Mahalik, Gautieri, & Mann, 1984) have shown that cocaine alters fetal oxygenation by reducing uterine blood flow and impairing oxygen transfer to the fetus due to elevated catecholamine levels and placental vasoconstriction. During pregnancy, uterine blood vessels supplying oxygen and nutrients to the developing fetus are maximally dilated, but they vasoconstrict in the presence of catecholamines. Cocaine blocks the re-uptake of catecholamines (Ritchie & Greene, 1985), thereby increasing their concentration, resulting in vasoconstriction of the uterine arteries and impaired oxygen delivery to the fetus.

In pregnant cocaine-abusing women, vasoconstriction, sudden hypertension, or cardiac arrhythmias may interrupt the blood supply to the placenta and reduce profusion to various fetal tissues in early gestation, causing deformation or disruption of morphogenesis in late gestation (Bingol et al., 1987). Vasoconstriction, tachycardia, and increased blood pressure caused by cocaine all increase the chance for intermittent intrauterine hypoxia, preterm labor, precipitous labor, and abruptio placenta followed by hemorrhage, shock, and anemia (Tarr & Macklin, 1987). Vasoconstriction at the uteroplacental complex coupled with anorexic effects of cocaine might explain the growth retardation that occurs in approximately 25% of the offspring of cocaine-abusing mothers (Fulroth et al., 1989; Hadeed & Siegel, 1989; Yoon, Kim, Mac Hee, Checola, & Nobel, 1989). Hypoxia by means of vasoconstriction has been shown to reduce fetal weight in animal studies (Mahalik et al., 1984). The relation between intrauterine growth retardation and behavior in cocaine-exposed infants has not been studied—specifically, the role of intrauterine growth retardation in mediating neurobehavioral effects of in utero exposure to cocaine.

We hypothesized that excitable behavior may be related to the direct neurotoxic effects of cocaine. These effects may be due to the action of cocaine in blocking re-uptake of norepinephrine and dopamine, resulting in increased synaptic availability of neurotransmitters. The persistence of vasoactive amines near the receptors of the effector organs can lead to an exaggerated responsiveness or supersensitivity to neurotransmitters (Smith, 1982). Preclinical research suggests that cocaine facilitates activity of a CNS reward system, presumably by increasing neurotransmission in mesolimbic and/or mesocortical dopaminergic tracts (Wise, 1984). The action of cocaine on mesolimbic and mesocortical systems could foster increased neurotransmission and CNS irritability (Doberczak et al., 1988), triggering the cry which is activated by the hypothalamic-limbic system and controlled by midbrain and brainstem regions (Lester & Boukydis, 1991; Lester et al., 1989).

Our hypothesis further suggests that depressed behavior may be due to the indirect effects of cocaine by altering the exchange of nutrients and oxygen between mother and fetus. This is explained by atecholamine-mediated vasoconstriction of the uterine arteries that decreases blood supply to fetal tissue, resulting in fetal hypoxia and intrauterine growth retardation. Thus, depressed behavior in cocaine-exposed infants is viewed as secondary to, or mediated by, IUGR.

Newborn Cry

In previous work, acoustic characteristics of the newborn cry, including measures of the frequency components of the cry sound (e.g., fundamental frequency or voice pitch), and measures of the temporal aspects of the cry (e.g., latency and duration) have been related to biological insult (Lester & Boukydis, 1985). This literature includes studies of low-birthweight and IUGR infants (Lester, 1979; Lester & Zeskind, 1978; Zeskind & Lester, 1981) and, more recently, studies of infants with prenatal exposure to marijuana (Lester & Dreher, 1989) and alcohol (Lester et al., 1989; Nugent, Lester, & Greene, 1990). It is interesting that although crying, including the high-pitched cry, is used in the scoring of neonatal abstinence scales (Finnegan, 1984), there have been no attempts to quantify cry characteristics in cocaine-exposed infants. Therefore, it seemed reasonable to use the acoustic characteristics of the cry to study the effects of cocaine on the neurobehavioral organization of the infant. Moreover, as a neurobehavioral assessment, cry analysis lends itself to the study of excitable and depressed dimensions of behavior. Although in previous work cry analysis has not explicitly been used to study these behavioral dimensions, cry characteristics that reflect excitable and depressed behavior and that presumably represent different CNS control mechanisms can readily be defined from acoustical measures of the cry.

The purpose of this study was to relate direct and indirect effects of prenatal cocaine exposure to specific acoustic characteristics of the newborn cry. We hypothesized that cocaine would affect excitable cry characteristics independent of the mediating effects of IUGR (direct effects), whereas the effects of cocaine on depressed cry characteristics would be mediated by IUGR (indirect effects). Excitable cry characteristics are seen as reflecting increased CNS reactivity, which results in a lower threshold for responsivity, higher levels of arousal, and increased tension in the laryngeal structures that control the frequency characteristics of the cry. These characteristics would include a shorter latency from stimulus to cry onset, more cry utterances, longer cry duration, and higher and more variable fundamental and formant frequencies. Depressed cry characteristics are seen as reflecting lower CNS arousal and decreased effort in producing the cry sound. These characteristics would include a longer latency, fewer cry utterances, a lower amplitude, and more turbulence (diminished voiced component) in the cry.

METHOD

The data base for this study was from a larger project on cry analysis and the sudden infant death syndrome (SIDS) conducted in 13 hospitals located in nine cities in the United States. As part of that study, informed consent was requested from parents of infants who were scheduled for their pre-discharge metabolic screening blood test. Following informed consent, the medical records of the mother and infant were abstracted onto standard data-collection forms. Data included mother's prepregnancy, pregnancy, and delivery histories as well as neonatal outcome, including physical growth. Substance use (cocaine, marijuana, cigarettes, alcohol, opiates, and others) was determined based on the information noted in the chart, including urine assays if ordered by the patient's physician. An initial report from this larger study showed that in this population, in which cocaine use was discovered during routine obstetrical care, cocaine use was related to reductions in birthweight, length, and head circumference (Corwin et al., 1990).

The cries of the infants were recorded on the second day following delivery for 30 sec with a Realistic SCT-35 cassette recorder and Realistic Cardioid Dynamic Microphone following either a heel stick performed for routine blood studies or a flick to the heel by the research assistant using a standardized procedure. A specially designed tone box was used to place a 3,300-Hz tone on the tape to mark the onset of the cry stimulus. For infants who required more than one stimulus, the tone marked the final stimulus applied to elicit the cry. The cries were analyzed using a high-speed computer system developed in collaboration with Cry Research, Inc. (Cambridge, MA) used in previous work (Golub & Corwin, 1982; Lester, 1987; Lester & Dreher, 1989; Lester et al., 1989).

The cry analysis system was specifically designed for infants based on the acoustic theory of speech production developed by Fant (1960) and Stevens (1964) and modified for the infant vocal tract. The system takes advantage of modern computer-assisted digital signal processing methods, includes the automatic detection of individual cry utterances, and uses the Fast Fourier Transform (FFT) to derive acoustic measures. The cry is played directly into the computer, low pass filtered at 5 KHz, and digitized at 10 KHz. The energy distribution of the digitized signal is plotted in 25-msec blocks. Utterances occur during the expiratory phase of respiration when the energy remains above a minimum threshold for at least .5 sec. The FFT is used to compute the log magnitude spectrum in 25-msec blocks for each cry utterance. The FFT is smoothed with a 20-point moving average. The ratio of distances between peaks in the smoothed and unsmoothed transform is used to determine if the block is harmonic or inharmonic.

The reliability of the system was determined by analyzing the same tape of 30 cries three times. The resolution of the utterance detection is 25 msec with a 2% error. There was a 2% error in the detection of a single 25-msec block. The resolution of the FFT is 5–10 Hz with a 1% error in the calculation of the acoustic measures.

A total of 12 summary cry variables were computed. Averages were based on the first two utterances. The summary variables include:

Latency—time from stimulus application to cry onset.

Number of cries—number of expiratory cry phonations that occurred during the 30-sec recording.

Duration—average length in msec of the cry utterance.

Amplitude—average energy in dB of the cry utterance.

Dysphonation—average percent of the cry utterance with turbulence (noise) or aperiodic sound.

Fundamental frequency (f0)—average median frequency in Hz of vocal fold vibration or what we hear as voice pitch.

f0 variability—average interquartile range of f0.

Hyperphonation—average percent of the cry utterance in which f0 exceeds 1,000 Hz.

Formant frequencies (two variables, F1 and F2)—average median frequencies in Hz of the resonance frequencies that occur as a result of the filtering of the vocal tract.

Formant variability—average interquartile range of F1 and F2 (also two variables).

To evaluate the effects of cocaine on cry characteristics, comparisons were performed on 80 cocaine-exposed infants and 80 controls. The two groups of cocaine-exposed and control infants were selected to be greater than 36 weeks gestational age at birth and stratified for maternal age, ethnicity, cigarette use, and the use of other drugs and alcohol. The two groups were also balanced for type of cry stimulus (stick or flick). Analysis of variance showed that the cry variables were unaffected by type of cry stimulus. Therefore, this variable was not included in the analyses that follow.

RESULTS

Characteristics of the cocaine-exposed and control groups are shown in Table 1. The cocaine-exposed infants had a significantly lower birthweight, shorter birth length, and smaller head circumference than the unexposed controls.

To test the hypothesis that cocaine exposure results in excitable cry characteristics independent of IUGR and that effects of cocaine on depressed cry characteristics are mediated by IUGR, we used the EQS structural equation modeling procedure (Bentler, 1989). The EQS implements a general mathematical and statistical approach to the analysis of linear structural equation systems. The advantage of

TABLE 1
Demographic and Medical Characteristics of Cocaine-Exposed and
Control Groups

	COCAINE		CONTROL		
	Mean	(SD)	Mean	(SD)	*p* <
Maternal:					
Age	25.60	(3.9)	25.20	(5.1)	. . .
Percent white	27.88		29.2		. . .
Percent black	42.3		45.1		. . .
Percent other	31.3		26.7		. . .
Percent cigarette use	65.1		60.6		. . .
Percent heroin use	3.4		2.6		. . .
Percent methadone use	2.1		1.8		. . .
Percent marijuana use	11.4		11.6		. . .
Percent alcohol use	17.2		15.4		. . .
Infant:					
Gestational age (wks)	38.90	(1.56)	39.20	(1.35)	. . .
Birthweight (gms)	2972.91	(452)	3172.95	(523)	.007
Length (cm)	48.72	(2.39)	50.24	(2.94)	.0006
Head circumference (cm)	33.23	(1.47)	33.96	(1.84)	.006
Ponderal index	2.57	(.33)	2.49	(.27)	. . .
Apgar (1 min)	7.98	(1.12)	8.10	(.98)	. . .
Apgar (5 min)	8.87	(.57)	8.88	(.39)	. . .
% Male	57		54		. . .

this approach, when used in an appropriate hypothesis-testing mode, is that structural parameters presumably represent relatively invariant parameters of a causal process and are considered to have more theoretical meaning than ordinary predictive regression equations, especially when the regression equation is embedded in a series of simultaneous equations designed to implement a substantive theory.

The general path diagram of the model from the present study is shown in Figure 1. Each measured variable is shown in a square. Cocaine (F1) is a latent variable based on the two estimates of cocaine use, self-report (V1) and positive urine assay (V2). The double arrow between V1 and V2 represents the covariance between these two variables. D1 is "disturbance" or error associated with the estimate of F1 (cocaine). V1, V2, and V3 (birthweight) are the same in each model tested with a different V4 (cry characteristic) variable. E3 and E4 represent, respectively, the variances of V3 and V4. The regression coefficients B1, B2, and B3 are represented as unidirectional arrows. The paths from V1 and V2 to F1 were fixed; the paths represented by B1, B2, and B3 were free parameters estimated by the model. The analysis was performed on the covariance matrix using maximum likelihood estimation.

A total of 12 models were tested, one model with each cry variable. A summary

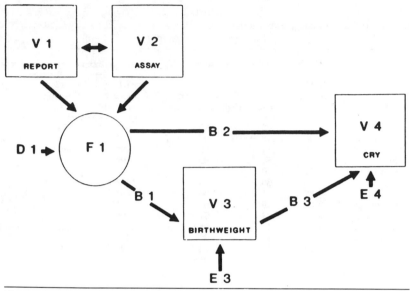

Figure 1. Structural equation model of cocaine effects on infant cry

of these 12 models is shown in Table 2. Two estimates are provided of the "goodness of fit" or adequacy of the model. The maximum likelihood (ML) chi-square is used to determine the probability of obtaining a chi-square value as large as or larger than the value actually obtained given that the model is correct. When the null hypothesis is true, the model should fit the data poorly and the chi-square probability should exceed the standard ($p < .05$) cut-off in the chi-square distribution. In a well-fitting model, the probability will be large ($p > .05$). The Bentler-Bonnet (1980) Fit Index is based on the fit function as well as an appropriate null model. Values of this index that exceed .9 indicate a good-fitting model.

Table 2 also shows the standardized parameter estimates for the B1, B2, and B3 regression coefficients. This provides a completely standardized path analysis type of solution with all variables rescaled to have unit variance. Statistical significance tests are performed on the unstandardized parameter estimates. The test statistic is the parameter estimates. The test statistic is the parameter estimate divided by the standard error and is a normal z test. Values that exceed the standard normal critical value of 1.96 associated with a .05 probability level indicate that the parameter is significantly different from zero. In Table 2, parameter estimates that were found to be statistically significant are indicated.

The most effective use of structural models is when competing models are compared directly. In the case where competing models are tested and where there is

TABLE 2
Summary of Structural Equation Models (EQS) of Cocaine Predicting Cry Characteristics
Mediated by Birthweight

	GOODNESS-OF-FIT SUMMARY			STANDARDIZED PARAMETER ESTIMATES		
	ML Chi-			B1	B2	B3
	Square		Bentler-Bonnet	Cocaine to	Cocaine	Birthweight
CRY MEASURE	($df = 2$)	$p <$	(Normed) Index	Birthweight	to Cry	to Cry
Latency	1.72	.42	.93	.49*	.24	−.41*
Number cries........	1.48	.48	.96	.49*	.28	.56*
Duration..............	1.36	.51	.98	.49*	.42*	.13
Amplitude............	1.28	.53	.96	.49*	.21	.40*
Dysphonation	1.01	.60	.96	.49*	.24	−.37*
f0...........................	.86	.65	.94	.49*	.44*	.21
f0 var	.87	.65	.96	.49*	.15	−.10
Hyperphonation ...	1.99	.39	.92	.49*	.10	.09
F1	2.96	.23	.91	.49*	.38*	−.34
F1 var....................	1.66	.43	.94	.49*	.43*	−.27
F2	1.78	.41	.92	.49*	.25	.12
F2 var....................	1.05	.59	.96	.49*	.10	.18

* Z score >1.96, $p < .05$.

a difference in the models of a single path being eliminated in the more restricted model, the significance of the path (in the unrestricted model) is equivalent to the chi-square difference test of the two competing modes (Bentler, 1989). Thus, in Table 2 the significance of B3 is equivalent to testing the comparison of the models with and without the birthweight to cry path, that is, with and without the indirect effect.

As shown in Table 2, the ML chi-squares for each of the 12 models showed a nonsignificant chi-square, indicating that each model provides an adequate fit to the data by p value. The Bentler-Bonnet Fit Indices for the 12 models are all >.9, suggesting that all models also fit by the Bentler-Bonnet criteria.

The standardized estimates for B1 are all the same since the relation between cocaine and birthweight is constant in all 12 models. This shows the association between cocaine use and low birthweight. Of the 12 models that were tested, statistically significant effects were observed on eight of the cry variables. Four of the effects were due to the direct effects of cocaine on cry characteristics (B2); the other four effects were due to birthweight (B3) mediating the effects of cocaine on cry characteristics.

The direct (B2) effects showed that cocaine use was associated with longer duration cries and cries with a higher fundamental frequency, higher first formant, and more variability in the first formant. None of the effects for birthweight (B3) were significant for these variables, suggesting that the effects were due only to cocaine.

The indirect effects indicated by statistically significant effects for birthweight

(B3) showed that lower birthweight infants had a longer latency from stimulus application to cry onset, fewer cry utterances, a lower amplitude cry, and more dysphonation or turbulence in the cry. These effects were due to the effects of cocaine use, resulting in lower birthweight infants (B1), with low birthweight in turn affecting the cry characteristics. None of the direct effects of cocaine were found to be significant in these analyses, showing the mediating effects of IUGR on cry characteristics.

DISCUSSION

Cocaine exposure in utero appears to affect the acoustic characteristics of the newborn infant cry through two different paths—a direct path and an indirect path mediated by birthweight. The first path, or direct effects of cocaine, resulted in newborn cries that were longer in duration with a higher fundamental frequency and a higher and more variable first formant. This constellation of cry characteristics is compatible with the construct of excitable behavior, and from a physiological point of view would be due to increased respiratory effort, increased laryngeal tension, and constriction in the upper airway. As mentioned earlier, high-pitched and excessive crying are part of the scoring of the neonatal abstinence scale (Finnegan, 1984) used to measure withdrawal effects. It is very likely that cries with a longer duration, a higher fundamental frequency and first formant, and a more variable first formant would be perceived as excessive and high pitched. It is also noteworthy that a higher first formant has been found in infants who died of sudden infant death syndrome, and fetal cocaine exposure has been associated with SIDS (Chasnoff et al., 1986; Chasnoff, Griffith, MacGregor, Dirkes, & Burns, 1989).

The second path is one in which cocaine results in low birthweight, which in turn affects a different set of cry characteristics. These indirect effects result in cries with a longer latency, fewer overall cry utterances, lower amplitude, and more dysphonation or turbulence. These cry characteristics suggest a decrease in functional activity or more depressed, underaroused behavior as a result of a hyporesponsive CNS with consequent poor respiratory effort.

These findings of two different pathways reflecting excitable and depressed cry characteristics in cocaine-exposed infants are compatible with previously mentioned neurobehavioral findings (Bingol et al., 1987; Chasnoff et al., 1985, 1986; Cherukuri et al., 1988; Dixon et al., 1987; Doberczak et al., 1988; Fulroth et al., 1989; LeBlanc et al., 1987; Madden et al., 1986; Oro & Dixon, 1987) and support the distinction between excitable and depressed neurobehavioral syndromes in these infants. We offer here a distinction between "type" and "syndrome." In contrast to *types*, where each infant has one distinct pattern of behavior, *syndromes* are patterns of behavior, of which any infant may have one or more of the syndromes.

Some infants may show a mixed syndrome consisting of elements of both excitable and depressed behavior, for example, infants who have an initially high threshold for reactivity and appear depressed but with stimulation become very reactive. It is likely that various combinations of excitable and depressed behavior will be observed in future studies of cocaine-exposed infants.

Physiological Mechanisms

The direct and indirect effects of cocaine that we observed support the hypothesis that these two paths may be due to different physiological mechanisms. Direct effects include the action of cocaine on the fetus consequent to transfer of the drug through the placenta and are probably due to alterations in synaptic transmission as cocaine blocks the retrieval of dopamine and norepinephrine after they are released across a synapse. This fosters increased neurotransmission and CNS irritability.

The action of cocaine on mesolimbic systems (Wise, 1984) may trigger the cry, which is activated by the hypothalamic-limbic system and controlled by midbrain and brainstem regions (Lester & Boukydis, in press; Lester et al., 1989). The effects of cocaine on the tegmentum and on the raphe nuclei (Wise, 1984) could directly affect midbrain and brainstem control of the cry. In previous work, cry characteristics were affected by prenatal exposure to marijuana (Lester & Dreher, 1989) and alcohol (Lester et al., 1989). In monkeys (McIssac, Fritchie, Idanpaan-Heikkila, Ho, & Englert, 1971) and rats (Landfield, Cadwallader, & Vinsant, 1987), THC causes changes in the limbic system. Ethanol and short-acting opiates have also been found to affect hypothalamic neuroendocrine function (Wise, 1984). In addition, if cocaine affects endorphin systems in the same region, irritability and excitability may be due to a lower pain threshold. It is interesting that in clinical descriptions of cocaine-exposed newborns, Chasnoff (Chasnoff & Griffith, in press) mentions that some of these infants have low thresholds and are easily overstimulated.

Indirect effects of cocaine can be attributable to changes in the fetal environment and effects on the mother's CNS. Cocaine causes vasoconstriction, and when blood vessels in the placenta are constricted, the supply of oxygen and other nutrients to the fetus is reduced, resulting in fetal hypoxia and IUGR. These may be chronic effects in which the effects of cocaine are secondary to IUGR. Depressed catecholamine responses have been found in IUGR rat pups (Shaul, Cha, & Oh, 1989). Depressed behavior in IUGR human infants has been reported in studies of cry characteristics (Lester & Zeskind, 1978), feeding behavior (Mullen, Garcia-Coll, Vohr, & Oh, 1988), and in studies using the Brazelton scale (Als, Tronick, Adamson, & Brazelton, 1976; Lester, Garcia-Coll, Valcarcel, Hoffman, & Brazelton, 1986; Picone, Allen, Olsen, & Ferns, 1982).

There are other explanations that may account for excitable and depressed behavioral patterns in cocaine-exposed infants. First, the administration of cocaine generally results in an initial arousal followed by depression, in which case the manifestation of these two syndromes may be a function of time from the last dose of cocaine (Gawin & Kleber; 1988; Gold, Washton, & Dackis, 1985). Second, excitable behavior may reflect an abstinence syndrome and be a function of time from last dose and the magnitude of drug exposure (Gawin & Kleber, 1988; Tarr & Macklin, 1987). Third, excitable behavior may be related to the kindling phenomenon described by Post (Post & Kopanda, 1972; Post, Panda, & Black, 1976) and others (Wise, 1984). This is an electrical phenomenon that can cause motor seizures and reflects long-term repetitive exposure to cocaine. However, while these mechanisms may explain the presence of excitable and depressed behavior in cocaine-exposed infants, they do not readily explain why depressed behavior is related to cocaine-exposed IUGR infants and excitable behavior to cocaine-exposed non-IUGR infants.

Timing of Insult

The cocaine-exposed infants in the present study had a lower birthweight, shorter length, and smaller head circumference than controls. Similar findings have been reported in other studies of cocaine-exposed infants (Bingol et al., 1987; Chasnoff & MacGregor, 1987; Cherukuri et al., 1988; Fulroth et al., 1989; Hadeed & Siegel, 1989; Livesay et al., 1987; Oro & Dixon, 1987; Ryan et al., 1987; Zuckerman et al., 1989). We did not observe effects of cocaine on the weight-for-length ratio of the ponderal index. These findings speak to the potential timing of the insult in utero since the growth of length begins to peak around week 26 of gestation, whereas weight begins to peak around 33 weeks. Decreased substrate availability that begins in the first trimester will produce reductions in weight and length as well as head circumference, and this is known as symmetric IUGR. Asymmetric IUGR occurs when the insult begins around week 27–30, with growth affected after the peak velocity in length but before the peak velocity in weight, producing reductions in weight and the ponderal index. In previous work, these patterns of atypical fetal growth were found to have unique effects on the Brazelton scale (Lester et al., 1986). In the current study, the reductions in weight, length, and head circumference with no reduction in the ponderal index suggest a pattern of symmetric growth retardation indicative of nutritional deprivation early in pregnancy, probably due to early and frequent cocaine use, and hence, chronic effects. In future studies it would be useful to compare symmetric and asymmetric IUGR cocaine-exposed infants.

The limitation of this study is the use of hospital records to determine substance abuse. Because of this limitation, it was not possible to determine frequency and timing of usage patterns that could determine if, in fact, the growth retardation was due to early and frequent cocaine use. Such data are also important to determine potential dose response relations. A dose response relation was reported between prenatal exposure to marijuana and newborn cry (Lester & Dreher, 1989). Such relations have not been reported in studies of the neurobehavioral effects of cocaine exposure. Hospital records are also of limited use because they may result in the underreporting of substance abuse. Thus, there may have been subjects in the control group with prenatal exposure to toxic substances who were not detected. However, this would only underestimate the observed effects.

Developmental Implications

There are several ways in which the effects observed in this study could have long-term developmental consequences for the infant. Acoustic characteristics of the cry are thought to reflect the neurophysiological status of the infant and have been related to developmental outcome in preterm infants (Lester, 1987; Lester et al., 1989). Therefore, the alterations in cry characteristic due to cocaine exposure could represent effects of the drug on the developing nervous system with long-term sequelae.

Effects may be long-lasting due to permanent changes caused by cocaine exposure, in which case excitable and depressed neurobehavioral syndromes may persist. However, with regard to our expectations about neurobehavioral sequelae, it is useful to keep in mind the fact that as a drug, cocaine is less potent than, for example, thalidomide, and even with thalidomide only 26% of the mothers who took the drug during the critical exposure period had babies that were affected (McBride, 1977). Excitable and depressed neurobehavioral syndromes due to cocaine may represent relatively subtle effects. In addition, studies have not determined the stability of neurobehavioral effects in cocaine-exposed infants; it is possible, therefore, that these effects are transient.

From a transactional perspective (Sameroff & Chandler, 1975), the "goodness of fit" between the infant's neurobehavioral syndrome and the response of the caregiving environment would be expected to determine developmental processes that influence the long-term outcome of the infant. The parenting ability of the cocaine-using mother may be compromised by her drug problem, associated personality characteristics, and a life-style that may not provide an adequate child-rearing environment. The interaction between these factors and the excitable or depressed neurobehavioral syndrome in the infant may cause a violation or mismatch in the early parent-infant relationship that leads to poor infant outcome. From this perspective, even short-term effects of cocaine on the neurobehavioral organization of the infant could affect infant outcome.

REFERENCES

Als, H., Tronick, E., Adamson, L., & Brazelton, T. B. (1976). The behavior of the full-term yet underweight newborn infant. *Developmental Medicine and Child Neurology,* **18,** 590–602.

Anday, E., Cohen, M., Schwartz, D., & Hoffman, H. (1989). Effect of in utero cocaine exposure on sensorineural processing. *Pediatric Research,* **25,** 206A.

Bauchner, H., Zuckerman, B., Amaro, H., Frank, D. A., & Parker, S. (1987). Teratogenicity of cocaine. *Journal of Pediatrics,* **111,**160–161.

Bentler, P. M. (1989). *EQS: Structural equations program manual.* Los Angeles: BMDP Statistical Software.

Bentler, P. M., & Bonnet, D. G. (1980). Significance tests and goodness of fit in the analysis of covariance structures. *Psychological Bulletin,* **88,** 588–606.

Bingol, N., Fuchs, M., Diaz, V., Stone, R. X., & Gromisch, D. S. (1987). Teratogenicity of cocaine in humans. *Journal of Pediatrics,* **110,** 93–96.

Chasnoff, I. J., Burns, W. J., Schnoll, S. H., & Burns, K. A. (1985). Cocaine use in pregnancy. *New England Journal of Medicine,* **313,** 666–669.

Chasnoff, I. J., Burns, W. J., Schnoll, S. H., & Burns, K. A. (1986). *Effects of cocaine on pregnancy outcome.* National Institute of Drug Abuse and Research Monograph Series (Vol. **7,** pp. 335–341). Rockville, MD: NIDA.

Chasnoff, I. J., & Griffith, D. R. (in press). Maternal cocaine use: Neonatal outcome. In H. Fitzgerald, B. M. Lester, & M. Yogman (Eds.), *Theory and research in behavioral pediatrics* (Vol. **5**). New York: Plenum.

Chasnoff, I. J., Griffith, D. R., MacGregor, S., Dirkes, K., & Burns, K. A. (1989). Temporal patterns of cocaine use in pregnancy. *Journal of American Medical Association,* **261,** 1741–1744.

Chasnoff, I. J., & MacGregor, S. (1987). Maternal cocaine use and neonatal morbidity. *Pediatric Research,* **21,** 356A.

Cherukuri, R., Minkoff, H., Feldman, J., Parekh, A., & Glass, L. (1988). A cohort study of alkaloidal cocaine ("crack") in pregnancy. *Obstetrics and Gynecology,* **72,** 147–151.

Clayton, R. R. (1985). Cocaine use in the U.S.: in a blizzard or just being snowed? In N. J. Kozel & E. H. Adams (Eds.), *Cocaine use in America: Epidemiologic and clinical perspectives.* National Institute on Drug Abuse Research Monograph (Vol. *61,* pp. 8–34). Rockville, MD: Department of Health and Human Services.

Corwin, M. J., Lester, B. M., Sepkoski, C., McLaughlin, S., Kayne, H., & Golub, H. (1990). Effects of in utero cocaine exposure on newborn acoustical cry characteristics. *Pediatric Research,* **27**(4, pt. 2).

Cregler, L. L., & Mark, H. (1986). Special report: Medical complications of cocaine abuse. *New England Journal of Medicine,* **315**(23), 1495–1500.

Dixon, S. D., & Behar, R. (1989). Echoencephalographic findings in neonates associated with maternal cocaine and methamphentamine use: Incidence and clinical correlates. *Journal of Pediatrics,* **115,** 770–778.

Dixon, S. D., Coen, R. W., & Crutchfield, S. (1987). Visual dysfunction in cocaine-exposed infants. *Pediatric Research, 21,* 359A.

Doberczak, T. M., Shanzer, S., Senie, R. T., & Kandall, S. R. (1988). Neonatal neurologic and electroencephalographic effects of intrauterine cocaine exposure. *Journal of Pediatrics,* **113,** 354–358.

Fant, G. (1960). *Acoustic theory of speech production.* The Hague: Mouton.

Finnegan, L. P. (1984). Neonatal abstinence. In M. Nelson (Ed.), *Current therapy in neonatal and perinatal medicine* (pp. 262–270). St. Louis: Mosby.

Frank. D. A., Zuckerman, B. S., Amaro, H., Aboagye, K., Bauchner, H., Cabral, H., Fried, L., Hingson, R., Kayne, H., Levenson, S. M., Parker, S., Reece, H., & Vinci, R. (1988). Cocaine use during pregnancy: prevalency and correlates. *Pediatrics,* **82,** 888–895.

Fulroth, R. F., Phillips, B., & Durant, D. J. (1989). Perinatal outcome of infants exposed to cocaine and/or heroin in utero. *American Journal of Diseases in Children,* **143,** 905–910.

Gawin, F. H., & Kleber, H. D. (1988). Evolving conceptualizations of cocaine dependence. *Yale Journal of Biology and Medicine,* **61,** 123–136.

Gold, M. S., Washton, A. M., & Dackis, C. A. (1985). *Cocaine abuse: Neurochemistry, phenomenology, and treatment.* National Institute of Drug Abuse Research Monograph Series (Vol. **61,** pp. 130–150). Rockville, MD: NIDA.

Golub, H. A., & Corwin, M. J. (1982). Infant cry: A clue to diagnosis. *Pediatrics,* **69,** 197–201.

Golub, H. A., & Corwin, M. J. (1984). A physioacoustic model of the infant cry. In B. M. Lester & C. F. Z. Boukydis (Eds.), *Infant crying: Theoretical and research perspectives* (pp. 59–82). New York: Plenum.

Hadeed, A. J., & Siegel, S. R. (1989). Maternal cocaine use during pregnancy: Effect on the newborn infant. *Pediatrics,* **84,** 205–210.

Inglass, T. H., Curley, F. J., & Prindle, R. A. (1952). Experimental production of congenital anomalies. *New England Journal of Medicine,* **247,** 758–768.

Jones, C. L., & Lopez, R. (1988). *Direct and indirect effects on infants of maternal drug abuse.* Washington, DC: Department of Health and Human Services/National Institute of Health.

Landfield, P. W., Cadwallader, L. B., & Vinsant, S. (1987). Quantitative changes in hippocampal structure following long-term exposure to tetrahydrocannabinol: Possible mediation by glucocorticoid systems. *Brain Research,* **443,** 47–62.

LeBlanc, P. E., Parekh, A. J., Naso, B., & Glass, L. (1987). Effects of intrauterine exposure to alkaloidal cocaine ("crack"). *American Journal of Diseases of Childhood,* **141,** 937–938.

Lester, B. M. (1979). A synergistic process approach to the study of prenatal malnutrition. *International Journal of Behavioral Development,* **2,** 377–393.

Lester, B. M. (1987). Prediction of developmental outcome from acoustic cry analysis in term and preterm infants. *Pediatrics,* **80,** 529–534.

Lester, B., Anderson, L. T., Boukydis, C. F. Z., Garcia-Coll, C. T., Bohr, B., & Peucker, M. (1989). Early detection of infants at risk for later handicap through acoustic cry analysis. In *Research in infant assessment* (pp. 99–117). New York: March of Dimes Birth Defects Foundation.

Lester, B. M., & Boukydis, C. F. Z. (Eds.). (1985). *Infant crying: Theoretical and research perspectives.* New York: Plenum.

Lester, B. M., & Boukydis, C. F. Z. (1991). No language but a cry. In H. Papousek (Ed.), *Origin and development of nonverbal and vocal communication.* Cambridge: Cambridge University Press.

Lester, B. M., & Dreher, M. (1989). Effects of marijuana use during pregnancy on newborn cry. *Child Development, 60,* 765–771.

Lester, B. M., Garcia-Coll, C. T., Valcarcel, M., Hoffman, J., & Brazelton, T. B. (1986). Effects of atypical patterns of fetal growth on newborn (NBAS) behavior. *Child Development, 57,* 11–19.

Lester, B. M., & Zeskind, P. S. (1978). Brazelton scale and physical size correlates of neonatal cry features. *Infant Behavior and Development, 49,* 589–599.

Livesay, S., Ehrlich, S., & Finnegan, L. P. (1987). Cocaine and pregnancy: Maternal and infant outcome. *Pediatric Research, 21,* 238A.

Madden, J. D., Payne, T. F., & Miller, S. (1986). Maternal cocaine abuse and effect on the newborn. *Pediatrics, 77,* 209–211.

Mahalik, M. P., Gautieri, R. F., & Mann, D. E. (1984). Mechanisms of cocaine induced teratogenesis. *Research Communications in Substances of Abuse, 5*(4), 279–303.

McBride, W. G. (1977). Thalidomide embryopathy. *Teratology, 16,* 79–82.

McIsaac, W. M., Fritchie, G. E., Idanpaan-Heikkila, J. E., Ho, B. T., & Englert, L. F. (1971). Distribution of marijuana in monkey brain and concomitant behavioral effects. *Nature, 230,* 593–594.

Mullen, M. K., Garcia-Coll, C. T., Bohr, B. R., & Oh, W. (1988) Mother-infant feeding interaction in full-term small for gestational age infants. *Journal of Pediatrics, 112,* 143–148.

Nugent, J. K., Lester, B. M., & Greene, S. (1990). *Maternal alcohol consumption during pregnancy and acoustic cry analysis.* Paper presented at the Seventh International Conference on Infant Studies, Montreal.

Oro, A. S., & Dixon, S. D. (1987). Perinatal cocaine and methamphetamine exposure: Maternal and neonatal correlates. *Journal of Pediatrics, 3,* 571–578.

Picone, T., Allen, L., Olsen, P., & Ferns, M. (1982). Pregnancy outcome in North American women: II. Effects of diet, cigarette smoking, stress, and weight gain on neonatal physical and behavioral characteristics. *American Journal of Clinical Nutrition, 36,* 1214–1224.

Post, R. M., & Kopanda, R. T. (1972). Cocaine, kindling, and psychosis. *American Journal of Psychiatry, 133,* 627–634.

Post, R. M., Kopanda, R. T., & Black, K. E. (1976). Progressive effects of cocaine on behavior and central amine metabolism in rhesus monkeys: Relationship in kindling and psychosis. *Biological Psychiatry, 11,* 403–419.

Ritchie, J. M., & Greene, N. M. (1985). Local anesthetics. In A. G. Gillman, L. S.

Goodman, T. W. Rall, & F. Murad (Eds.), *The pharmacological basis of therapeutics* (7th ed., pp. 309–310). New York: Macmillan.

Ryan, L., Ehrlich, S., & Finnegan, L. (1987). Cocaine abuse in pregnancy: Effects on the fetus and newborn. *Neurotoxicology Teratology, 9,* 295–299.

Sameroff, A. J., & Chandler, J. J. (1975). Reproductive risk, and the continuum of caretaking casualty. In F. D. Horowitz (Ed.), *Review of child development research* (Vol. **4,** pp. 187–244). Chicago: University of Chicago Press.

Shaul, P. W., Cha, C. M., & Oh, W. (1989). Neonatal sympathoadrenal response to acute hypoxia: Impairment after experimental intrauterine growth retardation. *Pediatric Research,* **25,** 472–477.

Shih, L, Cone-Wesson, B., Reddix, B., & Wu, P. Y. K. (1989) Effect of maternal cocaine abuse on the neonatal auditory system. *Pediatric Research,* **25,** 264A.

Smith, D. W. (1982). *Recognizable patterns of human malformations.* Philadelphia: Saunders.

Stevens, K. N. (1964). Acoustical aspects of speech production. In W. O. Fenn & H. Rahn (Eds.), *Handbook of physiology: A critical comprehensive presentation of physiological knowledge and concepts: Section 3. Respiration.* Washington, DC: American Physiological Society.

Tarr, J. E., & Macklin, M. (1987). Cocaine. *Pediatric Clinics of North America,* **34,** 319–331.

Wise, R. (1984). *Neural mechanisms of the reenforcing action of cocaine.* National Institute of Drug Abuse Monograph Series (Vol. **50,** pp. 15–53). Washington, DC: Government Printing Office.

Woods, J. R., Plessinger, M. S., & Clark, K. E. (1987). Effect of cocaine on uterine blood flow and fetal oxygenation. *Journal of the American Medical Association,* **257,** 957–961.

Yoon, J. J., Kim, Mac Hee, K., Checola, R. T., & Noble, L. M. (1989). Maternal cocaine abuse and microcephaly. *Pediatric Research,* **25,** 79A.

Zeskind, P. S., & Lester, B. M. (1981). Analysis of cry features in newborns with differential fetal growth. *Child Development,* **52,** 207–212.

Zuckerman, B., Frank, D. A., Hingson, R., Amaro, H., Levenson, S. M., Kayne, H., Parker, S., Vinci, R., Aboagye, K., Fried, L. E., Cabral, H., Timperi, R., & Bauchner, H. (1989). Effects of maternal marijuana and cocaine use on fetal growth. *New England Journal of Medicine,* **320,** 762–768.

28

The Impact of Homelessness on Children

Yvonne Rafferty

Advocates for Children, Long Island City, New York

Marybeth Shinn

New York University, New York City

This article reviews and critiques community-based research on the effects of homelessness on children. Homeless children confront serious threats to their ability to succeed and their future well-being. Of particular concern are health problems, hunger, poor nutrition, developmental delays, anxiety, depression, behavioral problems, and educational underachievement. Factors that may mediate the observed outcomes include inadequate shelter conditions, instability in residences and shelters, inadequate services, and barriers to accessing services that are available. Public policy initiatives are needed to meet the needs of homeless children.

Research on the impact of homelessness on children indicates that homeless children (generally identified as those in emergency shelter facilities with their families) confront serious threats to their well-being. Of particular concern are health problems, hunger and poor nutrition, developmental delays, psychological problems, and educational underachievement. This article examines the problems faced by homeless children in each of these areas. Where possible, we describe the extent

Reprinted with permission from *American Psychologist,* 1991, Vol. 46, No. 11, 1170–1179. Copyright ©1991 by the American Psychological Association, Inc.

Preparation of this article was supported in part by grants from the Edna McConnell Clark Foundation and the Robert Sterling Clark Foundation to Advocates for Children, and Grant RO1MH46116 from the National Institute of Mental Health to the second author.

The first author gratefully acknowledges numerous insightful discussions with Norma Rollins, which resulted in *Learning in Limbo: The Educational Deprivation of Homeless Children,* published in September of 1989. The authors thank Andrea Solarz for her helpful comments on an earlier draft of this article.

to which homeless children are at a disadvantage, relative not only to the population at large but to other poor children. That is, we attempt to understand to what extent problems are associated with homelessness per se and to what extent they are linked with extreme poverty.

A second task of this article is to understand how homelessness leads to the outcomes we document and to identify which conditions in the lives of homeless children lead to particular adverse effects. As Molnar and Rubin (1991) pointed out, homelessness is a composite of many conditions and events, such as poverty, changes in residence, schools, and services, loss of possessions, disruptions in social networks, and exposure to extreme hardship. Effects of homelessness on children may be mediated by any of these ecological conditions and by their affects on parents and the family system. Research on homeless children, however, has not generally examined mediating mechanisms. We focus on mechanisms that can be influenced by social policy, namely, inadequate shelter conditions, instability of shelters and residences, lack of adequate services, and barriers to accessing available services. A final section describes linkages among outcomes and discusses implications for public policy.

HEALTH PROBLEMS

Studies have consistently found that homeless children experience elevated levels of acute and chronic health problems. Risk for health problems begins before birth. Chavkin, Kristal, Seabron, and Guigli (1987) compared the reproductive experience of 401 homeless women in welfare hotels in New York City with that of 13,249 women in public housing and with all live births in New York City during the same time period. Significantly more of the homeless women (16%, compared with 11% of women in public housing and 7% of all women) had low-birth-weight babies. Infant mortality was also extraordinarily high: 25 deaths per 1,000 live births among the homeless women, compared with 17 per 1,000 for housed poor women and 12 per 1,000 for women citywide.

Wright (1987, 1990, 1991) examined the medical records of 1,028 homeless children under 15 years of age who were treated in the Robert Wood Johnson Health Care for the Homeless programs in 16 cities. He compared the occurrence of various diseases and disorders among homeless children with rates reported in the National Ambulatory Medical Care Survey for U.S. ambulatory patients ages 15 and under. All of the disorders studied were more common among homeless children, often occurring at double the rate observed in the general pediatric caseload. The most common disorders among homeless children were upper respiratory infections (42% vs. 22% in the national sample), minor skin ailments (20% vs. 5% in the national sample), ear disorders (18% vs. 12% in the national sample), chronic physical disorders (15% vs. 9% in the national sample), and gastrointestinal disorders (15%

vs. 4% in the national sample). Infestational ailments, although less common than other disorders among homeless children (7%), occurred at more than 35 times the rate of those in the national sample. The Health Care for the Homeless and National Ambulatory Medical Care Survey samples differ along several dimensions. Members of the homeless sample are more likely to be poor, members of minority groups, and urban dwellers. Also, both surveys assess prevalence among those who use health services rather than among the general population. Although one might expect homeless families to wait until problems become serious before seeking treatment (leading to higher prevalence rates for many disorders), differences in utilization patterns are unlikely to account for the high prevalences observed. As Wright (1987) concluded, "Among the many good reasons to do something about homelessness is . . . that homelessness makes people ill; in the extreme case, it is a fatal condition" (p. 80).

Alperstein and Arnstein (1988) and Alperstein, Rappaport, and Flanigan (1988) made several comparisons between the health of homeless children in New York City and that of poor housed children receiving health care there. Using clinic records, they found that 27% of 265 homeless children under the age of 5 who were living in a "welfare" hotel were late in getting necessary immunizations, compared with 8% of 100 poor children attending the same outpatient clinic. Twice as many homeless children (4%) as members of the population of 1,072 children whose blood was tested that year by the clinic (2%), had elevated lead levels in the blood. (The comparison group may have included some homeless children.) Rates of hospital admission among a larger sample of 2,500 homeless children under the age of 18 were almost twice as high as for 6,000 children of the same age living in the same area (11.6 vs. 7.5 per thousand, respectively).

Bernstein, Alperstein, and Fierman (1988) compared the clinic charts of 90 homeless children aged 6 months to 12 years with those of a matched cohort of housed children whose family incomes were below the federal poverty level. Nearly one half (48%) of the homeless children under age 2 were delayed in their immunizations, compared with 16% of the housed children. Fifty percent of the homeless children, compared with 25% of the housed group, had iron deficiencies, which may be related to other unmeasured nutritional deficiencies. Most of these studies are based on families who use health care services, so that differential patterns in the use of services could account for some of the differences in health status.

Other studies that are based on self-reported health status or that lack comparison groups paint a consistent picture. Homeless children's health problems include immunization delays, asthma, ear infections, overall poor health, diarrhea, and anemia (Dehavenon & Benker, 1989; Miller & Lin, 1988; New York City Department of Health, 1986; Paone & Kay, 1988; Rafferty & Rollins, 1989; Redlener, 1989; Roth & Fox, 1988; Wright, 1990, 1991; but not Wood, Valdez, Hayashi, & Shen, 1990a).

Both inadequate emergency shelter conditions and lack of adequate preventive and curative health services are prime mechanisms by which homelessness leads to poor health. A third factor, poor nutrition, is discussed in the next section.

The conditions in many private and public shelters place children at risk of lead poisoning and other environmental hazards. Congregate living environments in many shelters present optimal conditions for the transmission of infectious and communicable diseases such as upper respiratory infections, skin disorders, and diarrhea. These conditions include close proximity of beds, use of bathrooms by many people, inadequate facilities to change and bathe infants, unsanitary conditions, and noise and light that disrupt sleep (cf. Citizens Committee for Children, 1988; Gross & Rosenberg, 1987; Jahiel, 1987). According to the New York City Department of Health (1986), "There appears to be no basis for concluding that congregate family shelters can be operated in compliance with basic principles of public health" (p. 5). Regulations in 50% of cities require families to leave shelters during daytime hours (U.S. Conference of Mayors, 1989). This policy means that children are exposed to the elements, and it makes daytime naps for preschoolers and adequate care of sick children impossible.

Another important mediator of health problems is the lack of adequate primary and preventive health care services. Research has demonstrated that poor children have less access to quality health care than do middle-class children (Newacheck & Starfield, 1988); children who are both poor and homeless are at an even greater disadvantage. Access to timely and consistent health care is compromised by extreme poverty, removal from community ties, frequent disruptions in family life, and lack of health insurance (Angel & Worobey, 1988; Rafferty & Rollins, 1989; Roth & Fox, 1988).

The scarcity of adequate health care for homeless children begins with the paucity of prenatal care available to their mothers. Chavkin et al. (1987) found that 40% of 401 homeless women received no prenatal care compared with 14.5% of public housing residents and 9% of all women in New York who gave birth during the same period. This may help to explain the higher risk of negative birth outcomes, previously described, for homeless women.

As noted earlier, most research focuses on homeless children in emergency shelters because they are easier to study and identify. Many health problems may predate shelter entry, including crowding in doubled-up situations, as well as exposure and lack of sanitary facilities in public places.

HUNGER AND POOR NUTRITION

In their survey of 26 cities, the U.S. Conference of Mayors (1987) described a variety of negative effects of homelessness on physical and emotional well-being. The factors mentioned most frequently by city officials were lack of food and poor nutrition. The struggle to maintain an adequate and nutritionally balanced diet while living in a welfare hotel was described by Simpson, Kilduff, and Blewett (1984), who surveyed 40 heads of families (representing 194 people). Overall, 92% had no refrigerator in the hotel room, no family had a stove, 80% reported eating less food and food of lesser quality than they previously had, and 67% said they "felt hungrier" since moving to the hotel. Similarly, Wood et al. (1990a) compared the dietary intake and episodes of hunger among 192 homeless and 194 stably housed poor children in Los Angeles. Homeless children were significantly more likely to have gone hungry during the prior month (23% vs. 4%, respectively); more than one fifth (21% vs. 7%, respectively) did not have enough to eat because of lack of money.

Dehavenon and Benker (1989) found that nonpregnant adults in 202 families requesting shelter in New York City reported eating only once per day over the previous three days, on average; pregnant women ate twice per day. Although children were reported to have eaten three times per day, suggesting that adults gave up food for them, it appears unlikely that the children's food intake was adequate, given the bleak nutritional picture for their families. Among those in the shelter system for at least a week, nonpregnant women lost a median of eight pounds; of 98 pregnant women, 22% reported losing weight during their pregnancy and an additional 8% reported no weight gain. Nine of 26 families reported stretching infants' formula with water.

Anecdotal observations of homeless children in day care settings also suggest that they are hungry. Molnar (1988) reported that some homeless children threw tantrums until they were fed. Grant (1989) noted that most "ate enthusiastically, asking for second helpings" but "nearly all lacked previous experience in eating at a table and sharing food family-style" (p. 30). Many had not used utensils or cups.

Inadequate benefits and difficulties in accessing food and entitlements are the major mediators of hunger and poor nutrition. The vast majority of homeless families are headed by women who rely on Aid to Families with Dependent Children (AFDC) as their primary source of income (Bassuk & Rosenberg, 1988; Rafferty & Rollins, 1989). However, benefit levels have been described as "woefully inadequate" (National Coalition for the Homeless, 1988) and a main cause of hunger (U.S. Conference of Mayors, 1989).

The difficulties homeless families have in trying to manage on benefits that generally fall below 70% of the federal poverty line (Community Food Resource Center, 1989) are frequently compounded by failure to receive benefits to which they are entitled, erroneous case closings, and benefit reductions (National Coalition for the Homeless, 1988). The U.S. House of Representatives Select Committee on Hunger (1987) surveyed 2,112 individuals in emergency shelters in New York City in 1987 and found that 49% of those who were eligible for food stamps were not receiving them. In addition, more than 50% of all New York City residents who were eligible for the federally funded Special Supplemental Food Program for Women, Infants, and Children (WIC) in 1988 did not receive benefits (New York State Department of Health, 1988). Among New York City families with a pregnant mother or a newborn, only 44% of 385 families seeking shelter were receiving WIC benefits, compared with 60% of 83 families randomly sampled from the public assistance caseload (Knickman & Weitzman, 1989).

Homeless families are also more likely than housed families to have had their welfare (AFDC) cases closed and benefits reduced. In one study conducted in California, 43% of 196 homeless families reported losing or being removed from the welfare rolls during the past year, often contributing to their loss of housing. In contrast, 23% of 194 stably housed poor families had *ever* lost their AFDC benefits (Wood, Valdez, Hayashi, & Shen, 1990b). In addition, homeless families were less likely to be receiving food stamps or WIC (62% vs. 81%, respectively).

Families with limited resources are often left with no other alternative than emergency food assistance facilities. However, in almost 20 of 27 cities surveyed, emergency food programs reported that they turned away people in need because of lack of resources. Emergency food programs in 17 of the cities reported being unable to provide adequate quantities of food (U.S. Conference of Mayors, 1989).

DEVELOPMENTAL DELAYS

Molnar (1988) documented observational and teachers' anecdotal accounts of distressing behaviors of homeless preschoolers aged 2½ to 5 years. The behaviors most frequently mentioned include short attention span, withdrawal, aggression, speech delays, sleep disorders, "regressive" toddlerlike behaviors, inappropriate social interaction with adults, immature peer interaction contrasted with strong sibling relationships, and immature motor behavior.

Whitman and her colleagues (Whitman, 1987; Whitman, Accardo, Boyert, & Kendagor, 1990) observed severe language disabilities and impaired cognitive ability among 88 children living in a dormitory style shelter for homeless families in St. Louis. Overall, 35% of these children scored at or below the borderline/slow-earner range on the Slosson Intelligence Test (Jensen & Armstrong, 1985), and 57% were delayed in their capacity to use and produce language as judged by the Peabody Picture Vocabulary Test (Dunn & Dunn, 1981).

Using the Denver Developmental Screening Test (DDST; Frankenburg, Goldstein, & Camp, 1971), Bassuk and her colleagues (Bassuk & Rosenberg, 1988; Bassuk & Rubin, 1987; Bassuk, Rubin, & Lauriat, 1986) assessed the development of 81 children (age 5 or younger) living in family shelters in

Massachusetts. Overall, 36% of the children demonstrated language delays, 34% could not complete the personal and social developmental tasks, 18% lacked gross motor skills, and 15% lacked fine motor coordination. Almost one half (47%) manifested at least one developmental lag, 33% had two or more, and 14% failed in all four areas. A subgroup of the sample (those sheltered in the Boston area) was subsequently compared with poor housed children. When compared with 75 housed preschoolers, the 48 homeless preschoolers tested were significantly more likely to manifest at least one developmental lag (54% vs. 16%, respectively), to lack personal and social development (42% vs. 3%, respectively), to demonstrate language delays (42% vs. 13%, respectively), to lack gross motor skills (17% vs. 4%, respectively), and to lack fine motor skills (15% vs. 1%, respectively; Bassuk & Rosenberg, 1988, 1990).

In contrast, more recent studies of homeless children in Ohio, Los Angeles, Philadelphia, and New York City, have not found such severe developmental problems. Wagner and Menke (1990), also using the DDST to assess 162 homeless children age 5 or younger in Ohio, found that 23% demonstrated language delays, 12% could not complete the personal and social developmental tasks, and 17% lacked gross motor skills. However, twice as many children in this sample lacked fine motor coordination as in the Boston sample (30% vs. 15%, respectively). Although Wagner and Menke (1990) had not comparison group, overall, their homeless children were more similar to the homeless than to the housed children in Bassuk and Rosenberg's (1988) study. Of the Ohio children, 44% manifested at least one developmental lag and 24% had two or more.

Wood et al. (1990b) studied developmental lags (as assessed by the DDST) in a sample of preschoolers in Los Angeles. Although overall performance was worse than in the general child population, only 15% manifested at least one delay and 9% had two or more. The most common delay was language (13%), then the fine motor coordination (11%), gross motor coordination (6%), and personal-social development (5%).

Rescorla, Parker, and Stollely (1991) compared the cognitive ability of 40 homeless children between the ages of 3 and 5 with 20 housed children of the same age awaiting treatment at a pediatric clinic in Philadelphia. Significant delays were found for receptive vocabulary as assessed by the Peabody Picture Vocabulary Test (*M* score of 68 for homeless children vs. 78 for housed children) and visual motor development as assessed by the Beery (1989) Developmental Test of Visual Motor Integration (82 vs. 90, respectively). However, no differences were found for vocabulary (using the Stanford-Binet [Thorndike, Hagen, & Sattler, 1986]), visual motor development (using the Draw-a-Person clinical technique [Harris, 1973]), or developmental ability (using the Cubes Test [Yale Child Study Center, 1986]).

When they assessed speech, language, cognition, perception, and gross and fine motor coordination using the Early Screening Inventory (Meisels & Wiske, 1988), Molnar and Rath (1990) found no significant differences between 84 homeless and 76 poor housed children between the ages of 3 and 5. Children in both groups scored poorly. Note that the only significant difference to emerge in this New York City sample was between children who did and those who did not receive day care services.

Although many of the instruments used to assess development have not been standardized for poor and minority children, the strong differences between homeless and comparison samples in several studies suggests that the problems are significant. In fact, problems may be underestimated because the commonly used DDST is a conservative screening instrument and because families in some studies had been in shelters for only short periods of time.

The poor performance of both homeless and comparison samples suggests that poverty may be a key mediator of developmental problems. Other influential mediating factors include inadequate shelter conditions, lack of access to quality day care services, instability in child care arrangements, and effects of homelessness on parents.

Media accounts detail the brutal and shocking conditions in welfare hotels and in other shelters for homeless families (Kozol, 1988). Berezin (1988) described how restrictive physical environments in emergency shelters make physical exploration virtually impossible: "There is little opportunity for the kind of exploration and interactive play that we know lay the foundation for healthy physical, emotional, and cognitive growth" (p. 3).

Despite the abundance of literature documenting the importance of high quality day care services for social and intellectual stimulation (Consortium for Longitudinal Studies, 1983; Haskins, 1989; Phillips, McCartney, & Scarr, 1987; Scarr & Weinberg, 1986), there is a paucity of such programs for homeless children (Berezin, 1988; Molnar, 1988). In New York City, for example, the percentage of homeless children reported to be enrolled in early childhood programs ranges from 15% (Vanderbourg & Christofides, 1986) to 20% (Molnar, 1988). Similarly, 15% of 40 homeless preschoolers in Philadelphia were enrolled in early childhood programs, in contrast to 65% of the 20 housed children in the comparison group (Rescorla et al., 1991).

Instability in shelter placements and other disruptions in child care and schooling may also impede children's development. For example, stability in child care arrangements for domiciled children is related to competent play with papers and toys in day care settings and to academic competence in first grade (Howes, 1988; Howes & Stewart, 1987). Finally, Molnar and Rubin (1991) extrapolate from research on poverty to posit that effects of homelessness on children's development and psychological functioning (reviewed next) are mediated by parental distress and its effect on parenting behaviors.

PSYCHOLOGICAL PROBLEMS

Psychological problems identified most often among homeless children include depression, anxiety, and behavioral problems. Bassuk and her colleagues (Bassuk & Rubin, 1987; Bassuk et al., 1986) studied 156 children from 82 families sheltered in Massachusetts. On the Children's Depression Inventory (CDI; Kovacs, 1983), 54% of the 44 homeless children over the age of 5 scored above the cutoff score of 9, indicating a need for mental health evaluation; 31% were clinically depressed. In fact, the mean score of 10.4 was higher than the mean for six of the eight clinical comparison groups studied during the development of the test. In a subsequent comparison of a subgroup of this sample, 16 of 31 children (52%) sheltered in Boston scored in the clinical range, compared with 16 of 33 (48%) housed poor children. Although mean scores for the children who were homeless were higher than were those for the housed group (101.3 vs. 8.3, respectively), the difference was not significant (Bassuk & Rosenberg, 1990). The 50 school-aged children's average score on the Children's Manifest Anxiety Scale (Reynolds & Richmond, 1985) was 14.4, and 30% scored in the clinical range (a T score of 60 or higher), indicating a need for mental health evaluation. In a subsequent comparison of a subgroup of this sample, 9 of 29 children (31%) sheltered in Boston scored in the clinical range compared with 3 out of 34 (9%) housed children ($p = .06$). No mean scores are presented (Bassuk & Rosenberg, 1990).

Two other studies also used the CDI to assess depression. Wagner and Menke (1990) found that 50% of 76 homeless children between the ages of 7 and 12 years manifested a need for mental health evaluation, and 35% were clinically depressed; boys scored slightly higher than did girls (11.3 vs. 10.3, respectively). Masten (1990) found that 159 homeless children and 62 poor housed children ages 8–17 years did not differ significantly from each other (9.45 vs. 8.13, respectively) or from normative levels either in mean scores or in the proportion of children in the clinical range.

Several studies have examined parents' reports of their children's behavior using the Achenbach Behavior Problem Checklist (CBCL; Achenbach & Edelbrock, 1981, 1983). Overall, mean differences between homeless and poor housed children are somewhat elusive, but more homeless children tend to score in the clinical range. Wood, Hayashi, Schlossman, and Valdez (1989) found no differences between 194 homeless and 193 stably housed poor children on the Behavior Problems Scale (adapted from the CBCL). Mean scores were quite similar, and only a minority of both groups displayed a significant number of behavior problems, primarily aggressive behaviors. Similarly, Masten (1990) found no difference in mean scores of 159 homeless children between the ages of 8 and 17 years and 62 housed children, although both groups had mean scores above normative levels. Also, the means for the externalizing subscale (reflecting acting-out behavior problems were significantly higher for the homeless sample, and significantly more homeless children scored in the clinical range on both internalizing (reflecting emotional problems like anxiety and depression) and externalizing.

Rescorla et al. (1991) found marginally significant differences on the CBCL between 43 homeless and 25 housed children between the ages of 6 and 12 years. More homeless school-age children (30%) than housed children (16%) had scores above 65; however, differences between the proportions of extreme scores were significant only for externalization (35% vs. 12%, respectively). Finally, Bassuk and Rosenberg (1990) found that a greater proportion of 31 homeless children between the ages of 6 and 16 years exceeded the cutoff point than did a comparison group of 54 housed children (39% vs. 26%, respectively). However, this difference was not significant.

Only two studies have used the CBCL among preschool children. Rescorla et al. (1991) found that their sample of 40 preschoolers between the ages of 3 and 5 scored significantly higher than did the comparison group of 20 housed children of the same age, and 20% of the homeless children (vs. 5% of the housed children) had scores in the clinical range. Molnar and Rath (1990) found no mean differences on the CBCL between 84 homeless and 76 poor housed children between the ages of 3 and 5 years; neither group differed from a nonclinical, normative group. However, once again, significantly more homeless children than housed comparison peers scored above the clinical cutoff point (33% vs. 11%, respectively).

Other, primarily descriptive, studies of behavioral problems also yield inconsistent findings. Bassuk and Rosenberg (1988) found that 55 homeless preschool children scored significantly higher ($M = 5.6$) on the Simmons Behavior Checklist (Reinherz & Gracey, 1982) than did both a sample of 17 "normal" children, the homeless children had poorer attention, more trouble sleeping, delayed speech, and were more likely to exhibit aggressive behaviors, shyness, and withdrawal. The only area in which homeless children scored significantly lower than both comparison groups was in being less afraid of new things. Note that a subsequent analysis compared a subgroup of this sample ($n = 21$) with 33 permanently housed poor children and found no significant differences on any of the aforementioned measures (Bassuk & Rosenberg, 1990).

A study of 83 families sheltered in New York City (Citizen's Committee for Children, 1988) revealed that 66% of parents had observed adverse behavioral changes in their children since becoming homeless. Among the most frequent changes were increased acting out, fighting, restlessness, depression, and moodiness. Molnar, Rath, and Klein (1991) cited parent reports of withdrawal, exaggerated fears, disobedience, and destructiveness.

In sum, several studies show that homeless children are more likely than are housed poor children or normative groups to have clinical levels of depression, anxiety, or behavior problems. Research findings, however, have not been entirely consistent. Possible explanations include small sample sizes and the lack of adequate comparison groups in some studies. In addition, several researchers suggest that other methodological issues need to be considered. For example, Cohen and Schwab-Stone (1990) noted the inadequacy of available instruments to assess the mental health of children generally, and additional limitations in making valid assessments of homeless children (e.g., lack of appropriate places to carry out interviews, families' greater involvement in problems connected to daily living than to the interview). The fact that families are often in an acutely stressful situation may temporarily inflate children's scores on measures of depression and anxiety. Molnar and Rubin (1991) also discussed how the chaotic life arrangements of homeless families are not conducive to lengthy interviews. They also address the limitations of assessment instruments in ethnic minority groups and suggest the use of multiple informants.

Finally, the fact that both homeless and poor housed children perform poorly, relative to normative samples, in more recent studies also implicates poverty, as well as specific conditions of homelessness, in the development of psychological problems. In fact, many of the risk factors previously discussed also prevail in extremely poor families. Homeless families, however, are even more likely to be deprived of some essential requirements for child rearing. These include adequate health care, nutrition, housing, employment, and status for parenthood (Bronfenbrenner, 1986).

In addition, the emergency shelter needs of families frequently go unmet. For example, 21 of 27 cities turn away homeless families because of a lack of resources (U.S. Conference of Mayors, 1989). Birmingham, Alabama, for example, turns away 25% of the families requesting emergency shelter each day (National Coalition for the Homeless, 1989a). In other cases in which shelter is available, fathers and older boys are separated from their families. Overall, 17 of the cities reported being unable to keep homeless families intact in emergency shelters.

For families who manage to obtain emergency shelter, other obstacles prevail. Unsafe, chaotic, unpredictable shelter placements are not conducive to normal psychological development. Rafferty and Rollins (1989) found that families in New York City shelters were routinely bounced from one facility to another, compounding stress for children already struggling to master their environments. According to Neiman (1988), the resiliency literature indicates that children are not particularly at risk from any single stressor, but when two stressors occur together, the risk quadruples. Thus, she argued, if even a portion of the multiple stressors that plague homeless families were substantially alleviated, the psychological risk for children would be greatly reduced.

Finally, homeless parents often encounter difficulties balancing their own physical, social, and personal needs and those of their children. The loss of control over their environment and their lives place them at increased risk for learned helplessness and depression. Drawing on Maslow's hierarchy of needs, Eddowes and Hranitz (1989) suggested that deprivation of basic needs and lack of security often lead to mistrust, apathy, and despair in homeless parents. Maternal depression, in turn, places children at increased risk for depressive disorders, behavior problems, anxiety, attention problems, insecure attachment, and social incompetence (cf. Dodge, 1990; Rutter, 1990).

EDUCATIONAL UNDERACHIEVEMENT

Little research has focused on the educational achievement of homeless children. What has been undertaken, however, indicates that homeless children score poorly on standardized reading and mathematics tests and are often required to repeat a grade.

Rafferty and Rollins (1989) examined the educational records of the entire population of 9,659 homeless school-age children identified by the New York City Board of Education between September 1987 and May 1988. Of the 3,805 homeless children in Grades 3 through 10 who took the Degrees of Reading Power test in the spring of 1988, 42% scored at or above grade level, compared with 68% citywide. Although these findings may reflect effects of poverty as well as homelessness, findings in the three school districts that served the greatest numbers of homeless children (45% of the total) were consistent. The percentages of homeless children scoring at or above grade level were 36%, 40%, and 41%, compared with 57%, 74%, and 68% for all children. Furthermore, of the 73 schools composing these three school districts, only 1 school had a lower proportion of students reading at or above grade level than did the overall proportion for homeless children attending schools in that district.

Results were similar for the Metropolitan Achievement Test in mathematics, which 4,203 homeless children in Grades 2 through 8 took in the spring of 1988. Homeless students were less than half as likely to score at or above grade level as were all students both citywide (28% vs. 57%, respectively) and in the three districts with the most homeless children (22%, 24%, and 23% vs. 48%, 70%, and 60%, respectively).

Several other studies have found that homeless children are more likely than are housed poor children to have repeated grades (Masten, 1990: 38% vs. 24%, respectively; Wood et al., 1989: 30% vs. 18%, respectively) or to be currently repeating a grade (Rafferty & Rollins, 1989: 15% vs. 7%, respectively). Other studies without comparison groups also found high rates of grade retention (Dumpson & Dinkins, 1987: 50%; Maza & Hall, 1988: 30%). In contrast, Rescorla et al. (1991) found similar retention rates among homeless and housed children (35% vs. 32%, respectively). The excessive rate of holdovers among homeless children will, no doubt, have longterm repercussions. Students who are overage for their grade are more likely than are others to drop out of school, get into trouble with the law, learn less the following year, and develop negative self-concepts (Hess, 1987).

Several factors appear to mediate the educational underachievement of homeless children. These include poor school attendance, lack of adequate educational services, inadequate shelter conditions, and shelter instability.

Government estimates of the number of homeless school-aged children who do not regularly attend school range from 15% (U.S. General Accounting Office, 1989) to 30% (U.S. Department of Education, 1989). In contrast, the National Coalition for the Homeless (1987a) estimated that 57% of homeless school-aged children do not regularly attend school. Two additional studies have evaluated the school attendance of homeless children. Homeless students in Los Angeles (Wood et al., 1989) missed more days in the prior three months than did poor housed children (8–9 vs. 5–6, respectively), and were more likely to have missed more than one week of school (42% vs. 22%, respectively). For housed children, the primary reason for absence was illness; for homeless children, it was family transience. In a New York City study of 6,142 homeless students (Rafferty & Rollins, 1989), homeless high school students had the poorest rate of attendance (51% vs. 84% citywide), followed by junior high school students (64% vs. 86% citywide) and children in elementary schools (74% vs. 89% citywide).

Many homeless children experience difficulty obtaining and maintaining access to a free public education. Major barriers include residency requirements, guardianship requirements, special education requirements, inability to obtain school records, transportation problems, lack of clothing and supplies, inadequate health care services, and lack of day care for teenage parents (Center for Law and Education, 1987; National Coalition for the Homeless, 1987a; Rafferty, 1991; U.S. Department of Education, 1990).

School is especially crucial for homeless children because it may instill a sense of stability that they otherwise lack (National Coalition for the Homeless, 1987a). Given the disruptions associated with homelessness and the excessive number of school transfers, homeless children may also need remedial educational services to address academic deficits, preschool enrichment services to prevent academic failure, psychological support services to respond to emotional problems, and greater sensitivity from school personnel who often stigmatize them (cf. Eddowes & Hranitz, 1989; Gewirtzman & Fodor, 1987; Horowitz, Springer, & Kose, 1988; National Association of State Coordinators for the Education of Homeless Children and Youth, 1990). Despite these needs, homeless children are likely to lose educational services with the onset of homelessness. Of 97 children who were receiving remedial assistance, bilingual services, or gifted and talented programs in New York City prior to their loss of permanent housing, only 54% continued to receive them while they were homeless (Rafferty & Rollins, 1989).

Environmental conditions within emergency shelters are hardly conducive to education. In addition, families entering the emergency shelter system are often placed in temporary facilities without consideration of the educational needs of the children or the impact of their being moved to unfamiliar and often distant communities. For example, 71% of 277 homeless families interviewed by Rafferty and Rollins (1989) were in temporary shelter facilities in a different borough than that of their last permanent home. Bouncing families from one facility to another compounded the disruptions in their lives and in their children's schooling. Overall, 66% of families had been in at least two shelters, 29% in at least four, and 10% in seven or more. The resulting school transitions significantly hindered children's continuity of education and disrupted their social relationships with classmates and friends.

CONCLUSION AND SOCIAL POLICY IMPLICATIONS

Homeless children confront abject poverty and experience a constellation of risks that have a devastating impact on their well-being. The research reviewed here links homelessness among children to hunger and poor nutrition, health problems and lack of health and mental health care, developmental delays, psychological problems, and academic underachievement. These consequences of homelessness often compound one another as well. When young children's nutritional needs are not met, growth is affected (Jahiel, 1987), physical health deteriorates (Acker, Fierman, & Dreyer, 1987), mental health is adversely affected (Winick, 1985), behavioral problems increase (Lazoff, 1989), the ability to concentrate is compromised (Jahiel, 1987), and academic performance suffers (Galler, 1984).

The paucity of prenatal care available to homeless women places unborn homeless children at risk of low birth weight (Buescher et al., 1988), subsequent health problems and chronic diseases (Hack, Caron, Rivers, & Fanaroff, 1983), cognitive and developmental problems (Resnick, Armstrong, & Carter, 1988), and academic problems (Russell & Williams, 1988). Delays in language development, motor skills, cognitive ability, and personal and social development place children at risk for academic failure (Molnar, 1988). Health problems are associated with psychological problems, classroom performance and dropout rates (Needleman, Gunnoe, & Leviton, 1979; Needleman, Schell, Bellinger, Leviton, & Allred, 1990). Anxiety, depression, and behavioral problems engendered by destructive psychological problems, classroom performance and dropout rates (Needleman, Gunnoe, & Leviton, 1979; Needleman, Schell, Bellinger, Leviton, & Allred, 1990). Anxiety, depression, and behavioral problems engendered by destructive psychological environments interfere with one's capacity to learn (Jahiel, 1987). Thus, the risks we have identified may snowball to seriously compromise the future of homeless children.

Any list of solutions to homelessness must begin with decent, permanent, and affordable housing (National Alliance to End Homelessness, 1988; National

Coalition for the Homeless, 1987b; Partnership for the Homeless, 1989; U.S. Conference of Mayors, 1988). National policy must focus both on rehousing those who are currently homeless and on preventing additional homelessness (National Coalition for the Homeless, 1989b). However, although affordable permanent housing is the fundamental issue of homelessness, it is not the sole need of homeless families with children. The research we have surveyed suggests that homeless families also have special needs in the areas of adequate shelter facilities, stability, and adequate services without barriers to access.

At the very least, homeless children and their families need access to safe, clean emergency shelters for transitional use while they are without homes. Shelters must provide privacy so that children are not exposed to communicable disease, control over light and noise so that children can sleep and do homework, and enough space so that young children can explore their environments. Shelters must provide nutritious meals, or they must have refrigeration and cooking facilities so that families can prepare nutritious meals.

Emergency shelter placements must be designed to create stability, not chaos, in children's lives. Families and their children should not be required to leave shelters during the day or to move from shelter to shelter (or back to the street) because of administrative convenience or arbitrary limits on length of stay. Families must be accommodated as families and not be forced to separate in order to obtain shelter. To minimize disruptions in schools and services, shelters should be in the neighborhoods from which families came or in the neighborhoods in which they will be housed permanently.

In the realm of services, homeless families need adequate health care, including prenatal, mental health, pediatric, and preventive care, and they need continuity of care. Children need day care and early intervention programs (to prevent the onset of developmental delays), after-school programs, and the same or better standard of public education received by other children. Children should continue to receive the bilingual, special education, or gifted and talented services they obtained previously. They should have the option of continuing at the schools they attended before becoming homeless. By maintaining stability for children and offering new services to help them cope with the trauma of homelessness, schools can play an important role in tertiary prevention and in preventing residual damage from homelessness.

Our poorest families with children, inside or outside of shelter, also need adequate levels of benefits to meet basic needs—a public assistance grant at least at the federal poverty level, food stamps, the WIC program—and the assurance of receiving, without interruption, benefits to which they are entitled. More adequate and continuous benefits, along with an increase in the supply of affordable housing, would prevent many families from ever becoming homeless.

Recent studies have emphasized similarities, rather than differences, between homeless and poor housed children on measures of development and psychological problems. Both groups are at high risk. Even in health and education, where homeless children clearly fare worse than do their housed peers, the profile of both groups is grim. These findings indicate the need for a public policy agenda that addresses poverty among children, in addition to providing housing, stability, and services for those who are homeless.

In conclusion, an entire generation of children faces truly unacceptable risks that jeopardize their future potential. In the long run, the monetary costs of neglecting children's needs are likely to substantially exceed the costs of combating poverty and homelessness. The human costs will be much more tragic. Our cities and our nation must develop an appropriate and effective response.

REFERENCES

Achlenbach, T.M., & Edelbrock, C. S. (1981). Behavioral problems and competencies reported by parents of normal and disturbed children aged four through sixteen. *Monograph of the Society for Research in Child Development, 46,* 1–82.

Achenbach, T. M., & Edelbrock, C. S. (1983). *Manual for the Child Behavior Checklist and Revised Child Behavior Profile.* Burlington, VT: University of Vermont, Department of Psychiatry.

Acker, P. J., Fierman, A. H., & Dreyer, B. P. (1987). An assessment of parameters of health care and nutrition in homeless children. *American Journal of Diseases of Children, 141,* 388.

Alperstein, G., & Arnstein, E. (1988). Homeless children—A challenge for pediatricians. *Pediatric Clinics of North America, 35,* 1413–1425.

Alperstein, G., Rappaport, C., & Flanigan, J. M. (1988). Health problems of homeless children in New York City. *American Journal of Public Health, 78,* 1232–1233.

Angel, R., & Worobey, J. (1988). Single motherhood and children's health. *Journal of Health and Social Behavior, 29,* 38–52.

Bassuk, E. L., and Rosenberg, L. (1988). Why does family homelessness occur? A case-control study. *American Journal of Public Health, 78,* 783–788.

Bassuk, E. L., & Rosenberg, L. (1990). Psychosocial characteristics of homeless children and children with homes. *Pediatrics, 85,* 257–261.

Bassuk, E. L., & Rubin, L. (1987). Homeless children: A neglected population. *American Journal of Orthopsychiatry, 57,* 279–286.

Bassuk, E. L., Rubin, L., & Lauriat, A. (1986). Characteristics of sheltered homeless families. *American Journal of Public Health, 76,* 1097–1101.

Beery, K. E. (1989). *The Developmental Test of Visual Motor Integration.* Cleveland, OH: Modern Curriculum Press.

Berezin, J. (1988). *Promises to keep: Child care for New York City's homeless children.* New York: Child Care.

Bernstein, A. B., Alperstein, G., & Fierman, A. H. (1988, November). *Health care of home-*

less children. Paper presented at the meeting of the American Public Health Association, Chicago.

Bronfenbrenner, U. (1986). Ecology of the family as a context for human development: Research perspectives. *Development Psychology, 22,* 723–742.

Buescher, P. A., Meis, P. J., Ernest, J. M., Moore, M. L., Michielutte, R., & Sharp, P. (1988). A comparison of women in and out of a prematurity prevention project in a North Carolina perinatal care region. *American Journal of Public Health, 78,* 264–267.

Center for Law and Education (1987). Homelessness: A barrier to education for thousands of children. *Newsnotes, 38,* 1–3.

Chavkin, W., Kristal, A., Seabron, C., & Guigli, P. E. (1987). Reproductive experience of women living in hotels for the homeless in New York City. *New York State Journal of Medicine, 87,* 10–13.

Citizens Committee for Children (1988). *Children in storage: Families in New York City's barracks-style shelters*. New York: Author.

Cohen, P., & Schwab-Stone, M. (1990). Assessing mental health status among children who are homeless. In J. Morrissey & D. Dennis (Eds.), *Proceedings of a NIMH sponsored conference* (pp. 78–87). Rockville, MD: National Institute of Mental Health, Office of Programs for the Homeless Mentally Ill.

Community Food Resource Center (1989). *Who are New York City's hungry?* New York: Author.

Consortium for Longitudinal Studies. (1983). *As the twig is bent: Lasting effects of preschool programs*. Hillsdale, NJ: Erlbaum.

Dehavenon, A. L., & Benker, K. (1989). *The tyranny of indifference: A study of hunger, homelessness, poor health and family dismemberment in 818 New York City households with children in 1988–1989*. New York: East Harlem Interfaith Welfare Committee.

Dodge, K. (1990). Developmental psychopathology in children of depressed mothers. *Developmental Psychology, 26,* 3–6.

Dumpson, J. R., & Dinkin, D. N. (1987). *A shelter is not a home: Report of the Manhattan borough president's task force on housing for homeless families*. New York: Author.

Dunn, L., & Dunn, L. (1981). *Peabody Picture Vocabulary Test—Revised manual*. CIrcle Pines, MN: American Guidance Service.

Eddowes, A., & Hranitz, J. (1989). Childhood education: Infancy through early adolescence. *Journal of the Association for Childhood Education International, 65,* 197–200.

Frankenburg, W. K., Goldstein, A., & Camp, P. (1971). The revised Denver Development Screening Test: Its accuracy as a screening instrument. *Journal of Pediatrics, 79,* 988–995.

Galler, J. R. (Ed.). (1984). Human nutrition: A comprehensive treatise. *Nutrition and behavior*. New York: Plenum Press.

Gewirtzman, R., & Fodor, I. (1987). The homeless child at school: From welfare hotel to classroom. *Child Welfare, 66,* 237–245.

Grant, R. (1989). *Assessing the damage: The impact of shelter experience on homeless young children*. New York: Association to Benefit Children.

Gross, T., & Rosenberg, M. (1987). Shelters for battered women and their children: An underrecognized source of communicable disease transmission. *American Journal of Public Health, 77,* 1198–1201.

Hack, M., Caron, B., Rivers, A., & Fanaroff, A. (1983). The very low birth weight infant: The broader spectrum of morbidity during infancy and early childhood. *Developmental and Behavioral Pediatrics, 4,* 243–249.

Harris, D. B. (1963). *Children's drawings as measures of intellectual maturity.* New York: Harcourt, Brace & World.

Haskins, R. (1989). Beyond metaphor: The efficacy of early childhood education. *American Psychologist, 44,* 274–282.

Hess, G. A. (1987). *Schools for early failure: The elementary years and dropout rates in Chicago.* Chicago: Chicago Panel on Public School Finances.

Horowitz, S., Springer, C., & Kose, G. (1988). Stress in hotel children: The effects of homelessness on attitudes toward school. *Children's Environments Quarterly, 5,* 34–36.

Howes, C. (1988). Relations between early child care and schooling. *Developmental Psychology, 24,* 53–57.

Howes, C., & Stewart, P. (1987). Child's play with adults, peers, and toys. *Developmental Psychology, 23,* 423–430.

Jahiel, R. I. (1987). The situation of homelessness. In R. D. Bingham, R. E. Green, & S. E. White (Eds.), *The homeless in contemporary society* (pp. 99–118). Newbury Park, CA: Sage.

Jensen, J. A., & Armstrong, R. J. (1985). *Slosson Intelligence Test (SIT) for Children and Adults: Expanded norms, tables, application, and development.* East Aurora, NY: Slosson Educational Publications.

Knickman, J. R., & Weitzman, B. C. (1989). *Forecasting models to target families at high risk of homelessness* (Final report: Vol. 3). New York: New York University Health Research Program.

Kovacs, M. (1983). *The Children's Depression Inventory: A self-rated depression scale for school age youngsters.* Pittsburgh, PA: University of Pittsburgh, School of Medicine.

Kozol, J. (1988). *Rachel and her children: Homeless families in America.* New York: Crown.

Lazoff, B. (1989). Nutrition and behavior. *American Psychologist, 44,* 231–236.

Masten, A. S. (1990, August). *Homeless children: Risk, trauma and adjustment.* Paper presented at the 98th Annual Convention of the American Psychological Association, Boston.

Maza, P. L., & Hall, J. A. (1988). *Homeless children and their families: A preliminary study.* Washington, DC: Child Welfare League of America.

Meisels, S. J., & Wiske, M. S. (1988). *Early Screening Inventory: Test and manual (2nd ed.).* New York: Teachers College Press.

Miller, D. S., & Lin, E. H. B. (1988). Children in sheltered homeless families: Reported health status and use of health services. *Pediatrics, 81,* 668–673.

Molnar, J. (1988). *Home is where the heart is: The crisis of homeless children and families in New York City.* New York: Bank Street College of Education.

Molnar, J., & Rath, W. (1990, August). *Beginning at the beginning: Public policy and home-*

less children. Paper presented at the 98th Annual Convention of the American Psychological Association, Boston.

Molnar, J., Rath, W., & Klein, T. (1991). Constantly compromised: The impact of homelessness on children. *Journal of Social Issues, 46*, 109–124.

Molnar, J., & Rubin, D. H. (1991, March). *The impact of homelessness on children: Review of prior studies and implications for future research*. Paper presented at the NIMH/NIAAA research conferences organized by the Better Homes Foundation, Cambridge, MA.

National Alliance to End Homelessness. (1988). *Housing and Homelessness*. Washington, DC: Author.

National Association of State Coordinators for the Education of Homeless Children and Youth. (1990). *Position document on the re-authorization of Subtitle VII-B of the Stewart B. McKinney Homeless Assistance Act*. Austin, TX: State Department of Education.

National Coalition for the Homeless. (1987a). *Broken lives: Denial of education to homeless children*. Washington, DC: Author.

National Coalition for the Homeless. (1987b). *Homelessness in the United States: Background and federal response. A briefing paper for presidential candidates*. Washington, DC: Author.

National Coalition for the Homeless. (1988). *Over the edge: Homeless famliies and the welfare system*. Washington, DC: Author.

National Coalition for the Homeless. (1989a). *American nightmare: A decade of homelessness in the United States*. Washington, DC: Author.

National Coalition for the Homeless. (1989b). *Unfinished business: The Stewart B. McKinney Homeless Assistance Act after two years*. Washington, DC: Author.

Needleman, H. L., Gunnoe, C., & Leviton, A. (1979). Deficits in psychological and classroom performance of children with elevated dentine lead levels. *The New England Journal of Medicine, 300*, 689–695.

Needleman, H. L., Schell, A., Bellinger, D., Leviton, A., & Allred, E. N. (1990). The long-term effects of exposure to low doses of lead in childhood: an 11-year follow-up report. *The New England Journal of Medicine, 322*, 83–88.

Neiman, L. (1988). A critical review of resiliency literature and its relevance to homeless children. *Children's Environments Quarterly, 5*(1), 17–25.

Newacheck, P. W., & Starfield, B. (1988). Morbidity and use of ambulatory care services among poor and non-poor children. *American Journal of Public Health, 78*, 927–933.

New York City Department of Health. (1986). *Diarrhea in the family congregate shelters of New York City* (Draft No. 5). Unpublished manuscript, New York City Department of Health.

New York State Department of Health. (1988). *WIC state plan*. New York: Author.

Paone, D., & Kay, K. (1988, November). *Immunization status of homeless preschoolers*. Paper presented at the meeting of the American Public Health Association, Boston.

Partnership for the Homeless. (1989). *Moving forward: A national agenda to address homelessness in 1990 and beyond*. New York: Author.

Phillips, D. A., McCartney, K., & Scarr, S. (1987). Child care quality and children's social development. *Developmental Psychology, 23*, 537–543.

Rafferty, Y. (1991). *Homeless children in New York City: Barriers to academic achievement and innovative strategies for the delivery of educational services.* Long Island City, NY: Advocates for Children.

Rafferty, Y., & Rollins, N. (1989). *Learning in limbo: The educational deprivation of homeless children.* New York: Advocates for Children (ERIC Document Reproduction No. ED 312 363).

Redlener, I. (1989, October 4). *Unacceptable losses: The consequences of failing America's homeless children* (Testimony presented before the U.S. Senate Committee on Labor and Human Resources Subcommittee on Children, Family, Drugs and Alcoholism). Washington, DC: U.S. Government Printing Office.

Reinherz, H., & Gracey, C. A. (1982). *The Simmons Behavior Checklist Technical information.* Boston: Simmons School of Social Work.

Rescorla, L., Parker, R., & Stolley, P. (1991). Ability, achievement, and adjustment in homeless children. *American Journal of Orthopsychiatry, 61,* 210–220.

Resnick, M. B., Armstrong, S., & Carter, R. (1988). Developmental intervention program for high-risk premature infants: Effects on development and parent-infant interactions. *Developmental and Behavioral Pediatrics, 9*(1), 73–78.

Reynolds, C. R., & Richmond, B. O. (1985). *Revised Children's Manifest Anxiety Scale manual.* Los Angeles: Western Psychological Services.

Roth, L., & Fox, E. R. (1988, November). *Children of homeless families. Health status and access to health care.* Paper presented at the meeting of the American Public Health Association, Boston.

Russell, S., & Williams, E. (1988). Homeless handicapped children: A special education perspective. *Children's Environments Quarterly, 5*(1), 3–7.

Rutter, M. (1990). Commentary: Some focus and process considerations regarding effects of parental depression on children. *Developmental Psychology, 26,* 60–67.

Scarr, S., & Weinberg, R. (1986). The early childhood enterprise: Care and education for the young. *American Psychologist, 41,* 1140–1146.

Simpson, J., Kilduff, M., & Blewett, C. D. (1984). *Struggling to survive in a welfare hotel.* New York: Community Service Society.

Thorndike, R. L., Hagen, E. P., & Sattler, J. M. (1986). *Stanford Binet Intelligence Scale* (4th ed). Chicago: Riverside Publishing.

U.S. Conference of Mayors. (1987). *The continuing growth of hunger, homelessness and poverty in America's cities: 1987, A 26-city survey.* Washington, DC: Author.

U.S. Conference of Mayors. (1988). *A status report on the Stewart B. McKinney Homeless Assistance Act of 1987.* Washington, DC: Author.

U.S. Conference of Mayors. (1989). *A status report on hunger and homelessness in America's cities—A 27-city survey.* Washington, DC: Author.

U.S. Department of Education. (1989, February 15). *Report to Congress on state interim reports on the education of homeless children.* Washington, DC: Author.

U.S. Department of Education. (1990, March 29). *Report to Congress on state interim reports on the education of homeless children.* Washington, DC: Author.

U.S. General Accounting Office. (1989). *Children and youths: Report to congressional committees*. Washington, DC: Author.

U.S. House of Representatives Select Committee on Hunger. (1987). *Hunger among the homeless: A survey of 140 shelters, food stamp participants and homelessness*. Washington, DC: U.S. Government Printing Office.

Vanderbourg, K., & Christofides, A. (1986, June). *Children in need: The child care needs of homeless families in temporary shelter in New York City* (Report prepared for Ruth W. Messinger, New York City Council member, 4th District). (Available from office of the President of the Borough of Manhattan, Municipal Building, New York, NY 10007).

Wagner, J., & Menke, E. (1990). *The mental health of homeless children*. Paper presented at the meeting of the American Public Health Association, New York City.

Whitman, B. (1987, February 24). *The crisis in homelessness: Effects on children and families* (Testimony presented before the U.S. House of Representatives Select Committee on Children, Youth, and Families). Washington, DC: U. S. Government Printing Office.

Whitman, B., Accardo, P., Boyert, M., & Kendagor, R. (1990). Homelessness and cognitive performance in children: A possible link. *Social Work, 35,* 516–519.

Winick, M. (1985). Nutritional and vitamin deficiency states. In P. Brickner, L. Scharer, B. Conanan, A. Elvy, & M. Savarese (Eds.), *Health care of homeless people* (pp. 103–108). New York: Springer.

Wood, D., Hayashi, T., Schlossman, S., & Valdez, R. B. (1989). *Over the brink: Homeless families in Los Angeles*. Sacramento, CA: State Assembly Office of Research, Box 942849.

Wood, D., Valdez, R. B., Hayashi, T., & Shen, A. (1990a). The health of homeless children: A comparison study. *Pediatrics, 86,* 858–866.

Wood, D., Valdez, R. B., Hayashi, T., & Shen, A. (1990b). Homeless and housed families in Los Angeles: A study comparing demographic, economic and family function characteristics. *American Journal of Public Health, 80,* 1049–1052.

Wright, J. (1987, February 24). *The crisis in homelessness: Effects on children and families* (Testimony presented before the U.S. House of Representatives Select Committee on Children, Youth, and Families, pp. 73–85). Washington, DC: U.S. Government Printing Office.

Wright, J. (1990). Homelessness is not healthy for children and other living things. *Child and Youth Services, 14*(1), 65–88.

Wright, J. (1991). Poverty, homelessness, health, nutrition, and children. In J. H. Kryder-Coe, L. M. Salamon, & J. M. Molnar (Eds.), *Homeless children and youth: A new American dilemma* (pp. 71–104). New Brunswick, NJ: Transaction.

Yale Child Study Center. (1986). *Cubes test*. Unpublished manuscript. New Haven, CT: Author.

29

Children's Capacity to Consent to Participation in Psychological Research: Empirical Findings

Rona Abramovitch, Jonathan L. Freedman, Kirby Thoden, and Crystal Nikolich

University of Toronto, Ontario

This is a series of studies that attempted to obtain some systematic data on the capacity of children between the ages of 5 and 12 to consent to psychological research. Most of the children understood all or most of what they were asked to do in a psychology study, but few children below the age of 12 fully understood or believed that their performance would be confidential. Similarly, most children appeared to know that they could end their participation in the study, but younger children were not clear on the details of how to accomplish this, and many of all ages believed that there would be some negative consequences if they asked to stop. Moreover, obtaining prior permission from their parents, while providing protection for the children, appeared to introduce additional pressure on them to agree to participate in the research and to continue once they had agreed. It is concluded that in general children of these ages do have the capacity to meaningfully assent to participation in research, but that there are substantial problems in guaranteeing that they are able to make this decision freely.

Over the past few decades, psychologists have become increasingly concerned about the ethics of research with human subjects. Although there are, of course, many ethical issues involved, it is generally agreed that one basic requirement of

Reprinted with permission from *Child Development*, 1991, Vol. 62, 1100–1109. Copyright © 1991 by The Society for Research in Child Development, Inc.

Studies 1 and 3 were conducted by Kirby Thoden and Crystal Nikolich as undergraduate research projects. The authors would like to thank Caroline Brown, Geoffry Haddock, Viviane Paquin, and Craig Steverango for their help with Studies 2 and 4.

virtually all research is that the subjects freely give fully informed consent. This poses many problems, even with adults, but it is especially difficult when the research involves children (see Ferguson, 1978, for a discussion of some of the issues). Indeed, the term "consent" is not generally considered appropriate for minors, so their agreement to participate is now generally referred to as "assent" (or "dissent" if they refuse). The usual procedure to protect the rights of the children is to obtain the permission of the children's parents or legal guardians. In addition, as noted by the APA's committee for the protection of human participants in research (1982), children should be given the opportunity to assent or dissent if they are capable of making "some reasonable judgment concerning the nature of the research and of participation in it" (p. 34). Thus the general rule is that even if substitute consent has been given, the investigator is under some obligation to obtain the child's agreement as well.

This is a sound principle, but acting on its presents a number of difficulties. One basic problem is how to decide if children are competent to assent to participation in research. Roth, Meisel, and Lidz (1977), Weithorn and Campbell (1982), and others have described several possible criteria that have been used in treatment situations. These include simply the ability to make a choice between treatment alternatives, the ability to make a "reasonable" choice, the ability to give rational reasons for the choice, and the ability to understand both the facts and the implications of those facts. These standards represent a considerable range of stringency, and it is not clear which is most appropriate for agreeing to participate in research. Since psychological research is not usually for the benefit of the particular child, it would seem that relatively stringent criteria should be used. In any case, our experience has been that very few children have any difficulty making a choice regarding being in a research study, and that typically they assent to the research. Therefore, our focus has been on the extent to which the children know what they have been asked to do, because it would seem that their assent means little unless they have this knowledge. In addition, it seems important that the children understand the rules under which they would be participating, including confidentiality and the freedom to withdraw. Finally, to give their assent freely, the children must be under no undue pressure to agree to participate.

A great deal of work has dealt with the cognitive and moral development of children. This research provides some general information on their capacities, but as Keith-Spiegel (1983) notes, "child development research has provided little information about children's capacity to consent" (p. 204). In this same article, Keith-Spiegel maintains that there is some evidence that even very young children can correctly recall descriptions of studies in which they are asked to participate. Similarly, Stanley, Sieber, and Melton (1987) suggest that psychologists often underestimate children's ability to consent to research. They base this belief on a small body of research indicating that children are capable of expressing preferences and making decisions in the context of medical treatment (Melton, 1984; Melton, Koocher, & Saks, 1983; Weithorn & Campbell, 1982) and on one study (Lewis, Lewis, & Ifekwunigue, 1978) in which children appeared to understand the implications of participating in an influenza vaccine trial.

Both Keith-Spiegel (1983) and Stanley et al. (1987) note the paucity of research directly relevant to the issue of the ability of children to consent to psychological research. The present paper describes a series of studies that attempt to obtain such data. The research focused on the following questions: Do children understand what they will be doing? Do children understand the rules of the study, especially confidentiality and their freedom to withdraw? Do children feel free to refuse, and are they under undue pressure to agree? In addition, we explored the extent to which children noticed what we considered to be ethical problems in hypothetical research studies.

METHOD

Overview

Conducting research on these issues raises some difficult ethical problems of its own. The basic paradigm for the first three studies was to ask children to consent to participate in a research study and then to ask them about their understanding of the study and their reactions to it. However, for ethical reasons we felt that it was essential that once a study had been described, those children who were willing should, in fact, be in the study and that the study itself should be a legitimate piece of research, not one constructed for the sole purpose of investigating consent. Therefore, with the exception of Study 4, our investigations were "piggy-backed" onto developmental studies that were already being conducted. In other words, studies (which we shall term the "basic" studies) were run exactly as they would have been in terms of the instructions about the study and the procedures for obtaining the children's assent to participate. The only difference was that after an experimenter described a study to a child and/or after the child completed a study, we stepped in and asked a number of questions to determine the child's understanding of the situation. In all instances, the children were asked separately if they were willing to participate in the consent study. All agreed.

All of the children who served as subjects lived in or around Mississauga. Ontario, in Canada. This is a generally affluent suburban area, and information from previous studies indicates that most of the children come from middle- to upper-class homes. In all a total of 163 children, ranging in age from 5 to 12, participated. In each of the studies there was an approximately equal number of boys and girls. There were no sex differences for any of the issues that we investigated, and therefore the results for boys and girls will not be presented separately.

Study 1

Subjects. The subjects were 19 7-year-olds and 23 11-year-olds. They were recruited through the infant studies subject pool at Erindale College, which maintains a list of a large number of children in the area. The parents were contacted by phone and asked for permission to have their children participate in the research. The "basic" study was described in detail, as was the additional "consent" part of the study. If the parents agreed, they brought their children to Erindale College, where the studies were conducted.

Procedure. The procedure for the basic study consisted of asking the children to answer age-appropriate arithmetic questions, to give the definitions for words having to do with money, and to answer a question about stories in which children either did or did not get paid for doing something. The rationale for the study was to look at the relation between math and money skills.

The study was described to the children, who were told that their participation was entirely voluntary, that they could stop at any time, that in order to stop they simply had to tell the experimenter, and that their results would be kept confidential. All of this was put into very simple language in order to maximize understanding. For example, confidentiality was described by the experimenter saying that she would not tell anyone about what the child did except other people who were working with her.

After the experimenter had described the study to the children and received their consent, she told them that she had to collect the materials for the study and that a second person would be coming in to ask them some questions. The first experimenter left and a second experimenter came into the room and asked the children if they would be willing to answer some questions. She told them that they could stop if they wanted and did not have to answer all of the questions.

Once the children had agreed, they were asked the following questions: "What is going to happen to you in the study?" "Why is this study being done?" "What happens if you want to stop being in the study?" "How can you stop being in the study?" and "Who will find out what you did in the study?" After these questions, the first experimenter returned and the children participated in the study that had been described to them. When that study was completed, the second experimenter came back once more and asked only whether anything had happened in the study that they had not expected.

Study 2

Subjects. The subjects were 21 children in each of three age groups: 5–6, 7–8, and 9–10. They came from the same pool and were recruited in the same way as for Study 1.

Procedure. In the basic procedure, the children were asked to eat and then to indicate their liking of different foods, some of which were familiar and some of which were novel. The rationale for the study was to look at children's liking of various foods.

The procedure for the consent part of the study was the same as for Study 1, with several additions. First, to probe the children's understanding of confidentiality, they were asked specifically: "Will your mother find out what you did in the study?" Second, after the children had participated in the basic study, they were given descriptions of 14 hypothetical studies (see below) and were asked if they would be willing to participate in them. Each child was given half of the total set of hypothetical studies. Finally, the children were asked whether it would be all right for them to participate in a study (not specified) if they were willing but their parents did not think they should and vice versa. The exact questions were: "Should you be in a study if you didn't like it and your mother did?" and "Should you be in a study if you liked it and your mother didn't?"

Study 3

Subjects. The subjects were 32 8–9-year-olds and 26 10–11-year-olds. They were recruited in the same way as for Studies 1 and 2.

Procedure. This study was added to three different basic studies. Two involved memory and the other involved questions about the children's understanding of economic and monetary concepts. In Study 3, the consent part of the study was done only after the children had completed their participation in the basic studies. As in the previous studies, the children were asked whether anything had happened that they did not expect. Then the children were asked the following questions designed to probe their understanding of the rules of voluntary participation: "How could you have stopped being in the study?" "What would [the first name of the first experimenter] have done or said if you wanted to stop being in the study?" "Do you think [name of experimenter] would have been mad if you wanted to stop being in the study?" and "Do you think your mother would have been mad if you wanted to stop being in the study?"

In addition, they were asked a series of questions about the confidentiality of their performance. The basic question was the same as in Studies 1 and 2: "Who do you think will find out about how you did in the study?" This was followed by various probes that depended on their previous answers. If mother was not mentioned, they were asked whether their mother would know what they did. If they replied that she would, they were asked: "Who will tell her?" If they said that they would, they were asked: "If you didn't tell her, then who would?"

Study 4

Subjects. The subjects were recruited through a summer program conducted by the local school board. This program is designed for gifted children, who participate in a number of activities at Erindale College. As usual, their parents were asked for permission for their children to participate in this study. There were 27 of these gifted children in Study 4 (10 10-year-olds, 7 11-year-olds, and 10 12-year-olds).

Procedure. Study 4 was not added to another experiment. Rather, it consisted entirely of questioning the children about various issues dealing with consent and the ethics of research. First the children were given (one at a time) all of the hypothetical studies used in Study 2 and asked if there were problems with them. Then, as in Study 3, they were questioned about their understanding of confidentiality and the voluntary nature of their participation. Finally, as in Study 2, they were asked whether it was all right to participate in a study if their mother said no and they were willing and vice versa.

Materials for Hypothetical Studies

We composed descriptions of 12 hypothetical studies, each of which incorporated an ethical problem plus two control studies that did not include ethical problems. Each ethical problem was represented in two of the hypothetical studies. The six kinds of problems were: being watched without being told (while playing games, while interacting with another child); deception (being given a placebo without being told, being tested after being told there would not be a test); being subjected to an unpleasant event (a scary movie, a very loud and sudden noise); breaking promised confidentiality (results of a spelling test or a baking contest); being made to complete a study (watching movies for a very long time, completing a series of puzzles); and being asked to do something that might create a dilemma for the child (lie to parents, disobey one adult in order to obey another adult). The descriptions were brief. For example, the study involving being made to complete a study was described as follows: "We want to know which puzzles are easy and which puzzles are hard for children your age. We would give you some puzzles to try. You would have to try all of them. Even if you didn't want to try all of them, you would have to stay until you were finished." The studies were described to the children one at a time, and they were asked if they would want to participate in each of them and why.

Scoring

When there was a range of answers rather than just yes and no, the children's responses were coded as being adequate or not adequate. To be considered adequate, the answer did not have to include all possible information, but did have to indicate that the child knew and understood the main point or points of the question. For example, in describing what would happen in Study 2, an adequate response had to include both tasting foods and something about rating them or about liking or disliking them. However, the scoring was lenient so that all that was necessary was to give the general idea. "Eating and if I like it or not," "You're supposed to try foods and if you don't like them, you don't have to taste them," and "You could eat some stuff and some will be yummy and some will be yucky" were all scored adequate. Typically, inadequate responses were those in which the children said they did not know or said something irrelevant. One-quarter of the protocols for all of the consent studies were scored by two independent coders, whose agreement was above 90% on all questions.

RESULTS

The data from Studies 1 and 2 are shown in Table 1, and from Studies 3 and 4 in Table 2. Because the samples in each study are rather small and because the questions asked overlapped considerably, the results will be discussed in terms of the issues, combining the various studies. Whenever there were substantial differences among the studies, this will be noted, although few appeared.

Knowing the Content of the Study

These results are based on Studies 1 and 2, with a total of 105 subjects. Most children were able to describe what was going to happen in the study after it had been described to them and before they had participated. However, as might be expected, there were large age differences. All of the 11- and 9–10-year-olds gave adequate answers, while 12.5% of the 7–8-year-olds (16% in Study 1 and 10% in Study 2) and 38% of the 5–6-year-olds did not.

Children had more difficulty when asked why the study was being conducted. Combining across studies, only 10% of the 5–6-year-olds, 27.5% of the 7–8-year-olds, and 61.4% of the 9–11-year-olds were able to answer correctly. In addition, it was clear that they found the purpose of the second study easier to understand. Whereas almost half of the 7–8-year-olds knew that it was being done to see what foods children liked and did not like, only 5%; (one child in a group of 19) of the 7-year-olds were able to link math and money knowledge in the first study.

Finally, after they had participated in the study, the children were asked whether anything had happened that they did not expect. The only positive answers concerned the actual content of the materials used in the studies. Some children were surprised at how "weird" the foods tasted or that the stories in the first study were not exactly the same as the one they had been given as an example. Otherwise, the studies were apparently what they were expecting.

TABLE 1
Percentage of Correct or Affirmative Answers in Studies 1 and 2

	STUDY AND AGE GROUP				
	Study 1		Study 2		
QUESTIONS	7 (n = 19)	11 (n = 23)	5–6 (n = 21)	7–8 (n = 21)	9–10 (n = 21)
Content:					
What? (% correct)	84	100	62	90	100
Why? (% correct)	5	56	10	48	67,
Confidentiality:					
Who will know? (% correct)	75	100	33	52	76
Will mom know? (% yes)	na	na	67	67	90
Stopping:					
What happens? (% correct)	21	83	38	67	76
How? (% correct)	95	100	57	81	90
Surrogate consent:					
Mom likes, child doesn't (% yes)	na	na	37	32	24
Child likes, mom doesn't (% yes)	na	na	56	59	80

NOTE.—na = not asked.

TABLE 2
Percentage of Correct or Affirmative Answers in Studies 3 and 4

	STUDY AND AGE GROUP		
	Study 3		Study 4
QUESTIONS	8–9 (n = 32)	10–11 (n = 26)	10–12 (n = 27)
Confidentiality:			
Will experimenter tell? (% yes)	41	50	56
Stopping:			
How? (% correct)	75	87	85
What will experimenter do or say? (% correct)	56	50	70
Experimenter mad? (% yes)	16	5	22
Parent mad? (% yes)	22	18	26
Surrogate consent:			
Mom likes, child doesn't (% yes)	na	na	16
Child likes, mom doesn't (% yes)	na	na	52

NOTE.—na = not asked.

Stopping Their Participation

The children were asked two questions dealing with this. The first, which was asked only in Studies 1 and 2, was, "What happens if you want to stop being in the study?" Responses were considered correct if the children said that they would tell the experimenter and leave or simply leave and get their mother. Thirty-eight percent of the 5–6-year-olds, 45% of the 7–8-year-olds (but consisting of 21% in Study 1 and 67% in Study 2), and 79.5% of the 9–11-year-olds gave the correct answer. This question may have been somewhat ambiguous, and it was followed immediately by the more direct question "How can you stop being in the study?" which was also asked in Study 3. In Studies 1 and 2, 57% of the 5–6-year-olds, 87.5% of the 7–8-year-olds, and 95.5% of the 9–11-year-olds gave the right answer. In Study 3, 75% of the 8–9-year-olds and 87% of the 10–11-year-olds responded correctly. Thus, most of the children knew that if they wanted to stop they would just tell the experimenter and stop. Nevertheless, over 40% of the youngest group and a substantial number of the older children did not. In addition, several children said that they would be too shy to ask or indicated that they would find some excuse for stopping, such as having to go to the bathroom.

Moreover, answers to the more detailed probes in Study 3 suggested that even the older children might not be entirely clear that they had the right to stop whenever they wished. Some of the answers seemed to indicate that the children understood the question in terms of being able to stop only temporarily and that there might be some negative consequences if they stopped. When the children were asked what the experimenter would do or say if they wanted to stop, only 56% of the 8–9-year-olds and 50% of the 10–11-year-olds said that the experimenter would simply agree. Twenty-two percent of the younger children and 14% of the older children gave answers indicating that the "stopping" would only be temporary and that the experimenter would then continue with the study; 19% of the younger children and 27% of the older children said that they did not know. In addition, one child in each age group said that the experimenter would make the child continue.

The children were then asked if they thought that the experimenter or their parents would be mad if they wanted to stop. Sixteen percent of the 8–9-year-olds and 5% of the 10–11-year-olds thought that the experimenter might be mad; 22% and 18% of the children in the two age groups, respectively, thought that their parents would be mad at them.

The gifted children (Study 4) were clearer on their right to stop. Eighty-five percent (23 of 27) seemed to understand that they could simply say they did not want to continue, two said they would use the excuse of needing a bathroom, and two were unsure. In addition, 70% said there would be no consequences. On the other hand, even among this group of children, 22% thought that the experimenter would be mad at them for stopping (two said that she would be mad but would not show it) and, when asked specifically, 26% thought that their mothers would be mad or disappointed if they stopped.

Confidentiality

In Study 1, the only question regarding confidentiality was, "Who will find out what you did in the study?" All of the 11-year-olds and 75% of the 7-year-olds responded "the experimenter" or the "experimenter and people at the college." In the second study, the corresponding results were that 76% of the 9–10-year-olds, 52% of the 7–8-year-olds, and a third of the 5–6-year-olds gave that answer. However, we had the impression that many of the children just assumed that their parents would know. Therefore, in Study 2 we probed further by asking whether their mothers would know. Two-thirds of the two younger groups and 90% of the oldest group responded that she would. Unfortunately, the significance of this is not entirely clear because many of the children indicated that they would tell their parents, and we did not ask them what would happen if they didn't tell and their parents then asked the experimenter.

The degree of misunderstanding (or disbelief) of the rules of confidentiality became clear in Study 3 when we probed about whether the experimenter would tell their parents. Forty-one percent of the 8–9-year-olds and 50% of the 10–11-year-olds thought that the experimenter would tell their parents if their parents wanted to know; 37% and 39%, respectively, said that their performance was confidential and their parents would not be told; and the rest were not sure or refused to answer. The gifted children in Study 4 were no better at comprehending (or perhaps believing) what they had been told about confidentiality. A third of them seemed to understand it fully, but 56% did not and 11% were uncertain.

Thus, it appears that children as old as 12 did not fully understand or did not believe what they were told about the confidentiality of their responses. Although many of them did say that only the experimenter would now, it seems clear that they did not fully accept this. Rather, they thought that their parents would be told if they really wanted to know.

Surrogate Consent

Children who participated in Studies 2 and 4 were asked if they thought that they should participate in a study if they liked it and their mother didn't and vice versa. In Study 2, the majority of the children at all three ages (63%, 68%, and 76%) said that they should not be in a study if they did not like it even if their mother did. In Study 4, 84% of the children said they should not participate if they did not like the study and their mother did, and half of those who said they should participate said that they would do it to please their mothers. When they were asked to justify their answers, most of those who said they should not do it gave answers indicating an understanding of the principle that children should only participate voluntarily. Some typical responses were: "If I don't want to do it, I shouldn't be forced to do it." "It should be your choice."

The responses to these questions indicate that while some children did think that "mother knows best," there were many for whom surrogate parental consent was not a sufficient condition for their participation in a study. On the other hand, the pattern of answers makes it clear that once the mother has consented to the study, a substantial number of children (between 15% and 35%) felt that they should participate even if they would rather not.

When the question was phrased in terms of the child liking the study and the mother not liking it, the younger children were split about whether they should do it. Among the 5–6-year-olds, 44% said they should not, as did 41% of the 7–8-year-olds. However, the 9–10-year-olds were strongly in favor of participating under this condition (80%). Among the gifted children, a bare majority (52%) said they should participate, while only 8% gave a categorical no. The rest indicated that they would try to convince their mothers or that, while they should be able to, their mothers would not let them. A substantial number of the oldest children who said they should participate justified their answer in terms of "being their own person." ("It's your decision—they were asking me, not my mom." "You're the one who is going to do it.")

Hypothetical Studies

These data are based on the responses of 18 7–8-year-olds and 19 9–10-year-olds in Study 2 and the 27 gifted children (aged 10–12) in Study 4. Generally, the children were willing to participate in almost all of the studies and were not concerned with any of the problems in the procedures. Fewer than half of the children in Study 2 were concerned about even one of the studies, and overall the children identified only 11.7% of all of the possible problems. The 9–10-year-olds were somewhat more likely than the 7–8-year-olds to find problems (12.3% vs. 7.4%). The gifted children, who were also older (10–12), were a little more likely to be concerned about the studies. Overall, they noticed 23% of the possible problems, and only 27% failed to mention any.

Thus, the finding is that children in the age range 7–12 said that they would agree to participate in almost all of the hypothetical studies even though they contained what we considered to be serious ethical problems. Yet during debriefing, the children were asked specifically about each of the problems, and many of them seemed to understand them. In other words, even when they appeared to be capable of understanding the ethical problems in a study, most of the children were willing to participate in it.

DISCUSSION

Before considering the implications of these findings, let us put them in perspective. Obviously, the children in these studies were not a representative sample. They wcre from relatively affluent, suburban families and had parents who were willing to have them participate in psychological rescarch. In addition, the children were participating in particular studies and were given instructions for those studies. There is no reason to believe that the percentage of the subjects who gave the various responses would hold for other subject populations and other experimental instructions. That is, the precise figures should not be given much weight. On the other hand, it seems to us highly likely that regardless of variations in the population and the situation, the overall pattern of responses would be substantially the same as that found here. Thus, we would argue that the children's responses do provide some indication of both the capacity to assent to research and the limitations on that capacity of children of the ages from 5 to 12.

First, it was encouraging to find that understanding what they were being asked to do was not a major problem for most of the children. Almost all of the 7–11-year-olds and a clear majority of the 5–6-year-olds could tell us what the study involved. These figures may underestimate the degree of understanding, because many of those who did not give adequate answers may have had difficulty expressing what they knew or may have forgotten the details by the time we asked. Overall, it would seem that if the instructions are given clearly and the study is not excessively complex, most children as young as 5 are capable of understanding what they will be doing and therefore have the capacity to give their assent or dissent to the research.

In contrast, many of the children, even the 11-year-olds and the 10–12-year-old gifted children, did not understand or did not believe that their performance would be entirely confidential. This is not surprising. Children are accustomed from school and other testing situations to the fact that their parents can get their results if they wish. Psychology studies are unusual in that ordinarily the children's results can be kept confidential. However, even in this context there are circumstances (e.g., evidence of child abuse) in which the experimenter might be required by law to reveal the children's results either to the parent or some third party. Thus, the children's perception that their mothers would find out their results if they really wanted to is both understandable and not entirely inaccurate.

This does not indicate that the children lack the capacity to assent to the research. Some may be assenting to research having been told their results will be confidential but not believing or not understanding this. Yet, at the worst, this means that they have agreed to participate thinking that their performance is less confidential than it actually will be—that is, the experimenter is providing more protection of their privacy than they expect.

While the children's lack of acceptance of the instructions regarding confidentiality does not appear to limit their capacity to assent, it may have serious implications for the results of the research. If the study does not involve threatening or evaluative material, the children will probably react in the same way whether or not they think that their responses are entirely confidential. However, studies in which children are asked to provide information that is private—that concerns their feelings toward school or home or other sensitive matters—might be affected substantially. Indeed, we have data indicating that even older children who are involved in this kind of research tend to think that their parents could find out what they said. Seventeen children ranging in age from 12 to 17 were asked a series of questions about family relationships. The questions were somewhat sensitive and the children had been assured of confidentiality. Yet almost half, equally distributed across the age range, thought that the experimenter would tell their parents what they had answered if the parents really wanted to know. If the children believe that their parents will find out what they answered, they may be less honest and open in responding.

It may be quite difficult to explain confidentiality to younger children, or to convince older children that it will be maintained. But we would suggest that in these kinds of studies a special effort should be made to do so. In particular, it might be useful to say explicitly that their parents will not be told even if they ask, assuming, of course, that this degree of confidentiality can be assured.

The results concerning the freedom with which assent is given are less encouraging. We are assuming that the ideal is for consent or assent to be given without any pressure to comply. The study is described to the potential subjects, they are asked if they will participate, and their only considerations are whether they would like to take part and have the time for it. Of course, this is rarely if ever achieved in any research. Whether they are students in introductory psychology courses choosing to participate in a study rather than write a paper, or others who have signed up for a study and know that the experimenter will be disappointed if they decide not to participate, they are under some pressure to comply. Although there is almost no way to eliminate these kinds of pressures, they do not limit the person's freedom to any substantial degree. The potential subjects are still free to refuse, because the negative consequences are minor or nonexistent. On the other hand, as these pressures increase, they clearly reduce the freedom to refuse. For example, at many universities, introductory psychology students are required to participate in research, but are given the option of writing a paper instead. This maintains their freedom to consent to or refuse to participate in the research. However, if the paper were required to be 100 pages long, it would not be a viable option for most students, and they would not in practice have the freedom to refuse to be subjects. Similarly, students may feel some pressure to participate when asked by any experimenter, and this does not eliminate their freedom. But if the request is made by the students' professor, who implies that it may affect their grades, obviously this is undue pressure and does reduce or eliminate the freedom to refuse. Thus, it seems clear that when the negative consequences or difficulty of refusing become too great, consent is no longer given freely.

With sufficient safeguards, adults can be protected from these kinds of undue pressure. The problem is considerably more difficult when doing research with children. They are faced by an older person who is asking them to do something, and they believe, as do many adults, that the experimenter will be unhappy if they refuse to participate or decide to stop once they have agreed. This belief is almost certainly accurate in most situations. Indeed, the two children who said that the experimenter would be upset but would not show it may have been precisely correct. Although the children are theoretically free to refuse, most children are quite submissive when faced with an authority who will be upset if they do not agree.

In addition, the current research suggests another source of pressure that may often be overlooked. This is that the children's parents have already agreed to have the children participate and the children usually know this. If they refuse or stop after agreeing, the children may perceive (possibly correctly) that their parents will be upset. Indeed, quite a few subjects mentioned this in response to the question whether there would be any consequences if they stopped. Moreover, the fact that their parents have approved the study lends weight to the request, because the study is clearly acceptable to the parents. Again, the results of this study indicate that some children feel they should participate even if they do not like the study as long as their parents think it is all right.

Thus, ironically, while the substitute consent from their parents provides a necessary protection for the children, it may also reduce their freedom to refuse to participate and may make it harder for them to stop if they do not want to continue. Although it may be difficult to eliminate this source of pressure, perhaps its effect could be reduced by dealing with it explicitly. For example, the experimenter could ask the parents to make it clear that the children need not participate and the experimenter might repeat that the parents have given their consent but they will not mind if the children refuse.

One general implication of our findings is that many children feel that their parents are, in some sense, a party to the experiment. They expect their parents to get information about their performance if they want it, they think their parents may be disappointed if they stop participating, and they think that if their parents have approved of the study, they should agree even if they would rather not participate. This was true even for the children in Study 4, who were not brought to the school by their parents for the express purpose of participating in research and whose parents were not present during the research. Thus, it must be recognized that to some extent children who know that their parents have agreed to an experiment are not entirely free agents. This element should be taken into account when designing the consent instructions for each study and probably when interpreting the children's responses, especially when they involve sensitive material.

Finally, we should note that the findings presented here may have implications beyond the participation of children in psychological research. Similar questions are raised when children are asked to consent to medical research and treatment or become involved in legal proceedings such as custody cases. In discussing medical research with children, Langer (1985), a physician and lawyer, made precisely the same recommendation as the American Psychological Association. Langer wrote that children should be asked for their consent when they have the capacity to "understand the general purpose of the research and to indicate [their] wishes regarding participation" (p. 660), and added that children of 7 and older do have this capacity. The present findings suggest that 7-year-olds may have the capacity to understand certain aspects of psychological research (and presumably medical research and treatment), but that they and considerably older children do not fully understand or believe other essential elements of the situation. The implications of this may be considerably more serious in other situations. For example, that children do not accept the experimenter's guarantee of confidentiality may not affect their responses in most psychology studies. In contrast, when the child is being represented by a lawyer, the child, fearing that his or her parents might find out, might refuse to give the lawyer information that is vital to the child's interests. In addition, the data suggest that it may be very difficult to guarantee that children are making their decisions freely. This may be true (and perhaps more crucial) when consent is asked for procedures that are likely to have far greater consequences for the children than participation in psychological research.

REFERENCES

American Psychological Association (1982). *Ethical principles in the conduct of research with human participants* (rev. ed.). Washington, DC: Author.

Ferguson, L. R. (1978). The competence and freedom of children to make choices regarding participation in research: A statement. *Journal of Social Issues, 34,* 114–121.

Keith-Spiegel, P. (1983). Children and consent to participate in research. In G. B. Melton. G. P. Koocher, & M. J. Saks (Eds.), *Children's competence to consent* (pp. 179–211), New York: Plenum.

Langer, D. H. (1985). Children's legal rights as research subjects. *Journal of the American Academy of Child Psychiatry, 24,* 653–662.

Lewis, C. E., Lewis, M. A., & Ifekwunigue, M. (1978). Informed consent by children and participation in an influenza vaccine trial. *American Journal of Public Health, 68,* 1079–1082.

Melton, G. B. (1984). Developmental psychology and the law: The state of the art. *Journal of Family Law, 22,* 445–482.

Melton, G. B., Koocher, G. P., & Saks, M. J. (1983). *Children's competence to consent.* New York: Plenum.

Roth, L. H., Meisel, A., & Lidz, C. W. (1977). Tests of competency to consent to treatment. *American Journal of Psychiatry,* **134,** 279–284.

Stanley, B., Sieber, J. E., & Melton, G. B. (1987). Empirical studies of ethical issues in research: A research agenda. *American Psychologist,* **42,** 735–741.

Weithorn, L. A. (183)). Involving children in decisions affecting their own welfare. In G. B. Melton, G. P. Koocher, & M. J. Saks (Eds.), *Children's competence to consent* (pp. 237–260). New York: Plenum.

Weithorn, L. A., & Campbell, S. B. (1982). The competency of children and adolescents to make informed treatment decisions. *Child Development,* **53,** 1589–1598.